AF556682

# Childhood Asthma

# ALLERGIC DISEASE AND THERAPY

*Series Editor*

**DAVID G. TINKELMAN**

*Medical College of Georgia*
*Augusta, Georgia, and*
*Atlanta Allergy Clinic*
*Atlanta, Georgia*

1. Histamine and $H_2$ Antagonists in Inflammation and Immunodeficiency, *edited by Ross E. Rocklin*
2. Asthma as an Inflammatory Disease, *edited by Paul M. O'Byrne*
3. Childhood Rhinitis and Sinusitis: Pathophysiology and Treatment, *edited by Charles K. Naspitz and David G. Tinkelman*
4. Allergen Immunotherapy, *edited by Richard F. Lockey and Samuel C. Bukantz*
5. Clinical Management of Urticaria and Anaphylaxis, *edited by Alan L. Schocket*
6. Childhood Asthma: Pathophysiology and Treatment. Second Edition, Revised and Expanded, *edited by David G. Tinkelman and Charles K. Naspitz*

*Additional Volumes in Preparation*

Asthma and Allergy in Pregnancy and Early Infancy, *edited by Michael Schatz and Robert S. Zeiger*

# Childhood Asthma

## Pathophysiology and Treatment

Second Edition, Revised and Expanded

edited by

David G. Tinkelman

*Medical College of Georgia, Augusta, Georgia and Atlanta Allergy Clinic, Atlanta, Georgia*

Charles K. Naspitz

*Escola Paulista de Medicina São Paulo, Brazil*

Marcel Dekker, Inc. New York • Basel • Hong Kong

**Library of Congress Cataloging-in-Publication Data**

Childhood asthma : pathophysiology and treatment / edited by David G.
Tinkelman, Charles K. Naspitz. -- 2nd ed., rev. and expanded.
p. cm. -- (Allergic disease and therapy ; v. 6)
Originally published: New York : Dekker, 1987.
Includes bibliographical references and index.
ISBN 0-8247-8751-X
1. Asthma in children. I. Tinkelman, David G.
II. Naspitz, Charles K. III. Series.
RJ436.A8C48 1992
618.92'238--dc20 92-29092
CIP

This book is printed on acid-free paper.



MARCEL DEKKER, INC.
270 Madison Avenue, New York, New York 10016

Current printing (last digit):
10 9 8 7 6 5 4 3 2

PRINTED IN THE UNITED STATES OF AMERICA

# Foreword

It was not long ago that asthma was generally viewed as a disorder largely of childhood, frequently outgrown, completely reversible, and rarely fatal. This point of view unfortunately tended to trivialize the importance of asthma as a disorder to be reckoned with. Indeed, asthma is a leading cause of school absenteeism for all chronic conditions in children and is reponsible for much work loss in adults and interference with normal living at all ages. In recent years, despite what we consider to be great advances in understanding of asthma and how best to treat it, the incidence, morbidity, and mortality of asthma have grown significantly. In recognition of the importance of proper management of this disorder (actually, asthma most likely is a group of disorders), a National Asthma Education Program was organized under the auspices of the National Institutes of Health, and guidelines for the treatment of asthma were published in 1991 as the result of efforts of a national task force convened to address concerns about the diagnosis and treatment of asthma.

Asthma frequently begins in childhood, often within the first three years of life. Although the disorder is apparently "outgrown" by some children, particularly those who do not have a propensity to mount IgE-mediated allergic responses, there is evidence that asthma persists, in fact much more commonly than previously recognized, into and perhaps throughout adulthood. The refocusing of attention on the pathology of asthma with greater appreciation of an inflammatory basis for asthma, along with evidence that lung function may decrease abnormally rapidly in children and adults with asthma, has raised important questions concerning the potentially destructive nature of the disease, risk factors for its development, how best to treat the disorder, and how to prevent it. The greater appreciation of the morbidity associated with asthma and the small, but significant, mortality from this disease has focused attention on underdiagnosis and undertreatment of asthma yet, at the same time, has raised questions concerning the potential harmful effects of aggressive treatment with potent antiasthmatic agents commonly in use, especially in children.

Although it has long been accepted that genetic factors play a role in "predisposing" to asthma, it also is recognized that environmental factors play a critical role in originating and propagating the disorder. Many have been implicated, but viral infections and allergens assume particular prominence on the list. The earliest manifestations of asthma can be seen in infancy in some patients, most frequently in association with certain viral respiratory infections but even from allergic causes in this age group. Risk factors have been associated with the development of asthma and include heavy exposure to house dust mite allergens early in life. Because of the more limited environmental encounters of very young children in general, the possibility for intervention in the development and control of asthma beginning early in life, with identification and understanding of such environmental risk factors, makes attention to this whole disease process beginning at the earliest stages of life particularly important.

The recognition that children are not simply small adults led many years ago to specialization in pediatrics and eventually to subspecialization in pediatric allergy. The physiological changes in early life and special influences and needs of children through different phases of childhood have further led to other subspecialties focusing on the neonate and the adolescent, for example.

The editors of this book, Drs. David Tinkelman and Charles Naspitz, are eminent allergists and pediatricians who recognized the importance of addressing the subject of asthma with specific reference to childhood for the reasons cited. They have selected authoritative investigators and practitioners throughout the world to address asthma from fundamental considerations of pathophysiology and etiology as a prelude to therapeutic considerations of asthma in general, but especially in relation to its diagnosis and treatment in childhood, from infancy through adolescence. Although of particular value to those who care for asthmatic children, the information assembled in this volume is important and relevant to the care of asthma at any age.

*David S. Pearlman, M.D.*
Clinical Professor of Pediatrics
University of Colorado School of Medicine
Denver, Colorado

# Preface

In the last five years, since the publication of the first edition of *Childhood Asthma*, there have been significant advances in our understanding of the pathophysiology of asthma. This knowledge has been directly responsible for a major shift in emphasis from primarily treating a "bronchospastic disease" to treatment of a predominantly inflammatory disease with a bronchospastic component.

In an effort to keep up with the rapidly changing concepts and approaches to the diagnosis and management of asthma in children, the second edition of *Childhood Asthma* was conceived and developed. While the basic approach of establishing a balance in the dynamic relationship of the impact of asthma on the developing child and the influence of the developing child on asthma has been maintained, we have expanded our approach to delve into the effect of a variety of daily exposures on this balance. Therefore, chapters relating to exercise, common infections, school activity, and sinus disease have been added to the basic chapters dealing with pathophysiology, diagnosis, and treatment of children with asthma.

Again, chapter authors from around the world give varying, expert perspectives about a common problem. These individuals bring to this textbook a wealth of knowledge and a broad perspective from years of research and clinical experience. Each chapter reflects and maintains the authors' individuality and style, while being melded into the overall concept that childhood asthma is a disease which, while having the potential to be fatal, should be controlled to allow the child to develop and live as normal an existence as possible. The principles and procedures described in each chapter may actually apply to several situations, in children of different ages and those with both acute and chronic conditions. The fact that many of these important topics are discussed in more than one chapter does not necessarily imply a superfluous duplication of effort. On the contrary, the result is a multidimensional view of many problems, whereby the reader is provided with an opportunity to see how a number of authorities approach a situation. If the authors agree completely, the statements and recommendations become even stronger. However, where disagreement exists, it allows the reader to use the ability to assimilate alternative data, to reason, and to act according to his or her best judgment.

We have thoroughly enjoyed the challenge of not only assembling the work and knowledge of so many authorities into one text, but also negotiating the varying opinions and strategies of these experts into concepts that can be used on a daily basis by the physician treating children with asthma. We hope that our readers not only will benefit directly from these approaches to their patients, but will also see this text as a stimulus for further questioning and research to increase understanding of this complex, yet common, problem of childhood.

At this time we would like to acknowledge our contributing authors from around the globe. We value their expertise as well as their cooperation in meeting deadlines so that this book can present the latest information concerning pediatric asthma from around the world. We sincerely thank all contributors for their time and effort in writing their chapters, and also their concern for the well-being of children with asthma.

*David G. Tinkelman*
*Charles K. Naspitz*

# Contributors

**Againdra K. Bewtra, M.D.** Division of Allergy, Creighton University, Omaha, Nebraska

**S. Allan Bock, M.D.** National Jewish Center for Immunology and Respiratory Medicine and Department of Pediatrics, University of Colorado Health Sciences Center, Denver, Colorado

**William W. Busse, M.D.** Department of Medicine, University of Wisconsin Medical School, Madison, Wisconsin

**Gerard J. Canny, M.D., B.Ch., F.R.C.P.(C.), F.C.C.P.** Pulmonary Division, Department of Pediatrics, The Hospital for Sick Children and University of Toronto, Toronto, Ontario, Canada

**Kathleen Conboy, M.S., R.N., P.N.P.** Department of Pediatrics, Children's Hospital of Buffalo, Buffalo, New York

**David B. Coultas, M.D.** Department of Internal Medicine, University of New Mexico School of Medicine, Albuquerque, New Mexico

**Thomas L. Creer, Ph.D.** Department of Psychology, Ohio University, Athens, Ohio

**Johan C. de Jongste, M.D., Ph.D.** University Hospital Rotterdam/Sophia Children's Hospital, Rotterdam, The Netherlands

**Peyton A. Eggleston, M.D.** Department of Pediatrics, The Johns Hopkins Medical School, Baltimore, Maryland

**Alexander C. Ferguson, M.B., Ch.B., F.R.C.P.C.** Department of Pediatrics, University of British Columbia, Vancouver, British Columbia, Canada

**Enrique Fernandez-Caldas, Ph.D.** Division of Allergy and Immunology, University of South Florida College of Medicine, Tampa, Florida

**Thomas J. Fischer, M.D.** Division of Allergy/Immunology, Cincinnati Children's Hospital Medical Center, and Department of Pediatrics, University of Cincinnati College of Medicine, Cincinnati, Ohio

**Simon Godfrey, M.D.** Institute of Pulmonology, Hadassah University Hospital, Jerusalem, Israel

**Peter W. Heymann, M.D.** Division of Allergy and Clinical Immunology, Department of Medicine, University of Virginia Health Sciences Center, Charlottesville, Virginia

**Bettina C. Hilman, M.D.** Department of Pediatrics, Louisiana State University Medical Center, Shreveport, Louisiana

**S. T. Holgate, M.D., D.Sc., F.R.C.P.** Departments of Immunopharmacology and Medicine, University of Southampton and Southampton General Hospital, Southampton, England

**Setsuko Ito, M.D.** Department of Pediatrics, Faculty of Medicine, Kyoto University, Kyoto, Japan

**Roger M. Katz, M.D.** Allergy Research Foundation, Inc., and Department of Pediatrics, UCLA School of Medicine, Los Angeles, California

**Henry Levison, M.D.** Pulmonary Division, Department of Pediatrics, The Hospital for Sick Children and University of Toronto, Toronto, Ontario, Canada

**Eli O. Meltzer, M.D.** Allergy and Asthma Medical Group and Research Center and Division of Allergy/Immunology, Children's Hospital, San Diego, California

**Haruki Mikawa, M.D.** Department of Pediatrics, Faculty of Medicine, Kyoto University, Kyoto, Japan

**Kevin R. Murphy, M.D.** Department of Pediatric Pulmonology, Omaha Children's Hospital, Omaha, Nebraska

**Charles K. Naspitz, M.D.** Section of Allergy and Clinical Immunology, Escola Paulista de Medicina, São Paulo, Brazil

**Herman J. Neijens, M.D.** University Hospital Rotterdam/Sophia Children's Hospital, Rotterdam, The Netherlands

**Thomas C. Nilsson, M.D.** Midwest Allergy and Asthma Clinic, Omaha, Nebraska

**H. Alice Orgel, M.D., Ph.D.** Allergy and Asthma Medical Group and Research Center and Division of Allergy/Immunology, Children's Hospital, San Diego, California

**Nancy K. Ostrom, M.D.** Allergy and Asthma Medical Group and Research Center and Division of Allergy/Immunology, Children's Hospital, San Diego, California

**Thomas A. E. Platts-Mills, M.D., Ph.D.** Department of Medicine, University of Virginia Health Sciences Center, Charlottesville, Virginia

**Gary S. Rachelefsky, M.D.** Allergy Research Foundation, Inc., and Department of Pediatrics, UCLA School of Medicine, Los Angeles, California

**John Joseph Reisman, M.D., F.R.C.P.(C.)** Pulmonary Division, Department of Pediatrics, The Hospital for Sick Children and University of Toronto, Toronto, Ontario, Canada

**J. Alan Roberts, B.Sc., M.D., M.R.C.P.** Department of Medicine, University of Southampton and Southampton General Hospital, Southampton, England

**Jonathan M. Samet, M.D.** Department of Medicine and New Mexico Tumor Registry, University of New Mexico School of Medicine, Albuquerque, New Mexico

**Gail G. Shapiro, M.D.** Department of Pediatrics, University of Washington School of Medicine, Seattle, Washington

**Ketan K. Sheth, M.D.** Division of Allergy/Clinical Immunology, Departments of Medicine and Pediatrics, University of Wisconsin Medical School, Madison, Wisconsin

**Sheldon C. Siegel, M.D.** Allergy Research Foundation, Inc., and UCLA School of Medicine, Los Angeles, California

**R. Michael Sly, M.D.** Department of Allergy and Immunology, Children's National Medical Center, and Department of Pediatrics, The George Washington University School of Medicine and Health Sciences, Washington, D.C.

**Richard Sporik, D.Ch., D.R.C.O.G., M.R.C.P.** Department of Medicine, University of Virginia Health Sciences Center, Charlottesville, Virginia

**Margaret A. Springer, M.D.** Department of Pediatrics, Louisiana State University Medical Center, Shreveport, Louisiana

**David G. Tinkelman, M.D.** Section of Allergy and Immunology, Department of Pediatrics, Medical College of Georgia, Augusta, Georgia, and Atlanta Allergy Clinic, Atlanta, Georgia

**Robert G. Townley, M.D.** Division of Allergy, Creighton University, Omaha, Nebraska

**Frank S. Virant, M.D.** Department of Pediatrics, University of Washington School of Medicine, Seattle, Washington

**Michael J. Welch, M.D.** Allergy and Asthma Medical Group and Research Center and Division of Allergy/Immunology, Children's Hospital, San Diego, California

# Contents

# 1

# Asthma: Basic Mechanisms

**J. ALAN ROBERTS and S. T. HOLGATE**

*University of Southampton and*
*Southampton General Hospital*
*Southampton, England*

Asthma is a multifactorial condition determined by an interaction of genetic and environmental factors leading to chronic inflammatory state in the airways (Fig. 1). Inflammation seems to be the major feature, the importance of which was first suggested in the late 19th century by Sir Andrew Clark (1). Since then various topics have been fashionable in asthma research such as the mast cell, the eosinophil, bronchial hyperreactivity, but all are now thought to be factors producing or produced by airway inflammation (Fig. 1). In this chapter we will discuss the various aspects of the inflammatory response individually, although in practice each is interdependent on the others.

## CONCEPTS

The asthmatic response to an acute allergen challenge consists of two phases. The early response is an immediate, and short-lived bronchoconstriction lasting approximately 1 hr. This is thought to be due to release of bronchoconstrictor mediators by cross-linkage of IgE receptors on mast cells and basophils. As well as bronchoconstrictors such as histamine, prostaglandins, and leukotrienes, mast cell degranulation also releases chemotactic factors producing a secondary influx of inflammatory cells, which, in a proportion of asthmatic patients, produces a secondary bronchoconstriction 3–8 hr after the original stimulus (2,3). A secondary wave of chemotactic factors is released in parallel, and this continuing process is thought to result in the chronic inflammation seen in asthmatic airways.

Bronchial hyperreactivity is closely associated with the asthmatic state (4) and correlates with the presence of airway inflammation (5). It seems

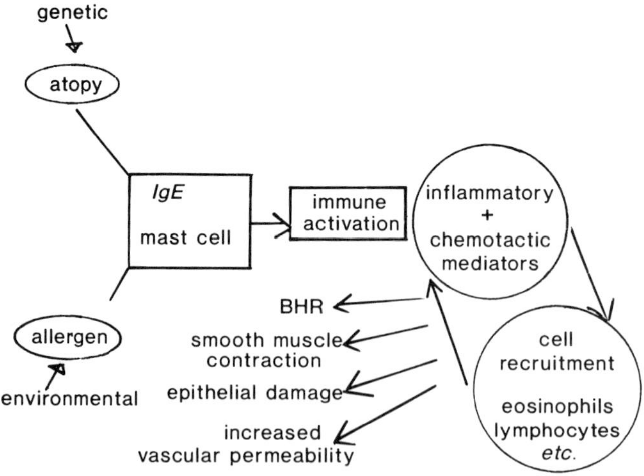


FIGURE 1 Scheme for the causes of allergic asthma.

likely that the inflammatory process not only releases mediators that may alter bronchial reactivity, such as platelet-activating factor (PAF) (6) and leukotrienes (LT) (7), but also damages mucosa, thereby increasing access of stimuli to airway smooth muscle and possibly reducing the production of epithelium-derived relaxant factor, a substance analogous to the better-characterized endothelium-derived relaxant factor found in blood vessels.

All the above relate to airway inflammation. We will now discuss evidence for the role of various cells and mediators in the inflammatory response.

## MEDIATORS

### Histamine

Histamine was the first bronchoconstrictor agent to be studied (8). Herxheimer in 1949 (2) demonstrated that histamine produced bronchoconstriction similar to that found in asthma and that this bronchoconstriction was prevented by treatment with antihistamines. Histamine is present in high concentrations in human mast cells. Histamine release has been demonstrated after acute bronchial provocation with allergen from peripheral blood cells (9) and in bronchoalveolar lavage fluid (BAL) (10), and histamine levels in BAL correlate with the degree of airflow obstruction (11). Histamine release may also occur during the late response (12). Potent antihistamines have been found to prevent 60% of the early response to allergen (13), but have been disappointing when used in clinical asthma, implying a limited role for histamine as a mediator in clinical asthma.

### Leukotrienes

Arachidonic acid, a major constituent of the cell membrane, is metabolized by cyclo-oxygenase to prostaglandin $PGD_2$, $PGF_{2\alpha}$ and thromboxane $A_2$ which are bronchoconstrictors, and $PGI_2$ and $PGE_2$, which have a bronchodilator effect, and by lipoxygenase to the leukotriene family of chemicals and platelet-activating factor. In the 1930s, slow-reacting substance of anaphylaxis (SRS-A) was described (14). This substance produced a slow-onset prolonged contraction of airway smooth muscle. More recently SRS-A has been shown to be a mixture of cysteinyl leukotrienes ($LTC_4$, $LTD_4$, and $LTE_4$) (Fig. 2). Lipoxygenase and cyclo-oxygenase are found in many cells participating in the inflammatory response and both PG (15) and LT (16) compounds are released following allergen challenge.

Leukotrienes are present in BAL from asthmatic patients (17), and urinary $LTE_4$ levels are elevated in asthmatic patients during acute exacerbations of their disease (18). Eosinophils synthesize $LTC_4$ (19), as do human mast cells (20) and monocytes (21). Leukotrienes increase in vitro reactivity of guinea pig smooth muscle to histamine and acetylcholine (22)

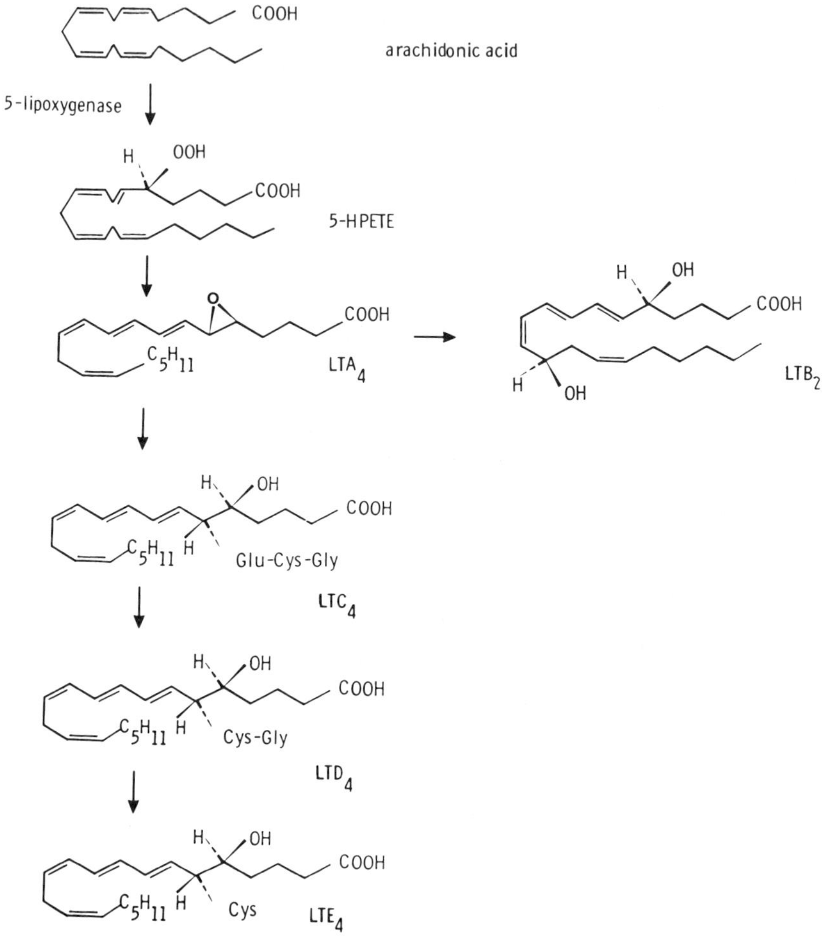

FIGURE 2 5-Lipoxygenase pathway of arachidonic acid metabolism.

and increase BHR to histamine (7). Experimental administration of leukotrienes produces many of the features of clinical asthma, including bronchoconstriction, mucus secretion, and increased vascular permeability (23). Leukotrienes also increase leucocyte adhesion to endothelium (24) and, in the form of $LTB_4$, are chemotactic to neutrophils (25) and eosinophils (26). Effective leukotriene antagonists such as ICI 204219 and MK571, which produce a 40–80-fold shift to the right in the leukotriene dose-response curve, are now available and have been reported to increase baseline airway caliber in asthmatic patients (25a). These drugs also afford appreciable protection against allergen-provoked early- and late-phase reactions and asthma provoked by exercise and inhaled PAF, indicating a role for leukotrienes in these responses. Further studies with potent antagonists will help to dissect out the role and importance of the leukotrienes in clinical asthma.

## Prostanoids

Prostaglandin D2 ($PGD_2$) is released from human lung fragments after IgE-dependent challenge (27) (Fig. 3). $PGD_2$ is the most abundant cyclooxygenase product released after immunologic challenge of mast cells (28) and is present in post-antigen-challenge BAL obtained from patients with allergic asthma challenged with the appropriate allergen (29). $PGD_2$ produces bronchoconstriction in both normal and asthmatic subjects (30). Cyclo-oxygenase inhibition reduced (by 25%) the bronchoconstrictor response to inhaled allergen (30a), which suggests that cyclo-oxygenase products play a part in the acute antigen-induced bronchoconstriction. Antagonism of $PGD_2$ and other contractile prostanoids at the level of $TP_1$ receptor with such drugs as GR32191 also modifies the early asthmatic response but has little effect on subsequent inflammation. The cyclo-oxygenase inhibitor indomethacin produced a decrease in airway sensitivity to histamine (31) and $PGD_2$ potentiated airway reactivity to histamine and methacholine (32). Thus, prostanoids can initiate and perpetuate an inflammatory response by both producing bronchoconstriction and sensitizing airway smooth muscle to the effects of other bronchoconstrictors. However, their role in "clinical" asthma seems limited.

## Platelet-Activating Factor

Like leukotrienes and prostaglandins, PAF is produced from arachidonic acid released from the cell membrane and is released by many inflammatory cells present in the asthmatic airway. As well as its action as a bronchoconstrictor (33), PAF increases microvascular permeability (33a), increases mucus secretion (34), is chemotactic for eosinophils (26), and has been reported to increase BHR in normal human subjects (6), although this has been disputed (35). Recent studies have demonstrated that as well as acting directly on airway smooth muscle, PAF induces bronchoconstriction in part by histamine release but does not involve cyclo-oxygenase or cholinergic pathways (36). Lipoxygenase metabolites also appear to play a part in an animal models of PAF-induced bronchoconstriction (37). In the skin the PAF-produced wheal and flare seems more histamine dependent (38).

PAF has many actions that appear to be important in clinical asthma. However, none of these effects is unique to PAF, and studies with effective and specific PAF antagonists such as WEB2086 will be necessary to clarify the role of PAF in asthma.

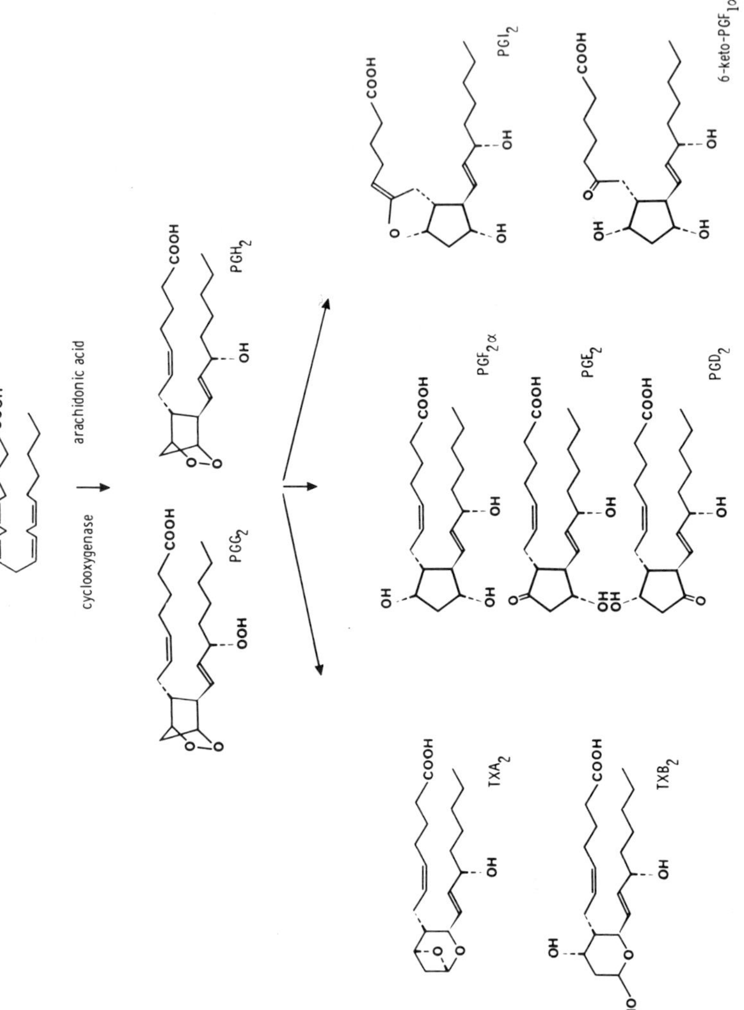


FIGURE 3 Cyclo-oxygenase pathway of arachidonic acid metabolism.

### Neuropeptides

Many neuropeptides and their receptors have been identified in human lung (39) (Table 1). The most abundant of these is vasoactive intestinal polypeptide (VIP), which is a bronchodilator in animal models but has little effect in humans when given by the inhaled (40) or intravenous routes (41,42).

Substance P has been difficult to demonstrate in human airway (43), although the related neurokinin A produces bronchoconstriction in humans (44). Calcitonin gene-related peptide (CGRP) has been isolated from human airway (45) and causes smooth muscle contraction of human airway smooth muscle in vitro. The present knowledge of the role of neurokinins is patchy. Many of the data available are derived from animal models of asthma. Although many neurokinins have been demonstrated in human lung, their role in the manifestations of clinical asthma is speculative.

The role of mediators of asthma has been a popular topic for study, in part because Koch's postulates can be applied in a structured way. It is difficult to assess the importance of individual bronchoconstrictor agents in the mix of mediators released during allergen-induced bronchoconstriction and present during exacerbations of clinical asthma. However, it seems more likely that improved control of asthma will come from a better understanding of the mechanisms controlling the source of these mediators (i.e., the cells of the inflammatory response). As with mediators, inflammatory cells do not act in isolation, but it is of interest to consider interactions between cells as we currently understand them.

## INFLAMMATORY CELLS

### Mast Cell

The mast cell has long been recognized as playing a major role in the acute asthmatic response. First described by Ehrlich in 1879, mast cells are found in the bronchial mucosa and submucosa (46). Elevated numbers of mast cells have been reported in asthmatic airway (47) and mast cell numbers are reduced by oral corticosteroid treatment of asthma (48). Furthermore, in patients who have died during an asthmatic attack there is evidence of degranulation of a large proportion of mast cells (48a), and continued mast cell degranulation has been demonstrated in mild asthma (Fig. 4).

Mast cells discharge contents of granules via a cross-linkage of cell surface IgE receptors (49), typically by specific allergen. Thus, stimulated mast cells release preformed mediators stored in cytoplasmic granules. These include histamine (50), tryptase (51), heparin (52), and chemotactic factors for both neutrophils and eosinophils (53). Furthermore, mast cell

TABLE 1 Effects of Neuropeptides on Human Airway

| Peptide | Smooth muscle | Mucus secretion | Vessels | Nerves | Other cells |
|---|---|---|---|---|---|
| VIP | Relax | ↑ or ↓ | Dilate | ↓ Chol/e-NANC | ↓ Mast cells/T lymphocytes |
| SP | (Contract) | ↑ | Dilate<br>↑<br>Leak | (↑ Chol) | ↑ Macrophage/monocytes |
| NKA | Contract | ↑ | (dilate) | ↑ Chol | ↑ Macrophage |
| CRGP | (Contract) | (↑) | Dilate | ? | ↓ Macrophage |
| NPY | (Contract) | ↑ | Constrict | ↓ Chol/e-NANC | ? |
| GRP | Contract | ↑ | Constrict | ? | ↑ Epithelial growth |
| $CCK_8$ | Contract | ? | ? | No effect | ? |
| Galanin | No effect | ? | No effect | ↓ e-NANC | ? |

VIP, vasoactive intestinal peptide; SP, substance P; NKA, neurokinin A; CGRP, calcitonin gene-related peptide; NPY, neuropeptide Y; GRP, gastrin-releasing peptide; $CCK_8$, cholecystokinin; e-NANC, excitatory nonadrenergic noncholinergic. Parentheses indicate small or uncertain effects.

*Source:* From Barnes PJ, Barniak JN, Belvisi ME. Neuropeptides in the respiratory tract. *Am Rev Respir Dis* 166:1187–1198, 1991.

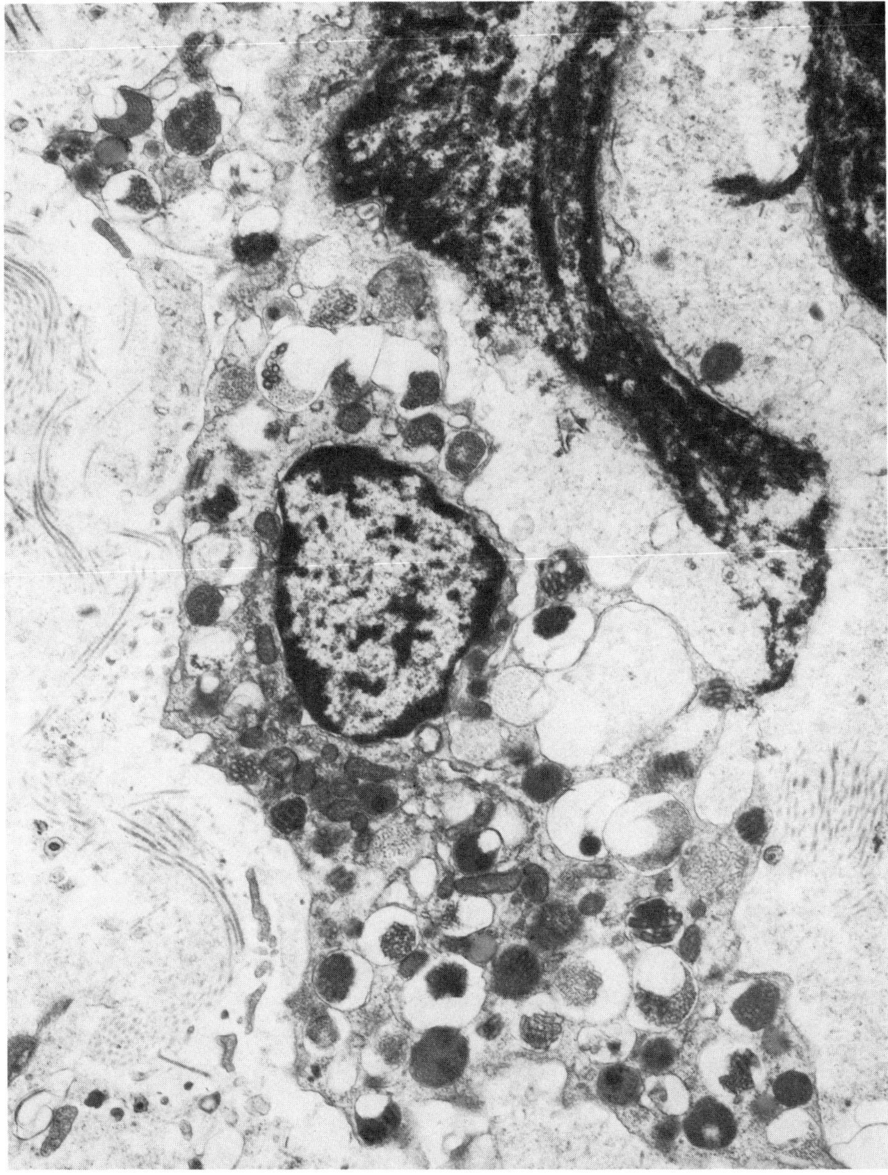

FIGURE 4 Electron micrograph shows degranulated human mucosal mast cell in bronchial mucosal biopsy.

degranulation leads to the appearance of newly synthesized mediators including bradykinin (54), prostaglandins (55), and leukotrienes (56) in addition to chemotactic factors, all of which may contribute to the late response. Until recently the mast cell was considered a cell that might initiate the immune response, but that other cells such as eosinophils and lymphocytes were more central to the maintenance of airway inflammation and its manifestations. However, recent evidence that cytokines influence mast cell growth and differentiation suggest that the mast cell may be more integral to continued inflammation than previously suspected (57). Indeed, both mouse and human mast cells are capable of generating and secreting IL-4, IL-5, IL-6, and TNFα, which cytokines are involved in IgE isotype switching (IL-4), eosinophil recruitment (IL-5), and leukocyte adhesion and chemotaxis (IL-4, IL-5, TNFα).

### Eosinophils

Eosinophilia, both in peripheral blood and sputum (Fig. 5) is closely associated with clinical asthma (58), and, more recently, increased eosinophil counts have been demonstrated both in bronchoalveolar lavage specimens (59) and bronchial biopsies from patients with mild bronchial asthma (60) (Fig. 6). The most effective treatment for asthma—corticosteroids—pro-

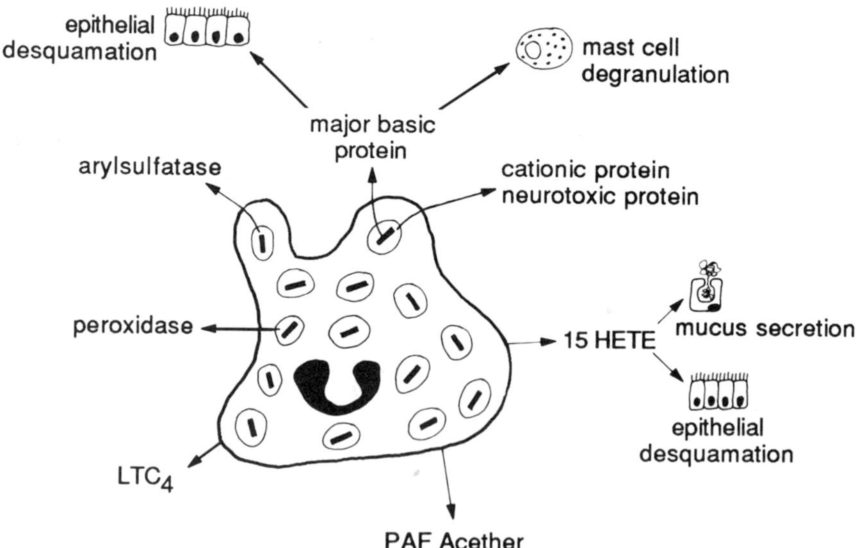


FIGURE 5 Diagram shows range of mediators released by activated human eosinophils.

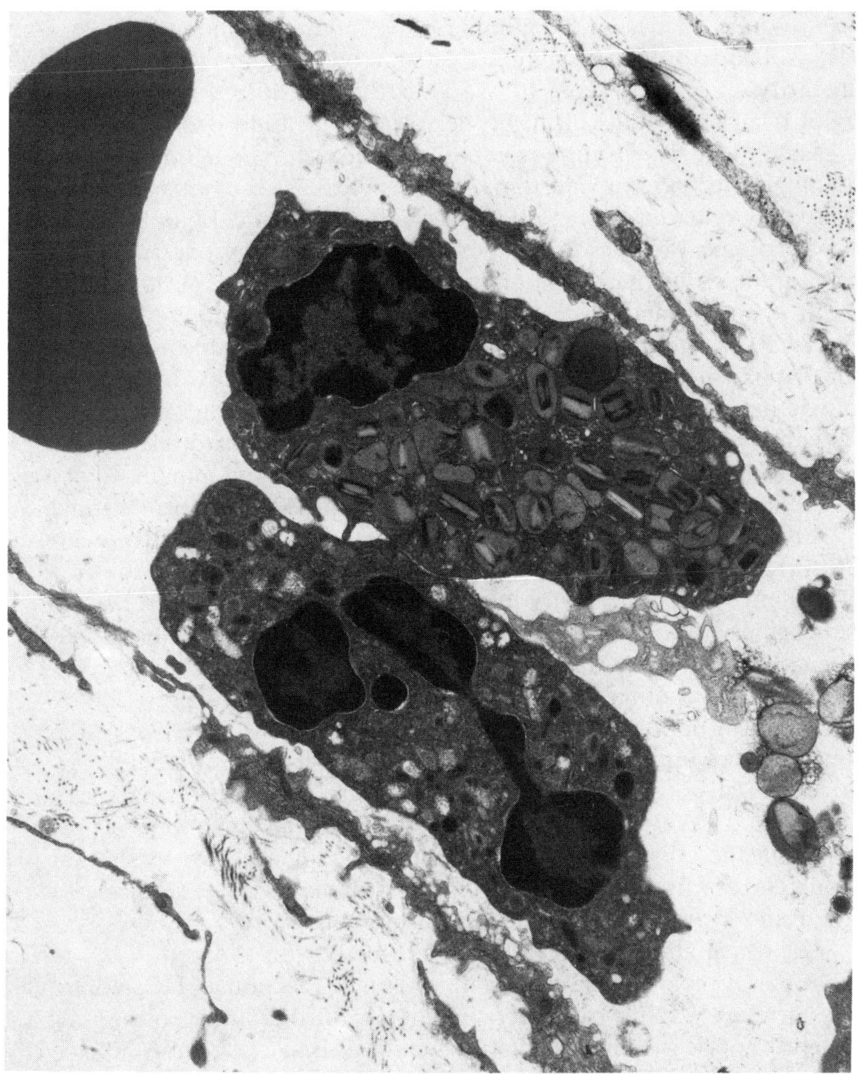

FIGURE 6 Electron micrograph from a patient with asthma shows intravascular eosinophils in a bronchial biopsy specimen.

duces a striking reduction in the number of eosinophils found in bronchial biopsies, probably through an inhibitory action on cytokines that maintain their integrity (IL-5, GM-CSF) (60a). Thus there is little doubt that the eosinophil is an important cell in bronchial asthma. Indeed, Barnes (61) has suggested the term *chronic eosinophilic bronchitis*, to take into account the pathologic mechanisms in asthma. PAF is a potent chemotactic factor for eosinophils released during allergen challenge (26). Eosinophils may have a physiological role in the response to infestation by parasites. Cytoplasmic granules in the eosinophil contain four cationic proteins that have both cytotoxic and noncytotoxic actions (62). Eosinophil cationic protein (ECP) is cytotoxic for mammalian cells, and is able to release histamine from mast cells and basophils (63). Eosinophil peroxidase (EPO) is cytotoxic but also is able to cause mast cell degranulation and can inactivate leukotrienes. Major basic protein (MBP) is also cytolytic to parasites (64), causes exfoliation of respiratory epithelium and impairs ciliary beating similar to the shedding of airway epithelium seen in clinical asthma (65,66). In patients who had died during an asthmatic attack, high levels of MBP were found in lung tissue (66a). An alternative pathway for eosinophil-mediated epithelial injury in asthma involves a cognate interaction between eosinophils and the epithelium, with induction of neuroendopeptidases such as gelatinase from the epithelial cells themselves (67).

In experimental asthma, eosinophil influx to the airway is preceded by a transient fall in peripheral blood eosinophil count (68), which suggests recruitment to the airway, followed by increased blood eosinophilia. Although eosinophils are able to suppress histamine release and inactivate leukotrienes and PAF (69), and were at one time thought to have a protective role in the allergic response, irrefutable evidence now exists that eosinophils have a proinflammatory function mediated by the release of preformed and synthesized chemicals. Eosinophils express an $Fc\varepsilon R_2$ receptor (70), which allows them to interact directly with allergen.

Eosinophils also participate in the late asthmatic reaction and eosinophil numbers correlate with bronchial reactivity (71). Furthermore, eosinophils in bronchial biopsies from patients with mild asthma have morphologic features suggestive of activation (60). Many eosinophil functions are controlled by T-cell-derived cytokines. Eosinophil production and differentiation are stimulated by IL-3, GM-CSF, and IL-5 sequentially (72,73). Corticosteroids reduce eosinophil numbers in parallel with clinical improvement (71). Thus the eosinophil is an important component of the continuing inflammatory response.

### Neutrophils

The neutrophil is an important cell in the allergic response in animal models (74). However, in human asthma neutrophils do not appear to play an important role. Neutrophils are present in bronchial biopsy specimens from patients with mild asthma, mainly in the perivascular area, in contrast to eosinophils, which were found in the mucosa of asthmatic patients (but not controls) (60). Like eosinophils, neutrophils contain cytoplasmic granules that contain numerous enzymes (53) and theoretically could have a cytotoxic action in the airways. There are no data to suggest that neutrophil numbers are increased in BAL obtained from asthmatic subjects, except in certain forms of occupational asthma. Thus, although neutrophils are present in the airway there is little hard evidence to suggest that they play a major role in airway inflammation.

## Monocytes/Macrophage

The alveolar macrophage is the predominant cell found in bronchoalveolar lavage from both normal and asthmatic subjects (75). These cells have low-affinity cell surface IgE receptors (76), and macrophages from atopic asthmatics have increased IgE on the cell surface (77).

Macrophages migrate to the lung after inhaled allergen challenge (78). They may release mediators including leukotrienes, prostanoids (79), and PAF (80). The macrophage plays a central and essential role in the immune response by presenting antigen to lymphocytes during the development of specific immunity (Fig. 7). Monocytes circulate in peripheral blood. They migrate to a site of inflammation where they transform to the macrophage and remain (81). Once in tissue, the macrophage is activated by T-cell-derived lymphokines (82). When an unrecognized antigen enters the lung, macrophages are attracted by a concentration gradient and will phagocytose the offending allergen. Macrophages may then present antigen to the T lymphocyte (83) and will also release the lymphocyte-stimulating factor interleukin 1 (IL-1), which stimulates T cell activation, B cell proliferation, and antibody production (84). Complex antigens are degraded into soluble immunogenic materials that can interact better with lymphocytes (85). In vitro, the macrophage is essential for the immune response to the majority of antigens. The counterpart of the macrophage in the epithelium is the dendritic cell, which forms a network on the surface of the airway to act in the antigen-presenting process. The cells are clearly important in the immune response to inhaled allergens, but relatively little is known about them.

Macrophages are exquisitely sensitive to the actions of anti-inflammatory steroids (85). In vivo treatment reduces circulating monocyte numbers and also the proportion with IgE receptors (87). Steroids also inhibit the release of mucous secretagogues by macrophages (88). Indirect evidence therefore suggests an important role for the monocyte/macrophage in the immune response.

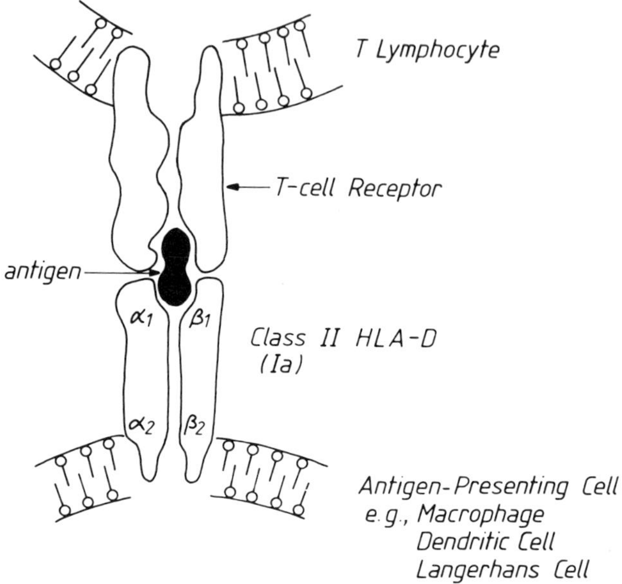


FIGURE 7 Diagram shows the interaction between antigen-presenting cells and T lymphocytes involving a cognate interaction between the T-cell receptor and the major histocompatibility class II molecule HLA-DR.

### Lymphocytes

Lymphocytes are prominent among the inflammatory cells infiltrating the bronchi in autopsy studies of asthma deaths (89,90). More recently, bronchial biopsies from patients with mild asthma have demonstrated the presence in the bronchial wall of lymphocytes (60,91).

The B lymphocyte has a well-defined role in atopic disease, namely the production of IgE (92). More recently interest has switched to the role of the T-lymphocyte, which, through release of immunomodulating lymphokines, is thought to control immune responses. Increased activation of T cells, demonstrated by increased receptor expression, has been shown in peripheral blood T cells of patients during an acute exacerbation of asthma (93). More recently, the degree of activation of blood T lymphocytes was found to decrease as asthma improved clinically (94).

Studies using allergen challenge have demonstrated an increase in lymphocyte numbers in postchallenge BAL at the time of the late response (59,95). Activation of T-lymphocytes in asthma has been shown by increased expression of receptors such as the $\alpha$ chain of the IL-2r (CD25) (96).

The increasing evidence for the importance of the T cell in asthma may relate to its effects on other cells involved in the inflammatory response in asthma. Recent work suggests that the $T_H2$ subtype of the $T_H$ cell is upregulated in asthma to secrete an array of cytokines involved in the allergic tissue response (Fig. 8). The $T_H2$ helper cell enhances the synthesis of IgE by B lymphocytes by means of secreted IL-4 (97). IL-5 is chemotactic for eosinophils (98). IL-3, IL-5, and GM-CSF initiate and support eosinophil production by bone marrow (72,99) and IL-3, IL-4, IL-5, and IL-10 regulate mouse mast cell differentiation (100,101). Corticosteroids, which are the most effective therapy for asthma, modify lymphocyte activation by inhibiting the production of IL-1 (102) and IL-2 (103), which could lead to downregulation of the T-lymphocyte-driven immune response.

Thus the T lymphocyte is present in asthmatic airway and its presence and activation mirror disease activity. Asthma treatment with corticosteroids modifies T-cell activation. Whether this is cause and effect is unproven to date.

## Platelets

In addition to their primary role in hemostasis there is now evidence for platelet participation in bronchoconstrictor (104) and inflammatory reactions (105). Platelet aggregation in pulmonary vessels has been demonstrated in acute fatal asthma (106). During antigen challenge in vivo, a transient thrombocytopenia occurs (107) and PAF is released by a number of inflammatory cells including basophils, macrophages, and neutrophils. Platelets possess low-affinity (Fc RII) IgE receptors (108). They are present in BAL from asthma patients (109) and on the mucosal surface of symptomatic asthmatic patients (91), which suggests that they undergo diapedesis when appropriately stimulated. Platelets can generate proinflammatory mediators (110) and so may play an important role in the inflammatory response. However, platelets are numerous in plasma and their presence at the site of inflammation cannot be assumed to indicate a major role in the process. The importance of platelets in clinical airway inflammation is speculative and further information as to their importance is awaited.

## Epithelium

The epithelial layer is the barrier between the atmosphere and lung parenchyma. For inflammatory cells to interact with inhaled allergen, they must migrate through the epithelium or the antigen must diffuse through the mucosal barrier. Epithelium may modify responses to allergen and moderate the inflammatory response by both a barrier effect and possibly by the release of endothelium-derived relaxant factor (EDRF) (111). In fact epithelium releases $PGE_2$ (112), which reduces smooth muscle tone

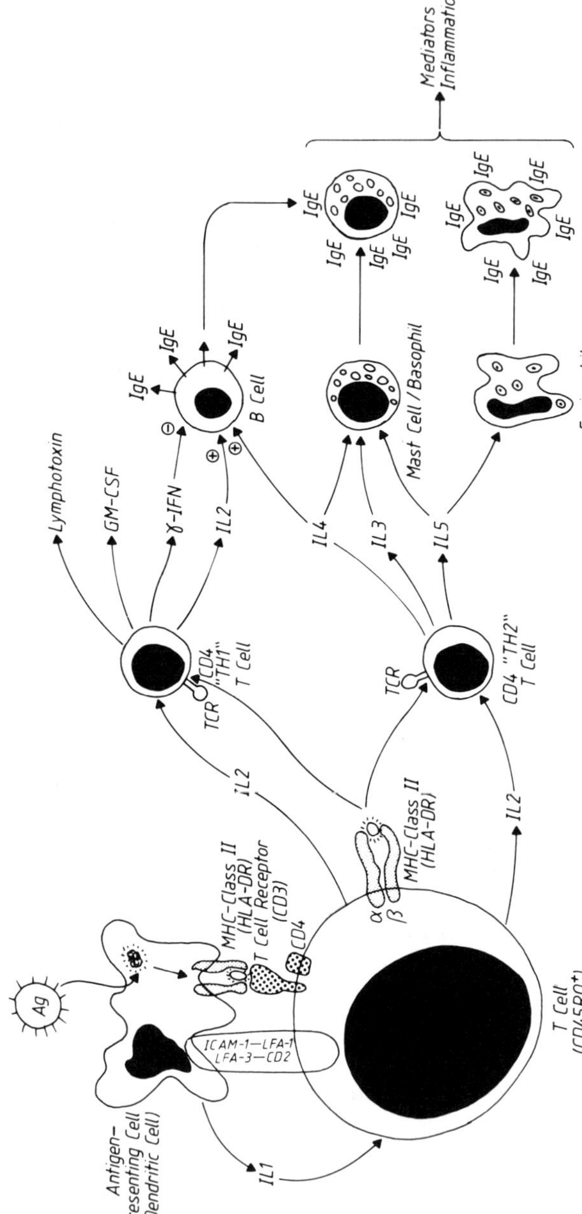


FIGURE 8 Diagram of the central role of the T lymphocyte in asthmatic airway inflammation demonstrates the cytokine profile of the two major subtypes of $T_H$ cell.

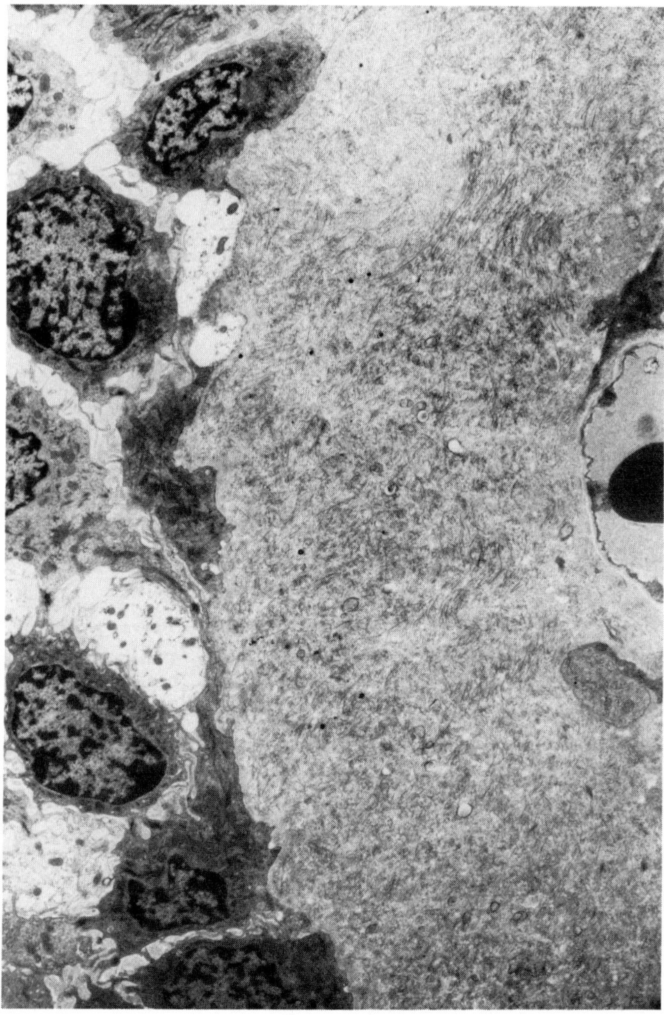

FIGURE 9 Electron micrograph shows sub-basement-membrane collagen in chronic asthma.

and contains neutral endopeptidase (113). This inactivates the neuropeptide bronchoconstrictors. Epithelium is often disrupted even in mild asthma (64). Activated eosinophils contain several cationic proteins within their granules (114) and one of these, major basic protein (MBP), produces damage to airway epithelium reminiscent of the pathologic changes seen in asthma (115).

Epithelial damage in vitro produced by gentle trauma increases smooth muscle responses to acetylcholine and histamine (116) without changing the maximum contraction, which suggests that the epithelium may be modifying bronchial reactivity (110). Evidence also exists for epithelial repair by laying down of collagen in the basement membrane (117) (Fig. 9). EDRF plays a significant role in the determination of tone in airways smooth muscle (118). However, some of the disruption of epithelium seen in mild asthma may be due to artifact induced by the fiberoptic bronchoscopy technique.

### Adhesion Molecules

Adhesion molecules are an important feature of epithelial cells. In addition to allowing cell to cell adhesion (118a), which maintains the epithelial layer integrity, adhesion molecules also fix epithelial cells to the underlying submucosa. Several families of receptors exist, including desmosomes, integrins (119), syndecan (120), and CD44 (121) (Fig. 10). Abnormal expression or function of these receptors could explain the increased shedding of bronchial mucosa found in asthmatic airway.

During inflammation, cells migrate from the vascular compartment to the submucosa and airway lumen. This occurs through interaction of inflammatory cells with endothelium and epithelium. The initial interaction is mediated by adhesion molecules found on the endothelial and/or epithelial surfaces (122). Adhesion molecules are present at low levels on resting tissue. Inflammation produces a marked increase in the expression of these integrins (123). Upregulation of ICAM-1 associated with an influx of eosinophils has been observed in an animal model of asthma and anti-ICAM-1 antibody inhibited eosinophil influx to the airway and reduced BHR (124). Although adhesion molecules are not the primary effector cells in the inflammatory process, they clearly have an important role in cell migration to sites of inflammation and cell-to-cell interaction.

## SUMMARY

In this chapter considerable emphasis has been placed on the components of the inflammatory process underlying much of the disordered function found in asthma. The various mediator components have overlapping effects and it is likely that their interaction produces many of the clinical features of asthma. The cellular components interact through a variety of cytokines that modulate IgE production and mast cell and eosinophil activity in the airways and hence the release of mediators. T lymphocytes also release cytokines, which modify their own behavior and so may maintain an inflammatory process once it is established.

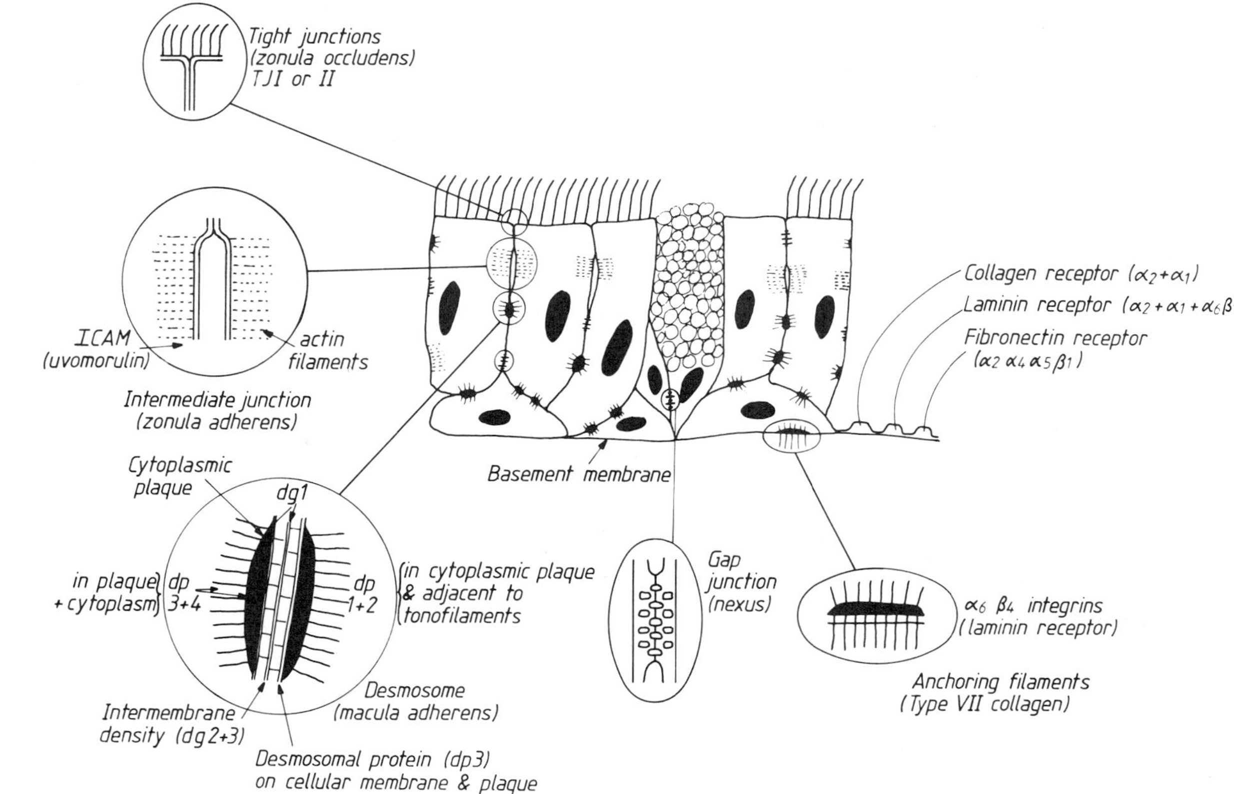


FIGURE 10 Diagram demonstrates the array of functional adhesion molecules that maintain epithelial integrity.

Consideration of asthma as a chronic inflammatory condition explains the increased airway lability and clinical features of the condition. Further advances in the knowledge of these interactions will improve our understanding of the asthmatic state and allow targeting of specific inhibitors and receptor blockers to dissect the components of the inflammatory response and perhaps produce specific therapies that will break the cycle of continued inflammation in the asthmatic airway.

We have discussed the role of mediators, inflammatory cells, and their interactions. As more evidence accumulates about the importance of inflammation in asthma, improved understanding of the process and interactions involved will allow scientists and clinicians to modify immune responses and control inflammation and asthma.

## REFERENCES


1. Clark A. Some observations on the theory of bronchial asthma. *Am J Med Sci* 91:104–112, 1886.
2. Herxheimer HGJ. Antihistamines in bronchial asthma. *Br Med J* 2:901–094, 1949.
3. Booij-Nord H, De Vries K, Sluiter JH, Oru NGM. Late bronchial obstructive reaction to experimental inhalation of house dust extract. *Clin Allergy* 2:43–61, 1972.
4. Hargreave FE, Ryan G, Thomson NC, et al. Bronchial hyperresponsiveness to histamine or methacholine in asthma: measurement and clinical significance. *J Allergy Clin Immunol* 68:347–355, 1981.
5. Nadel JA. Inflammation in asthma. *J Allergy Clin Immunol* 73:651–653, 1984.
6. Cuss FM, Dixon CMS, Barnes PJ. Effects of inhaled platelet activating factor on pulmonary function and bronchial responsiveness in man. *Lancet* 2:189–192, 1986.
7. Phillips GD, Holgate ST. Interaction of inhaled $LTC_4$ with histamine and $PGD_2$ in airway calibre in man. *J Appl Physiol* 66:304–312, 1989.
8. Dale HH, Laidlaw PP. Histamine shock. *J Physiol* 41:318–324, 1910.
9. Howarth PH, Durham SR, Kay AB, et al. Influence of albuterol, cromolyn sodium, and ipcatropium bromide on the airway and circulating mediator responses to antigen bronchial provocation in asthma. *Am Rev Respir Dis* 132:986–993, 1985.
10. Wanzel SE, Fowler AA, Schwartz LB. Activation of pulmonary mast cells by bronchoalveolar lavage allergen challenge: In vivo release of histamine and tryptase in atopic subjects with and without asthma. *Am Rev Respir Dis* 137:1002–1007, 1988.
11. Jarjour NN, Calhoun WJ, Schwartz LB, Busse WW. Elevated bronchoalveolar lavage fluid histamine levels in allergic asthmatics are associated with increased airway obstruction. *Am Rev Respir Dis* 144:83–82, 1991.

12. Durham SR, Lee TH, Cromwell O, et al. Immunologic studies in allergen induced late phase asthmatic responses. *J Allergy Clin Immunol* 74:47–54, 1984.
13. Rafferty P, Beasley CR, Holgate ST. The contribution of histamine to bronchoconstriction produced by inhaled allergen and adenosine 5′-monophosphate in asthma. *Am Rev Respir Dis* 136:369–373, 1987.
14. Kellaway CH, Trethewie ER. The liberation of a slow reacting smooth muscle stimulating substance of anaphylaxis. *Q J Exp Med* 30:131–145, 1940.
15. Adkinson NF, Newball HH, Findlay S, Adams K, Lichtenstein LL. Anaphylactic release of prostaglandins from human lung in vitro. *Am Rev Respir Dis* 121:911–920, 1980.
16. Sheard P, Killingback PG, Blair AMJN. Antigen induced release of histamine and SRS-A from human lung passively sensitised with reaginic serum *Nature* 216:283–284, 1967.
17. Lam S, Chan H, LeRiche JC, Chan-Yeung M, Salari H. Release of Leukotrienes in patients with bronchial asthma. *J Allergy Clin Immunol* 1:711–717, 1988.
18. Taylor GW, Taylor I, Black P, et al. Urinary leukotriene E4 after antigen $E_4$ challenge in acute asthma and allergic rhinitis. *Lancet* 1:584–587, 1989.
19. Shaw RJ, Cromwell O, Kay AB. Preferential generation of leucotriene $C_4$ by human eosinophils. *Clin Exp Immunol* 56:716–722, 1984.
20. Schleimer RP, MacGlasham DW, Peters SP, Pinckard RN, Adkinson NF Jr, Lichtenstein LM. Characterisation of inflammatory mediator release from purified human lung mast cell. *Am Rev Respir Dis* 133:614–617, 1986.
21. Czop JK, Austen KF. Generation of leukotrienes by human monocytes upon stimulation of their beta glucan receptor during phagocytosis. *Proc Natl Acad Sci USA* 82:2751–2755, 1985.
22. Creese BR, Bach MK. Hyperreactivity of airways smooth muscle produced in vitro by leukotrienes. *Prostaglandins Leukotrienes Med* 11:161–169, 1983.
23. Samuellson B. Leukotrienes: mediators of immediate hypersensitivity reactions and inflammation. *Science* 220:568–575, 1983.
24. Hoover RL, Karnovsky MJ, Austen KF, Corey EJ, Lewis RA. Leukotriene $B_4$ action on endothelium mediates augmented neutrophil/endothelial adhesion. *Proc Natl Acad Sci USA* 81:2191–2293, 1984.
25. Goetzl EJ, Pickett WC. The human PMN leukocyte chemotactic activity of complex hydroxyeicosotetraenoic acids (HETES). *J Immunol* 125:1789–1791, 1980.

25a. Kips JC, Joos G, DeLepeleive, et al. MK-571, a potent antagonist of Leukotriene $D_4$-induced bronchoconstriction in humans. *Am Rev Respir Dis* 144:617–621, 1991.

26. Wardlaw AJ, Moqbel R, Cromwell O, Kaye AB. Platelet activating factor: a potent chemotactic and chemokinetic factor for human eosinophils. *J Clin Inves* 78:1701–1706, 1986.
27. Schluman ES, Newball HH, Demers LM, Fitzpatrick FA, Atkinson NF. Anaphylactic release of thromboxane A2, prostaglandin D2 and prosta-

cyclin from human lung parenchyma. *Am Rev Respir Dis* 124:402–406, 1981.

28. Lewis RA, Soter NA, Diamond PT, Austen KF, Oates JA, Roberts LJ II. Prostaglandin $D_2$ generation after activation of rat and human mast cells with anti IgE. *J Immunol* 129:1627–1631, 1982.
29. Murray JJ, Tonnel AB, Brash AR, Roberts LJ II, Gosset P, Workman R, Capron A, Oates JA. Release of prostaglandin $D_2$ into human airways during acute antigen challenge. *N Engl J Med* 315:800–804, 1986.
30. Hardy CC, Robinson C, Tattersfield AE, Holgate ST. The bronchoconstrictor effect of inhaled $PGD_2$ in normal and asthmatic men. *N Engl J Med* 311:209–213, 1984.

30a. Curzen N, Rafferty P, Holgate ST. Effects of a cyclo-oxygenase inhibitor flurbiprofen and an H/histamine receptor antagonist, terfenadine, alone and in combination on allergen induced immediate bronchoconstriction in man. *Thorax* 42:946–952, 1987.

31. Walters EH. Prostaglandins and the control of airway responses to histamine in normal and asthmatic subjects. *Thorax* 38:188–196, 1983.
32. Fuller RW, Dixon CMS, Dollery CT, Barnes PJ. $PGD_2$ potentiates airway responsiveness to histamine and methacholine. *Am Rev Respir Dis* 133:252–254, 1986.
33. Rubin A, HE Smith LJ, Patterson R. The bronchoconstrictor properties of platelet activating factor in humans. *Am Rev Respir Dis* 136:1145–1151, 1987.

33a. Evans TW, Chung KF, Rogers DF, Barnes PJ. Effects of platelet activating factor on airway vascular permeability: possible mechanisms. *J Appl Physiol* 64:479–484, 1987.

34. Wittz H, Lang M, Sannwald U, Hahn H. Mechanisms of platelet activating factor (PAF)-induced secretion from tracheal submucous glands in ferrets. *Fed Proc* 45:418, 1986.
35. Lai CKW, Jenkins JR, Polosa R, Holgate ST. Inhaled PAF fails to induce airway responsiveness to methacholine in normal human subjects. *J Appl Physiol* 68:919–926, 1990.
36. Smith LJ, Rubin AE, Patterson R. Mechanisms of platelet activating factor induced bronchoconstriction in humans. *Am Rev Respir Dis* 137:1015–1019, 1988.
37. Anderson GP, White HL, Fennessy MR. Increased airways responsiveness to histamine induced by platelet activating factor in the guinea pig; possible role of lypoxygenase metabolites. *Agents Actions* 24:1–7, 1988.
38. Chung KF, Minette P, McCusker M, Barnes PJ. Ketotifen inhibits the cutaneous but not the airway responses to platelet activating factor in man. *J Allergy Clin Immunol* 81:1192–1198, 1988.
39. Polack JM, Bloom Sr. Regulatory peptides of the gastrointestinal and respiratory tracts. *Arch Int Pharmacodyn Ther* 280(Suppl:16–49), 1986.
40. Barnes PJ, Dixon CMS. The effect of inhaled vasoactive intestinal peptide on bronchial hyperresponsiveness in man. *Am Rev Respir Dis* 130:162–166, 1984.

41. Morice A, Unwin RJ, Sever PS. Vasoactive intestinal peptide causes bronchodilation and projects against histamine induced bronchoconstriction in asthmatic subjects. *Lancet* 2:1225–1226, 1983.
42. Palmer JBD, Cuss FMC, Warren JB, Barnes PJ. The effect of infused vasoactive peptide on airway function in normal subjects. *Thorax* 41:663–666, 1986.
43. Laitenen LA, Laitenen A, Panula PA, Partenan M, Tervo T. Immunochemical demonstration of substance P in the lower respiratory tract of the rabbit and not of man. *Thorax* 38:531–536, 1983.
44. Clarke B, Evans TW, Dixon CMS, Conradson TB, Barnes PJ. Comparison of the cardiovascular and respiratory effects of substance P and neurokinin A in man. *Clin Sci* 72,41P, 1987.
45. Palmer JBD, Cuss FMC, Mulderry PK, Barnes PJ. Calcitonin gene related peptide is localised to human airway nerves and potentially constricts airway smooth muscle. *Br J Pharmacol* 91:95–101, 1987.
46. Jeffrey PK, Corrin B. Structural analysis of the respiratory tract. In: Bienstock J (ed.), *Immunology of the Lung and Upper Respiratory Tract*. McGraw-Hill, New York and Toronto: 1984, pp. 1–27.
47. Tomiaka M, Ida S, Yuriko S, Ishizaka T, Takiskima Y. Mast cells in bronchoalveolar lumen of patients with bronchial asthma. *Am Rev Respir Dis* 129:1–27, 1984.
48. Wilson JW, Schrader JW, Pain MCF. Human bronchial mast cells. In *Proceedings of the 30th Congress of the International Union of Physical Sciences*, Vancouver, British Columbia, 1986, 123a (abs).
48a. Connell JT. Asthmatic deaths. The role of the mast cell. *JAMA* 215:769–776, 1971.
49. Ishizaka T, Ishizaka K, Tomioko H. Release of histamine and slow reacting substance of anaphylaxis (SRS-A) by IgE and anti-IgE reaction on monkey mast cells. *J Immunol* 108:513–518, 1971.
50. Agius RM, Godfrey RC, Holgate ST. Mast cell and histamine content of human bronchoalveolar lavage. *Thorax* 40:760–766, 1985.
51. Schwartz LB. Performed mediators of human mast cells. In: Holgate ST (ed.), *Mast Cells, Mediators and Disease*. Kluwer Academic Publishers, London, 1988, pp. 129–147.
52. Lison L. Etudes sur la metachromasie: colorants metachromatiques et substances chromotropes. *Arch Biol* 46:599–604, 1935.
53. Kay AB. Mediators and inflammatory cells in asthma. In: Kay AB (ed.), *Asthma, Clinical Pharmacology and Therapeutics Progress*. Blackwell Scientific, Oxford, 1986, pp. 1–10.
54. Proud D, Liekrerski ES, Bailey GS. Identification of human lung mast cell, kininogenase as tryptase and relevance of tryptase kininogenase activity. *Biochem Pharmacol* 78:1473–1480, 1988.
55. Fitzpatrick FA, Adkinson NF. Anaphylactic release of thromboxane $A_2$ prostaglandin from human lung parenchyma. *Am Rev Respir Dis* 124:402–406, 1981.
56. Lewis RA. Slow reacting substance of anaphylaxis: identification of leu-

kotrienes $C_1$ and D from human and rat sources. *Proc Natl Acad Sci* 77:3710–3718, 1980.

57. Yokota T, Otsuka K, Mossman T, Blancherean J, DeFrance T, Blanchard D, DeVries JE, Lee F, Arai K. Isolation and characterisation of a human interleukin cDNA clone, homologous to mouse. B-cell stimulatory factor 1 that expresses B cell and T cell stimulating activities. *Proc Natl Acad Sci* 83:5894–5898, 1986.
58. Horne BR, Robin ED, Theordore J, Vankissel A. Total eosinophil counts in the management of bronchial asthma. *N Engl J Med* 292:1152–1155, 1975.
59. De Monchy JGR, Kauffman H, Venge, P, et al. Bronchoalveolar eosinophilia during allergen induced late asthmatic reaction *Am Rev Respir Dis* 131;373–376, 1985.
60. Beasley CRW, Roche WR, Roberts JA, Holgate ST. Cellular events in the bronchi in mild asthma and after bronchial challenge. *Am Rev Respir Dis* 139:805–817, 1989.

60a. Djukanovic R, Wilson JW, Britlon KM, et al. The inhibitory affect of the inhaled corticosteroid, beclomethasone dipropionate on airway mucosal mast cell and eosinophil numbers relates to its clinical efficiency in asthma. *Am Rev Respir Dis* 1992 (in press).

61. Barnes PJ. New approaches to the treatment of asthma. *N Engl J Med* 321:1517–1527, 1989.
62. Venge P, Kakansson L. Current understanding of the role of the eosinophil granulocyte in asthma. *Clin Exp Allergy* 21:Supplement 3, 31–37, 1991.
63. Sanderson CJ, Campbell HD, Young IG. Molecular and cellular biology of eosinophil differentiation factor (IL5) and its effect on human and mouse B cells. *Immunol Rev* 102:29–53, 1988.
64. Wasson DL, Fleich GJ. Damage to *Trichinella spirilis* newborn larvae by eosinophil major basic protein. *Am J Trop Med Hyg* 28:860–863, 1979.
65. Laitenen LA, Heino M, Laitenen A, Kava J, Haahtela T. Damage of the airway epithelium and bronchial reactivity in patients with asthma. *Am Rev Respir Dis* 131:599–606, 1985.
66. Naylor B. The shedding of the mucosa of the bronchial tree in asthma. *Thorax* 17:69–72, 1962.

66a. Filley WV, Holley KE, Kephant GM, Gleich GJ. Identification by immunofluorescence of eosinophil granule major basic protein in lung tissues of patients with asthma. *Lancet* 1982;2:11–16.

67. Herbert CA, Edwards D, Boot JR, Robinson C. In vitro modulation of the eosinophil dependent enhancement of the permeability of the bronchial mucosa. *Br J Pharmacol* 104;391–398, 1991.
68. Durham SR, Cookson WO, Faux J, Craddock CF, Benson MK. Basic mechanisms in allergen induced late asthmatic responses. *Clin Exp Allergy* 19:117A, 1989.
69. Bass DA. The functions of eosinophils. *Ann Intern Med* 91:120–121, 1979.
70. Capron M, Capron A, Dessiant JP, Torpier G, Johannsen SG, Prin L. $F_c$ receptors of IgE on human and rat eosinophils. *J Immunol* 126:2087–2092, 1981.

71. Durham SR, Kay AB. Eosinophils bronchial hyperreactivity and late phase asthmatic reactions. *Clin Allergy* 15:411–418, 1985.
72. Sanderson CJ, Warren DJ, Strath M. Identification of lymphokine that stimulate eosinophil differentiation in vitro. *J Exp Med* 162:60–70, 1980.
73. Lopez AF, Sanderson CJ, Gamble JR, Campbell HD, Young IG, Vadas MA. Recombinant human IL5 is a selective activator of human eosinophil functions. *J Exp Med* 167:219–228, 1986.
74. Murphy KR, Wilson MC, Irvin CG, et al. The requirement for polymorphonuclear leukocytes in the late asthmatic response and heightened airways reactivity in an animal model. *Am Rev Respir Dis* 134:62–68, 1986.
75. Eshenbacher WL, Gravelyn TR. A technique for isolated airway segment lavage. *Chest* 92:105–109, 1987.
76. Joseph M, Tonnel AB, Torpier G, Capron A, Arnoux B, Benveniste J. Involvement of IgE in the secretory process of alveolar macrophages from asthmatic patients. *J Clin Invest* 71:221–230, 1983.
77. Capron M, Jouault T, Prin C, Joseph M, Ameisen JC, Butterworth AA, Papin JP, Kusneirz JP, Capron A. Functional study of a monoclonal antibody to IgE $F_c$ receptor of eosinophils platelets and macrophages. *J Exp Med* 164:72–89, 1986.
78. Kay AB, Henson PM, Hunninghake GW, Irvin C, Lichtenstein LM, Nadel JA. Cellular mechanisms In: Holgate ST et al. (eds.), *The Role of Inflammatory Processes in Airway Hyperresponsiveness* Blackwell Scientific Publications, Oxford, 1989, pp. 151–178.
79. Nathan CF. Secretory products of macrophages. *J Clin Invest* 79:312–326, 1987.
80. Arnoux B, Simoes-Chair MH, Landes A, Mathieu M, Doroux P, Benveniste J. Alveolar macrophages from asthmatic patients release PAF acether and lyso-PAF acether when stimulated with specific allergen. *Am Rev Respir Dis* 125:A70, 1982.
81. vanFurth R, Raeburn JA, vanZwet TL. Characteristics of human mononuclear phagocytes. Blood 54:485–500, 1979.
82. Nathan CF, Prendergast TJ, Weibe ME, et al. Activation of human macrophage: comparison of other cytokines with interferon gamma. *J Exp Med* 160:600–605, 1984.
83. Rosenthal AS. Regulation of the immune response role of the macrophage. *N Engl J Med* 20:1153–1159, 1980.
84. Dinarello CA. An update in interleukin 1: from molecular biology to clinical relevance. *J Clin Immunol* 5:287–297, 1985.
85. Shortman K, Palmer J. The requirement for macrophages in the in vitro immune response. 2:399–405, 1971.
86. Guyre PM, Munck A. Glucocorticoid actions on monocytes and macrophages. In: Schleimer RP, Glaman NH, Oronsky AR (eds.), *Anti Inflammatory Steroids: Basic and Clinical Aspects*. Academic Press, New York, 1988.
87. Speigelberg HL, O'Connor RD, Simon RA, Mathison DA. Lymphocytes with immunoglobulin $EF_c$ receptors in patients with atopic disorders. *J Clin Invest* 64:714–799, 1979.

88. Marom Z, Shelhamer J, Allurig D, Kaliner M. The effects of corticosteroids on mucous glycoprotein secretion from human airways in vitro. *Am Rev Respir Dis* 129:62–66, 1984.
89. Dunnill MS. The pathology of asthma with special reference to changes in the bronchial mucosa. *J Clin Pathol* 13:27–37, 1960.
90. Dunnill MS. The pathology of asthma. In: Middleton E Jr, Reed CE, Ellis EF (eds.), *Allergy, Principles and Practice.* CV Mosby, St Louis, 1978, pp. 678–686.
91. Jeffrey PK, Wardlaw AJ, Nelson FC, Collins JV, Kay AB. Bronchial biopsies in asthma. An ultrastructural quantitative study and correlation with hyperreactivity. *Am Rev Respir Dis* 140:1745–1753, 1989.
92. Tada K, Ishizaka K. Distribution of IgE forming cells in lymphoid tissues of the human and monkey. *J Immunol* 104:377–382, 1970.
93. Corrigan CJ, Hartnell A, Kay AB. T Lymphocyte activation in acute severe asthma. *Lancet* 1:1129–1132, 1988.
94. Corrigan CJ, Kay AB. CD4 T-lymphocyte activation in acute severe asthma. *Am Rev Respir Dis* 141:970–977, 1990.
95. Diaz P, Gonzules MC, Gallegullos FR, et al. Leukocytes and mediators in BAL during allergen induced late phase asthmatic reactions. *Am Rev Respir Dis* 1383–1389, 1989.
96. Azzawi M, Bradley B, Jeffrey PK, Frew AJ, Wardlaw AJ, Knowles J, Assoufi A, Collins JV, Durham S, Kay AB. Identification of activated T lymphocytes and eosinophils in bronchial biopsies in stable atopic asthma. *Am Rev Respir Dis* 142:1407–1413, 1990.
97. Romanagni S, Del Prete G, Maggi E, Parronchi P, Tiri A. Macchia D, Guidizz MG, Almerigogna F, Ricci M. Role of interleukins in induction and regulation of human IgE synthesis. *Clin Immunol Immunopathol* 50:S13–S23, 1989.
98. Wang JM, Rambaldi A, Biondi A, Chen AZ, Sanderson CJ, Mantorani A. Recombinant interleukin 5 is a selective eosinophils chemo-attractant. *Eur J Immunol* 19:701–705, 1989.
99. Vadas MA, Nicola NA, Metcalf D. Activation of an antibody dependent cell mediated cytotoxicity of human neutrophils and eosinophils by separate colony stimulating factors. *J Immunol* 130:795–799, 1983.
100. Hamaguchi Y, Kanakura Y, Futija J, et al. Interleukin 4 as an essential factor for in vitro clonal growth of human connective tissue type mast cells. *J Exp Med* 165:268–273, 1987.
101. Ihle JN, Keller J, Orsoszahn S, et al. Biologic properties of homogeneous interleukin 3. Demonstration of WEH1-3 growth factor activity, P cell stimulating factor activity, colony stimulating factor activity and histamine producing cell stimulating factor activity. *J Immunol* 131:282–287, 1983.
102. Snyder DS, Inanue ER. Corticosteroids inhibit murine Ia and Ihl production. *J Immunol* 129:1803–1809, 1982.
103. Smith KA. T cell growth factor. *J Immunol* 51:337–343, 1980.
104. Vargaftig BB, Lefort J, Chignard M, Benveniste J. Platelet activating factor induces a platelet dependent bronchoconstriction unrelated to the formulation of prostaglandin derivatives. *Eur J Pharmacol* 65:815–192, 1980.

105. Own RT. Platelets: a review of selected aspects of their physiology, pharmacology and pathology, with special reference to their role in inflammation and thrombogenesis. *Drugs Today* 15:487–503, 1979.
106. Schneider RC, Zapol WM, Carvatho AC. Platelet consumption and sequestration in severe acute respiratory failure. *Am Rev Respir Dis* 122:445–449, 1980.
107. Storck H, Hoigne R, Koller F. Thrombocytes in allergic reactions. *Int Arch Allergy* 6:372–378, 1955.
108. Joseph M, Capron A, Amiesen JC, et al. The receptor of IgE on blood platelets. *Eur J Immunol* 16:306–312, 1986.
109. Metzger WJ, Sjoerdsma K, Richerson HB, et al. Platelets in bronchoalveolar lavage from asthmatic patients and allergic rabbits with allergen induces late phase responses. *Agents Actions* 21(suppl):151–159, 1987.
110. Metzger WJ, Henriksen RA, Atkinson LB, Wirefel-Svet KL, Fisher RH. Bronchial challenge with platelet derived histamine releasing factor (PD-HRF) induces a pulmonary eosinophilic infiltrate. *J Allergy Clin Immunol* 5:262(abstr), 1990.
111. Vanhoutte PM. Epithelium derived relaxing factors and bronchial reactivity *Am Rev Respir Dis* 1988; 183(6)-Part 2.524–30.
112. Barnett K, Jacoby DB, Nadel JA, Lazanis SC. The effects of epithelial cell supernatant on contractions of isolated canine tracheal smooth muscle. *Am Rev Respir Dis* 136:780–783, 1988.
113. Sekizawa K, Tamaoki J, Graf PD, Basbaum CB, Borson DB, Nadel JA. Tachykinins inhibit encephalinase activity from tracheas and lungs of ferrets. *Physiologist* 29:174, 1986.
114. Gleich GJ and Adolphson CR. The eosinophil leucocyte: structure and function. In Dixon F (ed.), *Advances in Immunology*. Academic Press, New York, 1986, pp. 177–254.
115. Frigas E, Loegering DA, Gleich GJ. Cytotoxic effects of the guinea pig major basic protein on tracheal epithelium. *Lab Invest* 42:35–43, 1980.
116. Raeburn D, Hay DW, Farmer SG, Fedan JS. Epithelium removal increases the reactivity of human isolated tracheal muscle and reduces the effect of verapamil. *Eur J Pharmacol* 123:451–453, 1986.
117. Roche WR, Beasley R, Williams JH, Holgate ST. Subepithelial fibrosis in the bronchi of asthmatics. *Lancet* 1:520–523, 1989.
118. Flavahan NA, Vanhoutte PM. The respiratory epithelium releases a smooth muscle relaxing factor. *Chest* 87:189–190, 1987.
118a. Stephenson BR, Paul DL. The molecular constituents of intercellular junctions. *Curr Opin Cell Res* 1989:884–891, 1990.
119. Hynes RO. Integrins, a family of cell surface receptors. *Cell* 48:549–555, 1987.
120. Saunders S, Jalkanen M, O'Favvell S, Barnfield M. Molecular cloning of syndecan, an integral membrane glycoprotein. *J Cell Biol* 108:1547–1556, 1989.
121. Aruffo A, Stamenovic I, Melmck M, Underhill CB, Seed B. CD44 is the principal cell surface receptor for hyaluronidase. *Cell* 61:1303–1313, 1990.

122. Osborn L. Leukocytes adhesion to endothelium in inflammation. *Cell* 62:3–6, 1990.
123. Pober JS, Cotram RS. The role of endothelial cells in inflammation. *Transplantation* 50:537–544, 1990.
124. Wegner CD, Gundel RH, Reilly P, Haynes N, Letts LG, Rothlein. Intercellular adhesion molecule-1 (ICAM-1) in the pathogenesis of asthma. *Science* 247:456–459, 1990.

# 2

# Bronchial Hyperresponsiveness in Normal and Asthmatic Children

**AGAINDRA K. BEWTRA and ROBERT G. TOWNLEY**

*Creighton University*
*Omaha, Nebraska*



The precise definition of asthma is difficult in patients of any age group, but is even more difficult in children than in adults. There are several reasons for this. The causes and pathologic features of asthma are multifactorial. It is difficult to complete a comprehensive history in children and furthermore it may be impossible to do adequate testing. A history of wheezing and coughing and the occasional use of bronchodilators is very helpful in ascertaining the diagnosis of asthma, but in clinical medicine this is not always true. For the above reasons, pulmonary function testing has become an extremely important and valuable tool in the evaluation of the asthmatic individual. The diagnosis of bronchial asthma can be readily established if reversible bronchoconstriction can be demonstrated by routine spirometry. The diagnosis becomes difficult to establish if the patient has only intermittent symptoms of coughing, dyspnea, or wheezing and the baseline spirometry is normal. It is under these circumstances that bronchial provocation challenges are being increasingly performed to establish the diagnosis of asthma.

## DEFINITIONS

Curry in 1947 (1) first induced attacks of asthma in healthy persons and subjects with hay fever and asthma by challenging them with methacholine (acetyl-beta-methylcholine) and histamine in his office. It soon became clear that asthmatic subjects of all ages are exquisitively sensitive to bronchoconstrictive agents. However, only recently has this increased bronchial responsiveness been included in the definition of asthma (2,3). An exaggerated bronchoconstrictor response to methacholine or histamine is a uniform finding in patients with bronchial asthma. Several studies have shown that >80% of all subjects with a history of asthma and 98–100% of patients with currently symptomatic asthma have significantly increased bronchial responsiveness to methacholine or histamine challenges (1–12). However, increased bronchial responsiveness is not unique only to subjects with asthma. Enhanced bronchial responsiveness has been seen in subjects with allergic rhinitis (5,11,13), subjects with atopic family history (5), children (14–17), siblings of subjects with asthma (18), subjects with chronic pulmonary diseases (19), bronchopulmonary dysplasia (20), after respiratory tract infections (21–23), in young asymptomatic smokers (24), and in subjects with a history of atopic diseases but without asthma (5,11,13). Because of these conditions, it becomes imperative to establish the sensitivity and the specificity of this increased bronchial responsiveness in diagnosing asthma. Townley and his colleagues (5,25) did just that in a very large population (Fig. 1). Their studies helped to establish realistic cutoff values for the diagnosis of asthma without encountering significant false-positive or negative results. A realistic cutoff value for the diagnosis of asthma currently in use is approximately a provocative dose of methacholine producing a 20% decrease in forced expiratory volume in 1 sec ($FEV_1$)($PD_{20}$) of 100 breath units (bu). As can be seen from the data, at this cutoff value of 100 bu, the sensitivity and specificity are roughly 90% each. This means that a $PD_{20}$ of 100 bu could be associated with a 10% false-positive and a 10% false-negative result. Any methacholine challenge with a $PD_{20}$ close to a 100 bu should be cautiously interpreted in association with a clinical history and a physical examination.

## BRONCHIAL CHALLENGE MODALITIES

Bronchial hyperresponsiveness can be and has been induced by numerous means. These can be, for convenience and from a pathophysiological point of view, classified as pharmacologic, allergen, and natural challenges. Methacholine, histamine, acetylcholine, carbachol, pilocarpine, serotonin, prostaglandin F2a, leukotrienes, and platelet activating factor (PAF) have all been used as pharmacologic agents to induce bronchial constriction directly. Of these, methacholine and histamine are the agents most commonly used currently. The allergen challenges are performed to those allergens that the patient shows skin test sensitivity to and has a history of reacting to clinically. The natural challenges include mainly exercise (26), isocapneic cold air hyperventilation (27), and hypo- and hypertonic nebulized saline challenges (28). There is a good overall correlation between the various challenges, but in any given subject a certain challenge may be highly positive while another challenge is only weakly positive or, rarely, completely negative. These differences between the various challenges are extensively evaluated to allow us to understand the biochemical and immunologic mechanisms in asthma and airway hyperresponsiveness.

Methacholine inhalation challenge has been extensively undertaken in both research and clinical situations. Along with these studies methacholine challenges have also proved very useful in population, genetic, and epidemiologic studies (5,29–37).

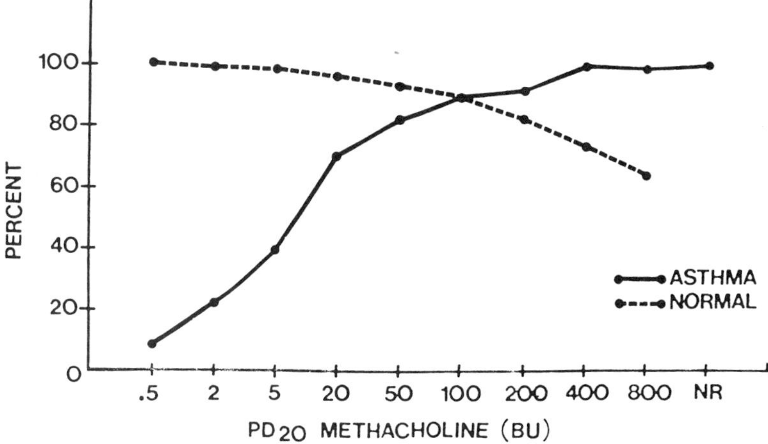


FIGURE 1 Comparing response to methacholine with clinical diagnosis we found that a $PD_{20}$ of 100 bu optimized both sensitivity and specificity at 90%. (Adapted from Ref. 25.)

## EFFECT OF AGE AND PREDICTIVE VALUE OF AIRWAY HYPERRESPONSIVENESS

In addition to all the factors and diseases that affect methacholine responsiveness and have been discussed earlier, age seems to have a very significant effect on the degree of responsiveness. This effect of age on methacholine sensitivity has been studied by us in a population study of over 750 individuals (14). When the methacholine responsiveness was plotted against age (Fig. 2) in subjects who have no history of asthma, it can be very easily appreciated that the very young and the very old have significantly increased bronchial responsiveness. If this factor is not taken into account in clinical practice there could be a tendency to suggest falsely the presence of hyperresponsive airways in these populations. Tepper and his colleagues (16) have suggested that increased airway responsiveness is common to many young infants. Dave et al. (38) have shown that allergic nonasthmatic children have increased nonspecific bronchial responsiveness and that this increased bronchial responsiveness persists over time in this group of children. They postulate that it is possible that individuals with allergies and

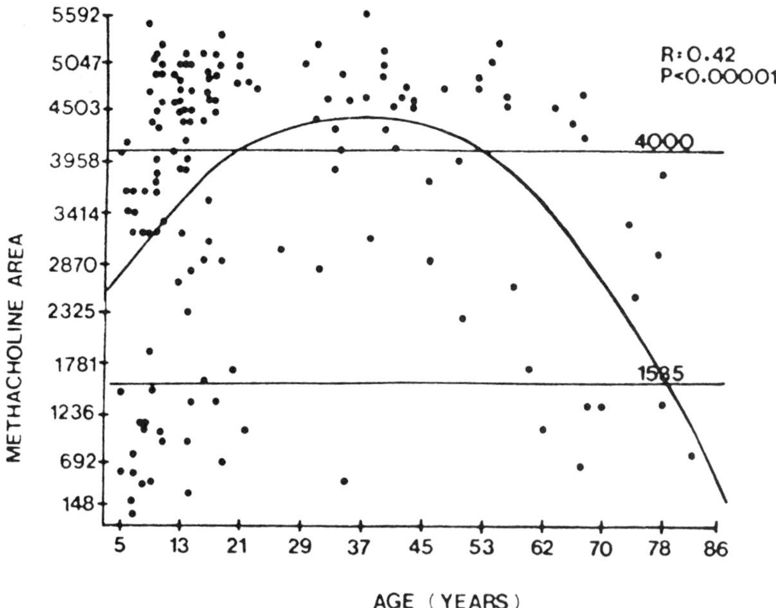


FIGURE 2 Methacholine responses of individuals studied. Results ≥4000 indicate normal responses. Values ≤1535 indicate responses that are ≤ breath units of methacholine. The best-fitting curve is superimposed. (Adapted from Ref. 14.)

family members of asthmatic subjects "retain" this enhanced bronchial responsiveness, thus increasing their chance of developing asthma. This would require that increased bronchial responsiveness precede the development of asthma symptoms. Very few large or small prospective studies have been undertaken to date to evaluate this. Hopp and colleagues (39) were able to evaluate 20 children with increased bronchial reactivity over several years and were able to show that 17 of them went on to develop symptoms of asthma years later. However, they also found three subjects from their population studies who developed asthma but had had a completely normal methacholine response before the development of the symptoms. Sears and colleagues (40) have also been able to show that increased airway responsiveness pre-existed in children who later became clinically asthmatic. Although not conclusive these studies suggest that airway hyperresponsiveness may be genetically determined.

## ASTHMA IN FAMILIES AND TWINS

The studies discussed above increased interest in the evaluation of genetic transmission of airway hyperresponsiveness. Genetic studies have been undertaken using either asthma as a diagnosis in family or twin studies or bronchial hyperresponsiveness as a genetic marker in these populations. Sibbald et al. (41,42) selected an asthmatic proband and studied the nuclear family of this person with questionnaires. They reported that asthma was more frequent in parents (13%) and offspring (9%) than the siblings (8%) of the probands and concluded from these data that atopic asthma appears to have genetic basis and that atopy enhances the development of asthma. Gerrard et al. (43) also used a questionnaire to study 176 families and were also able to show a significant association between asthma, hay fever, recurrent rhinitis, or bronchitis in parents and children. These authors suggested that there was an inherited component to end-organ hyperresponsiveness.

Edfors-Lubs (44) contacted the 7000 pairs of twins collected in the Swedish Twin Registry by questionnaire and was able to tabulate the data for zygosity and asthma history in this population. A current or former diagnosis of asthma was found in 3.8% of this population. The intrapair concordance rate was found to be 19% in the monozygous twins and only 4% in the dizygous twins. Falliers (45) reviewed all such studies and tabulated collective concordance rates. He found an intrapair concordance of 30–80% for monozygous twins and 4–45% for dizygous twins. Although all these studies used only histories and had no objective data they were able to show that the development of asthma may have a genetic and hereditary component.

### Airway Hyperresponsiveness in Families

To obtain objective data to determine the genetics of asthma, it became imperative that a genetic marker be established for the diagnosis of asthma. Skin tests and IgE levels have been tried but asthmatic subjects are not universally atopic. Since all patients with asthma have increased bronchial responsiveness and since this has been incorporated into the definition of asthma, we decided to determine if methacholine hyperresponsiveness could be used as a genetic marker for asthma.

We undertook family and twin studies. For the family studies we studied 750 individuals from 53 families with asthma and 26 control families (5,46). The asthmatic families had a proband with asthma and at least three generations of that family were studied. The control families had no history of atopic disease, atopic eczema, allergic rhinitis, or bronchial asthma for

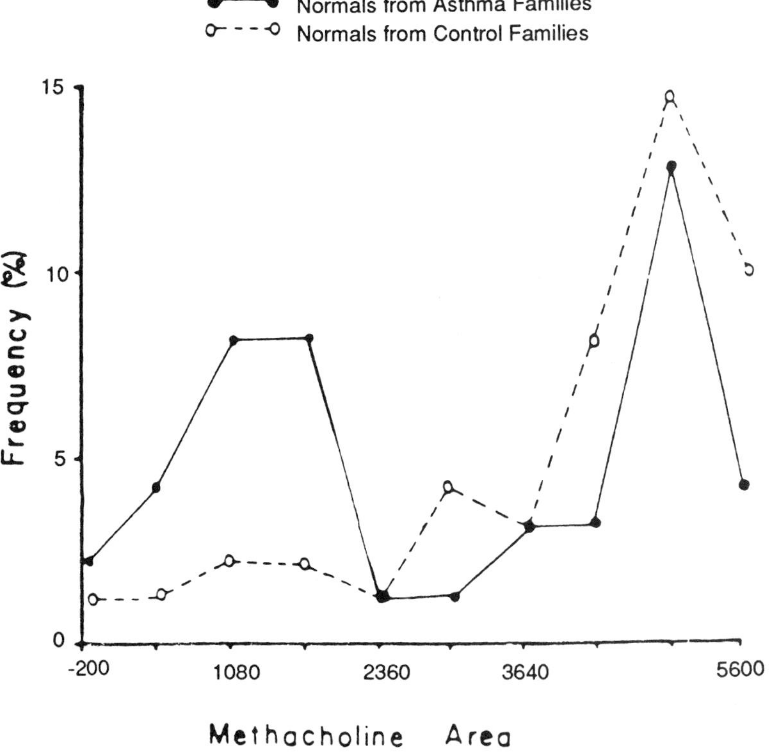


FIGURE 3 Frequency plot of age-corrected area under dose–response curves for methacholine in normal individuals from both asthmatic and control families. Left-hand mode shows excess number of positive responders from asthmatic families. (From Ref. 5.)

the three generations. The methacholine responsiveness of normal nonatopic individuals from asthmatic families compared to that of normal individuals from control families is shown in Figure 3. The normal subjects from control families essentially show a unimodal distribution. In contrast, normal subjects from asthmatic families show a bimodal distribution of methacholine responsiveness. Although these subjects were all clinically normal there was a subgroup with a positive methacholine response. These responders may be at greater risk of developing asthma at a later date. A similar bimodal distribution was also obtained in nonatopic parents of asthmatic children and not in the control parents (Fig. 4). This bimodal distribution of bronchial hyperresponsiveness could suggest a single physiological and perhaps a single genetic abnormality. However, when we undertook a segregation analysis of these data (46,47), although the anal-

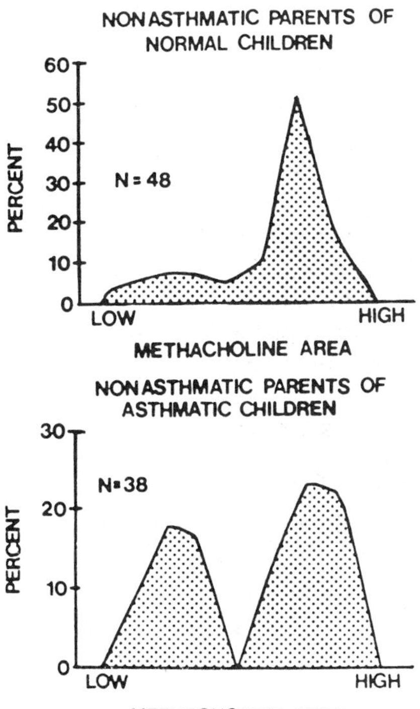


FIGURE 4 Distribution of methacholine area responses in the subjects studied. The four categories of responses were arbitrarily determined. Marked bronchial responsiveness up to 80 bu; moderate up to 340 bu; minimal bronchial up to 800 bu; negative, not more than a 19.9% fall in $FEV_1$ by 800 bu. (Adapted from Refs. 30 and 47.)

ysis showed that a familial component exists in the transmission of bronchial hyperresponsiveness, it failed to show a single autosomal transmission as responsible. This means that airway hyperresponsiveness appears to be determined both by genetic and environmental factors. The airway hyperresponsiveness could thus be transmitted by polygenetic mechanisms. More studies need to be undertaken for us to be able to state accurately the mode of genetic inheritance of asthma, atopic diseases, and bronchial hyperresponsiveness.

### Airway Responsiveness in Twins

There are significant limitations in using twins to evaluate the role of heredity. However, twins studies are an accessible and practical method for estimating the degree of genetic influence. Monozygous (MZ) twins should have the same gene pool and also have significantly similar environmental influences, whereas dizygous (DZ) twins should only have similar environmental factors. The comparison of intrapair correlation coefficient (r) provides an indicator of the role of heredity in atopic diseases and bronchial reactivity. A heritability estimate (H) = 2(rMZ − rDZ), where r is the intrapair correlation coefficient, has been described by Woolf (48). This provides an estimate of the contribution of heredity to the variance of the measured trait or marker. When H equals 1, the variation in the measurement is completely due to heredity. As H approaches 0, the measurement is due to environmental factors. We studied methacholine responsiveness in 61 pairs of monozygous and 47 pairs of dizygous twins (29). As shown in Figure 5, we obtained an intrapair correlation coefficient of 0.67 for monozygous twins and 0.34 for dizygous twins. These differences are statistically significant and the heritability estimated from this data is 0.66. These studies support the family studies and suggest that there is significant genetic influence in airway reactivity. Konig and Godfrey (49) studying 8 MZ and 7 DZ twins found a greater intrapair concordance in the monozygous twins, while Zamel et al. (50) found no evidence of genetic influence on nonspecific bronchial responsiveness in 10 pairs of monozygous and 10 pairs of dizygous twins. Thus it would be safe to conclude from current knowledge that there is significant genetic contribution to increased bronchial responsiveness in asthma and atopic diseases.

## SUMMARY

Bronchial hyperresponsiveness is an important test that can be safely and easily done to establish the diagnosis of bronchial asthma. Young children tend to have increased bronchial responsiveness compared to adults. A $PD_{20}$ of 100 bu for methacholine is a good cutoff value for the diagnosis

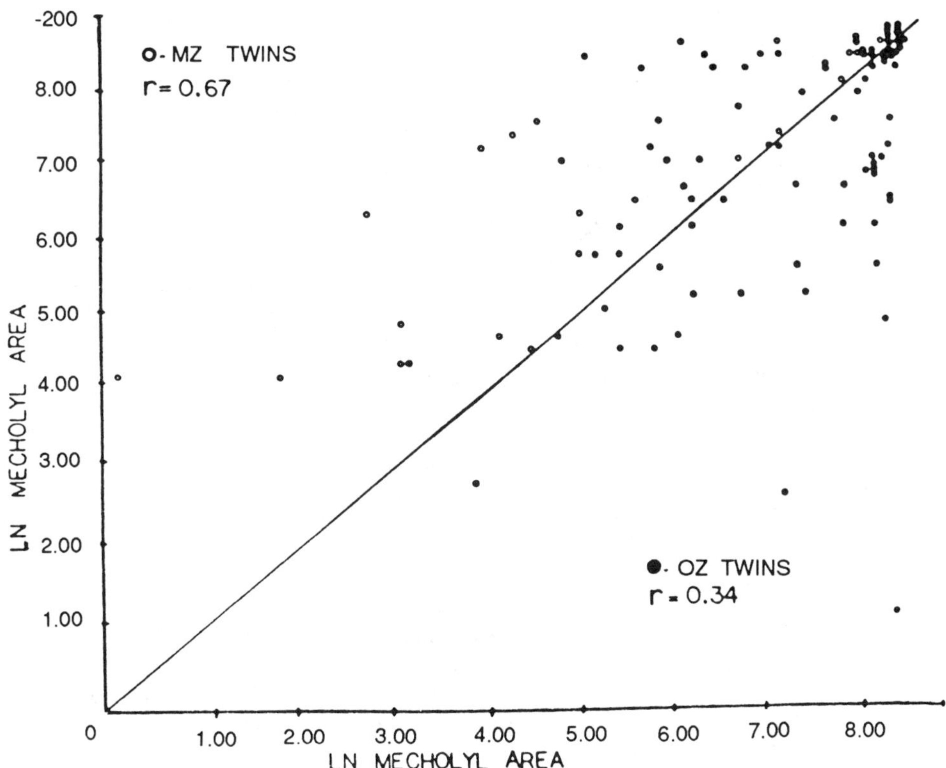


FIGURE 5 Intrapair correlation of methacholine (mecholyl) sensitivity as determined by the area under the dose–response curve. Methacholine area expressed as the natural log shows a correlation coefficient of 0.67 in monozygous (MZ) twins and 0.34 in dizygous (DZ) twins (From Ref. 47.)

of asthma. Bronchial hyperresponsiveness could be used as a genetic marker for asthma. There is evidence that asthma and bronchial hyperresponsiveness could be genetically transmitted, based on both family and twin studies. The mode of genetic inheritance remains to be determined.

## REFERENCES

1. Curry JJ. Comparative action of acetyl-beta-methylcholine and histamine on the respiratory tract in normals, patients with hay fever and subjects with bronchial asthma. *J Clin Invest* 26:430–435, 1947.

2. Rosenthal RR, Chai H, Mathison DA, et al. Indications for inhalation challenge. *J Allergy Clin Immunol* 64:603–605, 1979.
3. Reed C, Townley R: Asthma: classification and pathogenesis. In: Middleton E Jr, Reed CE, Ellis EF (eds.), *Allergy: Principles and Practice*, ed. 2, CV Mosby, St. Louis, 1983, pp. 811–832.
4. Juniper EF, Frith PA, Dunnett C, Cockcroft DW, Hargreave FE. Reproducibility and comparison of responses to inhaled histamine and methacholine. *Thorax* 33:705–710, 1978.
5. Townley RG, Bewtra AK, Nair NM, Brodkey FD, Watt GD, Burke KM. Methacholine inhalation challenge studies. *J Allergy Clin Immunol* 64(2):569–574, 1979.
6. Cockcroft DW, Killian DN, Mellon JJA, Hargreave FE. Bronchial reactivity to inhaled histamine: a method and clinical survey. *Clin Allergy* 7:235–243, 1977.
7. Parker CD, Bilbo RE, Reed CE. Methacholine aerosol as a test for bronchial asthma. *Arch Intern Med* 115:452–458, 1965.
8. Orehek J, Gayrard P, Smith AP, Grimand C, Charpin J. Airway response to carbachol in normal and asthmatic subjects. *Am Rev Respir Dis* 115:937–943, 1977.
9. Itkin IH. Bronchial hypersensitivity to mecholyl and histamine in asthma subjects. *J Allergy* 40:245–256, 1967.
10. Spector SL, Farr RS. A comparison of methacholine and histamine inhalations in asthmatics. *J Allergy Clin Immunol* 56:308–316, 1975.
11. Townley RG, Dennis M, Itkin IH. Comparative action of acetyl-beta-methylcholine, histamine and pollen antigens in subjects with hay fever and patients with bronchial asthma. *J Allergy* 36:121–137, 1965.
12. Mitchell I, Corey M, Woenne R, Krastins IRB, Levison H. Bronchial hyperreactivity in cystic fibrosis and asthma. *J Pediatr* 93(5):744–748, 1978.
13. Townley RG, Ryo UY, Kolotkin BM, Kang B. Bronchial sensitivity to methacholine in current and former asthmatics and allergic rhinitis patients and control subjects. *J Allergy Clin Immunol* 56:429–442, 1975.
14. Hopp RJ, Bewtra A, Nair NM, Townley RG. The effect of age on methacholine response. *J Allergy Clin Immunol* 76:609–613, 1985.
15. Hopp RJ, Bewtra AK, Nair NM, Watt GD, Townley RG. Methacholine inhalation challenge studies in a selected pediatric population. *Am Rev Respir Dis* 134:994–998, 1986.
16. Tepper RS. Airway reactivity in infants: a positive response to methacholine and metaproterenol. *J Appl Physiol* 62:1155–1159, 1987.
17. LeSouef PN, Geelhoed G, Turner DJ, Morgan SEG, Landau LI: Response of normal infants to histamine. *Am Rev Respir Dis* 139:62–66, 1989.
18. Hopp RJ, Bewtra AK, Nair NM, Biven RE, Townley RG. Pattern of methacholine induced bronchial reactivity in siblings of asthmatic subjects. *Pediatr Asthma Allergy Immunol* 1(2):103–109, 1987.
19. Bahous J, Cartier A, Ouimet G, Pineau L, Malo J. Nonallergic bronchial reactivity in chronic bronchitis. *Am Rev Respir Dis* 129:216–220, 1984.
20. Motoyama EK, Fort MD. Evidence of bronchial reactivity in premature

infants with BPD and related chronic respiratory disorders. Report of the Ninetieth Ross Laboratories Conference in Pediatric Research, Columbus, Ohio, March 1986.

21. Empey DW, Laitinen LA, Jacobs L, Gold WM, Nadel, JA. Mechanisms of bronchial hyper-reactivity in normal subjects after upper respiratory tract infection. *Am Rev Respir Dis* 113:131–139, 1976.
22. Gurwitz D, Mindorff C, Levison H. Increased incidence of bronchial reactivity in children with a history of bronchiolitis. *J Pediatr* 98(4):551–555, 1981.
23. Busse WW. The relationship between viral infections and onset of allergic diseases and asthma. *Clin Exp Allergy* 19:1–9, 1989.
24. Malo JL, Filiatrault S, Martin RR. Bronchial responsiveness to inhaled methacholine in young asymptomatic smokers. *J Appl Physiol* 52(6):1464–1470, 1982.
25. Hopp RJ, Bewtra AK, Nair NM, Townley RG. Specificity and sensitivity of methacholine inhalation challenge in normal and asthmatic children. *J Allergy Clin Immunol* 74(2):154–158, 1984.
26. Eggleston PA. Exercise challenge: indications, techniques and data analysis. *J Allergy Clin Immunol* 64(6):604–645, 1979.
27. Strauss RH, McFadden ER, Ingram RH, Jaeger JJ. Enhancement of exercise-induced asthma by cold air. *N Engl J Med* 297:743–747, 1977.
28. Anderson SD, Schoeffel RE, Finney M. Evaluation of ultrasonically nebulized solutions for provocation testing for patients with asthma. *Thorax* 38:284–291, 1983.
29. Hopp RJ, Bewtra AK, Watt GD, Nair NM, Townlet RG. Genetic analysis of allergic diseases in twins. *J Allergy Clin Immunol* 73:265–270, 1984.
30. Townley RG, Hopp RJ, Bewtra AK, Nair NM. Airway reactivity in asthmatic families and twins. In: Spector S (ed.), *Provocative Challenge Procedures: Background and Methodology*, Futura Publishing, Mount Kisco, NY, 1989.
31. Cockcroft DW, Bercheid BA, Murdock KY. Unimodal distribution of bronchial responsiveness to inhaled histamine in a random human population. *Chest* 83:751, 1983.
32. Malo JL, Cartier A, Pineau L, Martin R. Reference values of the provocative concentration of methacholine that causes 6% and 20% changes in forced expiratory volume in one second in a normal population. *Am Rev Respir Dis* 128:8, 1983.
33. Rachelefsky G, Park MS, Siegels S, et al. Strong association between beta-lymphocytes group-2 specificity and asthma. *Lancet* 2:1042–1044, 1976.
34. Easton J, Brady R, Kaplan M, et al. Studies on the relationship of bronchial reactivity to methacholine and HLA haplotypes in asthmatic families. *J Allergy Clin Immunol* 58(4):323, 1975.
35. Longo G, Strinati R, Poli F, et al. Genetic factors in nonspecific bronchial hyperreactivity. *Am J Dis Child* 141:331–334, 1987.
36. Clifford RD, Pugsley A, Radford M, et al. Symptoms, atopy and bronchial response to methacholine in parents with asthma and children. *Arch Dis Child* 62:66–73, 1987.

37. Anton-Guirgis H, Townley RG, Schanfield MS. Methacholine inhalation and Gm allotypes in familial asthma. *J Asthma* 21:1–8, 1984.
38. Dave, NK, Hopp RJ, Biven RE, Degan J, Bewtra AK, Townley RG. Persistence of increased nonspecific bronchial reactivity in allergic children and adolescents. *J Allergy Clin Immunol* 86(2):147–153, 1990.
39. Hopp RJ, Townley RG, Biven RE, Bewtra AK, Nair NM. The presence of airway reactivity before the development of asthma. *Am Rev Respir Dis* 141:2–8, 1990.
40. Sears MR, Holdaway MD, Hewitt CJ, Silva PA. Bronchial reactivity in children without asthma (abstract). *Aust NZ J Med* 14:542, 1984.
41. Sibbald B. Extrinsic and intrinsic asthma: influence of classification on family history and allergic disease. *Clin Allergy* 10:313–318, 1980.
42. Sibbald B, Horn MEC, Brain EA, et al. Genetic factors in childhood asthma. *Thorax* 35:671–674, 1980.
43. Gerrard JW, Ko CG, Vickers P, et al. The familial incidence of allergic disease. *Ann Allergy* 36:10–15, 1976.
44. Edfors-Lubs MI: Allergy in 7000 twin pairs. *Acta Allergol (Kbh)* 26:249–285, 1971.
45. Falliers CI, deACardoso RR, Bane HN, et al. Discordant allergic manifestations in monozygotic twins. Genetic identity versus clinical, physiological and biochemical differences. *J Allergy* 47:207–219, 1971.
46. Townley RG, Bewtra AK, Wilson AF, Hopp RJ, Elston RC, Nair NM, Watt GD. Segregation analysis of bronchial response to methacholine inhalation challenge in families with and without asthma. *J Allergy Clin Immunol* 77:101–107, 1986.
47. Hopp RJ, Bewtra AK, Biven R, Nair NM, Townley RG. Bronchial reactivity pattern in nonasthmatic parents of asthmatics. *Ann Allergy* 61:184–186, 1988.
48. Woolf CA. *Principles of Biometry*. Van Nostrand, Princeton, NJ, 1968, 14:230–231.
49. Konig P, Godfrey S. Exercise-induced bronchial lability in monozygotic (identical) and dizygotic (non-identical) twins. *J Allergy Clin Immunol* 54:280–287, 1974.
50. Zamel N, Leroux M, Vanerdoelen JL. Airway response to inhaled methacholine in healthy nonsmoking twins. *J Appl Physiol* 56:936–939, 1984.

# 3

# Lung Function in Infants and Children and the Effect of Asthma

**SIMON GODFREY**

*Hadassah University Hospital*
*Jerusalem, Israel*



The lungs have a number of functions, including metabolic functions, but as far as asthma is concerned the important aspects of lung function include the mechanics of breathing, gas transfer, and those immunologic, neural, and humoral functions that determine bronchial caliber. Since asthma is a disease par excellence of disturbed physiology, it is important to understand the normal physiology of the lungs in children and the way that this is altered by the disease if we are to understand the disease itself and make rational decisions about treatment.

The essential difference between the lungs of the asthmatic child and the normal child is the state of bronchial hyperreactivity that exists in the asthmatic: airway narrowing occurs readily in response to a variety of stimuli (1). This very marked difference is, however, an exaggeration of the normal physiological responses of the airways and the difference is one of quantity rather than quality. Moreover, increased bronchial reactivity occurs in diseases other than asthma, but there are some very important differences in reactivity between asthmatics and others in response to various stimuli (2).

## MECHANICAL FUNCTION OF THE LUNGS

At the simplest level, the lungs consist of a bellows system whose function is to exchange gas with the environment. Bellows are rather inefficient because part of each inspired breath consists of air expired in the previous breath that has remained in the tubing or dead space. Fish have a much more efficient system because they have countercurrent flow of blood and water over their gills. In order to effect adequate gas exchange, the lungs must ensure that the alveolar gas is replenished at a sufficient rate to allow oxygen uptake and carbon dioxide excretion to proceed normally, irrespective of the size of the child or the metabolic demands on the body due to physical exertion or other factors. The oxygen consumption of the newborn infant is about 30 ml/min, that of a child of 10 years at rest is about 150 ml/min, and that of a 16-year-old working at his or her maximal level is about 3000 ml/min (3). Thus it can be seen that the lungs are required to cope with a very considerable increase in demand both as a result of growth and as a result of activity. In order to follow the changes that occur in pulmonary physiology to cope with these factors, it is necessary to understand the essential functional parameters of the respiratory system and consider how they determine the pattern of breathing. Reverting to the bellows model, the performance of such a pump will depend essentially upon its volume, the depth and rate of its excursion, the resistance to airflow through its tubing, and the stiffness of the bellows material itself.

## LUNG VOLUME

The important subdivisions of lung volume are illustrated in Figure 1. The total volume of gas in the lungs after a maximal inspiration is known as

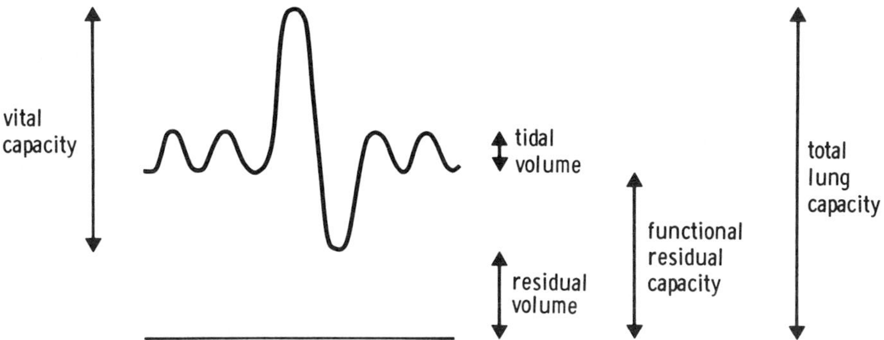


FIGURE 1 The basic subdivisions of lung volume. (From Godfrey S. In: Godfrey S, Baum JD (eds.), *Clinical Paediatric Physiology*. Blackwell Scientific Publications, Oxford, 1979.)

the total lung capacity (TLC) and this volume is limited by the absolute size of the lungs and thoracic cage and by the ability of the muscles of inspiration to overcome the inward elastic recoil of the lungs and chest wall. After a maximal expiration there remains a volume of gas in the lungs known as the residual volume (RV) that cannot be expelled because of the minimal size of the thoracic cage and the inability of the expiratory muscles to overcome the outward recoil of the lungs and chest wall. An important additional factor is that some of the small airways close off completely as lung volume is reduced, trapping the gas in the alveoli that they supply. The RV is 20–25% of the TLC.

The difference between TLC and RV (i.e., the size of the largest breath possible for the subject) is known as the vital capacity (VC). From the above it is clear that the VC is governed by the strength of the muscles of respiration, the elastic properties of the lungs and chest wall, and the degree of gas trapping. It is also governed by the time available for expiration, since if expiration is unduly slow, as it may be in severe asthma, the subject may simply be unable to continue expiring long enough to expel all the VC. The determination of the VC requires maximum cooperation on behalf of the child and hence it is an unreliable measure in the very young or uncooperative subject.

The volume of gas in the lungs in the resting position at the end of a normal expiration is known as the functional residual capacity (FRC), which is about 40% of the TLC. This is a much less well-defined volume since it varies with the pattern of breathing adopted. This is notoriously affected in conscious and alert subjects by having them breathe through respiratory apparatus. In infants and small children this is the only parameter of lung volume that can be measured reliably, because the measurement of TLC and RV require active cooperation on the part of the subject. The true FRC is the position of the lungs adopted at rest at the end of expiration with the muscles of breathing relaxed. At this volume there is an exact balance between the inward elastic recoil of the lungs and the outward elastic recoil of the chest wall. The actual end-expiratory position of the lungs in infants is usually somewhat greater than this true FRC, because of the interplay of a number of mechanical factors. In the infant and young child, the retractile force of the lung is weak and therefore there is a greater tendency for gas trapping at a relatively larger lung volume than in older children (4). The timing of breathing is also such that the infant begins to inspire before reaching the normal expiratory lung volume. The difference between actual end-expiratory volume and true FRC in infants becomes apparent when lung mechanics are measured by the passive expiration technique (5). The only other parameter of lung volume of importance is the volume of each normal breath, which is known as the tidal volume (VT). This is even more subject to variability for technical reasons than the FRC and is of little use as a measure of lung function. The other parameters of lung volume that are sometimes reported are merely subdivisions or composites of those described and are of no particular importance.

Lung volume and its various subdivisions grow in proportion to the increasing metabolic demand of the subject. In animals of different species, lung volume is closely related to body weight, the equation derived by Tenny and Remmers (6) for TLC being:

$$\mathrm{TLC} = \mathrm{WT}^{1.02}$$

In infants during the first year of life thoracic gas volume (Vtg) is also closely related to body weight (7), but in later childhood weight is a poorer base for prediction because, unlike animals, young humans may be relatively fat or thin. It is generally more convenient to relate lung volumes to height, as summarized in Figure 2. The relationship is nonlinear because of the nonlinear relationship between height and weight (or, more correctly, metabolic rate). In fact if the data for TLC shown in Figure 2 are converted to the equivalent for weight, the relationship between TLC and weight is very similar to that for animals of different species.

The normal growth of lung volume in childhood can be affected by disease. It will be hampered, for example, by a diaphragmatic hernia, scoliosis, or muscle weakness, and the earlier the abnormality is present the more it is likely to cause trouble. Contrary to popular belief, asthma does not affect lung growth, even though the lungs are hyperinflated during attacks.

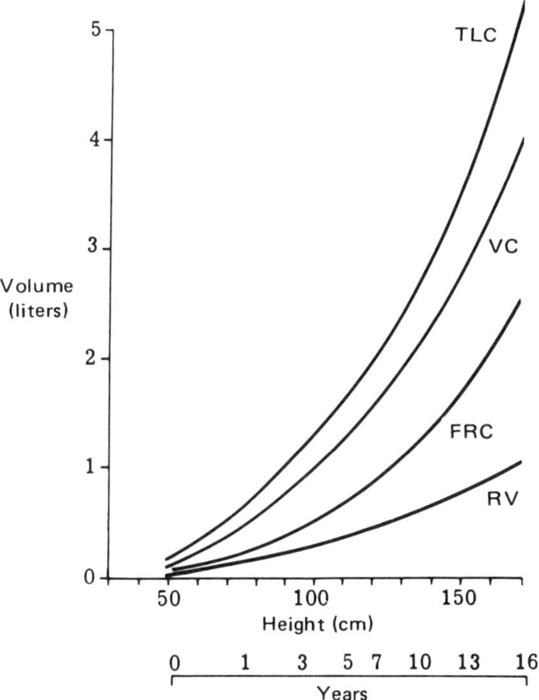


FIGURE 2 Relationship between various lung volumes and height throughout childhood. The age scale gives the approximate age based on the 50th percentile. Boys and girls combined. (From Ref. 3.)

## MEASUREMENT OF LUNG VOLUME

The volume of the lungs and their various subdivisions can be measured in a number of ways. VC and VT are measured by some form of spirometer. Originally, these were either water-filled or bellows instruments, but the modern electronic types are much more convenient. In these instruments airflow is measured in one way or another and this is integrated electronically to give volume. For children, it is important to ensure that the instrument is accurate in the range of values to be expected from small subjects.

The resting lung volume (FRC) can be measured most easily by the dilution of an inert gas such as helium. The subject breathes from a respiratory circuit containing a known volume of a helium–oxygen mixture. Over a few minutes of breathing, the gas in the lungs dilutes the helium while carbon dioxide is absorbed and oxygen added to keep the total volume constant. The FRC is determined from the change in helium concentration after thorough mixing. As an alternative, the naturally occurring inert gas, nitrogen, can be washed out from the lungs by having the subject inspire 100% oxygen with each breath through a one-way valve system. The total volume of nitrogen breathed out is determined and since the alveolar gas consisted originally of 80% nitrogen, FRC can be calculated. Once FRC is known, the other parameters TLC and RV can be determined by spirometry. The helium dilution technique has been used very successfully for years in infants and small children (8). The only limitation is that the child be willing to tolerate breathing through a face mask or mouthpiece for a few minutes to ensure adequate mixing. In normal children this only requires 3–5 min but in the presence of obstructive lung diseases, such as asthma, much longer may be needed.

An alternative to inert gas dilution is to use a whole-body plethysmograph (Fig. 3a) originally described by DuBois and colleagues (9). It operates on the principle of Boyle's law governing the relationship between the volume and pressure of a fixed mass of gas. The child sits (or lies, if an infant) within a closed chamber and breathes through a respiratory circuit containing a shutter that is closed at the end of a normal breath to trap the FRC within the lungs. The child continues to make respiratory efforts against the obstruction, thereby alternately compressing and rarefying the gas within the chest. This pressure change is sensed by a transducer connected to the mouth piece. The respiratory efforts against the obstruction change the volume of the gas trapped in the chest and this volume change is reflected by changes in the pressure of the air in the plethysmograph chamber surrounding the child. After appropriate calibration, this change in volume can be related to the change in pressure to give the volume of the gas trapped in the chest by the shutter. Because of its different mode of measurement, this volume is usually termed thoracic gas volume (Vtg) rather than FRC. If the shutter is closed at true end-expiration, FRC and Vtg are virtually identical in normal subjects, but in patients with poor gas mixing, gas trapping, or lung cysts, Vtg is usually greater than FRC. This is because its measurement depends solely on physical principles and not on the adequacy of gas equilibration. Unfortunately, some recent studies in infants with chronic postbronchiolitic airway obstruction have revealed problems with even the plethysmographic measurement of lung volume (10).

## RESISTANCE

Any tube through which gas flows has a resistance that can be quantitated by the pressure drop across the tube needed to produce a given flow. This

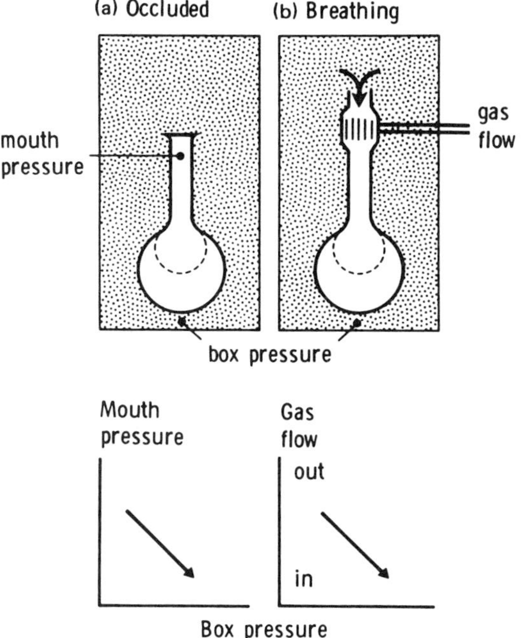


FIGURE 3 Theory of whole-body plethysmography. During an inspiratory effort against an occlusion (a) the pressure within the lungs as recorded at the mouth falls while the pressure in the chamber rises as the gas in the lungs is decompressed. During unobstructed inspiration (b) the inward flow of air is accompanied by a rise in chamber pressure that reflects the fall in alveolar pressure produced by the action of the inspiratory muscles. (From: Godfrey S. In: Godfrey S, Baum JD (eds.), *Clinical Paediatric Physiology*. Blackwell Scientific Publications, Oxford, 1979.)

resistance depends on both the length of the tube and its diameter and this latter term is particularly important since the resistance varies inversely to the fourth power of diameter. The resistance of the respiratory system as a whole, the total respiratory resistance (Rrs), is complex because it includes the resistance to movement (sliding) of the tissues of the chest wall and lungs, which is in series with the resistance due to airflow in the airways (Fig. 4). These resistances are additive but the tissue resistance is normally much less than the airway resistance (Raw). The Raw is itself rather complex since the airways consist of branching tubes that get narrower and shorter but far more numerous as one travels from the trachea to the periphery. The cumulative surface area of these branching tubes gets progressively greater and hence their resistance gets rapidly less towards the

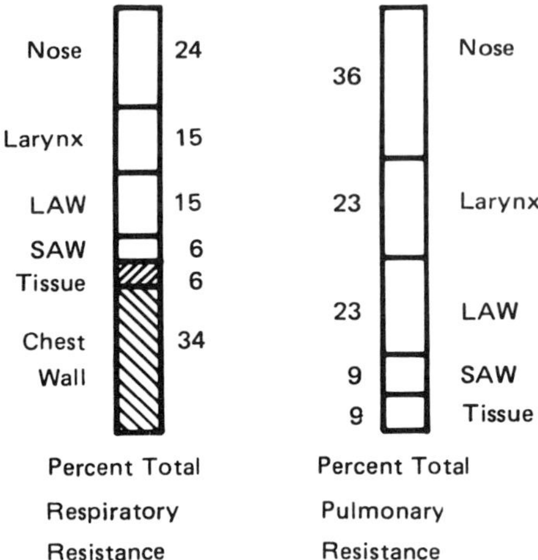


FIGURE 4 Approximate distribution of resistances in the respiratory system. If the measurements are made during open mouth breathing, the nasal resistance should be deducted. Note that the resistance of the small airways (SAW) is less than that of the large airways (LAW) and much less than the total upper airway and large airway combined.

periphery. This means that the total Raw (from alveoli to the mouth or nose) is dominated by the resistance of the more central airways. But what are these central airways? In adults and older children Raw is conventionally measured while the patient is panting through the mouth and in this situation the larynx is also widely open. Infants are obligatory nose breathers and almost certainly do not completely abduct their vocal chords during measurements made with normal tidal breathing, so that in these young patients the Raw includes a laryngeal and nasal component as well.

Except in rare diseases of the thoracic cage or interstitial lung tissue, the frictional resistance of the chest wall and lungs is fairly constant. Almost 50% of the total airway resistance is due to the nose, pharynx, and larynx and in children with upper airway disease this can be very important. Diseases affecting the lungs, such as asthma or cystic fibrosis, primarily cause alterations in the lower airways (below the larynx). These lower airways are generally considered in terms of large and small airways. There is no formal definition of where the boundary exists between them, but the larger airways include the trachea, main bronchi, and about four or five more generations of bronchi beyond. The small airways include all the remaining generations to the alveoli.

Raw is about 25 cm$H_2O$/liter/sec in the newborn infant and falls to about 2 cm$H_2O$/liter/sec in the young adult due to the increase in diameter of

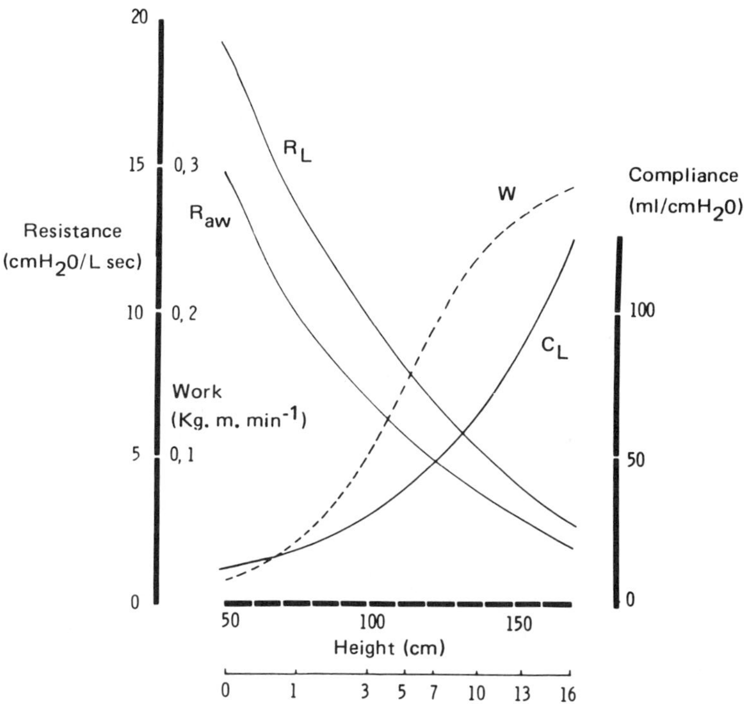


FIGURE 5 Relationship between airway resistance (Raw), pulmonary resistance ($R_L$), pulmonary compliance ($C_L$), work of breathing (W), and growth throughout childhood. (From: Ref. 3.).

the airways (Fig. 5). Even in a given subject, Raw varies with the volume at which it is measured in a curvilinear fashion. For this reason volume-independent parameters of resistance have been derived, such as specific resistance (SRaw = Raw × Vtg) or its reciprocal specific conductance (SGaw = 1/SRaw). In children this device is quite good because the normal SGaw is quite constant at 0.2–0.3 $cmH_2O^{-1} \cdot sec^{-1}$. An interesting finding is that SGaw is high in premature infants (11), possibly because their airways develop in advance of their lung volume. The main advantage of measuring Raw, as distinct from other types of lung function test, is that it is measured during quiet panting and is relatively independent of effort. This is particularly useful in cases where the degree of cooperation is in doubt.

## MEASUREMENT OF AIRWAY RESISTANCE

Raw can be measured in older children who can cooperate or in infants who are asleep using the whole body plethysmograph (Fig. 3b), which was originally developed by DuBois and colleagues (12). During unimpeded breathing from the chamber, the alternating rarefaction and compression of alveolar gas needed to draw air in and out of the lungs cause reciprocal pressure changes in the chamber. These pressure changes can be calibrated in terms of alveolar pressure changes from the measurements during temporary airflow obstruction used in the determination of Vtg. Relating plethysmograph pressure change to the air flow at the mouth after appropriate calibration gives airway resistance:

$$\text{Raw} = \frac{\Delta \text{Pbox}}{\Delta \text{Flow}} \times \text{CAL}$$

where ΔPbox = plethysmograph chamber pressure change, ΔFlow = change in flow rate at the mouth, and CAL = calibration factors.

For infants who cannot pant on demand, it is necessary to arrange for them to breathe warmed and humidified air from a bag within the plethysmograph to minimize exchange of temperature with the environment (13). Raw in children is conventionally measured at a specific inspiratory flow rate, usually 0.5 liters/sec, and in infants at two-thirds of their peak inspiratory flow rate. We have recently developed computer techniques that enable us to measure resistance at all points throughout the respiratory cycle (14). This has shown resistance to be far from constant, especially in infants with airway obstruction. The pattern of resistance changes throughout the respiratory cycle can provide important additional information as to the site of airway obstruction.

## FUNCTION OF THE SMALL AIRWAYS

The small airways contribute a relatively small amount to the total airway resistance even in disease and there can be considerable pathologic change in these small airways with little or no effect on total airway resistance or other tests that reflect chiefly the function of the larger airways. However, even though the resistance of the small airways is low in relation to the total airways resistance, it is important because it governs the maximum expiratory flow rate that can be achieved at low lung volumes.

The effect of the small airways on expiratory flow rates is illustrated by the model shown in Figure 6. During forced expiration, the pressure applied by the diaphragm and expiratory muscles to the thoracic contents also reaches the surface of the intrathoracic airways and alveoli. Within the alveoli, this applied pressure is added to the normal elastic retractile force of the lung tissue itself and this total pressure is then available to drive the forced expiration. The flow achieved depends upon this driving pressure

(P) and the resistance (R):

$$\text{Flow} = \frac{P}{R}$$

At large lung volumes, the resistance consists of the resistance of all the airways from the alveoli to the mouth and, since most of this resistance is in airways protected by cartilage from collapsing, the greater the force applied the greater the flow achieved. As the lung volume is reduced, the diameter of the smaller airways also reduces and at some critical point (usually after about one-third of the vital capacity has been expelled), the resistance of the small airways becomes the determining factor in the maximum flow rate that can be achieved. In this situation there will be a

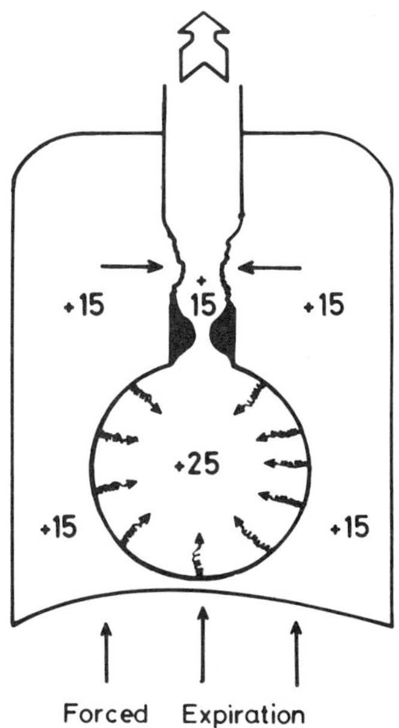


FIGURE 6 Model illustrates the equal pressure point concept of flow limitation during forced expiration in the presence of small airway obstruction. The pressure of the expiratory muscles is applied to the whole intrathoracic contents and the pressure within the alveoli is further increased by the retractile pressure of the lungs. This total pressure is partially dissipated across the small airway obstruction, so that there is equal pressure within and without the small, compressible intrathoracic airways. The remaining driving pressure for flow through the small airway is thus the retractile pressure of the lungs and remains constant at any given lung volume, whatever the applied pressure.

pressure drop across the small airways during flow; then the pressure within the small (and collapsible) airways is exactly equal to that surrounding them. At this stage the driving pressure producing flow across the small airways is the recoil pressure of the lungs, which is constant at any given lung volume. This driving pressure remains independent of the pressure applied by the diaphragm and therefore the maximum flow that can be obtained is constant and independent of effort. It depends only upon the resistance of the small airways and the recoil pressure of the lungs.

The maximum expiratory flow falls as lung volume is reduced further because the recoil pressure becomes less. This model suggests that maximum expiratory flow at low lung volume is largely independent of effort and also chiefly reflects the function of the smaller airways (15). It must be pointed out that this equal pressure point model is only one way of describing events in the airways. In another model the maximum flow rates are considered to be determined by the maximum speed of the propogation of a pressure wave in the airway (16), but for practical purposes the conclusions are very similar.

## LUNG FUNCTION TESTS EMPLOYING FORCED EXPIRATION

Tests employing forced expiration are commonly used to quantitate airways obstruction, because an increase in expiratory resistance is reflected in a decrease in forced expiratory flow rate. In the standard test of forced expiration, the subject takes a maximum inspiration and then expires as hard and fast as possible until no more air can be expelled. The maneuver is documented either by recording the forced expirogram in the form of a plot of volume against time (Fig. 7, below) or in the form of a plot of expiratory flow rate against volume expired (Fig. 7, above). For completeness, the inspiratory portions of the records are also shown, although inspiration is affected little by obstructive lung disease. The data in Figure 7 show schematically forced expiratory spirograms in health, and in mild and marked airways obstruction. It must be emphasized that the data in the two graphic representations (volume vs. time or flow vs. volume) are identical and it is possible to convert from one to the other.

The most commonly used parameters derived from the volume/time plot are the forced expired volume in the first second of expiration ($FEV_1$) and the forced vital capacity (FVC). The most commonly used parameters derived from the flow/volume plot are the peak expiratory flow rate (PEFR) and the maximum midexpiratory flow rate (MMEF). Since the PEFR is measured in the early part of forced expiration, it is very dependent on effort. However, the PEFR can be measured with very simple devices that can easily be used at home to monitor lung function and, in patients who

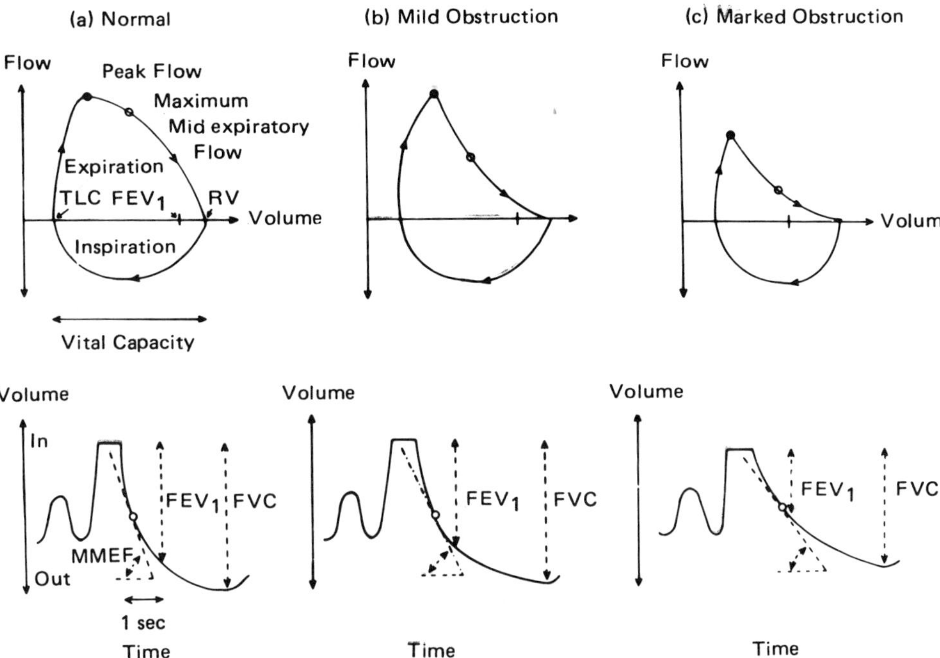


FIGURE 7 Diagram of forced expiratory flow–volume curves and the equivalent forced expiratory volume–time spirometry in normal subjects and those with mild or marked airway obstruction. The two graphic displays are different ways of showing the same data. The maximum midexpiratory flow rate (MMEF) is represented on the spirograms by the angle of a tangent to the curve drawn at mid-expiration.

cooperate properly, PEFR can be a very useful measure. Unfortunately, as discussed above, the early part of forced expiration is not only dependent on effort but also unrelated to small airway function. So it is possible for a patient to have considerable obstruction in the smaller airways without showing a reduction in PEFR (Fig. 7b). The volume of expiration represented by the $FEV_1$ includes a portion expired early on and a portion expired later. It is much less dependent on effort than the PEFR and reflects both large and small airway function, which makes it a most useful overall index of lung function. The MMEF is the least effort-dependent index of forced expiration. This parameter also primarily reflects small airway function.

The indices of lung function drived from forced expiration increase curvilinearly with increase in height during childhood in a similar fashion to the static lung volumes. In an attempt to standardize the MMEF (or other similar indices), the flow rate may be divided by the FRC (if known) and expressed as FRC/sec, which remains fairly constant at 1.8–2.0 throughout growth in normal children. When performing tests of forced expiration, it is usual to have the child make several attempts and to select the highest values for each parameter from technically adequate efforts. The recommendations of the American Thoracic Society are that the best test is that in which the sum of the $FEV_1$ and FVC are greatest provided that duplicate tests vary by less than 5% (17). This criterion is stringent for most studies in children and many prefer to take the highest value of each parameter, even if these results occur in different efforts, provided the expiration was performed correctly.

Until recently it was impossible to study small airway function by means of forced expiration in infants because they simply could not expire forcibly well. For this reason we developed a thoracoabdominal squeeze jacket that applies pressure suddenly around the chest and abdomen at end inspiration to produce a partial forced expiratory flow–volume curve (18,19) such as that shown in Figure 8. From this curve the forced expired flow corresponding to resting lung volume is obtained (VmaxFRC). This is numerically similar to the MMEF of older children when corrected for lung volume and expressed as FRC/sec. The shape of the curve in infants and its interpretation of the results are the same as for older children.

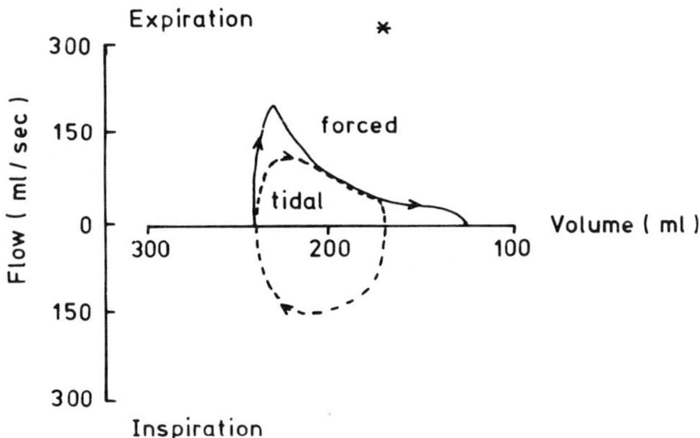


FIGURE 8 Partial forced expiratory flow–volume curve in an infant with bronchiolitis. The tidal breath before the application of the thoracic squeeze is shown by the dotted line. The star indicates the expected normal value for forced expiratory flow at a lung volume corresponding to the end-expiratory volume of the preceding breath.

Thus both in infants and in older children it is possible to measure large airway function in terms of Raw and small airway function in terms of MMEF or VmaxFRC. There remains the problem of the 1–6-year-old age group in whom such measurements are normally impossible, given the inability of the child to cooperate and the ethical problems posed by using very heavy sedation or anesthesia. However, noninvasive methods are available for measuring lung function and bronchial reactivity even in this age group, as will be discussed later.

## COMPLIANCE, ELASTANCE, STIFFNESS

The third element of mechanical function besides lung volume and airway resistance that is of importance involves the stiffness of the tissues of the lungs and chest wall. The former is significantly increased in interstitial lung diseases such as sarcoidosis and the latter in patients with scoliosis and other skeletal problems. Stiffness of the respiratory system is quantitated in terms of the pressure ($\Delta P$) that must be applied to produce a given volume change ($\Delta V$) under static conditions (i.e. after flow has ceased), which is termed elastance (E):

$$E = \frac{\Delta P}{\Delta V}$$

or its reciprocal, which is termed compliance (C):

$$C = \frac{\Delta V}{\Delta P}$$

Compliance, like resistance, reflects the properties of both the lungs and the chest wall. When expressed as elastance, these two components are simply additive. Normally, the elastance of the lungs is much less (greater compliance) than that of the chest wall. In infants with much more flaccid chest walls, the thoracic elastance may be comparable to that of the lungs. This explains why deformation of the thoracic cage is seen so readily in infants with respiratory distress. As the lungs grow during childhood, so the compliance apparently increases because a given change in pressure will produce a much greater change in volume. This is simply because there are more and larger lung units. However, if pulmonary compliance is standardized by dividing by resting lung volume (FRC) to obtain the specific compliance, this remains fairly constant at 0.05–0.06 $cmH_2O^{-1}$ throughout childhood.

The problem with compliance or elastance as indices is that they reflect only one small portion of the relation between volume and pressure of the lungs, normally in the tidal volume range. More informative is to present the whole relationship throughout the vital capacity as a pressure/volume (PV) curve (Fig. 9). From such a curve it is possible to obtain a measure of stiffness as the absolute pressure at any lung volume: the static recoil pressure. It is also possible to construct PV curves for the chest wall or the total respiratory system. The normal pulmonary static recoil pressure at FRC is about 5 $cmH_2O$ in older children and young adults and varies little in health. It is less in young children and in older subjects. As noted earlier, the pulmonary static recoil pressure is one of the determinants of forced expiratory flow at low lung volume and, unless compensated by changes in resistance, a low recoil pressure should result in a low MMEF. However, infants have a relatively low recoil pressure and yet they achieve relative flow rates similar to those of older children (20).

The volume at which the small airways begin to close off during expiration (the closing volume) also depends on the retractile forces of the surrounding lung tissue. In infants this force is less than in older subjects and it is likely that they have a relatively large closing volume. If the closing volume is similar to or greater than resting lung volume, some alveoli will be poorly ventilated. This could be why the resting arterial $PO_2$ is somewhat lower in infants (4).

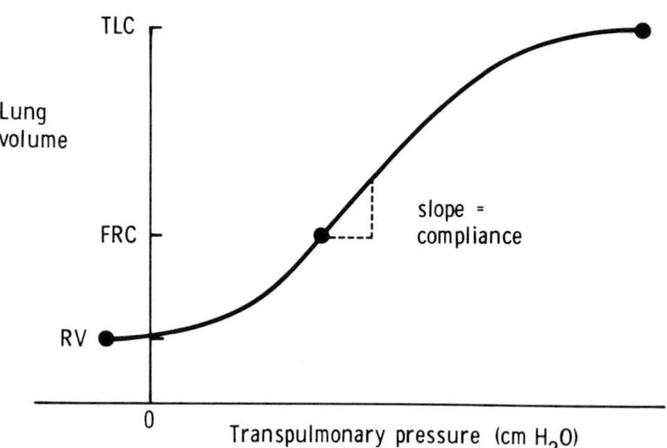


FIGURE 9 Schematic representation of the pressure–volume characteristics of the lungs. Compliance (1/elastance) is the slope of this line, which obviously varies with the region of measurement. The position of the curve with respect to the pressure axis depends on the static recoil pressure of the lungs. (From: Godfrey S. In: Godfrey S, Baum JD (eds), *Clinical Paediatric Physiology*. Blackwell Scientific Publications, Oxford, 1979).

The measurement of pulmonary compliance or the construction of a PV curve requires the positioning of a balloon in the midesophagus to measure pleural pressure. Besides the technical difficulties associated with esophageal balloons, they are very unpleasant for children to swallow. This makes the measurement of elastic properties of the lungs much less practical than other parameters of lung function, and they are used mainly as research tools. In recent years there has been considerable progress in the development of noninvasive techniques for the measurement of total respiratory mechanics, including total respiratory compliance (Crs) and total respiratory resistance (Rrs). These measurements are based on data obtained during complete relaxation of the respiratory muscles and completely passive expiration. They are only applicable in young infants in whom the Hering-Breur inflation reflex is still strong or in older subjects under anesthesia.

## PASSIVE EXPIRATORY MECHANICS

When the muscles of respiration are completely relaxed, the respiratory system as a whole (lungs and chest wall) can be considered as a mechanical system (21) in which passive expiration has a time constant ($\tau$) where

$$\tau = \text{Rrs} \times \text{Crs}$$

This time constant can be determined from the slope of a passive expiratory flow/volume curve, as shown in Figure 10a. The total respiratory compliance (Crs) can be determined separately by briefly obstructing a passive expiration at different lung volumes and relating the change in pressure at the mouth to the change in lung volume, as shown in Figure 10b. Once the time constant and Crs have been determined, Rrs can be calculated. Although this approach to the measurement of lung mechanics appears to be admirably simple, it depends critically upon obtaining complete relaxation and hence is only applicable to young infants and children who are anesthetized. Moreover, if Rrs and Crs vary during expiration, as certainly occurs in children with severe airways obstruction (14), the passive flow/volume curve is not linear and there is no single value for the time constant.

## GAS TRANSFER IN THE LUNGS

Having considered some of the mechanical properties of the lungs and the factors that govern them, we must now consider how oxygen and carbon dioxide are exchanged between the tissues and the environment through alveolar ventilation and the transport of gases in the blood. Both $O_2$ and $CO_2$ are relatively soluble in plasma, $CO_2$ more than $O_2$. The distribution of the molecules between the alveolar gas and the plasma in the pulmonary

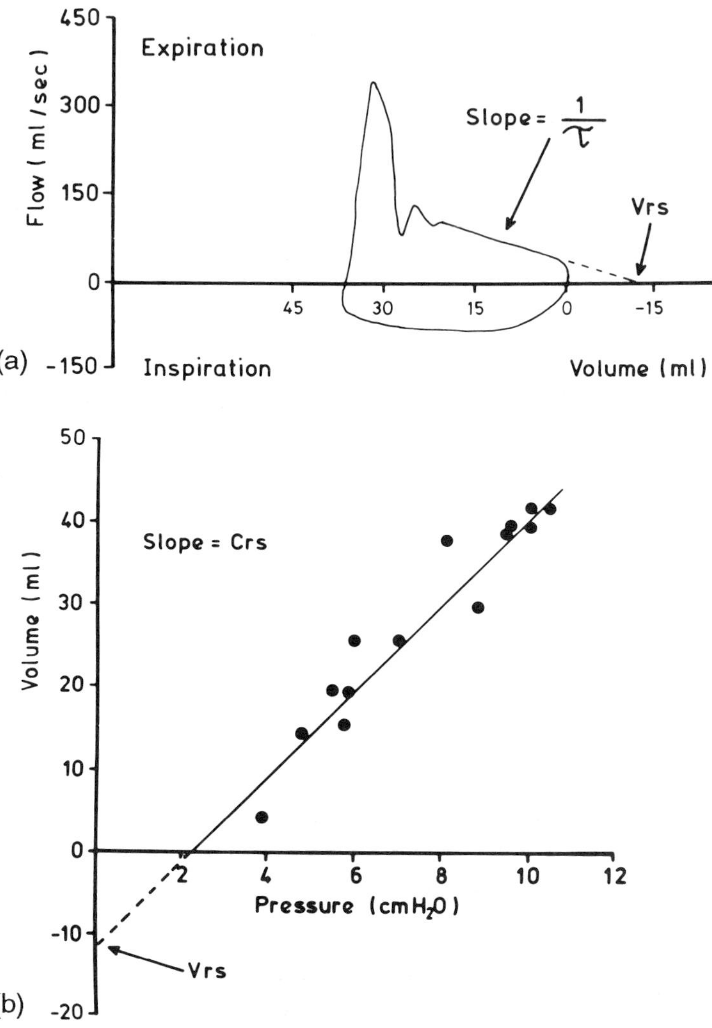


FIGURE 10 (a) Passive expiratory flow–volume curve. The airway is briefly occluded at end inspiration and then released. After the initial perturbations of flow there is a linear portion of the expiratory flow–volume curve the inverse of the slope of which is the time constant (τ) of passive expiration. Extrapolation of this portion to zero flow yields the true relaxed volume of the respiratory system (Vrs), which in this example is 12 ml below the end-expiratory volume. (b) Static volume–pressure relationship for the total respiratory system from the same subject obtained by a series of brief occlusions of the airway at different lung volumes. When the respiratory muscles are relaxed, the pressure recorded at the mouth reflects the total pressure of the respiratory system at the particular lung volume. The slope of regression line gives the compliance of the total respiratory system (Crs) and the intercept on the volume axis shows the true relaxed volume of the respiratory system (Vrs), which is identical to that obtained from (a).

capillaries depends upon the difference in partial pressure and the diffusion constant, which reflects the ease of passage of the molecules through the lung tissue. When a subject is breathing room air at sea level, the inspired gas contains $O_2$ at a partial pressure of about 150 mmHg and very little $CO_2$. Mixed venous blood in the resting subject arrives in the pulmonary capillaries with a $PO_2$ of about 40 mmHg and a $PCO_2$ of about 45 mmHg. $O_2$ is removed by the blood from the alveolar gas and $CO_2$ is added, which results in mean alveolar oxygen tension of about 100 mmHg and a mean alveolar carbon dioxide tension of about 40 mmHg. Because there is always a small obligatory right to left shunt of blood in the heart or small areas of complete atelectasis, the net result of gas exchange is that arterial blood has a $PO_2$ of about 90 mmHg and a $PCO_2$ of 35–40 mmHg. These values hold throughout life, except for young infants, who tend to have rather lower values for $PO_2$ for the reasons explained above. The constancy of arterial blood gases and pH attest to the remarkable adaptation that occurs in the respiratory system during growth and during transition from rest to exercise.

To achieve these optimal levels of gas exchange, it is essential that ventilation and perfusion be well matched at the alveolar level. If alveolar ventilation exceeds blood supply, some of the gas will be wasted and constitute extra dead space, while if blood supply exceeds ventilation some of the blood will not be oxygenated and cause an effective right to left shunt. The normal situation as well as the common types of deviation are illustrated in Figure 11. The effect of ventilation/perfusion (V/Q) mismatching on $O_2$ and $CO_2$ transfer is not symmetrical because of the different patterns of carriage of these gases in the blood. Within the physiological range there is a fairly linear relationship between the quantity (number of molecules) of $CO_2$ in the blood and the $PCO_2$. On the other hand, the $O_2$ dissociation curve is sigmoid shaped, so that above a $PO_2$ of about 80 mmHg there are very few additional molecules of $O_2$ added to the blood. In alveoli with a low V/Q ratio, the capillary blood leaving the region will have to carry an excess of $CO_2$ and less than normal $O_2$. In regions with a high V/Q, the blood leaves the alveoli with less than normal $CO_2$ but only the normal amount of $O_2$, despite the hyperventilation, because of the flat shape of the $O_2$ dissociation curve at high levels of $PO_2$. Thus, in the common situation of V/Q disturbance such as occurs in asthma, where there are both high and low V/Q regions, the net result on the arterial blood is a low $PO_2$ but a normal or even low $PCO_2$.

The carriage of $O_2$ and $CO_2$ in the blood is no different in children than in adults after the first week or two of life, during which any remaining fetal hemoglobin is replaced by adult hemoglobin. A small amount of the $O_2$ is carried dissolved in the plasma but the bulk is carried in chemical

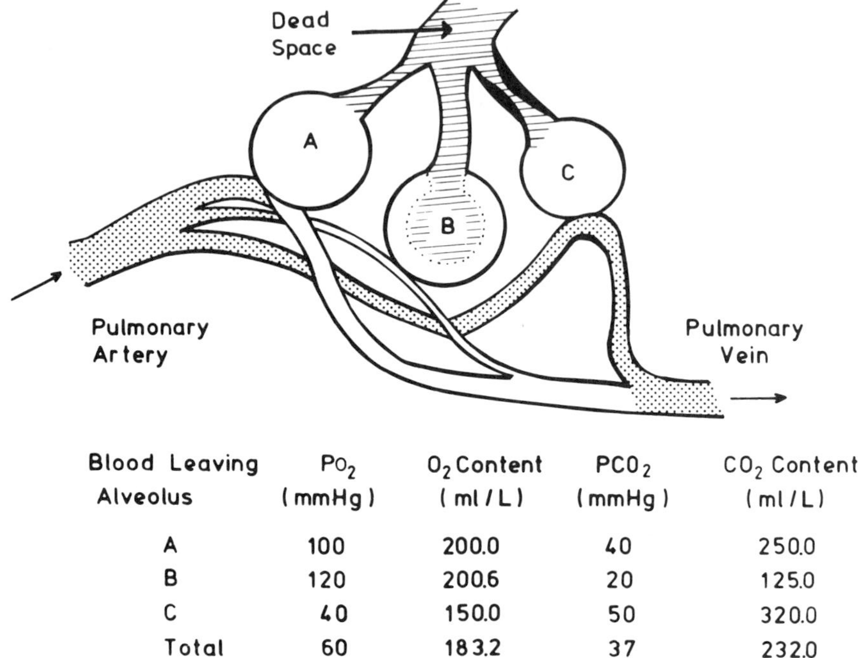


| Blood Leaving Alveolus | $Po_2$ (mmHg) | $O_2$ Content (ml/L) | $PCO_2$ (mmHg) | $CO_2$ Content (ml/L) |
|---|---|---|---|---|
| A | 100 | 200.0 | 40 | 250.0 |
| B | 120 | 200.6 | 20 | 125.0 |
| C | 40 | 150.0 | 50 | 320.0 |
| Total | 60 | 183.2 | 37 | 232.0 |

FIGURE 11 Diagram of ventilation–perfusion relationships in the lungs with a normal alveolus (A), an overventilated alveolus (B), and an underventilated alveolus (C). The effect of these ventilation–perfusion relationships on the blood leaving the alveoli individually and combined is shown below. Alveoli of types B and C can largely compensate each other in terms of $CO_2$, but because of the shape of the $O_2$ dissociation curve there is net hypoxia. (From: Godfrey S. In: Anderson RH, Macartney FJ, Shinebourne EA, Tynan M (eds.), *Paediatric Cardiology*. Churchill Livingstone, London, 1986.)

combination with the hemoglobin. The bulk of the $CO_2$ is transported in the plasma in the form of bicarbonate. The red blood cells play a critical role in $CO_2$ transport since the manufacture of bicarbonate in the tissue capillaries from $CO_2$ and the release of $CO_2$ in the lung capillaries from bicarbonate take place in the red cells with the help of the enzyme carbonic anhydrase. The lungs also form an important component of the regulatory system for acid–base balance in the body, since $CO_2$ can be readily removed or retained by alterations in alveolar ventilation. When metabolic acidosis is present, the normal response is hyperventilation with resultant hypocapnia and restoration of pH towards normal.

## PHYSIOLOGICAL CHANGES IN ASTHMA

Asthma is, almost by definition, a disease of function rather than structure. In most asthmatic subjects there is little if any evidence that the gross structure of the airways is abnormal and even the responsiveness of asthmatic airways to constrictor agents appears to be normal when removed from the body (22). There are obviously subtle differences in the airways of asthmatic subjects that render them susceptible to attacks of reversible airways obstruction. These changes may well lie in the structure and function of various cells in the epithelial layer (23). As a result of these subtle differences, the airways of the asthmatic subject respond to various stimuli by narrowing, which is brought about by contraction of the bronchial smooth muscle, accumulation of secretions within the lumen, and infiltration of the walls of the airways by inflammatory cells in the more persistent cases. These changes are described more fully in other chapters.

As far as lung function is concerned, the child with mild to moderate asthma may well be almost normal between attacks (Fig. 7). Sensitive tests may show a small reduction in forced expired flow rates at low lung volume and mild hyperinflation, reflecting some degree of small airways obstruction, but most other measurements, including the $FEV_1$, peak expiratory flow rate (PEFR), and airways resistance (Raw), will be normal. In such a patient, when a mild to moderate attack develops, there will be a further reduction in maximum midexpiratory flow (MMEF) and the indices of large airway function (Raw) or global tests, such as the $FEV_1$, will also become abnormal. As the obstruction worsens, so resting lung volume tends to increase because of gas trapped behind airways that close off at a greater than normal lung volume. Blood gases are normally well maintained in patients with mild to moderate asthma, although there is inevitably some hypoxia because of the ventilation–perfusion mismatching.

The patient with more severe asthma is much more likely to have abnormal lung function between attacks, although, again, this often involves the smaller airways more than the large. It is not at all uncommon for such a patient to have a normal PEFR, a nearly normal $FEV_1$, but a markedly reduced MMEF. This emphasizes the importance of using the flow–volume curve to evaluate lung function in asthma. Some patients are unaware of the severity of their asthma and unless lung function is measured as part of their evaluation, a potentially dangerous reduction in the functional reserve could be missed.

During an acute attack of asthma, there is widespread airways obstruction with a marked reduction in all parameters of lung function and the patient is often unable to perform lung function tests when first seen. Along with the airways obstruction, there is ventilation–perfusion imbalance resulting in hypoxia, which can be quite severe, but the $PCO_2$ usually remains on the low side for the reasons explained earlier. Only if respiratory failure supervenes due to exhaustion will the $PCO_2$ be elevated and this is an extremely serious finding in the patient with asthma. Indeed, any child with acute asthma who has an arterial $PCO_2$ over about 35 mmHg should be watched very carefully. As the acute attack wears off, there will be an improvement in lung function and the PEFR, which is the easiest bedside test, may increase rapidly. However, this test does not reflect the persisting severe small airways obstruction; a better index of this in the very sick patient is the level of hypoxia. Later, when the patient is able to perform lung function tests more adequately, the extent of large and small airway function can be judged from the flow–volume loop. It should also be remembered that hyperinflation can produce a spurious increase in simple tests of lung function, because the airways are also wider at large lung volume and static recoil pressure is greater. However, the hyperinflation subsides as the attack passes and by the time the patient is able to cooperate with the tests, it is not normally of clinical importance.

Asthma is normally thought of in terms of difficulty with expiratory airflow, because the airways narrow on expiration due to the falling lung volume and the pressure exerted upon them by the muscles of expiration. While it is undoubtedly true that expiratory resistance is higher than inspiratory resistance, it has been found that expiration is largely passive in asthma and the necessary pressure is produced by the elastic recoil of the lung and chest wall (24). This would be expected given that maximal expiratory flow rates in the presence of small airways obstruction are largely determined by the elastic recoil and additional expiration does not increase flow rates. The hyperinflation that accompanies the asthma attack helps in the sense that it increases the elastic recoil and the diameter of the airways to some degree. On the other hand, with the greater inward recoil of the lungs and chest wall, the muscles of inspiration (diaphragm, scaleni, sternomastoid, intercostals) have to work harder to fill the lungs. Thus in an asthma attack the resistance is greater during expiration but the fatigue occurs during inspiration.

An important sign reflecting the severity of an attack of asthma is pulsus paradoxicus. Studies in both adults and children have shown a correlation between the severity of the airways obstruction and the severity of the paradox (25). In particular, we noted that a difference greater than 25 mmHg in systolic blood pressure between inspiration and expiration was indicative of asthma severe enough to result in an elevated $PCO_2$ in more than half the children studied. From the other perspective, we found that whenever the $PCO_2$ was over 40 mmHg the paradox was always greater than 20 mmHg. The pulmonary circulation is also important for proper gas exchange but, as far as asthma is concerned, it only becomes a factor during severe attacks when the circulation may be impeded by the very large swings in intrathoracic pressure (26). In this situation there is an increase in right ventricular transmural pressure and movement of the intraventricular septum during inspiration that impedes left ventricular function. It is now believed that this interdependence of the ventricles is a major factor in the genesis of pulsus paradoxicus: the fall in systolic blood pressure during inspiration.

## BRONCHIAL REACTIVITY

The hallmark of asthma is the increased responsiveness of the airways to a variety of different stimuli so that airways obstruction is provoked more readily than in nonasthmatic subjects. It now appears to be certain that the difference between the asthmatic child and the normal child is one of quantity rather than quality. For example, Figure 12 shows the change in $FEV_1$ due to the inhalation of increasing dosages of histamine in normal and asthmatic children. The slopes of the dose–response curves are very similar, but the position of the asthmatic curve is well to the left, that is, asthmatic children are 10–20 times more sensitive than normal children on average. The bronchial reactivity to nonspecific challenges such as methacholine or histamine is conventionally expressed as the dosage that causes a 20% fall in $FEV_1$ ($PC_{20}$). There are various different methods of performing these challenges, but for children the simple steady-state technique (27) is the most practical. For this test the child breathes nebulized methacholine (or histamine) for 2 min followed by lung function tests over the following 3 min and then performs a repeat inhalation with an increase in concentrations until the required fall in $FEV_1$ occurs. Using this method, we found that for normal children the numeric equivalent of the geometric mean $PC_{20}$ less 1 SD was 5.2 mg/ml and less 2 SD it was 2.7 mg/ml. On the other hand, in children with active asthma the numeric equivalent of the geometric mean $PC_{20}$ plus 1 SD was 1.2 mg/ml and plus 2 SD it was 4.3 mg/ml, so that there was very little overlap (2).

Until recently it was impossible to undertake bronchial challenges with methacholine in children too young to cooperate with lung function tests. Yet about 40% of asthmatic children begin to have symptoms by the age of 2 years. To challenge young children we adapted the steady-state method so that the physician listens for wheezing or coughing as the end point of the test instead of performing lung function tests (28). The concentration of methacholine causing the first audible wheezing is termed the PCW. In young children able to cooperate with lung function tests we found an excellent correlation between the $PC_{20}$ and the PCW, as shown in Figure

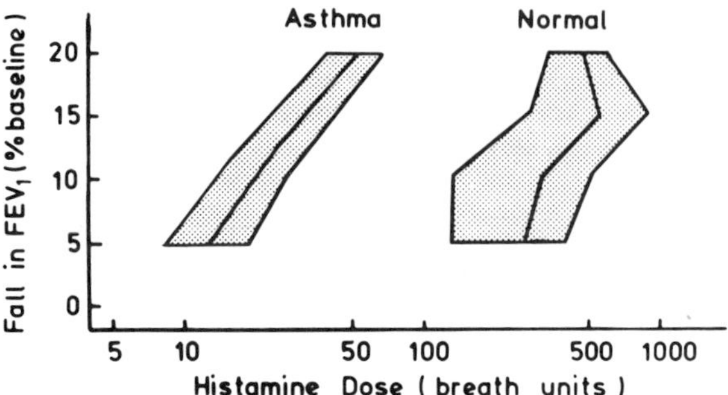


FIGURE 12 The mean and SE of the log dose–response curves to inhaled histamine in groups of healthy and asthmatic children. The histamine dosage is expressed in terms of a nominal number of standard breaths. The asthmatic children are 10–20 times more sensitive to histamine than the normal subjects.

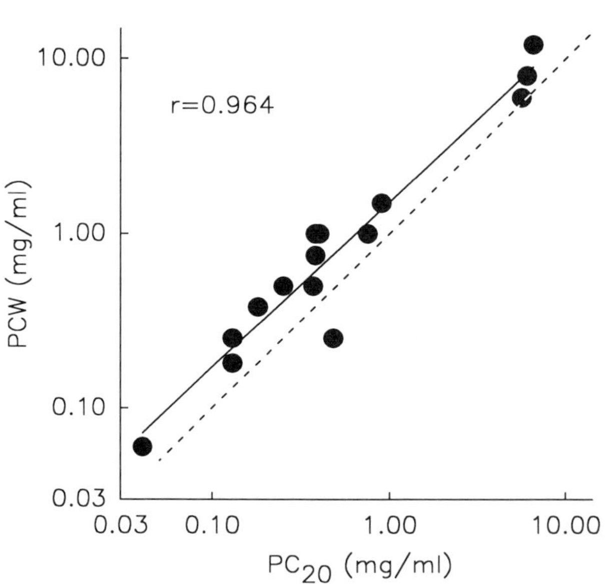


FIGURE 13 Relationship between PCW and $PC_{20}$ in individual children both plotted on logarithmic scales. The regression is shown by the solid line; the dashed line is the line of identity. The parallel shift of the regression line above the line of identity indicates that the PCW is, on average, 1.52 times as great as the $PC_{20}$. (From: Noviski et al. *Arch Dis Child*, 1991.)

13. The level of bronchial reactivity to methacholine or histamine reflects grossly the clinical severity of asthma (27) and we have now shown that this reactivity is similar for asthma of similar clinical severity at all ages (29).

The mechanisms underlying the bronchial responsiveness are still being actively investigated and are considered more fully elsewhere. Both chemical and neural pathways influence bronchial smooth muscle. The airways are supplied with mast cells and other inflammatory cells including eosinophils, macrophages, and lymphocytes, which are a very rich source of mediators. They may release prestored compounds or synthesize them for later release on appropriate allergic or nonallergic stimulation. These substances are not only capable of causing immediate bronchospasm but are also responsible for the delayed inflammatory response typical of the late phase of the asthmatic reaction (30).

Bronchial smooth muscle is innervated directly by parasympathetic (constrictor) and nonadrenergic, noncholinergic (dilator) efferent nerve endings. The adrenergic (dilator) system may well influence bronchial tone by a direct effect on parasympathetic ganglia or, indirectly, via circulating epinephrine and norepinephrine. It is very difficult to show whether these neural pathways are defective in some way in patients with asthma or even whether their role is primary or secondary in the asthmatic response. To complicate matters, mediator release can be influenced by neural activity and mediators can cause neural stimulation. Since it appears that the muscle itself is normal, it seems reasonable to assume that the neuromediator system is defective, possibly as a result of abnormal structure or function of cells in the epithelium lining the airways (23).

While methacholine or histamine can be used to demonstrate the difference between normal and asthmatic children in terms of bronchial responsiveness, they appear to act primarily at the final stage of the asthmatic process, that is, on the smooth muscle. More complex types of bronchial provocation that appear to resemble clinical asthma more closely are those due to specific antigen inhalation or to the nonspecific effects of physical exercise or hyperventilation. As far as allergen-induced asthma (AIA) is concerned, it seems that the allergen binds to specific IgE receptors on mast cells and possibly other mediator-containing cells lying in the lumen or just beneath the epithelium of the airway. The activation of these cells leads to an immediate attack of asthma within minutes that wears off over an hour or so and is generally thought to be due to bronchospasm. The muscle contraction may be due to the direct effect of the mediators or may be due to a reflex pathway mediated by the vagus. In many subjects there is also a late-phase reaction that occurs after a few hours and is much more persistent and less responsive to bronchodilator drugs. This late-phase reaction is now thought to be due to an inflammatory response triggered by the liberation of chemotactic mediators in response to the antigenic stimulation. Normal subjects and atopic subjects without asthma do not develop these responses, presumably because they lack the specific IgE-sensitized cells in their airways.

Exercise and isocapnic hyperventilation can trigger an attack of asthma in most, if not all, asthmatic persons (31). The exact mechanism of this nonspecific type of asthma is disputed but there is no doubt that cooling or, more probably, drying of the airways is an important triggering factor (32). Recent studies have shown that the severity of the exercise is also important even when the heat and water loss is kept constant (33). The intermediary pathway for exercise- (and probably for hyperventilation-) induced asthma appears to involve the liberation of mediator. This is because elevation of neutrophil chemotactic factor (NCF) has been detected in exercise-induced asthma and both its liberation and the asthma can be prevented by premedication with cromolyn sodium (34). Once an attack has occurred, most subjects are relatively refractory to a second attack for an hour or two and this refractoriness now appears to be due to the release of inhibitory prostaglandins (35). Normal subjects also show some changes in lung function in response to exercise but these are far less than those seen in asthmatic subjects. There is an interaction between allergic asthma and so called "nonspecific" bronchial reactivity: after an attack of antigen-induced asthma there is increased responsiveness to exercise and histamine (36).

Of particular interest is the responsiveness of children with asthma and other chronic respiratory diseases to bronchial provocation challenges with exercise and methacholine. It has long been known that children with cystic fibrosis demonstrate increased reactivity to methacholine and even to exercise (37). However, careful inspection of the data shows that the increased responsiveness to exercise consists of bronchodilatation during exercise rather than the bronchoconstriction after exercise that characterizes the response of the asthmatic. While most asthmatic persons respond abnormally to both exercise and methacholine, it is noteworthy that young adults who have grown out of the asthma they had as children often retain their increased responsiveness to methacholine (or histamine) while no longer responding to exercise (38). We have recently studied the response to exercise and methacholine in a group of asthmatic children, a group of children with other types of chronic lung disease including cystic fibrosis, and a group of children without any evidence of chronic lung disease (2). The results, which are shown in Figure 14, clearly demonstrate that both the asthmatic subjects and the children with chronic lung disease responded abnormally to methacholine, while only the asthmatic subjects responded

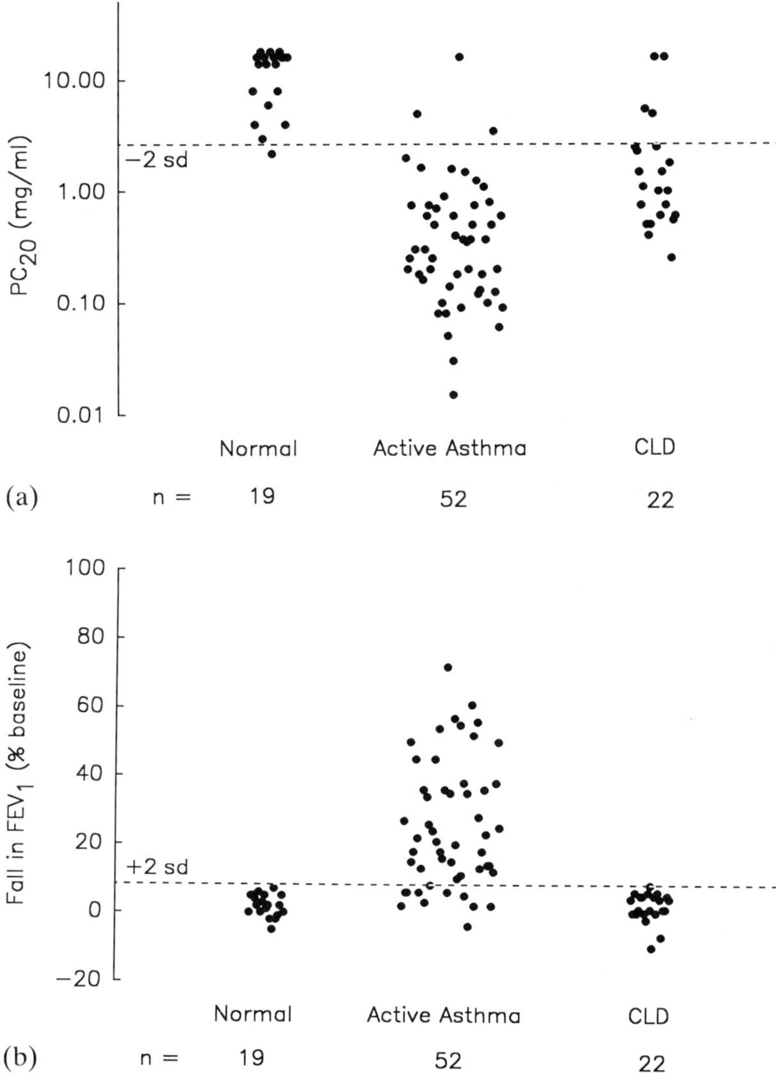


FIGURE 14 (a) Individual values for $PC_{20}$ plotted on a log scale in three groups of children: controls without lung disease, children with active asthma, and children with other types of chronic lung disease. The horizontal dashed line shows the lower limit of normal as the mean −2SD derived from the control group. (b) Individual values of postexercise fall in $FEV_1$ ($\Delta FEV_1$) in the three groups. The horizontal dashed line shows the upper limit of normal as the mean ±2SD derived from the control group. (From: Ref. 2.)

abnormally to exercise. This suggests that all kinds of chronic lung disease are capable of sensitizing the airways to methacholine but that only asthmatic subjects possess the type of trigger mechanism and intermediary pathway needed to respond to exercise.

## SUMMARY

There is an orderly adaptation of the physiology of the lungs of children to meet the demands of the growing body and to preserve the levels of arterial blood gases. This process results in changes in the mechanical properties of the lung tissues and resistance to airflow while ventilation/perfusion matching is maintained. In the asthmatic child the function of the lungs is disturbed by the airways obstruction, which is often most prominent in the smaller airways and is best detected from measurements of forced expiratory flow at low lung volume. When the obstruction is marked, it gives rise to ventilation/perfusion imbalance and resultant hypoxia. The asthmatic subject differs from the normal in that the airways are hyperreactive to specific (allergic) and nonspecific (pharmacologic or physical) stimuli. Since the bronchial muscle in vitro does not appear to be abnormal, the increased reactivity probably depends upon the release of specific mediators and upon local airway structure and function. While bronchial hyperreactivity to methacholine is found in other types of chronic lung disease of childhood, only asthmatic subjects possess the trigger sites and intermediate pathway needed to produce an abnormal response to physical exercise.

## REFERENCES

1. Townley RG, Bewtra AK, Nair NM, Brodky FD, Watt GD, Burke KM. Methacholine inhalation challenge studies. *J Allergy Clin Immunol* 64:569–574, 1979.
2. Godfrey S, Springer C, Noviski N, Maayan CH, Avital A. Exercise but not methacholine differentiates asthma from chronic lung disease in children. *Thorax* 46:488–492, 1991.
3. Godfrey S. Growth and development of the respiratory system, functional development. In: Davies JA, Dobbing J (eds.), *Scientific Foundations of Paediatrics*, 2nd ed. Heinemann Medical Books, London, 1981.
4. Mansell A, Bryan C, Levison H. Airway closure in children. *J Appl Physiol* 33:711–714, 1972.
5. Mortola JP, Fisher JT, Smith B, Fox G, Week S. Dynamics of breathing in infants. *J Appl Physiol* 52:1209–1215, 1982.
6. Tenney SM, Remmers JE. Comparative quantitative morphology of the mammalian lung: diffusing area. *Nature* 197:54–56, 1963.

7. Godfrey S. TGV or not TGV in WB?—that is the question. *Pediatr Pulmonol* 10:75–77, 1991.
8. Klaus M, Tooley WH, Weaver KM, Clements JA. Lung volume in the newborn infant. *Pediatrics* 30:111–116, 1962.
9. DuBois AB, Botelho SY, Bedell GN, Marshall R, Comroe JH Jr. A rapid plethysmographic method for measuring thoracic gas volume: a comparison with a nitrogen washout method for measuring functional residual capacity in normal subjects. *J Clin Invest* 35:322–326, 1956.
10. Godfrey S, Beardsmore CS, Maayan C, Bar-Yishay E. Can thoracic gas volume be measured in infants with airways obstruction? *Am Rev Respir Dis* 133:245–251, 1986.
11. Stocks J, Godfrey S. Specific airway conductance in relation to postconceptional age during infancy. *J Appl Physiol* 43:144–154, 1977.
12. DuBois AB, Botelho SY, Comroe JH Jr. A new method for measuring airway resistance in man using a body plethysmograph: values in normal subjects and in patients with respiratory disease. *J Clin Invest* 35:327–335, 1956.
13. Stocks J, Levy NM, Godfrey S. A new apparatus for the accurate measurement of airway resistance in infancy. *J Appl Physiol* 43:155–159, 1977.
14. Beardsmore CS, Godfrey S, Shani N, Maayan C, Bar-Yishay E. Airway resistance measurements throughout the respiratory cycle in infants. *Respiration* 49:81–93, 1986.
15. Mead J, Turner JM, Macklem PT, Little JB. Significance of the relationship between lung recoil and maximum expiratory flow. *J Appl Physiol* 22:95–108, 1967.
16. Mead J. Expiratory flow limitation: a physiologist's point of view. *Fed Proc* 39:2771–2775, 1980.
17. American Thoracic Society. Standardization of spirometry—1987 update. *Am Rev Respir Dis* 136:1285–1298, 1987.
18. Taussig LM, Landau LT, Godfrey S, Arad I. Determinants of forced expiratory flows in newborn infants. *J Appl Physiol* 53:1220–1227, 1982.
19. Godfrey S, Bar-Yishay E, Arad I, Landau LI, Taussig LM. Flow–volume curves in infants with lung disease. *Pediatrics* 72:517–522, 1983.
20. Hanrahan JP, Tager IB, Castile RG, Segal MR, Weiss ST, Speizer FE. Pulmonary function measures in healthy infants. Variability and size correction. *Am Rev Respir Dis* 141:127–1135, 1990.
21. Zin WA, Pengelly LD, Milic-Emili J. Single-breath method for measurement of respiratory mechanics in anesthetised animals. *J Appl Physiol* 52:1266–1271, 1982.
22. Roberts JA, Rodger IW, Thomson NC. Airway responsiveness to histamine in man: effect of atropine on in vivo and in vitro comparison. *Thorax* 40:261–267, 1985.
23. Gleich GJ. The eosinophil and bronchial asthma: current understanding. *J Allergy Clin Immunol* 85:422–436, 1990.
24. Pride NB. Physiology. In: Clark TJH, Godfrey S, Lee TH (eds.), *Asthma*, 3rd ed. Chapman and Hall, London, 1992.

25. Edmunds AT, Godfrey S. Cardiovascular response during acute severe asthma and its treatment in children. *Thorax* 36:534–540, 1981.
26. Scharf SM. Mechanical cardiopulmonary interactions with asthma. *Clin Rev Allergy* 3:487–500, 1985.
27. Cockcroft DW, Killian DM, Mellon JJA, Hargreave FE. Bronchial reactivity to inhaled histamine: a method and clinical survey. *Clin Allergy* 7:235–243, 1977.
28. Avital A, Bar-Yishay E, Springer C, Godfrey S. Bronchial provocation tests in young children using tracheal auscultation. *J Pediatr* 112:591–594, 1988.
29. Avital A, Noviski N, Bar-Yishay E, Springer C, Levy M, Godfrey S. Non specific bronchial reactivity in asthmatic children depends on severity but not on age. *Am Rev Respir Dis* 144:36–38, 1991.
30. Barnes PJ. New concepts in the pathogenesis of bronchial hyperresponsiveness and asthma. *J Allergy Clin Immunol* 83:1013–1026, 1989.
31. Godfrey S. Exercise induced asthma. In: Clark TJH, Godfrey S, Lee TH (eds.), *Asthma*, 3rd ed. Chapman and Hall, London, 1992.
32. Anderson SD. Is there a unifying hypothesis for exercise-induced asthma. *J Allergy Clin Immunol* 73:660–665, 1984.
33. Noviski N, Bar-Yishay E, Gur I, Godfrey S. Exercise intensity determines and climatic conditions modify the severity of exercise induced asthma. *Am Rev Respir Dis* 136:592–594, 1987.
34. Lee TH, Brown MJ, Nagy L, Causon R, Walport MJ, Kay AB. Exercise induced release of histamine and neutrophil chemotactic factor in atopic asthmatics. *J Allergy Clin Immunol* 70:73–81, 1982.
35. O'Byrne PM, Jones GM. The effect of indomethecin on exercise-induced bronchoconstriction and refractoriness after exercise. *Am Rev Respir Dis* 134:69–72, 1986.
36. Mussaffi H, Springer C, Godfrey S. Increased bronchial responsiveness to exercise and histamine after allergen challenge in asthmatic children. *J Allergy Clin Immunol* 77:48–52, 1986.
37. Counahan R, Mearns MB. Prevalence of atopy and exercise-induced bronchial lability in relatives of patients with cystic fibrosis. *Arch Dis Child* 50:477–481, 1975.
38. Martin AJ, Landau LI, Phelan PD. Lung function in young adults who had asthma in childhood. *Am Rev Respir Dis* 122:609–616, 1980.

# 4

# Epidemiology and Natural History of Childhood Asthma

**DAVID B. COULTAS and JONATHAN M. SAMET**

*University of New Mexico School of Medicine*
*Albuquerque, New Mexico*

Epidemiology is defined as the scientific methods used to study disease occurrence in human populations. Although formal definition of this discipline has been difficult, the emphasis on human populations differentiates epidemiology from conventional clinical research. Epidemiology may be considered to have two distinct components: description of disease occurrence, most often by person, place, or time; and the identification of risk factors for disease (1). Epidemiological study designs, such as the controlled clinical trial, are also used to evaluate therapeutic modalities and to conduct health services research.

The occurrence of disease in a population is described by incidence, mortality, and prevalence rates (1). The incidence rate during a specified time period is the ratio of the number of new cases to the population at risk. Mortality is a similar ratio, with the number of deaths as the numerator. Prevalence is either the proportion of diseased persons in a population at a particular time (point prevalence) or the proportion of persons ever having a disease in a population during a specified period of time (cumulative prevalence). Because prevalence is determined by both the incidence rate and the disease duration, it reflects the natural history of a disease. Diseases with a longer duration have a higher prevalence.

Cross-sectional surveys are used to measure disease prevalence. To identify risk factors for disease, epidemiologists conduct case–control and cohort studies. The case–control design involves the identification of a case series, such as persons with asthma, and an appropriate control group, followed by comparison of the proportions of cases and controls exposed to the risk factor of interest. In the cohort design, study subjects are followed over time and observations are made concerning risk factors for disease or concerning natural history. For example, a cohort study of atopy and asthma might involve follow-up of subjects with and without atopy and ascertainment of new cases of asthma in the two groups.

These epidemiological approaches have provided important information about the occurrence, causes, and natural history of childhood asthma. The epidemiological data complement data from clinical series, which are generally based on children who are ill or receiving medical care. This chapter reviews the epidemiology of childhood asthma and emphasizes accumulating evidence on the natural history and the risk factors of this disorder.

## PROBLEMS IN THE EPIDEMIOLOGICAL INVESTIGATION OF CHILDHOOD ASTHMA

### Definitions

Clinical, physiological, and questionnaire approaches can be used to identify subjects in the context of an epidemiological investigation. The difficulty of defining asthma in operational terms has frustrated the study of childhood asthma, regardless of the approach for identifying the disease. Both expert groups (Table 1) (2–9) and individuals have prepared definitions, but none of these have led to specific criteria for differentiating asthmatic from nonasthmatic children. In fact, participants in the 1971 Ciba Study Group on the Identification of Asthma concluded that the then available information was inadequate for developing a satisfactory definition of asthma (8); more recent information does not alter this conclusion.

The present terminology for major diseases associated with airflow obstruction follows that formulated in 1959 by participants in a Ciba symposium (2). That group addressed diseases in the adult and wrote a definition of asthma that emphasized varying physiological dysfunction (Table 1). More recent definitions have added hyperresponsiveness of the airways as a fundamental abnormality. Although not prepared specifically for childhood asthma, the widely used definitions of the American Thoracic Society and American College of Chest Physicians (3,4) are conceptually appropriate for children. Their application is difficult, however, because ventilatory function and airway responsiveness cannot be readily assessed in younger children.

## Questionnaires

Because children may be unable to cooperate adequately with physiological testing and, for reasons of feasibility, in epidemiological studies of childhood asthma, questionnaires are the most widely used method for classifying subjects as affected. At present, only one standardized respiratory symptoms questionnaire is available for children, developed by the American Thoracic Society (9). The questionnaire includes questions on major respiratory symptoms and diseases; some of the questions relate to asthma, but the questionnaire is not comprehensive in covering the symptoms of this disease.

In using questionnaires, epidemiologists usually consider a parent's report of asthma, with or without a physician's diagnosis, as affirmative evidence. This type of estimate of the disease occurrence is affected by patterns of use of medical care and the choice of diagnostic labels by individual physicians. For children, the terminology used by clinicians may not match that of epidemiologists. Taussig et al. (10) questioned physicians in Tucson, Arizona, about their diagnostic criteria for chronic bronchitis in children. For most of the physicians, wheezing and allergy were important considerations, and bronchodilator therapy was frequently given to children with chronic bronchitis. The authors concluded that the diagnoses of chronic bronchitis and asthma overlap considerably in children. In England, Speight et al. (11) identified children with a history of wheezing

TABLE 1 Definitions of Asthma

| Organization (Ref.) | Year | Definition of asthma |
|---|---|---|
| Ciba Guest Symposium (2) | 1959 | ". . . the condition of subjects with widespread narrowing of the bronchial airways which changes its severity over short periods of time either spontaneously or under treatment . . ." |
| American Thoracic Society (3) | 1962 | ". . . a disease characterized by an increased responsiveness of the trachea and bronchi to various stimuli and manifested by a widespread narrowing of the airways that changes in severity either spontaneously or as a result of therapy." |
| American College of Chest Physicians, American Thoracic Society (4) | 1975 | "A disease characterized by an increased responsiveness of the airways to various stimuli and manifested by slowing of forced expiration which changes in severity either spontaneously or as a result of therapy." |
| World Health Organization (5) | 1975 | ". . . a chronic condition characterized by recurrent bronchospasm resulting from a tendency to develop reversible narrowing of the airway lumina in response to stimuli of a level or intensity not inducing such narrowing in most individuals." |

| | | |
|---|---|---|
| American Thoracic Society (6) | 1987 | ". . . a clinical syndrome characterized by increased responsiveness of the tracheobronchial tree to a variety of stimuli. . . . symptoms of . . . paroxysms of dyspnea, wheezing, and cough, which may vary . . . physiological manifestation of . . . variable airways obstruction. Histologically, . . . evidence of mucosal edema of the bronchi; infiltration of the bronchial mucosa or submucosa with inflammatory cells, especially eosinophils; and shedding of epithelium and obstruction of peripheral airways with mucus." |
| National Asthma Education (7) | 1991 | ". . . a lung disease with the following characteristics: (1) airway obstruction that is reversible (but not completely so in some patients) either spontaneously or with treatment; (2) airway inflammation; and (3) increased airway responsiveness to a variety of stimuli." |

episodes and then confirmed the clinical significance of the wheezing by bronchial challenge testing with histamine, examination of school absenteeism, and treatment responses. Although most of the children with wheezing had been evaluated by a physician, only a small proportion had been diagnosed as having asthma.

In infants and younger children, the terms "wheezy bronchitis" and "asthmatic bronchitis" may be applied to patients who wheeze when provoked by a respiratory infection, but the labels do not differentiate these patients distinctly from those diagnosed with asthma. For example, Williams and McNicol (12) showed that the natural histories of disease in children diagnosed with asthma and wheezy bronchitis were the same. Thus, to assess completely the frequency of asthma, a questionnaire must include all labels that may be used by physicians. However, even a comprehensive questionnaire may not detect all cases of asthma, and some false-positive cases must be anticipated because of the imperfect sensitivity of questionnaires.

## DESCRIPTIVE EPIDEMIOLOGY

### Methods

Most of the information concerning the occurrence of asthma is prevalence data collected in cross-sectional surveys. In the United States, periodic surveys conducted by the National Center for Health Statistics provide prevalence estimates from nationwide probability samples. Numerous epidemiological surveys have been performed in the United States and elsewhere (13). In contrast to the abundant data on prevalence, only a few longitudinal studies provide incidence rates. Further insights into the occurrence of asthma may be gained from mortality and hospitalization rates. However, these measures integrate the frequency of the disease with variations in severity, diagnosis and treatment patterns, and classification.

### Prevalence

In the United States, data from nationwide samples and survey populations indicate that asthma is a common disease in children (Table 2). The community-based investigation of diseases in the population of Tecumseh, Michigan, provided one of the first comprehensive assessments of the prevalence of asthma (14). In this study, the classification of asthma was based on questionnaire information and physician evaluation. The cumulative prevalence was higher in males, a finding generally replicated in other populations, and increased with age. The high rates in Tucson may reflect migration of persons with respiratory disease (18). The nationwide esti-

TABLE 2 Prevalence of Childhood Asthma in Selected Studies in the United States

| Location and date (Ref.) | Criterion | Age | Findings (%) | |
|---|---|---|---|---|
| | | | Males | Females |
| Tecumseh, Michigan 1962–1965 (14) | Asthma or wheezing with appropriate characteristics at examination or during the last year | 0– 4 years | 4.6 | 2.7 |
| | | 5– 9 years | 5.3 | 3.0 |
| | | 10–15 years | 6.0 | 3.7 |
| Tucson, Arizona 1972–1973 (15) | Report of active asthma, diagnosed by a physician | 0– 4 years | 1.5 | 2.0 |
| | | 5– 9 years | 7.3 | 9.5 |
| | | 10–14 years | 8.9 | 8.1 |
| | | 15–19 years | 8.9 | 6.8 |
| | | | Both genders | |
| | | | Cumulative | Active |
| National sample, 1976–1980 (16) | Report of physician diagnosis of asthma | 6 months– 2 years | 4.0 | 2.3 |
| | | 3 years– 5 years | 6.5 | 3.9 |
| | | 6 years–11 years | 7.6 | 3.9 |
| | | 12 years–17 years | 6.6 | 3.2 |
| | | | Males | Females |
| Western Pennsylvania 1979 (17) | Report of ever receiving a physician diagnosis | 5– 9 years | 4.6 | 2.4 |
| | | 10–14 years | 4.4 | 2.9 |

mates, derived from the National Health and Nutrition Examination Survey II, confirm the findings of the smaller surveys (16). The data show that cumulative prevalence (the proportion ever affected) is greater than the point prevalence of active asthma at all ages. Cumulative prevalence varies with geographic region in the United States, from 8.3% in Midwestern children aged 3–11 years to 11.8% in Southern children of the same age. In this age group, 13.4% of black children and 9.7% of white children have ever had physician-diagnosed asthma or wheezing. Further analyses of these nationwide data have shown differences in asthma prevalence between urban and rural dwellers, 7.1% and 5.7%, respectively (19). In a survey of 4071 children in Western Pennsylvania (Table 2), Schenker et al. (17) used the new children's questionnaire developed by the American Thoracic Society.

Worldwide, data from cross-sectional surveys indicate a wide range for the prevalence of childhood asthma (13,18). Gregg (13) summarized the findings of surveys of children and adolescents and noted that the prevalence varied from near zero to 75%. Methodologic differences among the surveys may partially explain this range, but variation in the distributions of risk factors may also be important. Although prevalence estimates from other developed countries are generally similar to those listed in Table 2 for the United States (13), lower prevalence has been found in Scandinavian countries, ranging from 0.5% to 2.0% (20). Except for the United States, little information is available on the prevalence of asthma in different racial groups. In the United Kingdom, Johnston et al. (21) found that a history of asthma varied among Indian, African, and European children with prevalence estimates of 3%, 7%, and 5%, respectively. Compared with more developed countries, developing countries in general have an apparently lower prevalence of asthma that varies widely within their populations. The lowest prevalence has been found in poorer nonurban groups, and the highest in more urbanized populations (18).

Results from recent investigations of temporal trends in the prevalence of asthma have suggested increases in prevalence during the last 10–20 years (Table 3). While these increases in asthma prevalence may be attributed to rising incidence, increasing duration of disease, or increasing diagnosis of asthma, the available evidence suggests that the increased frequency is real and not simply increased recognition and diagnosis. For example, Burr et al. (23) in their surveys of schoolchildren (Table 3) found increases in the prevalence of wheezing, in the use of asthma medications, and in the proportion of children with greater than 25% decline in peak expiratory flow rate with exercise. All of these findings provide support for a true increase in the prevalence of asthma.

## Incidence Data

Incidence data are available from only a few cohort studies. In the United Kingdom, Leeder et al. (26) enrolled over 2000 newborns between 1963 and 1965 and evaluated them until age 5 years. During the follow-up period, 3.4% of boys and 2.9% of girls developed asthma, defined as wheezing episodes considered to be asthma by the parents. In a study of older children, Peat et al. (27) followed two cohorts of Australian schoolchildren with mean ages of 8.9 and 12.6 years at enrollment. Over the 6 year observation period, asthma occurred in 2.8% of boys and 1.7% of girls in the younger group and in 2.5 and 1.6%, respectively, in the older group. In the Tucson, Arizona, study the annual incidence of asthma was 1.4% for boys and 0.9% for girls in the 0–4 year age group, 1.0 and 0.7% in the 5–9 year age group, and 0.2 and 0.3% in the 10–14 year age group (15). When the follow-up period was extended from 3.5 to 8.2 years, the findings were similar (28). These incidence data confirm the more frequent occurrence of asthma in boys. They also show that incidence declines with increasing age, even though prevalence rates remain relatively constant (Table 2) (Fig. 1).

## Hospitalization Data

Hospitalization rates reflect disease prevalence, disease severity, and patterns of medical practice. Nationwide data from the National Hospital Discharge Survey show a recent dramatic increase in hospitalization among children younger than 15 years. The hospitalization rate for this age group had increased from 48:100,000 in 1965 to 166:100,000 in 1983 (16). Black children had a greater increase in hospitalization than white children (30), an increase that may reflect poverty more than race (31). Further analyses of nationwide data by Halfon and Newacheck (32) suggest that increased prevalence, increased severity of asthma, and improved access to hospital care all have contributed to rising hospitalization rates for asthma in the United States. Increases have also been reported for specific locales in the United States (33) and for other countries (34–37).

Other investigations to describe and to explain variations in hospitalization rates have been conducted in the United States (38), the United Kingdom (36,39), New Zealand (39–41), Australia (37,41), and Hong Kong (42). In all of these countries the greatest increase in hospitalization occurred in children aged 4 years and less. Differences in racial composition among populations may contribute to marked differences in hospitalization rates. For example, Mitchell et al. (40) found the increase in hospitalization among Polynesian children in New Zealand was twice that in European children. However, in a comparison of the prevalence of asthma in children from

TABLE 3 Changes in Prevalence of Childhood Asthma from Selected Studies Worldwide

| Country and date (Ref.) | Study population | Criterion | Findings | | |
|---|---|---|---|---|---|
| U.S., 1971–1974 and 1976–1980 (22) | Ages 6–11 years, nationwide sample | Report of a physician diagnosis of asthma | | 1971–1974 (%) | 1976–1980 (%) |
| | | | | 4.8 | 7.6 |
| U.K., 1973 and 1988 (23) | Age 12 years, living in same area, 1973 (n = 818) and 1988 (n = 965) | Parent's report of child ever having asthma | | 1973 (%) | 1988 (%) |
| | | | Males | 7.0 | 14.1 |
| | | | Females | 4.0 | 9.8 |
| | | | | 1973 | |
| U.K., 1973–1986 (24) | Ages 6–12 years, nationwide sample, 15,000 males and 14,156 females examined at least once | Patient's report of persistent wheeze | Age (yrs) | Males (%) | Females (%) |
| | | | 6 | 2.7 | 2.3 |
| | | | 7 | 2.8 | 2.0 |
| | | | 8 | 2.9 | 1.4 |
| | | | 9 | 1.6 | 1.4 |
| | | | 10 | 2.5 | 1.1 |
| | | | 11 | 3.6 | 1.6 |
| | | | 12 | 0.8 | 0.9 |

| | | | | 1986 | |
|---|---|---|---|---|---|
| | Ages 6–12 years, nationwide sample, 15,000 males and 14,156 females examined at least once | Patient's report of persistent wheeze | Age (yrs) | Males (%) | Females (%) |
| | | | 6 | 5.1 | 3.5 |
| | | | 7 | 4.8 | 2.4 |
| | | | 8 | 3.6 | 3.5 |
| | | | 9 | 2.9 | 2.0 |
| | | | 10 | 4.2 | 1.7 |
| | | | 11 | 2.5 | 1.9 |
| | | | 12 | 2.1 | 1.9 |
| New Zealand, 1979 and 1989 (25) | Ages 12–18 years, from a rural school, n = 499 | Self-reported asthma | | 1979 (%) | 1989 (%) |
| | | | | 8.0 | 13.3 |

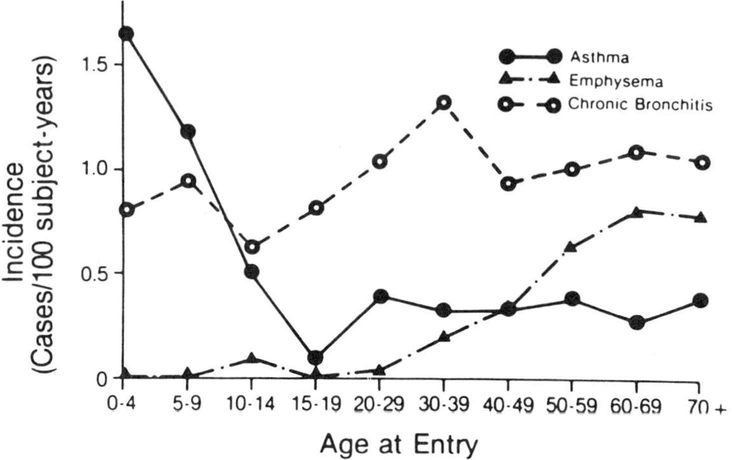


FIGURE 1 Incidence of asthma, emphysema, and chronic bronchitis according to age at entry into study. (From Ref. 29.)

New Zealand and from Australia, Asher et al. (41) were not able to explain differences in hospitalization rates simply by differences in asthma prevalence. Although increased prevalence (39), increased severity (30), or changes in diagnostic labeling (37) may all contribute to the increases in hospitalization rates, a consistent explanation has not emerged.

Seasonal variations in hospitalization rates have been examined in several locales (38,42–45). Using data from the National Hospital Discharge Survey, Weiss (38) found a peak in hospitalization for ages 5–34 years during September through November, with a trough in June through August. A similar pattern has been observed at two children's hospitals in the United Kingdom (44,45). Higher rates of hospitalization in Hong Kong were associated with decreases in relative humidity and increases in wind speed (42). Other possible explanations for seasonal variations in asthma hospitalizations include seasonal changes in the frequency of viral infections and in exposure to aeroallergens.

### Mortality Data

In the past, asthma was not considered to cause death (46). However, a well-documented increase in asthma mortality in certain countries during the late 1950s and 1960s showed that this clinical dictum was incorrect. In England and Wales between 1959 and 1966, the death rate from asthma among children and adults 5–34 years of age increased from approximately

0.6 to 1.5:100,000 annually (47). Increased mortality also occurred in this age group in Australia and New Zealand but not in the United States, Canada, or West Germany (48). The epidemic of asthma deaths abated during the late 1960s and 1970s, and was never fully explained. The most widely advanced hypothesis was overuse of sympathomimetic inhalers and their availability in high-dosage forms (49), but the relevant data have not been considered definitive (50).

The relative importance of asthma as a cause of death in childhood was described by Neuspiel and Kuller (51). These investigators reviewed death certificates of persons aged 1–21 years who died between 1972 and 1980 in Allegheny County, Pennsylvania. They identified 207 cases of sudden and unexpected deaths; 5% were from asthma. Although asthma is a cause of mortality in childhood, it leads to relatively few deaths.

A second epidemic of asthma deaths in children and young adults began in many countries in the mid to late 1970s (52). This epidemic has been documented in the United States (22,53,54), United Kingdom (55), Canada (56), New Zealand (39,57,58), and Hong Kong (59). One of the first indications of a new epidemic of asthma mortality came from New Zealand. Jackson et al. (57) reported mortality rates for young people aged 5–34 years increased from 1.3:100,000 in 1974 to 4.1:100,000 in 1979. An investigation of 271 asthma deaths from 1981 to 1983 in New Zealand did not satisfactorily explain the high mortality rate or the increase (60).

To characterize asthma mortality among young people aged 5–34 years, Weiss and Wagener (54) examined U.S. vital records for the period 1968 through 1987. From 1968 through 1977 asthma mortality in this age group declined by 7.8% per year (Fig. 2). Between 1978 and 1987, the death rate increased by an estimated 6.2% per year, with an overall mortality from asthma of 4.2 per million population in 1987 (Fig. 2). The greatest increase in mortality has been among children aged 5–14 years, with an average annual increase of 10.1%. Although the annual increase in asthma mortality has not been as great in nonwhite children (5.6%) as in white children (7.3%), the absolute mortality was markedly higher, especially among nonwhite boys. For white children there has been little difference in mortality rates between the sexes.

Other analyses of U.S. vital records have further characterized asthma mortality among children in the United States (38,53,61,62). Weiss (38, p. 2323) examined seasonal trends in asthma deaths during the period 1982 through 1986. For persons aged 5–34 years, mortality peaked in June through August. However, for children less than 15 years of age, Sly (53) did not find a consistent seasonal pattern for the years 1979–1984. Khot et al. (63) found a similar seasonal pattern for asthma mortality among persons aged 5–34 years in the United Kingdom.

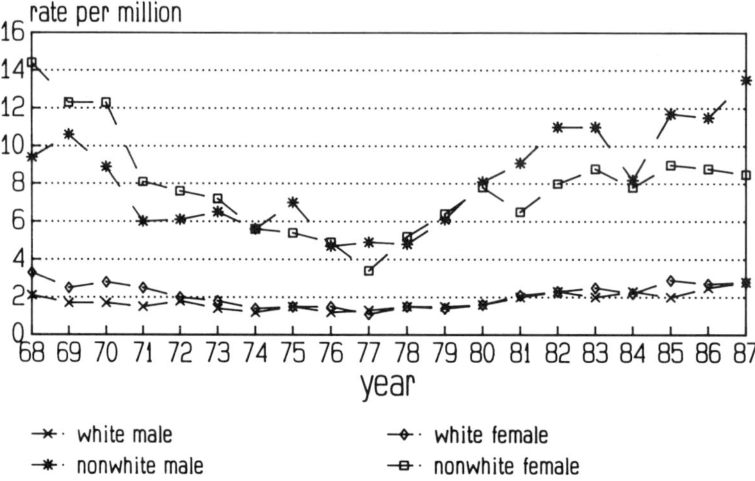


FIGURE 2 United States asthma mortality among persons aged 5–34 years, 1968–1987. Underlying cause of death data are from the National Center for Health Statistics, U.S. Vital Records. (Adapted from Ref. 54.)

In the United States asthma mortality varies widely by region (61,62) and race (62). For the period 1981–1985, Weiss and Wagener (61) examined geographic variations in asthma mortality for subjects ages 15–34 years and found increased mortality in four areas: the Central Plains states; New York, New York; Chicago, Illinois; and Phoenix, Arizona. Among racial groups, blacks have the highest mortality rates. Mortality for blacks is greatest in the Northeast and North Central regions (62).

Subsequent reports from the United Kingdom (55), Canada (56), and Hong Kong (59) have also documented increases in asthma mortality among children and young adults 5–34 years of age. However, mortality rates for children less than 5 years of age declined in the United Kingdom and Canada from 1974 through 1984.

Numerous international conferences and publications have addressed the increases in asthma mortality (64–67). Possible explanations include changes in diagnostic habits of physicians; improved diagnostic capabilities; increased prevalence; increased severity; changes in management; and changes in coding by the International Classification of Diseases (ICD). Although temporal trends must be interpreted cautiously because of changes in diagnostic habits and classification procedures that may alter mortality rates, there does not appear to be a systematic change in the diagnostic habits or capabilities of physicians that would explain the increase (52).

As described previously, mortality rates reflect the prevalence of a disease and the severity of the disease. The prevalence of asthma has increased worldwide in recent years, but the data on prevalence (23) and hospitalization for childhood asthma (30) suggest that in selected areas the severity of asthma also may be increasing and contributing to rising mortality rates. However, changes in prevalence and severity have not been documented to be of sufficient magnitude to explain entirely the rising mortality rates.

Mortality rates can also be affected by changes in the cause-of-death coding on death certificates. The cause of death is coded worldwide according to the International Classification of Diseases (ICD), which is revised approximately every 10 years. The Ninth Revision in 1979 introduced changes in the classification of respiratory diseases that increased the numbers of deaths classified as asthma (68). In the United States, use of the Ninth Revision in place of the Eighth Revision has been estimated to increase the overall number of deaths from asthma by 35% (68), but the increase is probably smaller in children (69). Most investigations of asthma mortality in children have been unable to attribute increases in mortality simply to changes in ICD coding (52).

Accuracy of death certificates also needs to be considered in interpreting mortality rates, although the error rate for children is probably small (70–71). The British Thoracic Association (70) recently reviewed 153 death certificates from 1979 that recorded the word asthma, and found 90% accuracy for subjects aged 15–44 years compared with 76% and 61% accuracy for subjects aged 45–54 years and 55–64 years, respectively. In New Zealand the overall accuracy of death certificates for patients less than 35 years of age was 97.8% (71).

Many investigations to determine risk factors for death from asthma, including case–series (58,72–78) and case–control studies (75,80–82), have been conducted worldwide. Results from these studies suggest that mortality from asthma is associated with a complex set of factors that vary among patients (Table 4). Because death from asthma is an infrequent occurrence, longitudinal studies have not been performed to evaluate the clinical usefulness of these factors for predicting and preventing death.

Given the rarity of asthma deaths, the case–control design is used to determine risk factors for dying. Several case–control studies have been conducted recently in New Zealand (75,81,82). Crane et al. (81) identified 117 patients aged 5–45 years who died from asthma between 1981 and 1983, and matched each case with 4 asthmatic subjects admitted to the hospital. For patients prescribed fenoterol by metered dose inhaler (MDI), the relative risk of death was 1.55 (95% confidence interval, 1.04–2.33). The increased risk was not confounded by severity of asthma. This finding has been the subject of extensive controversy (83,84), but the results were

TABLE 4 Factors Contributing to Death From Asthma

| |
|---|
| Patient-related |
| Severe, labile asthma |
| Poor chronic control of asthma |
| Reduced perception of severity of impairment |
| Specific allergies |
| Poor compliance with medical regimen |
| Discontinuity of medical care |
| Delay in seeking medical care |
| Psychosocial problems |
| Physician-related |
| Failure to recognize severity of asthma, acute and chronic |
| Failure to educate patient and family |
| Undertreatment of asthma, acute and chronic |
| Possible overtreatment with B-agonists, theophylline |
| Health care delivery |
| Poor access to care |

replicated by the same investigators in a subsequent study (82). Although the mechanism by which fenoterol increases risk of death from asthma is unknown, the drug's lack of beta-2 selectivity and its greater potency compared with other drugs administered by MDIs are proposed mechanisms.

Although deaths from asthma are uncommon in children, it should be possible to prevent many of those that do occur (75). To assist physicians to control the rise in mortality from asthma, physician education programs have been implemented in many countries including the United States (7).

## RISK FACTORS FOR CHILDHOOD ASTHMA

Risk factors are determinants of the risk of developing disease. Risk factors may increase or decrease the probability of disease, and are applied by epidemiologists to personal characteristics, acquired or genetic, and to environmental characteristics. Clinicians should use information on risk factors to identify patients at risk, and to counsel individual patients. This section reviews the major risk factors for childhood asthma.

### Familial and Genetic Factors

To determine the relative importance of genetic and environmental factors in the causes of asthma, studies have been made of familial aggregation, twins, and genetic markers, and analyses have been made of molecular genetic linkages. Studies of familial aggregation compare disease occurrence among family members, between parents and children, siblings, and spouses. The presence of aggregation may represent the effects of shared genes among household members or of the common household environment. In twin studies, disease frequency is compared in monozygotic twin pairs, whose genotypes are identical, and dizygotic twin pairs, who share only half their genes. A greater occurrence of disease in both twins (concordance) among monozygotic pairs than among dizygotic twin pairs provides evidence of heritability. The association of a disease with a genetic marker, such as human leukocyte antigen (HLA) type or an enzyme phenotype, suggests inheritance of the disease trait. Molecular genetic linkage analysis permits identification of chromosomal sequences and locations associated with specific diseases.

Studies of the familial aggregation of asthma in general population samples and in selected populations have shown an increased prevalence of asthma among first-degree relatives of an index subject. In the Tecumseh survey, Higgins and Keller (85) found that the prevalence of asthma increased among children younger than 16 years when one or both parents had asthma. The prevalence increased in boys from 7.4% when neither parent had asthma to 18.3% when one or both parents had asthma, and in girls from 4.1% to 11.7%. Similar findings were reported by Lebowitz et al. (86) in a study of 344 nuclear families from Tucson, Arizona. When neither parent had asthma, 6.5% of the children had physician-diagnosed asthma; when one or both parents had asthma, 19.7% and 63.6% of the children had asthma, respectively. Investigations of families in Connecticut and South Carolina provided similar results (87). Leeder et al. (26) evaluated a cohort of 2000 children from birth to age 5 years and found that the incidence of asthma increased from 2.5% if neither parent had asthma to 5.4% if one parent had asthma. In a birth cohort of 1265 children evaluated for 6 years, Horwood et al. (88) found that parental asthma increased risk only for asthma among males. Sibbald et al. (89) reported an increased prevalence of asthma among first-degree relatives of asthmatic children compared with relatives of nonasthmatic children evaluated in a general practice. These studies of familial aggregation in general population samples indicate a strong familial influence on the prevalence of childhood asthma, but do not separate genetic from environmental effects.

Twin studies provide more direct evidence on the heritability of asthma. In 6996 twin pairs from the Swedish twin register, Edfors-Lubs (90) found a prevalence of asthma of 3.8%. The higher concordance of asthma in monozygotic twins (19.0%) than in dizygotic twins (4.8%) implies that hereditary factors contribute to the causes of asthma. Under a single dominant or recessive gene model, the risk of asthma in the offspring of two affected parents was estimated to be approximately 30%. Between 1972 and 1982, Hopp et al. (91) enrolled 61 monozygotic and 46 dizygotic twin pairs; 14.7% of monozygotic and 8.7% of dizygotic twin pairs were concordant for a history of asthma. Among 256 monozygotic twins and 158 dizygotic twins from the Greater Boston Twin Registry, the concordance of a past history of asthma was 36% for monozygotic twins and zero for dizygotic twins (92). These studies of twin pairs show an increased concordance of asthma among monozygotic twins but do not quantify the relative importance of genetic and environmental factors.

To characterize further the role of genetic factors in the pathogenesis of asthma, other investigators have measured genetic markers in asthmatic subjects and performed molecular genetic linkage analyses. Turton et al. (93) tissue typed 122 asthmatic subjects for the HLA A, B, and C loci and compared the frequencies with those in 167 healthy controls; no significant differences were found. More recently, Ronchetti et al. (94) demonstrated reduced 2-1 adenosine deaminase phenotype among asthmatic children 5–15 years of age compared with children under 5 years and normal controls. Because adenosine modulates the release of histamine on antigenic challenge (94), the finding of different adenosine deaminase phenotypes suggests a mechanism for genetic modulation in the development of asthma. After identifying index cases with asthma or allergic rhinitis, Cookson et al. (95) performed molecular genetic linkage analyses on family members and found that atopy was inherited as an autosomal dominant trait localized to chromosome 11.

## Male Sex

Descriptive studies of childhood asthma have consistently shown an increased prevalence in boys. Before the age of 14 years, the prevalence may be as much as doubled in boys (88,96), but the differential narrows among older children (12,15). Differences in airway geometry in boys and girls offer one explanation for the male excess. Taussig (97) measured expiratory flow rates in 65 normal children aged 4–6 years and found lower flow rates in boys. This finding, together with the observation of lower airway resistance in girls (98), suggests that boys tend to have smaller airways at a given lung size than girls. This anatomical difference could predispose boys to more lower respiratory illnesses with wheezing. In addition, boys have a higher incidence of both upper and lower respiratory tract infections (99,100).

Although differences in airway geometry between boys and girls may contribute to a higher risk of asthma in boys, recent findings suggest that reduced lung function is the important factor for predicting development of a wheezing illness in boys or girls. Martinez et al. (101) measured lung function in 124 healthy infants before 6 months of age and found the risk for a subsequent wheezing illness was increased in boys with high respiratory resistance and in girls with a low functional residual capacity.

## Atopy

Atopic individuals characteristically have enhanced formation of specific IgE antibody after exposure to antigens (102). In the context of an epidemiological investigation, atopic status may be assessed by measuring skin test reactivity to common local antigens, by measuring serum levels of IgE, by questionnaire evaluation of diseases associated with atopy, such as infantile eczema and allergic rhinitis, and by assessment of parental history of illnesses associated with atopy as a marker of genetic predisposition.

Regardless of the index used, epidemiological studies indicate that asthma and atopy are linked (103), although the magnitude of the association has varied with the index and study population. For example, Burrows et al. (104) used skin tests with local antigens to assess the atopic status of subjects selected at random in Tucson, Arizona. In children 3–14 years old, skin test reactivity was strongly associated with attacks of wheezing with dyspnea, regardless of whether asthma had been diagnosed. Further analyses of data from the Tucson population show that the prevalence of asthma is more strongly associated with level of IgE than skin-test reactivity (105). When self-reports from a population sample in western Pennsylvania were used (15), hay fever had been diagnosed much more often in asthmatic than in nonasthmatic children (25.0 vs. 3.8% in boys and 22.2 vs. 2.5% in girls). In a longitudinal study, Fergusson et al. (106) evaluated the relationships among parental asthma, parental eczema, and the occurrence of asthma and eczema in children evaluated from birth through age 4 years. The results demonstrated complex interactions among those factors that depended on the child's sex. In boys, both parental asthma and eczema were associated with asthma, but only the latter association was statistically significant in girls. Davis and Bulpitt (107) found a similar interaction among parental atopy, sex, and childhood asthma.

The results of such studies demonstrate the complex relationship between atopy and asthma; however, the mechanistic pathways, either causal or noncausal, that link atopy and asthma are not well defined. Research in this area must also address the consequences of lower respiratory tract infections, which may be more severe and more common in atopic children (108). Nevertheless, atopy in parents or children does predict increased risk of asthma, and its presence or absence may be used as an empiric predictor.

## Environmental Factors

Although genetic factors may define the child most susceptible to developing asthma, this susceptibility may only manifest as asthma after exposure to evironmental triggers. The major environmental factors that have been investigated as risk factors for asthma include aeroallergens, respiratory tract infections, ambient air pollution, and environmental tobacco smoke.

### *Aeroallergens*

Allergens are well-known causes of asthma exacerbations, but their role in the development of asthma has been only recently examined. Using parents' reports of dampness and mold in the home as surrogates for allergen exposure, Brunekreef et al. (109) found among a cohort of 4625 children 8–12 years of age, living in six U.S. cities, relative risks of 1.42 (95% confidence interval, 1.04–1.94) and 1.27 (95% confidence interval 0.93–1.74), respectively, for doctor-diagnosed asthma. A more direct examination of the role of allergens was conducted by Sporik et al. (110) who enrolled 93 infants who had 1 parent with asthma or hay fever, and obtained baseline measurements of house-dust mite antigen in their homes. After 11 years, 67 children were re-evaluated, and 17 had asthma. The relative risk for development of asthma was 19.7 for children with skin-test sensitivity to house-dust mite, and 4.8 among children with high levels of exposure to the mite antigen during infancy. These results suggest that allergen exposure may be an important risk factor for development of childhood asthma.

### *Respiratory Tract Infection*

During childhood, the incidence of lower respiratory tract infections is high and all children have illnesses caused by respiratory syncytial virus, the parainfluenza viruses, or other pathogens. A community-based surveillance program in Tecumseh, Michigan, demonstrated that infants averaged 2.1 episodes of lower respiratory tract illness during the first year of life; the average dropped to only 1.5 at 1–2 years of age (100,111). Surveillance through a pediatric group practice, which detects more severe episodes, showed that 25% of children were affected during the first year of life; by age 5 years, about 12% of children had a lower respiratory illness annually; and by ages 6–8 years, about 8% annually visited the practice for a lower respiratory illness (99).

Investigations of lung function abnormalities in children with documented histories of lower respiratory infection suggest that these common illnesses may predispose to the later development of asthma (112). Most of these studies have been retrospective in design, with subjects identified by previous hospitalization. The results of these studies may not extend to the majority of children, who do not require hospitalization when ill with lower respiratory tract infections.

As a risk factor for asthma, the evidence is strongest for bronchiolitis, an illness most often associated with respiratory syncytial virus (Table 5). Each of the series based on hospitalized subjects showed abnormalities of lung function on follow up. The patterns of dysfunction were consistent with airflow obstruction: hyperinflation, increased respiratory resistance, and reduced spirometric flow rates. Nonspecific airway reactivity was assessed in four of the studies by exercise, by cold air inhalation, or by inhalation of histamine or methacholine. Increased airway responsiveness occurred in excess in each of the series based on hospitalized subjects (115–

TABLE 5 Long-Term Functional Sequelae of Bronchiolitis

| Study population (Ref.) | Follow-up interval | Findings |
|---|---|---|
| Hospitalized for bronchiolitis, n = 22 (113) | 13 months | 7/18 hyperinflation, ↑ total respiratory resistance |
| Hospitalized for bronchiolitis, n = 23 (114) | 10 years | 9/22, ↑ RV/TLC<br>18/23, ↓ $PaO_2$<br>12/16, ↑ Viso v |
| Hospitalized for RS virus bronchiolitis n = 35 (115) | 8 years | ↓ $FEV_{0.75}$/VC<br>↑ exercise-induced bronchial lability |
| Hospitalized for bronchiolitis n = 48 (116) | 9–10 years | 42% ↑ RV/TLC<br>56%, positive methacholine challenge |
| Hospitalized for RS virus lower respiratory tract infection, n = 130 (117) | 10 years | ↓ $FEV_1$, FVC, and expiratory flows, ↑ bronchial lability |
| Hospitalized for bronchiolitis, n = 55 (118) | 2 years | 60% with hyperinflation |
| Hospitalized for RS virus lower respiratory tract infection, n = 29 (119) | Up to 8 years | 55% with ↓ $SaO_2$ |
| Outpatient diagnosis of bronchiolitis, n = 25 (120) | Aged 8–12 years | Airway reactivity to cold air not increased |

Source: Adapted from 108.

117), but this was not the finding in the study reported by McConnochie et al. (120), which drew subjects from an outpatient practice. This discrepancy in findings illustrates the potentially limited generality of results obtained from more severely ill children. In contrast, however, Weiss et al. (103) found that a history of croup or bronchiolitis was a predictor of increased airway responsiveness in a population-based sample of children. In hospital and community-based series, croup has also been associated with increased airway reactivity (121–123).

Several of these follow-up studies indicate increased frequency of asthma and wheezing after episodes of bronchiolitis. Of the 35 children evaluated by Sims et al. (115), 18 gave a history of wheezing episodes in contrast to 1 of 35 controls. The findings from follow-up studies in Toronto (116) and in Tyneside (117) were similar. In each of these studies the wheezing episodes reported tended to be mild. Other longitudinal studies also document the increased occurrence of asthma and wheezing after hospitalization for bronchiolitis (Table 6). These findings, based on hospitalized children, are supported by a similarly designed study that drew subjects from a pediatric group practice. McConnochie and Roghmann (129) found that children who had bronchiolitis in early childhood had a threefold excess of wheezing 8 years later.

The data demonstrating an association between lower respiratory tract infections and subsequent asthma and increased airway reactivity are convincing, although they apply only to more severe illness episodes. Mechanisms by which viral infections might cause asthma are uncertain (130,131). Viral infections might be indirectly rather than directly associated with asthma. Children with atopy are more likely to have severe lower respiratory tract infections and to develop asthma (108). Thus, a severe lower respiratory tract infection may be only a marker for a genetic predisposition

TABLE 6 Attack Rate of Asthma and Wheezing in Children Hospitalized with Bronchiolitis

| Number of subjects (ref) | Length of follow-up (year) | Asthma on follow-up (%) | Wheezing on follow-up |
|---|---|---|---|
| 100 (124) | 1– 7 | 32 | Not stated |
| 63 (125) | 4–14 | 25 | 21% with respiratory infections |
| 24 (126) | 3– 4 | Not stated | 46% |
| 62 (127) | 2– 7 | Not stated | 44% >5 episodes |
| 35 (128) | 5 | Not stated | 50% |

Source: Adapted from 108.

to asthma. Recent data from a prospective study of infants suggest that infants who wheeze with a lower respiratory tract infection have lower premorbid lung function than children who do not wheeze (101). Regardless of the underlying mechanism, a history of hospitalization for bronchiolitis does predict a clinically important increase in the risk of asthma.

### *Ambient Air Pollution*

Because of difficulties in measuring personal exposure to air pollutants and controlling for other potential risk factors for asthma, limited epidemiological data are available on the role of air pollution in the development of asthma. Laboratory exposure studies demonstrate that asthmatic subjects may be adversely affected by exposure to common atmospheric pollutants, including nitrogen dioxide, sulfur oxides, respirable particulate matter, and ozone. Epidemiological studies provide further evidence that air pollution may exacerbate asthma (132–134).

Results from two recent cross-sectional surveys in Israel (135) and in Sweden (136) suggest that ambient air pollution increases the prevalence of asthma. Goren and Hellmann (135) compared the prevalence of asthma among second and fifth graders from an industrialized city (n = 1672) with high levels of sulfer oxides and nitrogen oxides with that among children from a city with lower levels of these pollutants (n = 1702). After potential risk factors were controlled for, the relative risk for asthma was 2.66 comparing the polluted with the unpolluted city. Similar results were found among children in Sweden (136).

### *Passive Exposure to Cigarette Smoke*

The nonsmoking child is exposed to environmental tobacco smoke, a mixture of the sidestream smoke released by the smoldering cigarette with mainstream smoke exhaled by the smoker (137). Exposure to environmental tobacco smoke is often referred to as "passive" or "involuntary" smoking. Smoking contributes respirable particles and gaseous compounds to indoor air; it represents one of the major sources of inhalable particles in U.S. homes (137,138). Thus, in comparison with children residing in homes without smokers, children living in homes with smokers would be anticipated to have substantially greater personal exposures to particles. Studies using the biological marker of exposure, cotinine, document uptake of environmental tobacco smoke by children (139,140).

Exposure to environmental tobacco smoke (ETS) could plausibly contribute to the causes of asthma or worsen the clinical status of children with asthma. Several mechanisms, not necessarily exclusive, can be postulated by which passive smoking could cause asthma. First, passive smoking increases the risk for more severe lower respiratory tract infections during the first years of life (137); respiratory infections increase airways responsiveness and may possibly trigger the development of asthma (141). Second, direct toxicity of environmental tobacco smoke components might induce and sustain the heightened nonspecific airways responsiveness found in asthmatic children. Third, many children who are exposed to environmental tobacco smoke after birth have also been exposed during gestation. In utero exposure to circulating tobacco smoke components might affect airways responsiveness after birth. In children with established asthma, irritant components of environmental tobacco smoke might exacerbate the disease and chronically increase the level of nonspecific airways responsiveness.

Evidence that involuntary smoking causes childhood asthma has been conflicting. Increased airway responsiveness has been associated with parental smoking even in infancy. Young et al. (142) assessed nonspecific airway responsiveness using histamine challenge in 63 normal infants at a mean age of 4.5 weeks. Parental smoking and a family history of asthma were both associated with an increased level of airway responsiveness. It will be important to determine if this increased responsiveness predisposes to subsequent asthma.

In older children, the role of passive smoking has been examined in cross-sectional studies or surveys and in longitudinal studies. Gortmacker

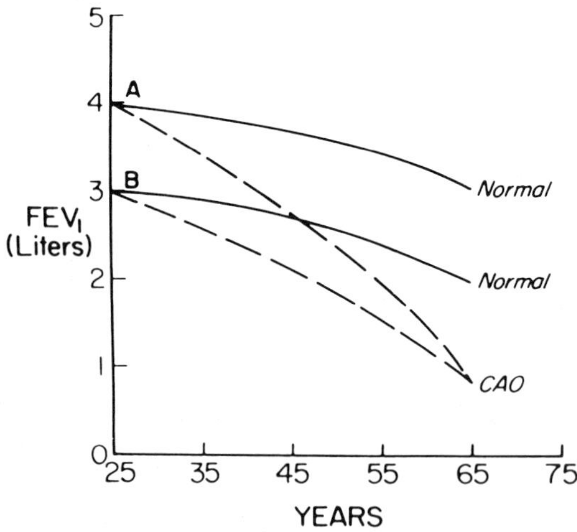


FIGURE 3 Decline of $FEV_1$ at normal rate (solid line) and at an accelerated rate (dashed line). A. A person who has attained a "normal" maximal $FEV_1$ during lung growth and development. B. A person whose maximal $FEV_1$ has been reduced by childhood respiratory infection. CAO, chronic airflow obstruction.

et al. (143) collected data from 2 U.S. population samples of children aged 0–17 years. The relative risk for asthma associated with maternal smoking was 1.5 in a Midwestern urbanized county and 1.8 in a more rural Eastern county. In a longitudinal study of children in Tecumseh, Michigan, aged 0–19 years on enrollment, parental smoking increased the prevalence of asthma at the first examination and was associated with a doubling of the risk for developing asthma during a 15-year follow-up period (144,145). A case–control study of children aged 5 and under in the United Kingdom also showed increased risk for moderately severe asthma in association with exposure to ETS at home (146). In a 1981 national U.S. sample of 4331 children aged 0–5 years, maternal smoking of one-half pack or more of cigarettes per day doubled the risk of asthma (147). The findings were similar for the 15,416 children aged 0–17 years in the entire sample.

In contrast, in a longitudinal study in New Zealand, parental smoking habits were not found to affect the incidence of asthma during the first 6 years of life (88). Through age 6 years, 11.0% of children with neither parent smoking and 10.1% of children with two parents smoking had two or more consultations for asthma. In another longitudinal study of over 2000 children in Harrow, England, parental smoking was not a significant predictor of the development of asthma during a 5 year follow-up period (26). Maternal smoking likewise did not predict a report of asthma by age 10 years in 9670 British children followed from birth through that age, although it was significantly associated with a report of wheezy bronchitis (148). Some cross-sectional studies have also failed to demonstrate a relationship between parental smoking and asthma (15,149,150). The inconsistencies among these investigations cannot be readily explained by differences in methodology or among the populations.

While involuntary exposure to tobacco smoke has not yet been established as a cause of asthma, evidence indicates that involuntary smoking worsens the status of patients with asthma. The possibility that ETS adversely affects children with asthma was described as early as 1950 in a case report entitled "Bronchial asthma due to allergy to tobacco smoke in an infant" (151). More recently, Murray and Morrison (152) evaluated 94 asthmatic children aged 7–17 years. Level of lung function, symptom frequency, and responsiveness to inhaled histamine were adversely affected by maternal smoking. Subsequently, Murray and Morrison (153) described the effects of passive smoking on 415 asthmatic children presenting to a clinic. This larger series confirmed the adverse effect of maternal smoking on asthmatic children and suggested that boys may be more susceptible than girls.

In a study of 21 asthmatic subjects aged 6–21 years in a population sample, O'Connor and colleagues (154) also found that maternal smoking increased the level of airways responsiveness. Male 9-year-old Italian schoolchildren had greater bronchial responsiveness if their parents smoked; the association with smoking was strongest for children with asthma (101). The increased level of airways responsiveness associated with maternal smoking in these studies would be expected to increase the clinical severity of asthma. In this regard, exposure to smoking in the home has been shown to increase the number of emergency room visits made by asthmatic children (22). Asthmatic children with mothers who smoke are also more likely to use asthma medications (147), a finding that confirms the clinically significant effects of ETS on children with asthma. In a New York City cohort of 276 New York City children with asthma from 259 low-income families, children from households that included a smoker had 3.1 annual visits while children from households with no smoker had only 1.8. In surveys, children from households with smokers had a higher frequency of function-impairing asthma (143). However, in the 1981 nationwide data for children aged 0–5 years analyzed by Weitzman et al. (147), maternal smoking was not associated with the number of hospitalizations for asthmatic children.

While uncertainty remains concerning the role of passive smoking in causing asthma, the evidence on exacerbation of asthma by passive smoking is more convincing. Pediatricians should caution the parents of asthmatic children that their smoking may have adverse effects on their children's disease.

## Bronchial Hyperreactivity

Bronchial hyperreactivity refers to increased responsiveness of the airways to specific or nonspecific stimuli (155,156). Nonspecific reactivity is usually assessed by inhalation of methacholine, histamine, or cold air. Although increased reactivity fulfills the definitional criterion for asthma, "increased responsiveness" of the airways, as specified by the American Thoracic Society and the American College of Chest Physicians (Table 1), may have limited diagnostic usefulness that is dependent on the study population. In a survey of 2053 7–10-year-old schoolchildren from New Zealand, Pattemore et al. (17) found that 53% of those with bronchial hyperreactivity had no asthma diagnosis, and 48% of those with an asthma diagnosis did not have bronchial hyperreactivity. Worldwide, similar results have been found in other population-based studies (158,159). In contrast, clinical studies with methacholine challenge testing of children from selected populations show that nearly all asthmatic subjects have increased reactivity, but some nonasthmatic children are equally responsive (160,161). Increased bronchial responsiveness may result from recent respiratory tract infection, allergic rhinitis, atopic family history, and chronic pulmonary disease.

Because of lack of information on the onset and natural history of bronchial hyperreactivity, the relationship between bronchial hyperreactivity and the development of asthma has created a great deal of debate. However, recent findings begin to provide insight into the role of bronchial hyperreactivity in asthma. Infants without a history of respiratory tract infection have been found to have bronchial hyperresponsiveness to histamine as early as 4.5 weeks of age, and the degree of responsiveness is increased with a family history of asthma and parental smoking, which suggests that both genetic and environmental factors are important in its development (142). Furthermore, in the majority of children and young adults bronchial hyperreactivity precedes the development of asthma (162). These findings suggest that bronchial hyperreactivity occurs early in life and may progress to clinical asthma. However, the factors determining the outcome of bronchial hyperreactivity from infancy through childhood remain to be determined.

The development of asthma probably results from a complex interaction of a genetic predisposition with many environmental exposures. To understand better the independent effects of these risk factors and others, several multiple regression analyses have been recently conducted using data from different groups of children in the United Kingdom (163) and the United States (147,164,165). Although the risk factors examined in these investigations are not identical, in general the findings provide further support for many of the risk factors discussed previously. Other factors that have been identified in these analyses as independent risk factors for childhood asthma incude maternal age less than 20 years (147,163,164), history of pneumonia (163,165), history of bronchitis (165), poverty (147,164), and black race (147,164).

## NATURAL HISTORY

### Descriptive Data on the Clinical Course of Asthma

To describe the natural history of childhood asthma, investigators have identified cohorts of asthmatic children and monitored their clinical status as they age. Most studies have been retrospective and based on follow-up of patients from office practices or hospital clinics (166–170). Only two longitudinal studies of children from general population samples have been carried out (Table 7) (96,171). These studies have shown that between 30 and 70% of asthmatic children improve by adolescence or early adulthood (Table 7). Differences in the study populations along with differing criteria for clinical outcome probably contribute to the wide range of reported improvement, and the studies cannot readily be compared. In some studies the categories of symptom status were not explicitly defined (166,167), and

TABLE 7 Selected Studies Describing the Clinical Course of Childhood Asthma

| Population (ref) | Average duration of follow-up years | Outcome (%) | | | Dead from asthma |
|---|---|---|---|---|---|
| | | Asymptomatic or improved | Symptomatic | | |
| | | | Mild | Chronic/ severe | |
| 688 with onset of asthma before age 13 years from a private office (166) | 20 | 66 | 14 | 17 | 1.5 |
| 236 less than 14 years seen at pediatric allergy clinic (167) | 5 | 44 | 36 | 20 | 1.0 |
| 1000 referred to author for care after 1935 (168) | 11 | 48 | 26 | 19 | 7 |
| 518 treated at a private office before 1956 (169) | 10 | 41 | 52 | 6 | 1 |
| 244 under 12 years of age seen 1948–1952 in a group practice (170) | 20 | 27 | 49 | 21 | 1 |
| 314 age 7 years old sampled from public schools beginning in 1964 (171) | 7 | 48 | 52 | | — |
| 25 ages 7–17 years from a general population sample beginning in 1972 (96) | 7 | 72 | 28 | | — |

in others the criteria were not compatible (96,168–171). For example, Ogilvie (168) considered a subject to be in "good" health if either asymptomatic for 2 years or with moderate continuous dyspnea. This classification may explain the high proportion of "asymptomatic" individuals in this study compared with that of Blair (170), who counted as in "good" health only those subjects who were asymptomatic for 2 years. Other differences among the studies that may underlie the variation in results include different periods of study and varying durations of follow-up. However, no major trends in outcome are obvious from the 1930s to the 1960s.

These studies of the natural history of childhood asthma provide some information on characteristics that predict outcome. In this section we review the available literature concerning sex, age, and severity of onset, atopic disorders, family history, smoking, level of pulmonary function, and treatment as determinants of clinical course.

### *Gender*

Investigations to date do not provide consistent results concerning child's gender as a predictor of outcome. In 1952, Rackemann and Edwards (166) described the clinical course of 688 asthmatic children selected from a private practice and followed over 20 years. Boys and girls did not differ in the severity of asthma. Blair's (170) findings in a study of 244 children also evaluated over 20 years were similar. In 1964, Williams and McNicol (12) studied a sample of 7-year-old asthmatic and normal children from 30,000 Australian schoolchildren. At ages 14 and 21 years, the clinical status of these subjects was determined by McNicol and Williams (171) and Martin et al. (172), respectively. At age 14 years a higher proportion of boys had severe asthma, and from 14 to 21 years boys had a greater relative improvement of their asthma. In 1972, Schachter et al. (96) identified 25 asthmatics aged 7–17 years; after 8 years of follow-up, 67% of boys and 86% of girls had experienced improvement of symptoms.

### *Age and Severity of Onset*

The available data are conflicting regarding age of onset and the course of childhood asthma. Buffum and Settipane (169) evaluated 518 asthmatic children from a private practice for 10 years and 136 for 20 years. At 10 years of follow-up, no difference in prognosis was found for those whose asthma began by age 2 years in comparison to those with later onset. However, at 20 years of follow-up, a higher proportion were asymptomatic if their asthma began after 2 years of age. Conflicting data were reported by Foucard and Sjoberg (173), who evaluated 81 children with wheezy bronchitis for 12 years. Of those whose wheezing began after 12 months of age, 42% had asthma 12 years later compared with only 21% who had wheezing before 1 year of age. Among asthmatic schoolchildren evaluated from age 7 to 21, Martin et al. (172) did not find onset before 12 months to be predictive of a more severe form of asthma. After 20 years of follow-up, Blair (170) likewise found no difference in prognosis for those whose asthma started before age 2 compared with onset after age 2.

Although age of onset may not predict the course of a child's asthma, the initial severity of wheezing may be a more useful predictor. Blair (170), during the first 5 years of follow-up, identified 126 children with severe asthma, defined as more than 3 attacks per year, with some attacks requiring hospitalization or persisting for more than 5 days. After 20 years, these children were more likely to develop chronic asthma than those with mild asthma. Similar conclusions have been reached by McNicol and Williams (171).

### *Atopic Disorders*

Several investigators have examined whether evidence of eczema, allergic rhinitis, and skin test reactivity to antigens alters the prognosis of children with asthma. Buffum and Settipane (169) in the study cited above found that 11.4% with eczema had severe asthma compared with 2.4% of those without. Likewise, 15.4% of those with a positive skin test reaction to whole-egg extract had severe disease after 10 years of follow up compared with only 3.5% of nonreactors. Blair (170) found that persistence of infantile eczema was associated with chronic or recurrent asthma in 88% of subjects. In contrast, only 27% of children whose eczema cleared had chronic or recurrent asthma. He did not find an association between skin test reactivity and prognosis, but he did show that perennial or seasonal rhinitis worsened prognosis. In contrast, allergic rhinitis was of no predictive value at age 21 years among the asthmatic children evaluated by Martin et al. (172). However, they did find that eczema and skin test reactivity at ages 10 and 14 years predicted a more severe form of asthma at age 21. These findings suggest that eczema is associated with persistence of asthma into young adulthood, but the predictive value of skin test reactivity and rhinitis is of less value.

### *Family History*

A family history of asthma or atopy among first-degree relatives increases a child's risk for developing persistent asthma. Of 244 children with asthma evaluated by Blair (170), 75 had first-degree relatives with a history of asthma or atopy. After 20 years of follow-up 73% had chronic or recurrent asthma and 27% had no asthma or mild asthma. Foucard and Sjoberg (173) found that infants and children with wheezy bronchitis and a family history of asthma or allergy had twice the risk of developing persistent asthma of those without such a family history.

### *Smoking*

Despite the persistent and common smoking of cigarettes by children (174), few epidemiological investigations of the natural history of childhood asthma have included data concerning smoking habits. Martin et al. (172) obtained smoking histories from 21-year-olds who wheezed before age 7; of those who had a current history of frequent or persistent wheezing during the last year, 46% smoked 5 or more cigarettes a day compared with 33% among those who had not wheezed for 3 years. More detailed analysis showed that between the ages of 14 and 21 years increased smoking decreased the probability for improvement in asthmatic symptoms. These data reinforce the need to counsel patients and families concerning the adverse effects of smoking on the prognosis of childhood asthma.

### *Level of Pulmonary Function*

Although airway obstruction is a hallmark of asthma, little is known about the natural history of childhood asthma and lung function. In their follow-up of Australian schoolchildren, Martin et al. (172) found that about 60% of children who had an abnormal forced expiratory volume in 1 sec ($FEV_1$) at ages 10 and 14 years had continued infrequent or frequent wheezing at age 21 years. However, the proportions of children with a reduced $FEV_1$ at 10 and 14 years were similar among those with no wheezing after age 18 and those who currently were wheezing frequently. These data suggest that a reduced $FEV_1$ during childhood predicts continued wheezing in early adulthood but does not predict the severity of symptoms.

### *Bronchial Hyperreactivity*

As for level of pulmonary function, few data are available on the degree of bronchial reactivity and prognosis of childhood asthma. Gerritsen et al. (175) examined 119 asthmatic children 6–14 years of age, and re-evaluated 85% of these subjects 14–20 years later. Of the 101 subjects examined as adults, 43% were currently having symptoms suggestive of asthma. The degree of bronchial hyperreactivity and reduced $FEV_1$ in childhood were independently associated with current symptoms as an adult.

### *Treatment*

The use of bronchodilators, corticosteroids, and disodium cromoglycate greatly reduces morbidity from asthma. Speight et al. (11) found that school absenteeism fell 10-fold after effective treatment among 31 asthmatic children with more than 12 attacks per year. However, most studies of the natural history of childhood asthma have not addressed the long-term effects of treatment. During their 14-year follow-up of asthmatic schoolchildren, Martin et al. (172) obtained data about drug treatment at ages 10 and 14 years. The authors then categorized the subjects according to the severity of their asthma into undertreated or appropriately treated groups. Severity of asthma at age 21 years was not influenced by undertreatment at ages 10 or 14 years. Further studies are needed to determine whether pharmacologic treatment alters the natural history of childhood asthma. A new clinical trial addressing this issue has been initiated by the National Heart, Lung, and Blood Institute.

## Relationship to Chronic Obstructive Pulmonary Disease

Cigarette smoking has been established as the cause of most cases of Chronic obstructive pulmonary disease (COPD) in adults (176), but the factors that place individual smokers at risk remain largely unknown (177). Longitudinal studies have partly described the development of chronic airflow obstruction in adults and provide a conceptual framework for considering the potential role of childhood factors, such as asthma, in the pathogenesis of COPD (Fig. 1) (176,178). Ventilatory function, as measured by the $FEV_1$ or other spirometric parameters, increases with lung growth and development during childhood and attains a maximum during early adulthood. Environmental exposure during childhood, respiratory infections, and respiratory diseases, such as asthma, may determine the level that is achieved, and some individuals may enter adulthood with less functional capacity than others, after this is standardized for body size. From the peak, the $FEV_1$ gradually and progressively declines. In those persons who develop COPD, a similar progressive decline takes place, but at an accelerated pace.

Childhood respiratory illnesses have been proposed as a risk factor for the development of COPD (179–181). Respiratory infections, particularly with respiratory syncytial virus, have been emphasized (108), but childhood asthma is also a biologically plausible risk factor. In fact, over 20 years ago, Dutch investigators postulated that an asthmatic predisposition increased risk for COPD (182). Supporting evidence for this hypothesis can be found in case series of nonsmoking asthmatic persons who develop a clinical picture compatible with COPD (183) and in epidemiological data that show accelerated decline of the $FEV_1$ in smokers with increased airway reactivity (184–186). However, these studies have not specifically addressed childhood asthma. Furthermore, the effects of asthma on lung growth and development have not been characterized (187).

The complicated relationship among lower respiratory infections, atopy, and airway reactivity is an additional barrier in investigating childhood asthma as a risk factor for COPD. Numerous investigations have established that a high proportion of children with severe lower respiratory tract infections during infancy have lung function abnormalities that include increased airway reactivity (108). Some studies suggest that the incidence of respiratory infection is increased in atopic children (108) and atopic status is associated with airway hyperresponsiveness (155,188). Thus, in assessing childhood asthma as a risk factor for COPD, the effects of childhood asthma cannot readily be separated from those of lower respiratory infection and atopy. Because of the prevalence of childhood asthma and the possibility of therapeutic intervention, the role of childhood asthma in the causes of COPD warrants further investigation.

## CLINICAL APPLICATIONS

In the United States and other countries, asthma is a frequent cause of morbidity but it is less frequently a cause of mortality. However, epidemiological investigations have shown that physicians often fail to diagnose asthma in children (11). Thus, awareness of the presentations of childhood asthma is important for proper management. Key historical features include persistent wheezing, chronic cough, and/or breathlessness (11,17), and in children able to perform a forced vital capacity maneuver, the finding of intermittent airflow obstruction is strongly suggestive of the presence of asthma. Appropriate treatment of asthmatic children significantly decreases school absenteeism (11) and, presumably, mortality. However, longitudinal data concerning treatment of asthma and death from asthma are unavailable. Treatment is not without hazard; recent observations suggest that overuse of theophyllines and beta agonists may contribute to increases in death from asthma (49,74,81,82). Factors that specifically identify the child at risk of dying from asthma have not been characterized.

In addition to diagnostic and therapeutic considerations, epidemiological investigations have provided data concerning risk factors for the development and persistence of childhood asthma. Awareness of these factors may offer further historical evidence supportive of the diagnosis of asthma. For example, a family history of asthma or atopy, a child's history of other atopic disorders, and a history of severe viral respiratory infections increase the risk for development of asthma. These same factors also affect the clinical course of childhood asthma, and knowledge of their presence or absence may be important in counseling a child's family and guiding long-term follow-up by a physician. For example, a family history of asthma in an asthmatic child with eczema is more likely to predict a more persistent form of asthma. Of particular importance is the need to identify the teenager who smokes cigarettes and advise cessation, because smoking is the major risk factor for the development of COPD in adulthood.

## ACKNOWLEDGMENTS

This work was supported in part by contract no. N01-CN-55426 from the Biometry Branch, National Cancer Institute. Dr. Coultas is a recipient of a Preventive Pulmonary Academic Award, K07 HL 02474, from the Division of Lung Diseases, National Heart, Lung, and Blood Institute.

## REFERENCES

1. Lilienfeld AM, Lilienfeld DE. *Foundations of Epidemiology*, 2nd ed., Oxford University Press, New York, 1980.

2. Ciba Foundation Guest Symposium. Terminology, definitions, and classification of chronic pulmonary emphysema and related conditions. *Thorax* 14:286–299, 1959.
3. American Thoracic Society. Chronic bronchitis, asthma, and pulmonary emphysema. *Am Rev Respir Dis* 85:762–768, 1962.
4. American College of Chest Physicians, American Thoracic Society. Pulmonary terms and symbols. *Chest* 67:583–593, 1975.
5. World Health Organization. Epidemiology of chronic nonspecific respiratory diseases. *Bull WHO* 52:251–259, 1975.
6. American Thoracic Society. Standards for the diagnosis and care of patients with chronic obstructive pulmonary disease (COPD) and asthma. *Am Rev Respir Dis* 136:225–243, 1987.
7. National Institutes of Health. Expert panel report on guidelines for diagnosis and management of asthma. National Heart, Lung, and Blood Institute Information Center, Bethesda, MD, 1991.
8. Ciba Foundation Study Group No. 38. *Identification of Asthma*, Churchill Livingstone, Edinburgh, 1971.
9. Ferris BG. Epidemiology standardization project. *Am Rev Respir Dis* 188:1–53, 1978.
10. Taussig LM, Smith SM, Blumenfeld R. Chronic bronchitis in childhood: what is it? *Pediatrics* 67:1–5, 1981.
11. Speight ANP, Lee DA, Hey EN. Underdiagnosis and undertreatment of asthma in childhood. *Br Med J* 286:1253–1256, 1983.
12. Williams H, McNicol K. Prevalence, natural history, and relationship of wheezy bronchitis and asthma in children. *Br Med J* 4:321–325, 1969.
13. Gregg I. Epidemiological aspects. In: Clark TJH, Godfrey S, (eds.), *Asthma*, Chapman and Hall, London, 1983, pp 242–284.
14. Broder I, Higgins MW, Mathews KP, Keller JB. Epidemiology of asthma and allergic rhinitis in a total community, Tecumseh, Michigan. III. Second survey of the community. *J Allergy Clin Immunol* 53:127–138, 1974.
15. Schenker MB, Samet JM, Speizer FE. Risk factors for childhood respiratory disease. The effect of host factors and home environment exposures. *Am Rev Respir Dis* 128:1038–1043, 1983.
16. Lebowitz MD, Burrows B. Tucson epidemiologic study of obstructive lung diseases. II. Effects of in-migration factors on the prevalence of obstructive lung diseases. *Am J Epidemiol* 102:153–163, 1975.
17. Dodge RR, Burrows B. The prevalence and incidence of asthma and asthma-like symptoms in a general population sample. *Am Rev Respir Dis* 122:567–575, 1980.
18. Cookson JB. Prevalence rates of asthma in developing countries and their comparison with those in Europe and North America. *Chest* 91(suppl):97S–103S, 1987.
19. Gergen PJ, Mullally DI, Evans R III. National survey of prevalence of asthma among children in the United States, 1976 to 1980. *Pediatrics* 81:1–7, 1988.

20. Charpin D, Vervloet D, Charpin J. Epidemiology of asthma in Western Europe. *Allergy* 43:481–492, 1988.
21. Johnston IDA, Bland JM, Anderson HR. Ethnic variation in respiratory morbidity and lung function in childhood. *Thorax* 42:542–548, 1987.
22. Evans R, Mullally DI, Wilson RW, Gergen PJ, Rosenberg HM, Grauman JS, Chevarley FM, Feinlab M. National trends in the morbidity and mortality of asthma in the US. Prevalence, hospitalization, and death from asthma over two decades: 1965–1984. *Chest* 91 (suppl):65S–74S, 1987.
23. Burr ML, Butland BK, King S, Vaughan-Williams. Changes in asthma prevalence: two surveys 15 years apart. *Arch Dis Child* 64:1452–1456, 1989.
24. Burney PGJ, Chinn S, Rona RJ. Has the prevalence of asthma increased in children? Evidence from the national study of health and growth 1973–1986. *Br Med J* 300:1306–1310, 1990.
25. Shaw RA, Crane J, O'Donnell TV. Prevalence of asthma in children. *Br Med J* 300:1652–1653, 1990.
26. Leeder SR, Corkhill RT, Irwig LM, Holland WW. Influence of family factors on asthma and wheezing during the first five years of life. *Br J Prev Soc Med* 20:213–218, 1976.
27. Peat JK, Woolcock AJ, Leeder SR, Blackburn CRB. Asthma and bronchitis in Sydney schoolchildren. I. Prevalence during a six-year study. *Am J Epidemiol* 111:721–727, 1980.
28. Barbee RA, Dodge R, Lebowitz ML, Burrows B. The epidemiology of asthma. *Chest* 87 (Suppl.):21S–25S, 1985.
29. Dodge R, Cline MG, Burrows B. Comparisons of asthma, emphysema, and chronic bronchitis diagnoses in a general population sample. *Am Rev Respir Dis* 133:981–986, 1986.
30. Gergen PJ, Weiss KB. Changing patterns of asthma hospitalization among children: 1979–1987. *JAMA* 264:1688–1692, 1990.
31. Wissow LS, Gittelsohn AM, Szklo M, Starfield B, Mussman M. Poverty, race, and hospitalization for childhood asthma. *Am J Public Health* 78:777–782, 1988.
32. Halfon N, Newacheck PW. Trends in the hospitalization for acute childhood asthma, 1970–1984. *Am J Public Health* 76:1308–1311, 1986.
33. Mullally DI, Howard WA, Hubbard TJ, Grauman JS, Cohen SG. Increased hospitalizations for asthma among children in the Washington, D.C. area during 1961–1981. *Ann Allergy* 53:15–19, 1984.
34. Jackson RT, Mitchell EA. Trends in the hospital admission rates and drug treatment of asthma in New Zealand. *NZ Med J* 96:728–730, 1983.
35. Mitchell EA. International trends in hospital admission rates for asthma. *Arch Dis Child* 60:376–378, 1985.
36. Anderson HR. Increase in hospital admissions for childhood asthma: trends in referral, severity, and readmissions from 1970 to 1985 in a health region of the United Kingdom. *Thorax* 44:614–619, 1989.
37. Carman PG, Landau LI. Increased paediatric admissions with asthma in Western Australia—a problem of diagnosis? *Med J Aust* 152:23–26, 1990.

38. Weiss KB. Seasonal trends in US asthma hospitalization and mortality. *JAMA* 263:2323–2328, 1990.
39. Mitchell EA, Anderson HR, Freeling P, White PT. Why are hospital admission and mortality rates for childhood asthma higher in New Zealand than in the United Kingdom? *Thorax* 45:176–182, 1990.
40. Mitchell EA, Borman B. Demographic characteristics of asthma admissions to hospitals. *NZ Med J* 99:576–579, 1986.
41. Asher MI, Pattemore PK, Harrison AC, Mitchell EA, Rea HH, Stewart AW, Woolcock AJ. International comparison of the prevalence of asthma symptoms and bronchial hyperresponsiveness. *Am Rev Respir Dis* 138:524–529, 1988.
42. Tseng RYM, Lo CN, Li CK, Ling TWC, Mok MMC. Seasonal asthma in Hong Kong and its management implications. *Ann Allergy* 63:247–250, 1989.
43. Khot A, Burn R, Evans N, Lenney C, Lenney W. Seasonal variation and time trends in childhood asthma in England and Wales 1975–81. *Br Med J* 289:235–237, 1984.
44. O'Halloran SM, Heaf DP. Accident and emergency department attendance by asthmatic children. *Thorax* 44:700–705, 1989.
45. Storr J, Lenney W. School holidays and admissions with asthma. *Arch Dis Child* 64:103–107, 1989.
46. Benatar SR. Fatal asthma. *N Engl J Med* 314:423–429, 1986.
47. Speizer FE, Doll R. A century of asthma deaths in young people. *Br Med J* 3:245–246, 1968.
48. Stolley PD. Asthma mortality. Why the United States was spared an epidemic of deaths due to asthma. *Am Rev Respir Dis* 105:883–890, 1972.
49. Stolley PD, Schinner R. Association between asthma mortality and isoproterenol aerosols: a review. *Prev Med* 7:519–538, 1978.
50. Lanes SF, Walker AM. Do pressurized bronchodilator aerosols cause death among asthmatics? *Am J Epidemiol* 125:755–760, 1987.
51. Neuspiel DR, Kuller LH. Sudden and unexpected natural death in childhood and adolescence. *JAMA* 254:1321–1325, 1985.
52. Jackson R, Sears MR, Beaglehole R, Rea HH. International trends in asthma mortality: 1970–1985. *Chest* 94:914–919, 1988.
53. Sly RM. Mortality from asthma in children 1979–1984. *Ann Allergy* 60:433–443, 1988.
54. Weiss KB, Wagener DK. Changing patterns of asthma mortality. Identifying target populations at high risk. *JAMA* 264:1683–1687, 1990.
55. Burney PGJ. Asthma mortality in England and Wales: evidence for a further increase, 1974–84. *Lancet* 2:323–326, 1986.
56. Mao Y, Semenciw R, Morrison H, MacWilliams L, Davies J, Wigle D. Increased rates of illness and death from asthma in Canada. *Can Med Assoc J* 137:620–624, 1987.
57. Jackson RT, Beaglehole R, Rea HH, Sutherland DC. Mortality from asthma: a new epidemic in New Zealand. *Br Med J* 285:771–774, 1982.
58. Sears MR, Rea HH, Fenwick J, Beaglehole R, Gillis AJD, Holst PE, O'Don-

nell TV, Rothwell RPG, Sutherland DC. Deaths from asthma in New Zealand. *Arch Dis Child* 61:6–10, 1986.

59. So SY, Ng MMT, Ip MSM, Lam WK. Rising asthma mortality in young males in Hong Kong, 1976–85. *Respir Med* 84:457–461, 1990.
60. Sears MR, Rea HH, Beaglehole R, Gillies AJD, Holst PE, O'Donnell TV, Rothwell RPG, Sutherland DC. Asthma mortality in New Zealand: a two year national study. *NZ Med J* 98:271–275, 1985.
61. Weiss KB, Wagener DK. Geographic variations in US asthma mortality: small-area analysis of excess mortality, 1981–1985. *Am J Epidemiol* 132:S107–S115, 1990.
62. Sly RM, O'Donnell R. Regional distribution of deaths from asthma. *Ann Allergy* 62:347–354, 1989.
63. Khot A, Burn R. Seasonal variation and time trends of death from asthma in England and Wales 1960–82. *Br Med J* 289:233–234, 1984.
64. Robin ED. Death from bronchial asthma. *Chest* 93:614–618, 1988.
65. Buist AS. Is asthma mortality increasing? (Editorial). *Chest* 93:449–450, 1988.
66. Buist AS, Vollmer WM. Reflections on the rise in asthma morbidity and mortality (Editorial). *JAMA* 246:1719–1720, 1990.
67. Shaffer AL, Buist AS. Preface to asthma mortality task force report. *J Allergy Clin Immunol* 80(s):361, 1987.
68. Klebba AJ, Scott JH. Estimates of selected comparability ratios based on dual coding of 1976 death certificates by the Eighth and Ninth Revisions of the International Classification of Diseases, DHEW Publication No. (PHS) 80-1120, Vol. 28, No. 11, Supplement, February 29, 1980.
69. Lambert PM. Letter. *Lancet* 2:200–201, 1981.
70. British Thoracic Association. Accuracy of death certificates in bronchial asthma. *Thorax* 29:505–509, 1984.
71. Sears MR, Rea HH, deBoer G, Beaglehole R, Gillies AJD, Holst PE, O'Donnell TV, Rothwell RPG. Accuracy of certification of deaths due to asthma. A national study. *Am J Epidemiol* 124:1004–1011, 1986.
72. Carswell F. Thirty deaths from asthma. *Arch Dis Child* 60:25–28, 1985.
73. Strunk RC, Mrazek DA, Wolfson Fuhrmann GS, LaBrecque JF. Physiologic and psychological characteristics associated with deaths due to asthma in childhood. A case–controlled study. *JAMA* 254:1193–1198, 1985.
74. Wilson JD, Sutherland DC, Thomas AC. Has the change to beta-agonists combined with oral theophylline increased cases of fatal asthma? *Lancet* 1:1235–1237, 1981.
75. Rea HH, Sears MR, Beaglehole R, Fanwick J, Jackson RT, Gillies AJD, O'Donnell TV, Holst PE, Rothwell RPG. Lessons from the national asthma mortality study: circumstances surrounding death. *NZ Med J* 100:10–13, 1987.
76. Zach MS, Karner V. Sudden death in asthma. *Arch Dis Child* 64:1446–1451, 1989.
77. Molfino NA, Nannini LJ, Martelli AN, Slutsky AS. Respiratory arrest in near-fatal asthma. *N Engl J Med* 324:285–288, 1991.

78. O'Hallaren MT, Yaninger JW, Offord KP, Somers MJ, O'Connell EJ, Ballard DJ, Sachs MI. Exposure to an aeroallergen as a possible precipitating factor in respiratory arrest in young patients with asthma. *N Engl J Med* 324:359–363, 1991.
79. Rea HH, Scragg R, Jackson R, Beaglehole RT, Fenwick J, Sutherland DC. A case–control study of deaths from asthma. *Thorax* 41:833–839, 1986.
80. Miller BD, Strunk RC. Circumstances surrounding the deaths of children due to asthma. *Am J Dis Child* 143:1294–1299, 1989.
81. Crane J, Flatt A, Jackson R, Ball M, Pearce N, Burgess C, Kwong T, Beasley R. Prescribed fenoterol and death from asthma in New Zealand, 1981–83: case–control study. *Lancet* 1:917–922, 1989.
82. Pearce N, Grainger J, Atkinson M, Crane J, Burgess C, Culling C, Windom H, Beasley R. Case–control study of prescribed fenoterol and death from asthma in New Zealand, 1977–81. *Thorax* 45:170–175, 1990.
83. Buist AS, Burney PGJ, Feinstein AR, Horwitz RI, Lanes SF, Rebuck AS, Spitzer WO. Evaluation of a draft report on fenoterol. *Lancet* 1:1071, 1989.
84. Sackett DL, Shannon HS, Browman GW. Fenoterol and fatal asthma. *Lancet* 335:45–46, 1990.
85. Higgins M, Keller J. Familial occurrence of chronic respiratory disease and familial resemblance in ventilatory capacity. *J Chron Dis* 28:239–251, 1975.
86. Lebowitz MD, Barbee R, Burrows B. Family concordance of IgE, atopy, and disease. *J Allergy Clin Immunol* 73:259–264, 1984.
87. Schilling RSF, Letai AD, Hui SL, Beck GJ, Schoenberg JB, Bouhuys A. Lung function, respiratory disease, and smoking in families. *Am J Epidemiol* 106:274–283, 1977.
88. Horwood LJ, Fergusson DM, Shannon FT. Social and familial factors in the development of early childhood asthma. *Pediatrics* 75:859–868, 1985.
89. Sibbald B, Horn MEC, Gregg I. A family study of the genetic basis of asthma and wheezy bronchitis. *Arch Dis Child* 55:54–57, 1980.
90. Edfors-Lubs ML. Allergy in 7000 twin pairs. *Acta Allergol* 26:249–285, 1971.
91. Hopp RJ, Bewtra AK, Watt GD, Nair NM, Townley RG. Genetic analysis of allergic disease in twins. *J Allergy Clin Immunol* 73:265–270, 1984.
92. Redline S, Tishler PV, Lewitter FI, Tager IB, Munoz A, Speizer FE. Assessment of genetic and nongenetic influences on pulmonary function. A twin study. *Am Rev Respir Dis* 135:217–222, 1987.
93. Turton CWG, Morris L, Buckingham JA, Lawler SD, Turner-Warwick M. Histocompatibility antigens in asthma: population and family studies. *Thorax* 34:670–676, 1979.
94. Ronchetti R, Lucarini N, Lucarelli P, Martinez F, Macri F, Carapella E, bottini E. A genetic basis for heterogeneity of asthma syndrome in pediatric ages: adenosine deaminase phenotypes. *J Allergy Clin Immunol* 74:81–84, 1984.
95. Cookson WOCM, Sharp PA, Faux JA, Hopkin JM. Linkage between immunoglobulin E responses underlying asthma and rhinitis and chromosome 11 q. *Lancet* 1:1292–1295, 1989.

96. Schachter EN, Doyle CA, Beck GJ. A prospective study of asthma in a rural community. *Chest* 85:623–630, 1984.
97. Taussig LM. Maximal expiratory flows at functional residual capacity: a test of lung function for young children. *Am Rev Respir Dis* 116:1031–1038, 1977.
98. Doershuk CF, Fisher BJ, Matthews LW. Specific airway resistance from the perinatal period into adulthood. Alterations in childhood pulmonary disease. *Am Rev Respir Dis* 109:452–457, 1974.
99. Glezen WP, Denny FW. Epidemiology of acute lower respiratory disease in children. *N Engl J Med* 288:498–505, 1973.
100. Monto AD, Ullman BM. Acute respiratory illness in an American community. The Tecumseh Study. *JAMA* 227:164–169, 1974.
101. Martinez FD, Morgan WJ, Wright AL, Holberg CJ, Taussig LM, and the Group Health Medical Associates' Personnel. Diminished lung function as a predisposing factor for wheezing respiratory illness in infants. *N Engl J Med* 319:1112–1117, 1988.
102. Marsh DG, Meyers DA, Bias WB. The epidemiology and genetics of atopic allergy. *N Engl J Med* 305:1551–1559, 1981.
103. Weiss ST, Tager IB, Munoz A, Speizer FE. The relationship of respiratory infections in early childhood to the occurrence of increased levels of bronchial responsiveness and atopy. *Am Rev Respir Dis* 131:573–578, 1985.
104. Burrows B, Lebowitz MD, Barbee RA. Respiratory disorders and allergy skin-test reactions. *Ann Intern Med* 84:134–139, 1976.
105. Burrows B, Martinez FD, Halonen M, Barbee RA, Cline MG. Association of asthma with serum IgE levels and skin-test reactivity to allergens. *N Engl J Med* 320:271–277, 1989.
106. Fergusson DM, Horwood LJ, Shannon FT. Parental asthma, parental eczema and asthma, and eczema in early childhood. *J Chron Dis* 36:517–524, 1983.
107. Davis JB, Bulpitt CJ. Atopy and wheeze in children according to parental atopy and family size. *Thorax* 36:185–189, 1981.
108. Samet JM, Tager IB, Speizer FE. The relationship between respiratory illness in childhood and chronic air-flow obstruction in adulthood. *Am Rev Respir Dis* 127:508–523, 1983.
109. Brunekreef B, Dockery DW, Speizer FE, Ware JH, Spengler JD, Ferris BG. Home dampness and respiratory morbidity in children. *Am Rev Respir Dis* 140:1363–1267, 1989.
110. Sporik R, Holgate ST, Platts-Mills TAE, Cogswell JJ. Exposure to house-dust mite allergen (Der pI) and the development of asthma in childhood. A prospective study. *N Engl J Med* 33:502–507, 1990.
111. Monto AS, Napier JA, Metzner HL. The Tecumseh study of respiratory illness. I. Plan of study and observation on syndromes of acute respiratory disease. *Am J Epidemiol* 94:269–279, 1971.
112. Tager IB. Epidemiology of respiratory infections in the development of airway hyperreactivity. *Semin Respir Med* 11:297–305, 1990.
113. Stokes GM, Milner AD, Hodges IGC, Groggins RC. Lung function abnormalities after acute bronchiolitis. *J Pediatr* 98:871–884, 1981.

114. Kattan M, Keens TG, Lapierre J-G, Levison H, Bryan AC, Reilly BJ. Pulmonary function abnormalities in symptom-free children after bronchiolitis. *Pediatrics* 59:683–688, 1977.
115. Sims DG, Downham MAPS, Gardner PS, Webb JKG, Weightman D. Study of 8-year-old children with a history of respiratory syncytial virus bronchiolitis in infancy. *Br Med J* 1:11–14, 1978.
116. Gurwitz D, Mindorff C, Levison H. Increased incidence of bronchial reactivity in children with a history of bronchiolitis. *J Pediatr* 98:551–555, 1981.
117. Pullan CR, Hey EN. Wheezing, asthma, and pulmonary dysfunction 10 years after infection with respiratory syncytial virus in infancy. *Br Med J* 284:1665–1669, 1982.
118. Henry RL, Hodges IGC, Milner AD, Stokes GM. Respiratory problems 2 years after acute bronchiolitis in infancy. *Arch Dis Child* 58:713–716, 1983.
119. Hall CB, Hall WJ, Gala CL, MaGill FB, Leedy JP. Long-term prospective study in children after respiratory syncytial virus infection. *J Pediatr* 105:358–364, 1984.
120. McConnochie KM, Mark JD, McBride JT, Hall WJ, Brooks JG, Klein SJ, Miller RL, McInerny TK, Nazarian LF, MacWhinney JB. Normal pulmonary function measurements and airway reactivity in childhood after mild bronchiolitis. *J Pediatr* 107:54–58, 1985.
121. Loughlin GM, Taussig LM. Pulmonary function in children with a history of laryngotracheobronchitis. *J Pediatr* 94:365–369, 1979.
122. Gurwitz D, Corey M, Levison H. Pulmonary function and bronchial reactivity in children after croup. *Am Rev Respir Dis* 122:95–99, 1980.
123. Zach M, Erben A, Olinsky A. Croup, recurrent croup, allergy, and airways hyperreactivity. *Arch Dis Child* 56:336–341, 1981.
124. Wittig HJ, Cranford NJ, Glaser J. The relationship between bronchiolitis and childhood asthma. *J Allergy* 30:19–23, 1959.
125. Eisen AH, Bacal HL. The relationship of acute bronchiolitis to bronchial asthma. A 4-to-14-year follow-up. *Pediatrics* 31:859–860, 1963.
126. Zwieman B, Schoenwetter WF, Hildreth EA. The relationship between bronchiolitis and allergic asthma. *J Allergy* 37:48–53, 1966.
127. Rooney JC, Williams HE. The relationship between proved viral bronchiolitis and subsequent wheezing. *J Pediatr* 79:744–747, 1971.
128. Zwieman B, Schoenwetter WF, Pappano JE, Jr., Tempest B, Hildreth EA. Patterns of allergic respiratory disease in children with a past history of bronchiolitis. *J Allergy Clin Immunol* 48:283–289, 1971.
129. McConnochie KM, Roghmann KJ. Bronchiolitis as a possible cause of wheezing in childhood: new evidence. *Pediatrics* 74:1–10, 1984.
130. Hall WJ, Hall CB. Alterations in pulmonary function following respiratory viral infection. *Chest* 76:458–565, 1979.
131. Sherter CB, Polnitsky CA. The relationship of viral infections to subsequent asthma. *Clin Chest Med* 2:67–78, 1981.
132. Anto JM, Sunyer J, Rodriguez-Roisin R, Suarez-Cervera M, Vazquez L, and the Toxicoepidemiological Committee. Community outbreaks of asthma associated with inhalation of soybean dust. *N Engl J Med* 320:1097–1102, 1989.

133. American Thoracic Society. *Health Effects of Air Pollution*, American Lung Association, New York, 1978.
134. American Thoracic Society. Health effects of atmospheric acids and their precursors. Report of the A.T.S. workshop. *Am Rev Respir Dis* 144:464–467, 1991.
135. Goren AI, Hellmann S. Prevalence of respiratory symptoms and diseases in school children living in a polluted and in a low polluted area in Israel. *Environ Res* 45:28–37, 1988.
136. Andrae S, Axelson O, Bjorksten B, Fredriksson M, Kjellman N-I M. Symptoms of bronchial hyperreactivity and asthma in relation to environmental factors. *Arch Dis Child* 63:473–478, 1988.
137. U.S. Department of Health and Human Services. The Health consequences of involuntary smoking. U.S. Government Printing Office, Washington, DC, 1986. DHHS, PHS Publication No. (CDC) 87-8398.
138 Coultas DB, Samet JM, McCarthy JF, Spengler JD. Variability of measures of exposure to environmental tobacco smoke in the home. *Am Rev Respir Dis* 142:602–606, 1990.
139. Coultas DB, Howard CA, Peake GT, Skipper BJ, Samet JM. Salivary cotinine levels and involuntary tobacco smoke exposure in children and adults in New Mexico. *Am Rev Respir Dis* 136:305–309, 1987.
140. Samet JM, Cain WS, Leaderer BP. Environmental tobacco smoke. In: Samet JM, Spengler JD (eds). *Indoor Air Pollution. A Health Perspective*, Johns Hopkins University Press, Baltimore, MD, 1991, pp 131–169.
141. Busse WW. Pathogenesis and sequelae of respiratory infections. *Rev Infect Dis* 13:S477–485, 1991.
142. Young S, Le Souef PN, Geelhoed GC, Stick SM, Turner KJ, Landau LI. The influence of a family history of asthma and parental smoking on airway responsiveness in early infancy. *N Engl J Med* 324:1168–1173, 1991.
143. Gortmaker SL, Walker DK, Jacobs FH, Ruch-Ross H. Parental smoking and the risk of childhood asthma. Am J Public Health 72:574–579, 1982.
144. Burchfiel CM III. Passive smoking, respiratory symptoms, lung function and initiation of smoking in Tecumseh, Michigan. Unpublished Ph.D. dissertation. Ann Arbor, MI, University of Michigan, 1984.
145. Burchfiel CM, Higgins MW, Keller JB, Howalt WF, Butler WJ, Higgins IT. Passive smoking in childhood. Respiratory conditions and pulmonary function in Tecumseh, Michigan. *Am Rev Respir Dis* 133:966–973, 1986.
146. Kershaw CR. Passive smoking, potential atopy and asthma in the first five years. *J R Soc Med* 80:683–688, 1987.
147. Weitzman M, Gortmaker S, Sobol A. Racial, social, and environmental risks for childhood asthma. *Am J Dis Child* 144:1189–1194, 1990.
148. Neuspiel DR, Rush D, Butler NR, Golding J, Bijur PE, Kurzon M. Parental smoking and post-infancy wheezing in children: a prospective cohort study. *Am J Public Health* 79:168–171, 1989.
149. Tashkin DP, Clark VA, Coulson AH, Simmons M, Buerque LB, Reems C, Detels R, Souyre JW, Rokaw SN. The UCLA population studies of chronic obstructive respiratory disease. VIII. Effects of smoking cessation on lung

function: a prospective study of a free-living population. *Am Rev Respir Dis* 130:707–715, 1984.

150. Somerville SM, Rona RJ, Chinn S. Passive smoking and respiratory conditions in primary school children. *J Epidemiol Commun Health* 42:105–110, 1988.
151. Rosen FL, Levy A. Bronchial asthma due to allergy to tobacco smoke in an infant. A case report. *JAMA* 143:620–621, 1950.
152. Murray AB, Morrison BJ. The effect of cigarette smoke from the mother on bronchial responsiveness and severity of symptoms in children with asthma. *J Allergy Clin Immunol* 77:575–581, 1986.
153. Murray AB, Morrison BJ. Passive smoking by asthmatics: its greater effect on boys than on girls and on older than on younger children. *Pediatrics* 84:451–459, 1989.
154. O'Conner GT, Weiss ST, Tager IB, Speizer FE. The effect of passive smoking on pulmonary function and nonspecific bronchial responsiveness in a population-based sample of children and young adults. *Am Rev Respir Dis* 135:800–804, 1987.
155. Boushey HA, Holtzman MJ, Sheller JR, Nadel JA. Bronchial hyperreactivity. *Am Rev Respir Dis* 121:389–413, 1980.
156. Hargreave FE, Ryan G, Thomson NC, O'Bryne PM, Latimer K, Juniper EF, Dolovich J. Bronchial responsiveness to histamine or methacholine in asthma: measurement and clinical significance. *J Allergy Clin Immunol* 68:347–355, 1981.
157. Pattemore PK, Asher MI, Harrison AC, Mitchell EA, Rea HH, Stewart AW. The interrelationship among bronchial hyperresponsiveness, the diagnosis of asthma, and asthma symptoms. *Am Rev Respir Dis* 142:549–554, 1990.
158. Weiss ST, Tager IB, Weiss JW, Munoz A, Speizer FE, Ingram RH. Airways responsiveness in a population sample of adults and children. *Am Rev Respir Dis* 129:898–902, 1984.
159. Schembri DA, Crockett AJ, Alpers JH, Latimer KM. Bronchial hyperresponsiveness in two populations of South Australian rural school children. *Med J Aust* 152:578–582, 1990.
160. Hopp RJ, Bewtra AK, Nair NM, Townley RG. Specificity and sensitivity of methacholine inhalation challenge in normal and asthmatic children. *J Allergy Clin Immunol* 74:154–158, 1984.
161. Hopp RJ, Bewtra AK, Nair NM, Watt GD, Townley RG. Methacholine inhalation challenge studies in a selected pediatric population. *Am Rev Respir Dis* 134:994–998, 1986.
162. Hopp RJ, Townley RG, Biven RE, Bewtra AK, Nair NM. The presence of airway reactivity before the development of asthma. *Am Rev Respir Dis* 141:2–8, 1990.
163. Anderson HR, Bland JM, Peckham CS. Risk factors for asthma up to 16 years of age. *Chest* 91(suppl):127S–130S, 1987.
164. Schwartz J, Gold D, Dockery DW, Weiss ST, Speizer FE. Predictors of

asthma and persistent wheeze in a national sample of children in the United States. *Am Rev Respir Dis* 1990 142:555–562, 1990.
165. Sherman CB, Tosteson TD, Tager IB, Speizer FE, Weiss ST. Early childhood predictors of asthma. *Am J Epidemiol* 132:83–95, 1990.
166. Rackemann FM, Edwards MC. Asthma in children. A follow-up study of 688 patients after an interval of twenty years. *N Engl J Med* 246:815–823, 1952.
167. Dees SC. Development and course of asthma in children. *Am J Dis Child* 93:228–233, 1957.
168. Ogilvie AG. Asthma: a study in prognosis of 1000 patients. *Thorax* 17:183–189, 1962.
169. Buffum WP, Settipane GA. Prognosis of asthma in childhood. *Am J Dis Child* 112:214–217, 1966.
170. Blair H. Natural history of childhood asthma. 20-year follow-up. *Arch Dis Child* 52:613–619, 1977.
171. McNicol KN, Williams HB. Spectrum of asthma in children. I. Clinical and physiological components. *Br Med J* 4:7–11, 1973.
172. Martin AJ, Landau LI, Phelan PD. Predicting the course of asthma in children. *Aust Pediatr J* 18:84–87, 1982.
173. Foucard T, Sjoberg O. A prospective 12-year follow-up study of children with wheezy bronchitis. *Acta Pediatr Scand* 73:577–583, 1984.
174. U.S. Department of Health, Education, and Welfare. *Smoking and Health: A Report of the Surgeon General.* U.S. Department of Health, Education, and Welfare, Public Health Service, Office of the Assistant Secretary for Health, Office on Smoking and Health, DHEW Publication No. (PHS) 79-50066, 1979.
175. Gerritson J, Koeter GH, Postma DS, Schouten JP, Knol K. Prognosis of asthma from childhood to adulthood. *Am Rev Respir Dis* 140:1325–1330, 1989.
176. U.S. Department of Health and Human Services. *Chronic Obstructive Lung Disease: A Report of the Surgeon General.* U.S. Department of Health and Human Services, Public Health Service, Office of the Assistant Secretary for Health, Office on Smoking and Health, DHHS Publication No. (PHS) 84-50205, 1984.
177. O'Conner GT, Sparrow D, Weiss ST. The role of allergy and nonspecific airway hyperresponsiveness in the pathogenesis of chronic obstructive pulmonary disease. *Am Rev Respir Dis* 140:225–252, 1989.
178. Fletcher CM, Peto R. The natural history of chronic airflow obstruction. *Br Med J* 1:1645–1648, 1977.
179. Reid DD. The beginning of bronchitis. *Proc R Soc Med* 62:311–316, 1969.
180. Burrows B, Knudson RJ, Lebowitz MD. The relationship of childhood respiratory illness to adult obstructive airway disease. *Am Rev Respir Dis* 115:751–760, 1977.
181. Burrows B, Taussig LM. "As the twig is bent, the tree inclines" (perhaps). *Am Rev Respir Dis* 122:813–816, 1980.

182. Orie NGM, Sluiter HJ, DeVries K, Tammeling GJ, Witkop J. The host factor in bronchitis. In: Orie NGM, Sluiter HJ (eds.), *Bronchitis*, Royal Vangorcum, Assen, Netherlands, 1961, pp 43.
183. Brown PJ, Greville HW, Finucane KE. Asthma and irreversible airflow obstruction. *Thorax* 39:131–136, 1984.
184. Barter CE, Campbell AH. Relationship of constitutional factors and cigarette smoking to decrease in 1-second forced expiratory volume. *Am Rev Respir Dis* 113:305–314, 1976.
185. Britt EJ, Cohen B, Menkes H, Bleecker E, Permutt S, Rosenthal R, Normal P. Airways reactivity and functional deterioration in relatives of COPD patients. *Chest* 77 (suppl):260S–261S, 1980.
186. Taylor RG, Joyce H, Gross E, Holland F, Pride NB. Bronchial reactivity to inhaled histamine and annual rate of decline in $FEV_1$ in male smokers and ex-smokers. *Thorax* 40:9–16, 1985.
187. Buist AS, Vollmer WM. Prospective investigations in asthma: what have we learned from longitudinal studies about lung growth and senescence in asthma. Transcript of Proceedings, NIH International Workshop on Etiology of Asthma, June 25–27, 1985, Bethesda, Maryland.
188. Bryant DH, Burns MW, Lazarus L. The correlation between skin tests, bronchial provocation tests and the serum level of IgE specific for common allergens in patients with asthma. *Clin Allergy* 5:145–157, 1975.

# 5

# Defense Mechanisms of the Lung

**SETSUKO ITO and HARUKI MIKAWA**

*Kyoto University*
*Kyoto, Japan*

The entire respiratory tract acts as the defense organ against noxious foreign agents to perform its task of gas exchange adequately. Defense mechanisms include filtrative clearance, mucociliary clearance, coughing reflexes, phagocytic clearance, mucosal proteins, and local immunity (Fig. 1).

## NONIMMUNOLOGIC DEFENSE MECHANISMS

### Filtrative Clearance of Particles

The fundamental defense mechanism of the respiratory tract derives from the anatomical characteristics of the nose, trachea, and bronchial tree, all of which are arranged to minimize the exposure of the lung to noxious agents, including infectious micro-organisms and biologically active and inactive particles.

As the air is inhaled through the nares, large particles (10 μm in diameter) are removed by impaction as they go through the nasal passage

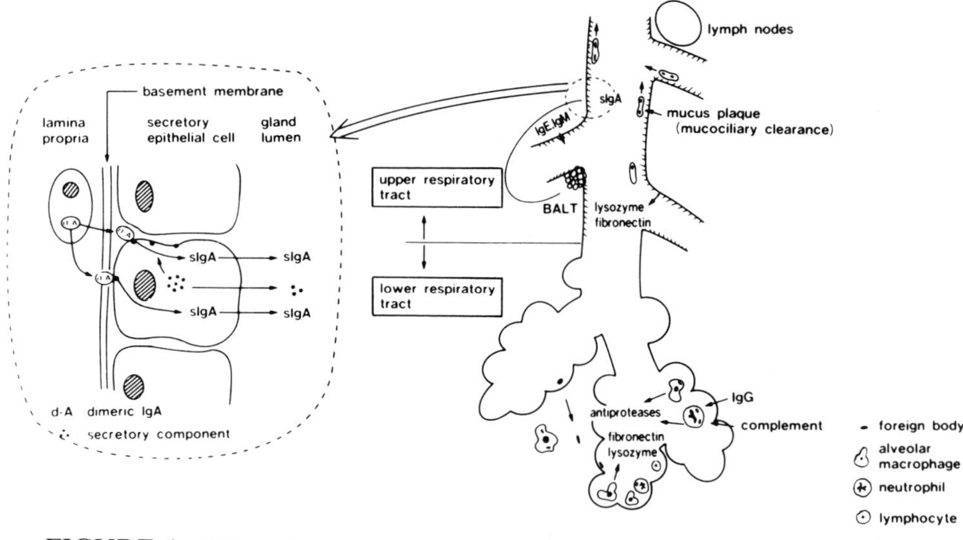


FIGURE 1 Schematic representation of the lung indicates the defense mechanisms of the lung. Filtrative clearance of particles (Fig. 2), mucociliary clearance, coughing reflexes, phagocytic clearance, lysozyme, fibronectin, and antiproteases are the representative nonimmunologic defense mechanisms. Immunologic defense mechanisms consist of the lymphoid system, complement system, and immunoglobulins, especially sIgA. Dimeric IgA with J chain binds to secretory component, which is produced by secretory epithelial cells and becomes sIgA and is secreted into the gland lumen.

with its sharp curves and interior nasal hairs. Most of the remaining large particles are impacted on the posterior wall of the pharynx, where the direction of the airflow is changed. Therefore, only a few particles larger than 10 μm can pass through the nasal passage and upper respiratory tract and enter the trachea when the air is inhaled through the nares. On the other hand, if the nose is bypassed either by mouth breathing or by intubation, large particles enter the trachea without undergoing the first efficient aerodynamic filtration and result in inflammation. Particle size can be changed by a number of environmental factors. Humidification of the incoming air, for example, allows hygroscopic particles to grow and to impact at a higher proportion in the respiratory tract.

Particles between 2 and 10 μm in diameter are trapped on the bifurcating bronchial trees. These particles adhere to the mucosal surface and are cleared by the mucociliary transport system and coughing reflexes. Smaller particles (0.5–2 μm) reach the terminal airways and alveolar surface and are subjected to phagocytic clearance (Fig. 2). Whereas insoluble external agents are removed in this way, soluble agents may be absorbed across the mucosal surface. The integrity of the epithelial mucosal surface is critical to clear noxious external agents effectively.

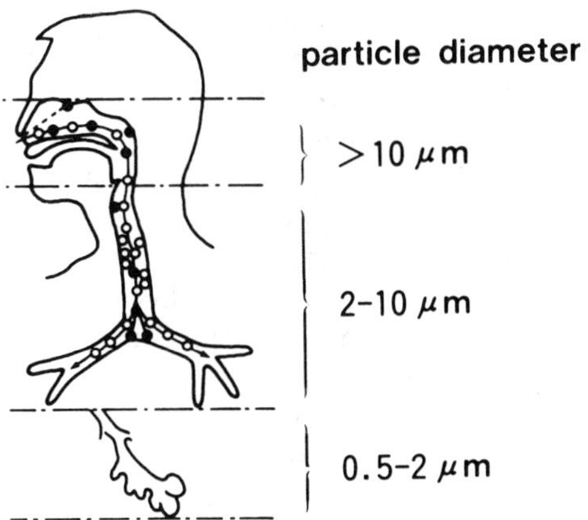


FIGURE 2 Deposition of various sizes of particles breathed in from the nose and the mouth in the respiratory tract (filtrative clearance of particles). More than 90% of particles with a diameter greater than 2–3 μm are deposited in the upper respiratory system, covered with a ciliated respiratory epithelium that extends from the nares down the terminal airways and alveolar surface, and are subjected to phagocytic clearance.

## Mucociliary Clearance

### *Mucociliary Clearance Mechanism*

Mucus-coated ciliated cells line the airways from the posterior two-thirds of the nasal passage, nasopharynx, and larynx all the way to terminal bronchioles (17th airway division) and provide the main clearance mechanism of the particles in the respiratory tract. Particles and micro-organisms landing on mucus-coated ciliated cells are escalated up to the posterior pharynx by ciliary action in the form of mucus plaques, which are formed at intervals in variable lengths instead of in the form of a continuous sheet, as was originally suggested by Lucas and Douglas (1). To perform effective clearance, ciliated cells, which are the most common cells in the trachea and bronchi, must have an adequate number of cilia beating in a coordinated direction and manner at a constant rate. Each cell has approximately 200 cilia on the surface (2), and these cilia beat at a rate of 1000–1500 cycles/min. Cilia do not all beat simultaneously but beat one after another in a metachromic way and propel mucus plaque upward (3). There is a progressive increase in the clearance rate and velocity of mucus transport from peripheral to central airways. If the amount of mucus is not excessive and the mucociliary clearance system is functioning well, the clearance of the plaque from the lung and upper respiratory tract is accomplished by unconscious swallowing. If the clearance mechanism does not work adequately, mucus clearing may be augmented by the coughing reflex or, in the upper respiratory tract, rhinorrhea may develop.

The mucus-coated epithelial surface is covered by two layers (3): a low-viscosity pericilliary fluid and a viscoelastic mucus layer of variable depth. The latter is penetrated by the tips of mucus-propelling cilia during their effective strokes to a depth of about 0.5 μm. The recovery strokes take place in the periciliary fluid layer and carry back the pericilliary fluid that has been moved by a previous effective stroke and result in little or no net movement of the periciliary fluid; only mucus plaques are propelled upward (Fig. 3). To propel mucus plaque effectively, both adequate penetration of the mucus layer by ciliary tips with a crown of projections, which enhances propulsion, and adequate quantity of periciliary fluid are required. If the periciliary layer becomes too deep, the cilia do not reach the mucus layer, and if the periciliary layer becomes too shallow, the cilia cannot complete their beat.

### *Constituents of Airway Mucus*

Airway mucus consists of water, contributing up to 95% of the total airway mucus, dialyzable material, and macromolecular constituents (Table 1) (4). Macromolecular constituents are composed of mucus glycoprotein (25–50%), lipids (20–30%), and proteins (10–25%). Protein includes locally produced secretory IgA (sIgA), IgM, IgE, lysozyme, bronchotransferrin,

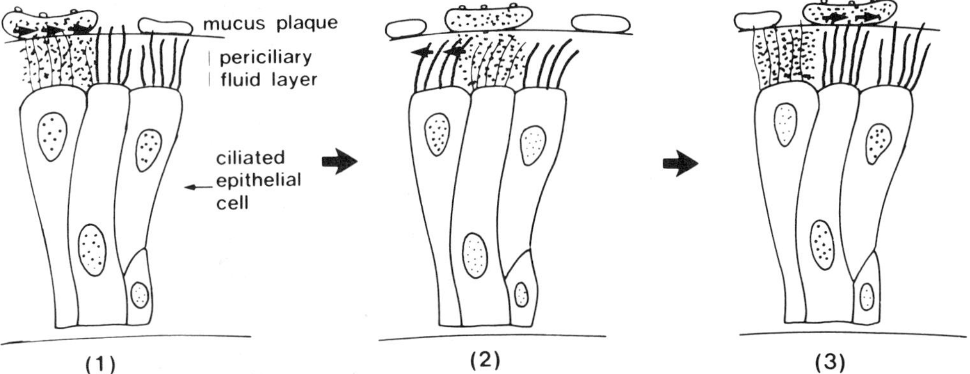


FIGURE 3 Mucociliary transport system. The mucus-coated epithelial surface is covered by a low-viscosity periciliary fluid layer and viscoelastic mucus layer. (1) The mucus layer is penetrated by the tips of mucus-propelling cilia. (2) The recovery strokes take place in the periciliary fluid layer, and the periciliary fluid, which has been moved by the previous effective stroke, is carried back. (3) Only mucus plaques on which particles are deposited are propelled upward.

and tissue fluid transudate. These proteins, particularly sIgA and protein-rich peptides, not only play an important role in host defense mechanisms but also contribute to the rheologic properties of airway mucus (5). Lipids contribute to one-third of the total macromolecular material of normal airway mucus and up to 40% in disease. Neutral lipids, phospholipids, and glycolipids have been identified in secretions of healthy individuals and patients with bronchial asthma. They are both locally produced and transudated from tissue fluid. Lipids are suggested to contribute to the organization of mucus fibrillar structure (6). Mucus glycoprotein is the main macromolecular constituent of airway mucus. The native mucus glycoprotein is a homogeneous polydispersed macromolecule with a molecular weight of 3–7 million daltons. It is made up of a polypeptide core with sugar chains studded along its length. Carbohydrate contributes 50–80% of the total weight with oligosaccharide side chains (4).

All the constituents of airway mucus are present in a soluble and gel form. The proportion of soluble components in the airway can modify its rheologic properties.

### *Control of Mucus Production*

Control of airway mucus production depends mostly on the control of mucus glycoprotein production. Mucus glycoprotein is supposed to be secreted from mucus cells of the surface epithelium and from the mucus and serous cells of the submucosal glands by histochemical analysis. The se-

TABLE 1 Constituents of Airway Mucus

| Constituent | Percentage |
|---|---|
| Water | 95 |
| Dialysable material | 1 |
| Macromolecular material | 4 |

cretory cycle is consisted of four stages: uptake of precursors, synthesis, transport, and discharge. Synthesis and discharge occur simultaneously in serous cells, while they occur alternately in mucous cells.

From short- and long-term experiments in various animal models, it has been shown that both α- and β-adrenergic agents increase secretion by increasing mucus glycoprotein and/or ion and water transport (4). Clinical mediators released during allergic reactions increase the release of mucus glycoprotein in vivo (7), while histamine, serotonin, and slow-reacting substance of anaphylaxis (SRS-A) failed to induce mucus secretion during in vitro studies using human tissue (8).

Further studies are expected to be pursued to develop a better understanding of the mucociliary clearance mechanisms, particularly in peripheral airways.

### *Anatomy of Cilium*

Ultrastructural studies of the cilium on cross-section (Fig. 4) reveal that a matrix containing nine microtubular doublets (A and B microtubules) surrounds two central microtubules enclosed in a sheath. The nine microtubular doublets have protrusions called dynein arms extending from the outer pairs of the peripheral microtubules. ATP has been shown to induce active sliding of adjacent microtubular doublets and is considered to be the energy source for ciliary beating (9, 10). The required ATP hydrolysis is accomplished by an ATPase system located in the dynein arms from outer pairs (Fig. 4) of the microtubular doublets. The A microtubules are jointed to each other at intervals along the cilium by nexin links and to the central microtubular doublets by radial spokes. A microtubule sliding along the side of the adjacent B (inner) microtubule results in ciliary movement.

### *Abnormality of Mucociliary Clearance Mechanism*

Both primary (congenital) and secondary (acquired) abnormalities of the mucociliary clearance mechanism result in disease. The clearest example of the ciliary abnormality causing human disease is primary ciliary dyskinesia, including the so-called immotile cilia syndrome. The first reported case (11) was the observation of immotile spermatozoa in a patient with infertility and Kartagener's syndrome (12) characterized by situs inversus,

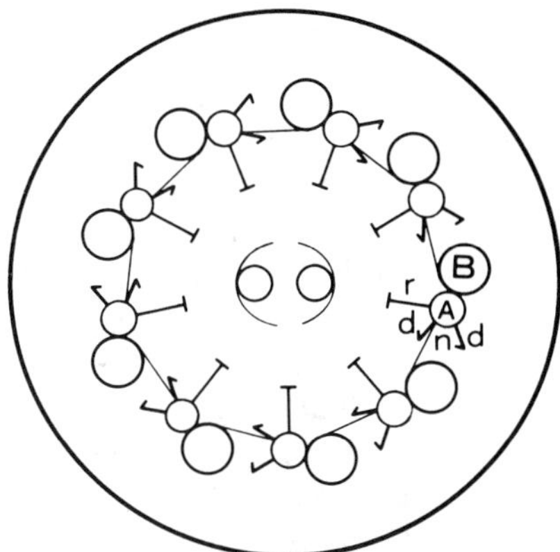


d : dynein arm
n : nexin link
r : radial spoke

FIGURE 4 Diagram of cross-section of a cilium. Nine microtubular doublets (A and B microtubules) surround two central microtubules enclosed in a sheath. The nine microtubular doublets have dynein arms (d) extending from outer pairs (A) of the microtubular doublets. The A microtubules are joined to each other at intervals along the cilium by nexin links (n) and to the central microtubular doublets by radial spokes (r).

bronchiectasia, and chronic sinusitis. Ultrastructural study of his sperm tails showed the absence of dynein arms. Since the cilium had the same ultrastructure as the sperm tail, a coexistent abnormality of ciliary motility was postulated, and this was proved to be true in two patients with this condition by demonstrating the absence of effective mucociliary transport (13). A female patient with Kartagener's syndrome with impaired nasal mucociliary transport was also found to lack dynein arms in nasal cilia (14). Studies on patients with primary ciliary dyskinesia suggest that an intact mucociliary clearance mechanism is important in protecting the lung from infection. The mucociliary clearance mechanism is modified by various external agents that cause degenerative changes. Acquired mucociliary dysfunction of this mechanism includes changes in beat frequency, development of abnormal cilia, or shedding of the entire cell with replacement of squamous epithelium. Viral infection is known to depress mucociliary clearance mechanism in humans and result in predisposition to bacterial infection (15). Mucociliary clearance is depressed in chronic smokers. This is consistent with the in vitro study that cigarette smoke contains ciliostatic components, such as phenols, which inhibit ciliary beat frequency and coordination (16).

## Mucociliary Dysfunction in Bronchial Asthma

The tracheal mucus velocity (TMV) in asymptomatic asthmatic nonsmokers with ragweed hypersensitivity was reported to be reduced to 54% of those in age-matched nonasthmatic nonsmokers (17). Inhalation challenge with ragweed extract produced a rapid decrease of TMV, and this decrease persisted longer than the bronchospasms: 1 hr after antigen challenge, when specific airway conductance had returned to baseline, mean TMV was 47% of baseline. Impairment of mucociliary transport mechanism after a single antigen challenge was observed for as long as 7 days in allergic sheep (18). Cromolyn sodium, which itself had no significant effect on mucociliary transport, prevented the expected decrease of mucus velocity in trachea after antigen challenge (17). These data suggested that acute mucociliary dysfunction after antigen challenge was related to airway anaphylaxis. Among many chemical mediators, SRS-A, but not histamine, which stimulates tracheal mucociliary transport instead of inhibition (19), is considered to play an important role in causing antigen-induced mucociliary dysfunction. Pretreatment of lung tissue with the SRS-A antagonist not only prevented the antigen-induced decrease of mucus transport but also converted it to significant stimulation (20). The most probable mechanism of mucociliary dysfunction caused by SRS-A is considered to be alteration in respiratory secretions, both qualitative and quantitative: biosynthetic and synthetic LTC4 and LTD4 produced a dosage-related increase in mucus production in cultured human airways. This enhancing effect was blocked by a specific SRS-A antagonist (21). Hypersecretion of the respiratory tract alters the depth of the periciliary fluid layer, which results in impairment of mucociliary function. Histamine, which has no direct inhibitory effect on cilia, also facilitates water transport system. With respect to the management of patients with bronchial asthma, the use of antiallergic agents or antagonists of mediators seems to be justified to avoid inhibition of the mucociliary transport system.

## Reflexes

Filtrative clearance and mucociliary clearance are facilitated by such reflexes as sneezing, coughing, and bronchoconstriction. Physicochemical stimulation of nasal cilia and mucosa induces sneezing, and physicochemical stimulation of mucosal epithelium from the oropharynx to bronchus induces coughing reflexes and bronchoconstriction. Receptors for these reflexes are located within and under the mucosal epithelium throughout the respiratory tract, from the nares to the alveoli, and make possible a prompt response to external noxious agents and minimize their invasion deep into the lung.

## Phagocytic Clearance

### *Alveolar Macrophages*

The analysis of bronchoalveolar lavage (BAL) fluids leads us to an increased awareness of the role of inflammatory cells in the defense mechanisms of the lung. About 90% of BAL cells in nonallergic nonsmokers are alveolar macrophages (22). Alveolar macrophages are considered to be the first line of defense against inhaled particles that have reached the alveoli. They are found both within the interstitium and at the epithelial surface of the alveoli. Alveolar macrophages are derived from blood monocytes and share many properties with macrophages in other parts of the body, including the possession of Fc(γ) receptors and C3b receptors. Their roles in lung defense mechanisms are phagocytosis of foreign materials, which undergo degradation of oxidative phosphorylation; transporting vehicle for elimination of foreign materials through the mucociliary transport system; and enhancing the immunologic activation of lymphocytes and neutrophils (23). Alveolar macrophages are activated through Fc(γ) and C3b receptors by numerous factors, including micro-organisms, immune complexes, and endotoxin. Once activated, they produce potent oxygen radicals, such as superoxide anion, hydrogen peroxide, and hydroxy radicals, which play an important role in the bactericidal capacity of macrophages but may cause tissue damage at the same time. Alveolar macrophages, however, also have high concentrations of superoxide dismutase and glutathion peroxide, which detoxify oxidants within themselves. Other important products of macrophages are proteases, including plasminogen activator, collagenase, elastase, kallikrein, and alpha-2-macroglobulin, which inhibits the activity of these proteases.

### *Neutrophils*

Neutrophils reside in the circulation and adhere to the vascular epithelium; they make up less than 1% of BAL cells in the normal lung (22). They might migrate rapidly from the marginal pool toward chemotactic factor on invasion of micro-organisms and other particles to pursue their bactericidal activity against microorganisms. Lung tissue injury may also result from oxidative metabolites released by neutrophils. Major neutrophil defense mechanisms against infection are composed of chemotaxis, phagocytosis, and intracellular bacterial killing. Neutrophils ingest a greater number of bacteria, and show more potent bactericidal capacity than macrophages, probably due to the higher density of Fc(γ) receptors on their surface and to a larger quantity of oxygen radicals produced by them (24). Neutrophils as well as macrophages also have a harmful effect on the cellular and noncellular constituents of the lung parenchyma by producing oxygen radicals and proteases, such as elastase, collagenase, neutral protease, acid protease, and glucuronidase. Neutrophil chemotaxis is induced not only by complement-derived chemotactic factor but also by macrophage-derived chemotactic factor (25) and is modified by various factors, including immune complexes (26, 27).

### Others

Lysozyme is produced by epithelial cells, glands of large airways, and alveolar macrophages and has bacteriolytic activity that is enhanced by secretory IgA and complement (28). It also has an inhibitory activity on neutrophil functions, such as chemotaxis and production of oxygen radicals, and acts to lessen the inflammatory response (29).

Fibronectin is a glycoprotein of large molecular weight and plays a nonspecific role in the defense mechanism of the lung by competitively blocking adherence and colonization of bacteria to the epithelial cells. It also has opsonic activity and enhances binding of particles to phagocytic cells. Fibronectin is not only present on the surface of normal oropharyngeal epithelial cells, in plasma, and in other body fluid, but also is synthesized and secreted by macrophages and fibroblasts and is considered to play an important role in the defense mechanisms of the lower respiratory tract.

Macrophages and neutrophils secrete proteases that may cause lung tissue injury, as described above. But these proteases are neutralized by antiproteases, such as alpha-1-antitrypsin and alpha-2-macroglobulin. The former diffuses from serum into the alveolus and forms a complex with neutrophil elastase (30), and the latter is produced by macrophages and is considered to bind to neutrophil elastase. These antiproteases are important in regulating lung tissue injury by enzymes released from alveolar macrophages and neutrophils.

## IMMUNOLOGIC DEFENSE MECHANISMS

### Lymphoid System

#### *Lymphoid Organs*

The respiratory tract is lined by many lymphoid tissues: fixed lymphoid tissue in nasopharynx (Waldeyer's ring), more diffusely distributed bronchus-associated lymphoid tissue, and lymphoid aggregates.

The immune system of the lung is considered to be divided into four compartments (31). The first compartment of lymphocytes resides in the epithelium of the respiratory tract. These lymphocytes appear to have T-cell phenotype and activity and to play an important role in defending against the invasion of phagocytic organisms because they have cytotoxic activities. The second compartment of lymphoid tissue is called bronchus-associated lymphoid tissue (BALT), which lies within the bronchial wall, consisting of solitary lymphoid follicles or lymphoid aggregates, just like Peyer's patches in the intestine. BALT is morphologically and probably functionally analogous to gut-associated lymphoid tissue (GALT). It is covered by a lymphoepithelium that appears to have pinocytic activity for both soluble and particulate substances in the lumen of the respiratory tract. BALT contains predominantly B cells and is considered to be a repository for immunoglobulin-secreting cells, particularly IgA-secreting cells, which may move to lamina propria along the respiratory tract and produce local antibody that protects the mucosal surface. The third compartment of lymphoid tissue is loosely organized in the lamina propria of the mucosal tissue and contains both T and B cells. IgA is synthesized by these B cells in the form of dimeric IgA and transported into the lumen across the mucosal epithelium, where mucosal glandular epithelial cells synthesize the polypeptide chain called secretory component with which dimeric IgA is transported in the form of secretory IgA. The last compartment is bronchoalveolar free lymphocytes that may be obtained by BAL from the peripheral airways. In normal subjects, about 90% of BAL cells are macrophages (32), which are responsible both for clearance of antigen and for processing of antigen for its presentation to lymphocytes to initiate immune response. Lymphocytes make up about 10% of BAL cells and have characteristics similar to those found in peripheral blood.

### *Lymphokines*

Stimulated lymphocytes release lymphokines, such as migration inhibitory factor and macrophage-activating factor, and enhance phagocytosis and intracellular killing of macrophages.

The lung may be organized into two major compartments from both a physiological and an immunologic point of view: the upper respiratory tract and the lower respiratory tract. The upper respiratory tract is the air-conducting portion of the lung extending from the nares down to the terminal bronchioles. This area corresponds anatomically to mucosal gland-containing tissue, and provides a mucosal immune response in which the secretory IgA system predominates. The lower respiratory tract includes the region of the lung from the bronchioles out to the alveoli and reflects a systemic immune response in which IgG predominates. Upper respiratory tract disease refers clinically only to the lesion above the pharynx, and lower respiratory tract disease includes lesions of the larynx, trachea, bronchus, bronchioles, alveoli, and lung parenchyma (31a).

IgA is synthesized by plasma cells in the lamina propria of the respiratory tract and other mucosal tissues. IgA-producing cells originate in the bone marrow and reside in GALT or BALT. It is considered that specific IgA-producing cells derived from GALT or BALT may seed in a variety of mucosal tissues, including the gut, salivary gland, parotid gland, lacrimal gland, and the respiratory tract. Antigen-trapping nonciliated cells are found in the respiratory epithelium and tonsillar crypts as well as in the Peyer's patches and appendix and they facilitate contact of these B cells with antigens. Antigens incorporated into GALT or BALT not only initiate an immune response but also work as the second signal that causes differentiation of B cells that arrive at the particular glandular tissues with the help of T cells (Fig. 5).

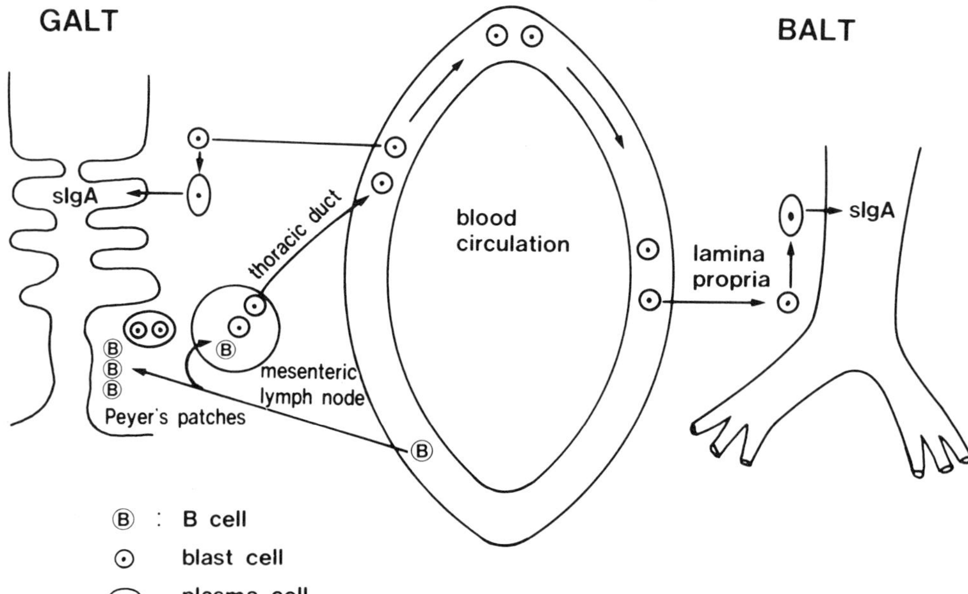


FIGURE 5 The relationship between BALT and GALT. The BALT is morphologically and functionally analogous to the GALT and contains predominantly B cells, most of which express IgA and are considered precursors of IgA-producing cells. Antigens incorporated by the GALT and BALT not only initiate immune responses but also act as the second signal and cause differentiation of B cells. Specific IgA-producing cells derived by GALT of BALT may seed into the lamina propria of a variety of mucosal tissues and differentiate into plasma cells and produce IgA, which is secreted into the gland lumen in the form of sIgA.

## Immunoglobulins

### *Secretory IgA and IgM: First Line of Local Humoral Immunity*

IgA is the major immunoglobulin in bronchial secretions and plays an important role in local mucosal defense mechanisms in the respiratory tract. IgA is found in the form of monomer and dimer. The latter dimeric form of IgA, with secretory component covalently bound to it, is the predominant type of immunoglobulin in respiratory secretions above the larynx and is called secretory IgA (sIgA). SIgA acts as an initial immunologic barrier against micro-organisms at the portal of entry. IgA also acts as an agglutinator of micro-organisms and a neutralizer of toxin and thus inhibits viral and bacterial binding to mucosal surfaces and therefore inhibits their replication. IgA is also considered to act as a blocking antibody in local allergic reactions. Platts-Mills et al. (32) reported that concentrated nasal washings from ragweed-allergic patients contained significantly higher levels of IgA and IgG antibodies to AgE (main allergen of ragweed) than those from normal individuals and that those specific antibodies had inhibitory activity on leukocyte histamine release. It has recently been reported that dimeric IgA without secretory component increases in serum after mucosal inflammation (33), especially in bowel inflammatory disease, such as anaphylactoid purpura (34) and elevation of specific IgA against external agents is seen in patients with anaphylactoid purpura and bronchial asthma (35, 36). Dimeric IgA and immune complexes consisting of dimeric IgA and antigen in the circulation are known to be selectively taken up by parenchymal cells and transferred across the liver into the bile and invasive antigen is cleared. IgA, in the form of both polymeric IgA (37) and IgA immune complex (26) with antigen against which it is directed, may have a noxious effect on the defense mechanisms by depressing neutrophil chemotaxis.

In patients with selective IgA deficiency, IgM seems to play an important role in mucosal immunity, although relatively small amounts of 19S IgM show a better affinity for secretory component and bind to it with stronger covalent forces than dimeric IgA in vitro (38). This suggests that IgM may have served as the protector of the mucosal surface before the evolution of dimeric IgA. IgM antibody has complement-mediated opsonic and bacteriolytic activity and, together with sIgA, contributes to the first line of defense mechanisms.

### *IgD, IgG, and IgE in Secretions and Role in the Defense Mechanism*

Local production of IgD is increased in respiratory mucosa and lacrimal and salivary glands in selective IgA deficiency, although only a trace amount of IgD is detected in serum. IgD has no affinity for secretory component, and there is no evidence of the active transport of IgD through the secretory epithelium.

Although the IgG/IgA ratio of the serum is 6.4 ± 0.6, that of the bronchial fluid is 0.19 ± 0.04 (22). IgG, however, is sometimes found in large amounts in secretions of the upper respiratory tract during infection, and this is considered to be derived from transudation from serum to the alveolus. Local production of IgG does occur in the respiratory tract. The percentage of IgG-producing cells in the glandular tissues of bronchial mucosa is as much as 29%, a much higher percentage than that of intestine (39). IgG plays an important role in the defense mechanisms of the lung, as opsonin for bacteria to facilitate elimination of bacteria by macrophages and neutrophils. IgG antibody also plays an important role in the elimination of antigen entering the circulation in the form of immune complexes with antigen (40). When polyclonal antibody formation is induced by the antigen with heterogeneous antigenicity, insoluble immune complexes are likely to be formed and are easily eliminated from the circulation by the reticuloendothelial system. On the other hand, when antigen with more homogeneous antigenicity induces oligoclonal antibody formation, antigen may remain in the circulation in the form of soluble immune complexes. This provides a greater opportunity to induce IgE formation, and may then cause an allergic response. The formation of IgG antibody and IgE antibody by human mononuclear cells is influenced by many environmental factors, such as mercuric chloride, lambda-carrageenan, and lipopolysaccharide in vitro (41–43). Ishizaka et al. showed that the predisposition to produce IgG antibody and IgE antibody was influenced by the kind of adjuvant used at the time of immunization in the rat (44).

IgE is formed in BAL fluid, and it has been suggested that when there is a relative enrichment of IgE in some exocrine fluids compared with serum, this may reflect local synthesis of IgE rather than passive effusion. IgE has no affinity for secretory component. The biological significance of exocrine IgE is unknown, but it seems to play an important role in allergic diseases, such as bronchial asthma. Mucosal lymphoid cells producing IgE have been identified in trachea and bronchial mucosa, among luminal cells, and in draining bronchial lymph nodes, but these cells are rarely formed in the lower respiratory tract in healthy individuals. Local synthesis of IgE in the respiratory tract increases following intratracheal and lung immunization. The specific IgE synthesized in the respiratory tract after infection can trigger an allergic reaction, including the release of chemical mediators and bronchospasm, and cause wheezing and dyspnea in young children (45, 46).

In recent years, attention has been paid to IgG subclass deficiency in relation to recurrent infections. Shackelford et al. reported that 7 of 30 children with recurrent infection had a low IgG2 concentration (<3 SD below the geometric mean for age). Five of 7 IgG2-deficient children had sinopulmonary infections (47). Ishizaka et al. also reported 4 IgG2-deficient children out of 100 children with recurrent sinopulmonary infections (48). In both reports, IgG2 was deficient alone or combined with other IgG subclass deficiency, especially IgG4 deficiency, and/or IgA deficiency. Sinusitis, one of the most common symptoms of IgG subclass deficiency, is known to provoke asthma exceptionally among bacterial respiratory infections. Rachelefsky and associates reported that antibiotic treatment of sinusitis reduced the severity of asthma in 48 children (49). The measurement of IgG subclasses has become available in recent years, and the association of IgG subclass deficiency with sinopulmonary infection as a provocative factor of asthma will be clarified in the near future.

### Complement System

The complement system is a complex series of proteins that plays an important role in host-defense mechanisms. The complement system has chemotactic activity (especially in the form of C5a) and opsonic activity for bacteria and promotes the bactericidal capacity of macrophages and neutrophils. Alveolar macrophages produce C5 (activated as C5a), which promotes neutrophil chemotaxis into the lung parenchyma and alveoli where they perpetuate their influx by self-generating C5a. Particles that can activate the complement system become coated with C3b and antibodies. These opsonized particles bind to C3b receptors of macrophages and neutrophils and facilitate their ingestion by Fc ($\gamma$) receptors.

Gross et al. showed inhibition of the clearance of aerosol *Streptococcus pneumoniae* and *Pseudomonas aeruginosa* from the murine lung but not that of *Staphylococcus aureus* and *Klebsiella pneumoniae* in cobra venom factor-induced complement-deficient mice (50). They further showed that augmentation of clearance of pneumococci from the lung was caused by complement-derived neutrophil chemotactic factor, but that of *P. aeruginosa* was caused by the opsonic activity of complement for macrophages and neutrophils (51).

Complement also plays a harmful role in the defense mechanisms of the lung by causing aggregation and degranulation of neutrophils and allows them to destroy the lung tissue by oxygen radicals and proteases.

## VIRAL INFECTIONS AND ASTHMA

### Respiratory Viral Infections as a Provoking Factor of Asthma

The relationship of respiratory infections to the development of airway hypersensitivity has been recognized for decades and some prospective studies led clinicians to the confirmation that viral but not bacterial infections trigger wheezing during upper respiratory illnesses.

McIntosh et al. (52) conducted a 2 year prospective study of 32 asthmatic children aged 1–5 years. There were 102 confirmed viral respiratory infections and 139 episodes of wheezing in these 32 children. Of the episodes of wheezing, 42% occurred in relationship to viral respiratory infections. Respiratory syncytial virus (RSV) was proved to be the most prevalent cause by serologic testing. The presence of bacterial respiratory infection did not correlate with asthmatic attacks.

Henderson et al. evaluated 6165 lower respiratory infections during an 11 year study in a pediatric outpatient clinic and found that 1851 (30%) episodes of respiratory infections were associated with wheezing and that half of the episodes of wheezing occurred in children less than 2 years of age (53). In 21% of children with wheezing, a nonbacterial pathogen was isolated: RSV, parainfluenza virus, adenovirus, and *Mycoplasma pneumoniae* accounted for more than 80% of the isolated organisms.

RSV proved to be the most common cause of wheezing in children less than 5 years of age. Wheezing in school-age children was more commonly associated with *M. pneumoniae*.

There is little evidence that bacterial respiratory infections other than sinusitis can be a major precipitant of asthma.

As for the possibility of a certain viral respiratory tract infection having a causal relationship to airway hypersensitivity, confirmative results were obtained by prospective studies.

Pullan and Hey evaluated 130 children who were admitted to the hospital with RSV lower respiratory tract infection during the first 5 years of life. Forty-two percent of them experienced wheezing later in life, while only 19% of the controls experienced wheezing by the age of 10 (54).

A higher prevalence of a family history of allergy was also observed by prospective studies. Zweiman et al. made a 5 year follow-up study of 25 children after hospitalization for acute bronchitis. Five years later, the incidence of persistent wheezing remained at about 50% and the children with wheezing had a higher prevalence of a family history of allergy (55). Rooney and Williams also reported that nearly 60% of children who had additional episodes of wheezing during 2–7 years after an episode of RSV bronchiolitis had a family history of asthma (56).

### Virus-Induced Airway Hypersensitivity

There are reports suggesting that viral respiratory infections themselves can cause transient airway hypersensitivity even in normal subjects (57). The persistence of increased airway resistance for 3–5 weeks after uncomplicated influenza virus type A infection (58) and 8 weeks after RSV infection in adults has been documented (59). Moreover, the possibility of the respiratory mucosal barrier becoming more permeable to allergen, such as mites, after viral respiratory infection is suggested as one of the mechanisms of the development of asthma after viral infection (60).

### Virus-Specific IgE

Although there is no direct evidence of virus-specific IgE on mast cells reacting with virus to release chemical mediators resulting in airway obstruction, some reports suggest the possibility that virus-specific IgE may contribute to the pathogenesis of bronchial asthma. IgE attached to exfoiliated nasopharyngeal epithelial cells was detected in 70–80% of patients with RSV infection (45). Clinical observation of these patients revealed that all of the patients with asthma or bronchiolitis had cell-bound IgE, while only 33% of patients with pneumonia or upper respiratory infection had detectable cell-bound IgE. They also detected higher titers of IgE antibodies specific to RSV in patients with wheezing than in those without wheezing during documented RSV infection (46).

### Inflammatory Cells

Enhancement of basophil histamine release was reported to be induced by interferon both exogeneously added and produced by virus (61), suggesting the possibility of respiratory viruses influencing mediator release. As for the participation of leukocytes in airway inflammation during viral infection, enhanced chemotaxis of basophils incubated with parainfluenza virus is reported (62). Respiratory viruses thus promote basophil accumulation in airways, resulting in airway obstruction caused by increased release of chemical mediators.

### Diminished Adrenergic Function During Viral Infections

Another mechanisms of asthma induced by respiratory viral infection is the diminished adrenergic responsiveness, which is known to be characteristics of asthma (63). As an in vitro model, granulocytes are often used to study responsiveness to isoproterenol in order to evaluate the subject's adrenergic function. There are reports that isolated granulocyte response to isoproterenol is diminished during viral upper respiratory tract infection that provokes asthma (64), and that granulocytes treated with certain virus particles, such as influenza type A virus and rhinovirus, became less responsive to isoproterenol (65, 66).

## REFERENCES


1. Lucas AM, Douglas LC. Principles underlying ciliary activity in the respiratory tract. II. A comparison of nasal clearance in man, monkey and other mammals. *Arch Otolaryngol* 20:518, 1934.
2. Rhodin JAG. Ultrastructure and function of the human tracheal mucosa. *Am Rev Respir Dis* 93(Suppl.3):1, 1966.
3. Sleigh MA. Movement and coordination of tracheal cilia and the relation of these to mucus transport. *Cell Motility Suppl* 1:19, 1982.
4. Lopez-Vidriero MT. Airway mucus. *Chest* 80:799, 1981.
5. Puchelle E, Zahm JM, Havez R. Biochemical and rheological data in sputum: III. Relationship between biochemical constituents and the rheological properties of sputum. *Bull Physiopathol Respir* 9:237, 1973.
6. Lhermitte M, Lambin G, Degand P, Roussel P, Mazzuca M. Affinity of bronchial secretion glycoproteins and cells of human bronchial mucosa for *Ricinus communis* lectins. *Biochemie* 59:611, 1977.
7. Richardson P, Phipps RJ, Balfre K, Hall RL. The role of mediators and allergens in causing mucin secretion from the trachea. In: *Respiratory Tract Mucus*, Ciba Foundation Series no. 54, Elsevier Excerpta, North-Holland, 1979, pp. 111–131.
8. Sturgess J, Reid L. An organ culture study of the effect of drugs on the secretory activity of the bronchial submucosal gland. *Clin Sci* 43:533, 1972.
9. Summers KE, Gibbons IR. Adenosine triphosphate induced sliding of tubules in trypsin treated flagella of sea urchin sperm. *Proc Natl Acad Sci USA* 68:3092, 1971.
10. Satir P. Studies on cilia. II. Examination of the distal region of the ciliary shaft and the role of the filaments in motility. *J Cell Biol* 26:805, 1965.
11. Pedersen H, Rebbe H. Absence of arms in the axoneme of immotile human spermatozoa. *Biol Reprod* 12:541, 1975.
12. Kartagener M. Zur Pathogenese der Bronchiektasien: Bronkiektasien bei Situs Viscerm inversus. *Beitr Klin Tuberk* 83:489, 1933.
13. Camner P, Mossberg B, Afzelius BA. Evidence for congenitally nonfunctioning cilia in the tracheobronchial tract in two subjects. *Am Rev Respir Dis* 112:807, 1975.
14. Pederson H, Mygind N. Absence of axonemal arms in nasal mucosal cilia in Kartagener's syndrome. *Nature* 262:494, 1976.
15. Camner P, Jarstrand C, Philipson C. Tracheobronchial clearance in patients with influenza. *Am Rev Respir Dis* 108:131, 1973.
16. Wanner A. Clinical aspects of mucociliary transport. *Am Rev Respir Dis* 116:73, 1977.
17. Mezey RJ, Corn MA, Fernandez EJ, Januszkiewicz AJ, Wanner A. Mucociliary transport in allergic patients with antigen-induced bronchospasms. *Am Rev Respir Dis* 118:677, 1978.
18. Allergra L, Abraham WM, Chapman GA, Wanner A. Duration of mucociliary dysfunction following antigen challenge in allergic sheep. *J Appl Physiol* 55:726, 1983.

19. Wanner A, Zarzeki S, Hirsch J, Epstein S. Tracheal mucous transport in experimental canine asthma. *J Appl Physiol* 39:950, 1975.
20. Ahmed T, Greenblatt DW, Birch S, Marchette B, Wanner A. Abnormal mucociliary transport in allergic patients with antigen-induced bronchospasm: role of slow reacting substance of anaphylaxis. *Am Rev Respir Dis* 124:110, 1981.
21. Marcom ZVI, Shelhamer JH, Bach MK, Morton DR, Kaliner M. Slow-reacting substances, leukotriens C4 and D4, increase the release of mucus from human airways in vitro. *Am Rev Respir Dis* 126:449, 1982.
22. Gee JBC. Bronchoalveolar lavage. *Thorax* 35:1, 1980.
23. Pennington JE, Rossig TH, Boerth LW, Lee TH. Isolation and partial characterization of a human alveolar macrophage-derived neutrophilactivating factor. *J Clin Invest* 75:1230, 1985.
24. Alexander EL, Titus JA, Segal DM. Human leukocyte Fc(IgG) receptors: quantitation and affinity with radiolabeled affinity cross-linked rabbit IgG. *J Immunol* 123:295, 1979.
25. Dauber JG, Daniele RP. Release of phagocyte and leukocyte chemotactic factors by alveolar macrophages. *Am Rev Respir Dis* 119(Suppl.):64, 1979.
26. Ito S, Mikawa H, Shinomiya K, Yoshida T. Suppressive effect of IgA soluble immune complexes on neutrophil chemotaxis. *Clin Exp Immunol* 37:436, 1979.
27. Ito S, Shinomiya K, Mikawa H. Suppressive effect of IgE soluble immune complex on neutrophil chemotaxis. *Clin Exp Immunol* 51:407, 1983.
28. Hill IK, Porter P. Studies in the bactericidal activity to *E. coli* of porcine serum and colostral immunoglobulins and the role of lysozyme with secretory IgA. *Immunology* 26:1239, 1974.
29. Gordon LI, Douglas DS, Kay NE, Yamada O, Osserman EF, Jacob HS. Modulation of neutrophil function by lysozyme. *J Clin Invest* 64:226, 1979.
30. Gadek JE, Fells GA, Zimmerman RL, Rennard SI, Crystol RG. Antielastases of the human alveolar structures. *J Clin Invest* 68:889, 1981.
31. Bienenstock J. The lung as an immunologic organ. *Am Rev Med* 35:49, 1984.
31. a. Boat TF, Doershuk CF, Stern RC. Diseases of the respiratory system. In: Behrman RE, Vaugham VC (eds.), *Nelson Textbook of Pediatrics*, W. B. Saunders, Philadelphia, 1983, p. 1008.
32. Platts-Mills TAE, von Maur RK, Ishizaka K, Norman PS, Lichtenstein LM. IgA and IgG anti-ragweed antibodies in nasal secretions: quantitative measurements of antibodies and correction with inhibition of histamine release. *J Clin Invest* 57:1041, 1976.
33. Bienenstock J, Befus AD. Some thoughts on the biologic role of immunoglobulin A. *Gastroenterology* 84:178, 1983.
34. Ito S, Mikawa H, Shinomiya K, Yoshida T, Hosoi S. Neutrophil chemotactic inhibitor insera of patients with acute stage of Schönlein-Henoch purpura. *Ann Paediatr Jpn* 27:60, 1981.
35. Hirao T, Mikawa H, Shinomiya K, Yoshida T. Antigen-specific IgA antibodies. I. Determination of antigen-specific IgA antibodies in human sera. *Ann Paediatr Jpn* 24:215, 1978.

36. Hirao T, Mikawa H, Shinomiya K, Yoshida T. Antigen-specific IgA antibodies. II. Antigen-specific IgA antibodies in sera of children with anaphylactoid purpura. *Ann Paediatr Jpn* 25:15, 1979.
37. Van Epps DE, Williams RC Jr. Suppression of leukocyte chemotaxis by human IgA myeloma components. *J Exp Med* 144:1227, 1976.
38. Brandtzaeg P. Human secretory component. VI. Immunoglobulin-binding properties. *Immunochemistry* 14:179, 1977.
39. Hanson LA, Brandtzaeg P. The mucosal defense system. In: Stiehm ER, Fulginiti VA (eds.), *Immunological Disorders in Infants and Children*, W. B. Saunders, Philadelphia, 1980, p. 137.
40. Hosoi H, Shinomiya K, Mikawa H. The use of monoclonal antibodies in demonstrating the effect of antibody heterogeneity on immune complex size. *Clin Immunol Immunopathol* 32:378, 1984.
41. Kimata H, Shinomiya K, Mikawa H. Selective enhancement of human IgE production in vitro by synergy of pokeweed mitogen and mercuric chloride. *Clin Exp Immunol* 53:183, 1983.
42. Kimata H, Hosoi S, Shinomiya K, Mikawa H. Pokeweed mitogen-induced human IgE production in vitro. I. Enhancing effect of $\gamma$ carrageenan. *Ann Paediatr Jpn* 30:50, 1984.
43. Kimata H, Hosoi S, Shinomiya K, Mikawa H. Pokeweed mitogen-induced human IgE production in vitro. II. Synergy of pokeweed mitogen and lipopolysaccharide. *Ann Paediatr Jpn* 30:57, 1984.
44. Ishizaka K. IgE-binding factors from rat T lymphocytes. *Lymphokines* 8:41, 1983.
45. Welliver RC, Kaul JN, Ogra PL. The appearance of cell-bound IgE in respiratory-tract epithelium after respiratory syncytial-virus infection. *N Engl J Med* 303:1198, 1980.
46. Welliver RC, Wong DJ, Sun M, Middleton E, Jr, Vaughan RS, Ogra PL. The development of respiratory syncytial virus-specific IgE and the release of histamine in nasopharyngeal secretions after infection. *N Engl J Med* 305:841, 1981.
47. Shackelford PG, Polmar SH, Mayus JL, Johnson WL, Corry JM, Nahm MH. Spectrum of IgG2 subclass deficiency in children with recurrent infections: prospective study. *J Pediatr* 108:647, 1986.
48. Ishizaka A, Kojima K, Tomizawa K, Nakanishi M, Sakiyama Y, Matsumoto S, Otsu M, Ozutsumi K. Clinical observations of four patients with IgG2 deficiency. *Acta Paediatr Jpn* 95:1168, 1991.
49. Rachelefsky GS, Katz RM, Siegel SC. Chronic sinus disease associated with reactive airway disease in children. *Pediatrics* 73:526–529, 1984.
50. Gross GN, Rehm SR, Pierce AK. The effect of complement depletion on lung clearance of bacteria. *J Clin Invest* 62:373, 1978.
51. Heidbrink PJ, Toews GB, Gross GN, Pierce AK. Mechanisms of complement mediated clearance of bacteria from the murine lung. *Am Rev Respir Dis* 125:517, 1982.
52. McIntosh K, Ellis EF, Hoffman LS, Lybass TG, Eller JJ, Fulginiti VA. The

association of viral and bacterial respiratory infections with exacerbations of wheezing in young asthmatic children. *J Pediatr* 83:578–590, 1973.
53. Henderson FW, Clyde WA Jr, Collier AM, Denny FW, Senior RJ, Sheaffer CI, Conley WG III, Christian RM. The etiology and epidemiologic spectrum of bronchiolitis in pediatric practice. *J Pediatr* 95:183–190, 1979.
54. Pullan CR, Hey EN. Wheezing, asthma, and pulmonary dysfunction 10 years after infection with respiratory syncytial virus in infancy. *Br Med J* 284:1665–1669, 1982.
55. Zweiman B, Schoenwetter WF, Pappano JE, Tempest B, Hildreth EA. Patterns of allergic respiratory disease in children with a past history of bronchiolitis. *Allergy* 48:283–289, 1971.
56. Rooney JC, Williams HE. The relationship between proven viral bronchiolitis and subsequent wheezing. *J Pediatr* 79:744–747, 1971.
57. Empey DW, Laitinen LA, Jacobs L, Gold WM, Nadel JA. Mechanisms of bronchial hypereactivity in normal subjects after upper respiratory tract infection. *Am Rev Respir Dis* 113:131–139, 1976.
58. Walsh JJ, Dietlein LF, Low FN, Burch GE, Mogabgab WJ. Tracheobronchial response in human influenza. *Arch Intern Med* 108:376–388, 1961.
59. Hall WJ, Hall CB, Speers DM. Respiratory syncytial virus infection in adults. Clinical, virologic, and serial pulmonary function studies. *Ann Intern Med* 88:203–295, 1978.
60. Sakamoto M, Ida S, Takishima T. Effect of influenza virus infection on allergic sensitization to aerosolized ovalbumin in mice. *J Immunol* 132:2614–2617, 1984.
61. Ida S, Hooks JJ, Siraganian, Notkins AL. Enhancement of IgE-mediated histamine release from human basophil by viruses: role of interferon. *J Exp Med* 145:892–906, 1977.
62. Lett-Brown MA, Aelvoet M, Hooks JJ, Georgiades JA, Thueson DO, Grant JA. Enhancement of basophil chemotaxis *in vitro* by virus-induced interferon. *J Clin Invest* 67:547–552, 1981.
63. Szentivanyi A. The beta-adrenergic theory of atopic abnormality in asthma. *J Allergy* 42:203–232, 1968.
64. Busse WW. Decreased granulocyte response to isoproterenol in asthma during upper respiratory infections. *Am Rev Respir Dis* 115:783–791, 1977.
65. Busse WW, Cooper W, Warshauer DM, Dick EC, Wallow IHC, Albrecht R. Impairment of isoproterenol, H2 histamine, and prostaglandin $E_1$ response of human granulocytes after incubation *in vitro* with live influenza vaccines. *Am Rev Respir Dis* 119:561–569, 1979.
66. Busse WW, Anderson CL, Dick EC, Warshauer D. Reduced granulocyte response to isoproterenol, histamine, and prostaglandin E, after *in vitro* incubation with rhinovirus 16. *Am Rev Respir Dis* 122:641–646, 1980.

# 6

# Lung Injury and Repair

**BETTINA C. HILMAN and MARGARET A. SPRINGER**

*Louisiana State University Medical Center*
*Shreveport, Louisiana*

The lungs, as the organ responsible for pulmonary gas exchange, interface with the environment and the circulation and are at risk of injury from both the air and the blood. Lung injury, a term used to describe the response of the airways and the lung parenchyma to insults, includes a range of phenomena that can be characterized both physiologically and pathologically. Some of the physiological responses to lung injury include alterations in gas exchange, lung water, vascular permeability, and pulmonary hemodynamics (1). Lung injury can be demonstrated pathologically by examination of tissues directly or indirectly from the analysis of bronchoalveolar lavage fluid. Injury can be characterized histologically by evidence of tissue/cell damage, other structural alterations of pulmonary architecture or by derangements in the number, types, and location of cells. The unique low-pressure characteristics of the pulmonary circulation may also contribute to inflammatory injury in the lung, particularly with regard to capillary localization of inflammatory cells (1).

The airways and lung parenchyma respond to insults by evoking inflammatory and immune effector cells as a part of the process of inflammation. Inflammation, a nonspecific reaction of vascularized tissues to injury from a variety of stimuli, is a complex process directed toward the resolution or repair of the injured tissue(s). Events during the inflammatory process include local circulatory changes, the influx of phagocytes, the release of vasoactive and inflammatory mediators, and the recruitment and stimulation of cells of the immune system. The inflammatory process is redundant (2), and is usually self-limited; however, it can be self-perpetuating. The outcome of the inflammatory response depends on the nature and intensity of the injurious stimuli and the ability of the host to limit the inflammation and complete the repair process, returning the injured tissue to its normal structure and function. Injury to the lung parenchyma and airways can be direct or a consequence of inflammation or immune reactions that share two common mechanisms: oxidant injury from the generation of oxygen radicals and proteolytic injury through the activation of hydrolytic enzymes. For inflammation to resolve, the influx of inflammatory cells must cease, the oxygen radicals and proteases must be inactivated, and the damaged cells replaced (2).

The lung can respond to insults with repair of structural damage and resolution of the physiological abnormalities or with the perpetuation of structural and/or functional abnormalities. The final outcome to any given lung injury is determined by the interaction of inflammatory cells (as a part of the nonspecific immune host defense system), specific immune host defense mechanisms, and the appropriate balance of pulmonary host protective mechanisms such as the oxidant–antioxidant and protease–antiprotease systems. The use of the terms *inflammation* and *injury* interchangeably as synonyms should be strongly discouraged, since injury is not an inevitable consequence of the presence of inflammatory cells. Inflammatory cells play a dual role in response to injury, that is, one of "protector" of the host and the other of the perpetuator of tissue damage or altered physiological functions. The term *lung injury* should be restricted to the inflammatory responses that initiate or perpetuate injury or result in sequelae that are harmful to the host. A basic knowledge of the characteristic histologic features and physiological actions of the resident cells of the airways or lung and the inflammatory or immune effector cells recruited in response to injury help in our understanding of the processes of inflammation, injury, and repair.

Injury to the host tissues can occur when inflammatory cells such as the neutrophil and mononuclear phagocytes elaborate proteases, cationic proteins, and oxidants. Other toxic agents such as cytotoxic cytokines (e.g., tumor necrosis factor) and lysosomal enzymes may also injury host tissues (2). The inflammatory cell types involved in injury will be discussed separately. Agents that induce lung injury and initiate inflammation are diverse and include infectious agents, physical agents, chemical agents, ischemic injury, and immunologic reactions (Table 1).

## MECHANISMS OF LUNG INJURY

### Proteases and Protease-Antiprotease Imbalance

#### *Proteases*

Proteases, enzymes that degrade proteins by hydrolyzing peptide bonds, can injure host tissues (3,4). These proteolytic enzymes vary in their substrate specificity and in the types of their protein targets. Proteases are classified as exopeptidases (enzymes whose function is restricted to N or C terminal peptide linkages) or endopeptidases (proteases that are not so restricted in their action) (5). Proteases can also be designated on the basis of the critical components of the catalytic mechanisms used to cleave peptide bonds, such as serine, cysteine, aspartic, metallo, and unclassified (3–5). In the lung, some proteases function within cells, while others are released by cells into the local milieu, where they are capable of modifying the extracellular matrix components and/or cells of the lung parenchyma or proteins in the complement or coagulation cascade systems (5). In general, proteases in the lung are endopeptidases and their catalytic function can be classified as the serine or metallotype processes (5).

Because of the abundance of plasma antiproteases, proteases released outside the lung normally do not reach the lung. The predominant source of proteases involved in the destruction of lung parenchymal components

TABLE 1 Agents Inducing Lung Injury

| |
|---|
| Infectious agents |
| Bacteria |
| Viruses |
| Parasites |
| Physical agents |
| Burns |
| Radiation |
| Trauma |
| Chemical agents |
| Drugs |
| Toxins |
| Industrial agents |
| Ischemic injury to tissues |
| Immunologic reactions |
| Allergy |
| Autoimmunity |

is inflammatory cells within or recruited to the lung from the pulmonary capillaries (5,6).

At least six extracellular proteases are found in neutrophils: neutrophil elastase, cathepsin G, collagenase, gelatinase, proteinase 3, and plasminogen activator. With the exception of the latter protease, the others are all stored within the granules of the cell (azurophilic or primary granules, specific or secondary granules, and tertiary granules). Table 2 lists characteristics of the proteases relevant to the lung.

Proteolytic destruction of the lung connective tissue contributes to the pathologic changes in the airways in bronchiectasis and is part of the progressive endobronchial and pulmonary parenchymal disease in patients with cystic fibrosis (CF) (7). Elastase of neutrophil origin has been identified in sputum samples from patients with CF (8,9). Bruce et al. (7) found uninhibited elastases of both neutrophil and bacterial origins in sputum samples of patients with CF chronically infected with *Pseudomonas aeruginosa*. Degradation of elastin produces amino acids that can be quantitated in the urine. Desmosine (cross-linking amino acids unique to elastin) has been found in urine of patients with CF with chronic severe lung infections (7). These observations, together with pathologic evidence of fragmented and distorted elastic fibers, indicate that destruction and resynthesis of elastic fibers is a chronic process in the patient with CF (7).

Elastase levels are higher in purulent than in mucoid sputum in patients with CF (10,11). Neutrophils recovered from bronchoalveolar (BAL) fluid

TABLE 2 Characteristics of Protease Relevant to the Lung

| Protease | Category | Cell source | Substrate |
|---|---|---|---|
| Neutrophil elastase | Serine | Neutrophil, basophil, mast cell | Elastin, type I-IV collagen, fibronectin, laminin, proteoglycans |
| Cathepsin G | Serine | Neutrophil | Fibronectin, proteoglycans, elastin, type IV collagen |
| Collagenase | Metalloprotease | Neutrophil, fibroblast, macrophage | Type I, III-V, and VII collagen; gelatin; fibronectin |
| Gelatinase | Metalloprotease | Neutrophil, fibroblast, macrophage | Laminin, elastin, fibronectin, gelatin, type V and VII collagen |
| Proteinase-3 | Serine | Neutrophil | Type I and III collagen |
| Plasminogen activator | Serine | Neutrophil, macrophage | Elastin |
| Cathepsin D | Aspartic | Monocyte, neutrophil fibroblast, macrophage | Proteoglycans, type IV collagen, fibronectin |
| Cathepsin L | Cysteine | Macrophage | Type IV collagen, fibronectin |
| Cathepsin B | Cysteine | Macrophage | Elastin |
| Granzymes 1-6[a] | Serine | T cell | Cellular matrix |

[a]Several human granzymes have been reported, but the biological function of only granzyme 1 has been evaluated.
*Source*: Modified from Ref. 5.

of patients with CF have marked down regulation of CR1 (the C3b receptor), which appears to be due to exposure to neutrophil elastase activity (12).

### *Antiproteases*

Antiproteases are proteins that inhibit proteases, preventing the protease from acting on its natural substrates and forming tight bonds with the protease at the catalytic site (3). Antiproteases usually function because the concentration–time kinetics of their interaction with the protease is more favorable than that of the protease with tissue components. (5,13,14). The protease cleaves a peptide bond at the reactive site of the antiprotease; however, the cleavage is slower and the protease–antiprotease binding is tight enough to inhibit the protease. The kinetics of protease inhibition is related to the concentration of the antiprotease (13,15).

Extracellular antiproteases that protect the lung from proteases capable of attacking lung components include alpha-1 antitrypsin, secretory leukoprotease inhibitor (SLPI), alpha-1 antichymotrypsin, alpha-2 macroglobulin, and tissue inhibitor of metalloprotease (TIMP) (13). In normal individuals, alpha-1 antitrypsin is the principal inhibitor of neutrophil elastase (NE) and contributes approximately 90% of the anti-NE activity (16,17). Alpha-1 antitrypsin, a serine protease, is coded by a single gene on chromosome 14 and consists of 7 exons and 6 introns. Advances in molecular biology have provided insights into the regulation of antiproteases and have led to the development of recombinant forms of alpha-1 antitrypsin produced in *Escherichia coli* or yeast that can inhibit NE similarly to the natural molecule (18–20).

Secretory leukoprotease inhibitor (SLPI), often called bronchial mucus inhibitor, is a serine antiprotease produced by mucosal cells in large and small airways whose major role is to protect the respiratory tract from neutrophil elastase (13,21). SLPI is coded for by a single gene spanning 2.6 kilobases (kb), which consists of four exons and three introns; exon III contains the sequences for the active inhibitory site (21). In the central airway, SLPI has been histochemically localized to the serous and goblet cells of the submucosal glands and to the surface epithelium (13). In the distal airways, SLPI is found in the nonciliated (Clara) epithelial cells (13). SLPI is present in 10-fold concentration in larger airways compared to the alveoli. A variety of serine proteases are inhibited by SLPI, including neutrophil elastase, cathepsin G, trypsin, chymotrypsin, and mast cell chymase. However, the rate of association is highest with neutrophil elastase. SLPI is acid stable, which enables it to retain its function in an acid environment such as the vicinity of activated neutrophils.

Other serine antiproteases are alpha-1-antichymotrypsin, TIMP, and alpha-2-macroglobulin (Table 3).

TABLE 3 Major Antiproteases Relevant to the Lung

| Antiprotease | Disulfide bonds | Antiprotease spectrum relevant to the lung extracellular matrix | Concentration in normal plasma (μM) | Concentration in ELF (μM) |
|---|---|---|---|---|
| $Alpha_1$-Antitrypsin | No | NE, cathepsin G, NE, | 20–53 | 2–6 |
| SLPI | Yes | cathepsin G, chymase | 0.004–0.007 | 1–1.2 |
| $Alpha_1$-Antichymotrypsin | Yes | Cathepsin G | 6–8 | 0.5–1 |
| TIMP | Yes | Collagenases, stromolysins, PUMP-1 | 0.03 | Not determined |
| $Alpha_2$-Macroglobulin | Yes | All classes of proteases | 2.5–5 | 0.01 |

ELF, epithelial lining fluid; NE, neutrophil elastase; PUMP-1, putative, metalloproteinase 1; SLPI, secretory leukoprotease inhibitor; TIMP, tissue inhibitor of metalloproteinase.
*Source*: Modified from Ref. 15.

## Oxidants and Antioxidants

### *Oxidants*

The breakdown products of oxygen metabolism, called oxygen free radicals or reactive oxygen species, are toxic to cells and have been implicated in oxidant-induced cellular damage in many pathologic processes. The lung can defend itself from oxidant injury by a variety of antioxidant mechanisms; however, when oxygen free radical production is increased, the detoxifying capacity of these antioxidant defenses may be overwhelmed, resulting in cellular injury and functional impairment.

Free radicals are the species of oxygen capable of independent existence and have one or more unpaired electrons (22). The unpaired electron(s) tend to cause instability and high chemical reactivity in these oxygen radicals. Fortunately, most of cellular oxygen reduction takes place without any substantial release of the free radical intermediates (23). When molecular oxygen is reduced by a univalent pathway, free radicals (superoxide radical, hydrogen peroxide, and the hydroxyl radical) are produced. The transfer of one electron to oxygen forms the superoxide radical ($O_2^{\bullet -}$); the addition of a second electron generates hydrogen peroxide ($H_2O_2$). Enzymatic and nonenzymatic reactions can produce these oxidants. In the presence of iron and other metals, superoxide and hydrogen peroxide may react to form the hydroxyl radical ($OH^-$) via the Haber–Weiss and Fenton reactions. Interactions between superoxide and other radicals can result in the formation of singlet oxygen. Although hydrogen peroxide and singlet oxygen do not have unpaired electrons and technically are not radicals, they are usually referred to as oxygen free radicals (24).

Oxygen radicals can be produced in many intracellular locations, such as mitochondria, endoplasmic reticulum, peroxisomes, plasma and nuclear membranes, and cytoplasm (25). Depending on the production site, free radicals can react with proteins or enzymes or damage membranes. These oxygen species are highly reactive, short-lived molecules with diverse activities that include an increase in membrane permeability (26), inhibition of calcium-mediated signal transduction (27), inactivation of cytosolic and membrane-imbedded enzymes (28), alteration of DNA formation and prevention of protein DNA interactions that regulate gene expression (29), initiation of lipid peroxidation chain reactions (30), a change of harmless drugs into harmful drugs (31), generation of vasoactive arachidonic acid metabolites (32), and degradation of carbohydrates within the extracellular matrix (33).

Enzymatic sources of these oxygen radicals include the xanthine oxidase reaction, aldehyde and amine oxidases, cytochrome b5, the cytochrome P450 mono-oxygenase system, and prostaglandin synthetase (24). Oxygen-derived oxidants are also produced within neutrophils and monocytes during the phagocytic respiratory burst and the myeloperoxidase reactions. The two main sources of oxygen radicals in the lungs are respiratory bursts in phagocytosing cells and the hypoxanthine–xanthine oxidative system (34). The latter is of special interest, since large amounts of hypoxanthine accumulate in the body during hypoxia.

Tissue injury triggered by immune complexes is closely related to the influx of neutrophils (34). The inflammatory reaction induced by immune complexes appears to be related to the production of superoxide, hydrogen peroxide, and the hydroxyl radical (35). An interaction occurs between the neutrophil and the immune complexes on the surface of the cell, resulting in superoxide production (36). If the phagocytic cell contains the appropriate Fc receptor, an immune complex can activate the cells to generate reactive oxygen products (34). Chemotactic factors such as complement components (C3b and C5b) and the leukotriene LTB4 can activate the phagocytic cell to produce the oxygen radicals (37–40).

Under normal conditions, approximately 90% of cellular oxygen reduction takes place via the mitochondrial cytochrome oxidase pathway; four electrons are transferred in sequential steps from reduced cytochrome c, through cytochrome oxidase, to molecular oxygen without any substantial release of free oxidants (23). Only 1–2% of the mitochondrial oxygen consumed in this process forms superoxide and hydrogen peroxide in nonpathologic states (41). However, under certain conditions, the production of free radicals increases and the body's defenses against these radicals are overwhelmed resulting in tissue damage (see Figs. 1–3, Table 4).

Superoxide ($O_2^{\bullet -}$) is generated both by enzymatic and nonenzymatic reactions. Enzymatic reactions include those in plasma membranes in leukocytes and macrophages by NADPH oxidase (42) and the cytosolic xanthine oxidase reaction (43). Superoxide is also formed by nonenzymatic reactions such as autooxidation of a variety of cellular components (e.g., catecholamines) by molecular oxygen (44). Ferrous ions can take part in electron transfer reactions with molecular oxygen to yield superoxide anions (45). Superoxide can be reduced to hydrogen peroxide spontaneously or catalyzed by superoxide dismutase (SOD). At a physiological pH, the dismutation of superoxide catalyzed by SOD is approximately $10^4$ times faster than spontaneous dismutation (46).

The hydroxyl radical, another free radical that is important in tissue damage, is formed from hydrogen peroxide catalyzed by metal salt (e.g., copper) via the Haber–Weiss reaction. If the metal salt involved is iron, this reaction is referred to as the Fenton reaction and can be accelerated by the presence of ascorbic acid (47). Usually the hydroxyl radicals are produced in very small quantities and can be neutralized by the body's defenses; this oxygen radical is more likely to react rapidly with molecules

**Univalent pathways of $O_2$ reduction**

$O_2 \xrightarrow{e^-} O_2^{\cdot -}$ (superoxide radical)

$O_2^{\cdot -} \xrightarrow{e^- + 2H^+} H_2O_2$ (hydrogen peroxide)

$H_2O_2 \xrightarrow{e^- + 2H^+} OH^{\cdot} + H_2O$ (hydroxyl radical)

$OH^{\cdot} \xrightarrow{e^- + 2H^+} H_2O$

**Other sources of oxygen radicals**

Haber-Weiss Reaction

$O_2^{\cdot -} + H_2O_2 \xrightarrow{Cu,\ Fe} OH^{\cdot} + OH^- + O_2$

Fenton reaction

$H_2O_2 + Fe^{2+} \longrightarrow OH^{\cdot} + OH^- + Fe^{3+}$

Oxygen radicals formed by enzymatic reaction

hypoxanthine + $O_2 \xrightarrow{\text{xanthine oxidase}}$ urate

$\searrow O_2^{\cdot -}$

FIGURE 1 Reactive oxygen species. Univalent pathways of oxygen reduction lead to the formation of reaction oxygen species: superoxide radical, hydrogen peroxide, and hydroxyl radical. Other sources of oxygen radicals include Haber–Weiss reaction, the Fenton reaction, and xanthine oxidase.

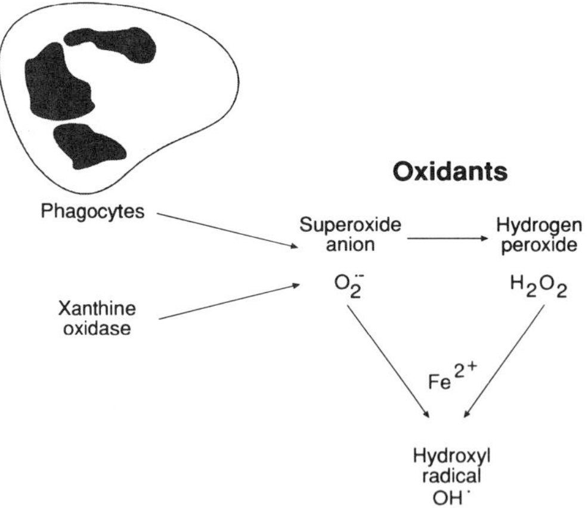


FIGURE 2 Two sources of oxidants are phagocytes and xanthines oxidase.

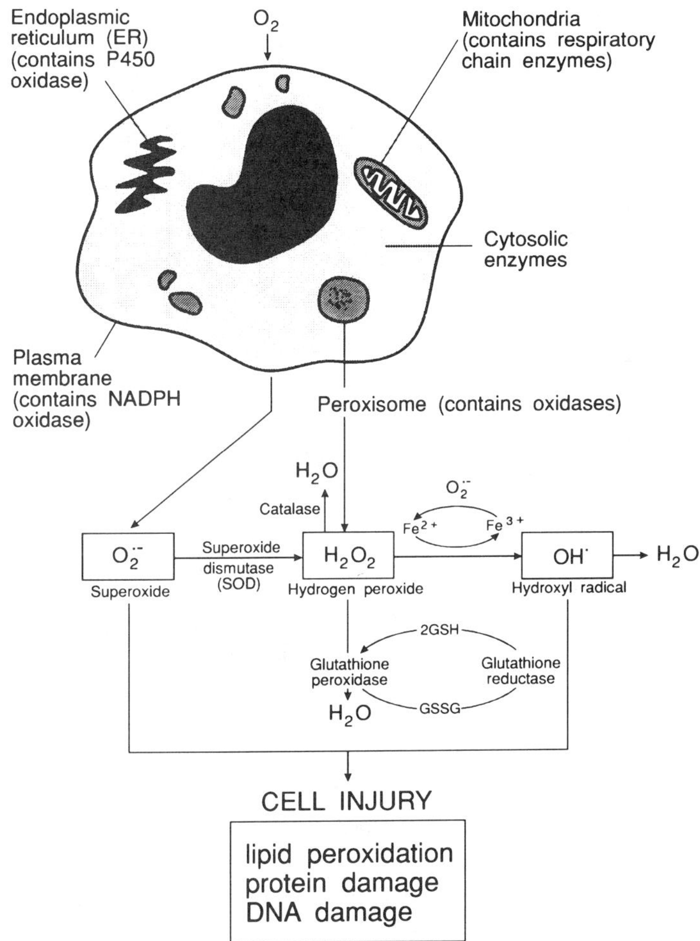


FIGURE 3 Formation of reactive oxygen species and antioxidant mechanisms.

in its immediate environment. In contrast to the hydroxyl radical, superoxide and hydrogen peroxide are able to diffuse away from their site of formation (48). Hydrogen peroxide is also able to cross cell membranes directly, while superoxide can cross via anion channels (49).

### *Antioxidants*

The antioxidant enzymes are the first line of defense against free radicals and can be classified as primary or secondary and categorized as enzymatic and nonenzymatic antioxidants (24,50). Superoxide dismutase, catalase,

TABLE 4 Body's Defenses Against Free Radicals

| Enzyme | Location | Function | Reaction | Comment |
|---|---|---|---|---|
| Superoxide dismutase | Cytosol<br>Mitochondria | Reduces superoxide radical | $O_2^{\cdot -} + O_2^{\cdot -} - 2H+$<br>$\longrightarrow H_2O_2 + O_2$ | Requires trace metal coenzymes |
| Catalase | Highly compartmentalized in peroxisomes | Reduces hydrogen peroxide | $2H_2O_2 \xrightarrow{\Delta}$<br>$2H_2O + O_2$ | Effective only against small molecule |
| Glutathione peroxidase | Widely available throughout cytosol | Reduces hydrogen peroxide<br>Detoxifies toxic intracellular hydroperoxide in membrane lipids | $2H_2O \xrightarrow{\Delta} 2H_2O_2 + O_2$<br>$LOOH + 2GSH \rightarrow$<br>$GSSG + LOH + H_2O$ | Requires glutathione reductase + GGPD to regenerate GSSG; effective against larger peroxides |

LOOH, lipid hydroperoxide; LOH, nontoxic lipid alcohol; GSH, reduced glutathione; GSSG, oxidized glutathione.

and the glutathione redox cycle (glutathione peroxidase, glutathione reductase, and glucose-6-phosphate dehydrogenase) are the three primary intracellular antioxidant defense mechanisms (51) (Fig. 4). These antioxidants must be present at the site of oxygen radical production to be effective (24). Secondary enzymatic antioxidants function by restoring peroxidized lipid membranes and oxidized protein sulfhydryl groups once the damage has occurred (24).

Superoxide dismutase (SOD) occurs in multiple forms, each utilizing a different metal as a coenzyme. The form containing copper and zinc is found in the cytoplasm and in small amounts in the plasma (52). The form containing manganese is found in the mitochondria (24). This enzyme

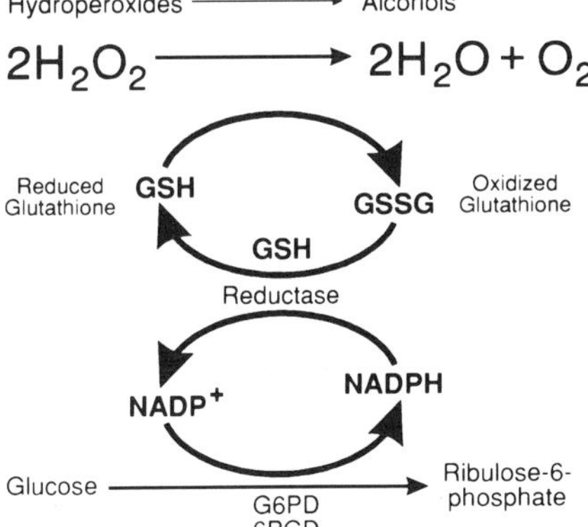


FIGURE 4 Antioxidant enzyme systems in the lung. The three major intracellular antioxidant systems are shown. Extracellular antioxidants include ceruloplasmin, beta carotene, bilirubin, albumin, and lactoferrin.

reduces the superoxide radical to form hydrogen peroxide and water. The hydrogen peroxide produced in this reaction is detoxified by the two remaining enzymes, catalase and glutathione peroxidase.

Catalase, a highly compartmentalized antioxidant enzyme, is found primarily in the peroxisomes (51). It is effective only against small molecules and reduces hydrogen peroxide to water and molecular oxygen.

Glutathione peroxidase, in contrast to catalase, is found intracellularly throughout the cytosol and can catalyze the reduction of hydrogen peroxide to water (50). Glutathione peroxidase has a greater affinity than catalase for $H_2O_2$ and is thought to be the preferred enzyme for handling low concentrations of hydrogen peroxide. It also detoxifies large molecular peroxides such as lipid hydroperoxides (50). Catalase becomes more important as rates of hydrogen peroxide formation increases.

During the reactions catalyzed by glutathione peroxidase, reduced glutathione (GSH) is converted to its oxidized form (GSSG), which then can be reduced back to GSH by the enzyme glutathione reductase (50). Glutathione reductase is required to maintain GSH (24). NADPH is generated by the action of the enzyme glucose-6-phosphate dehydrogenase (G-6 PD) and the hexose monophosphate shunt (50).

$$\text{GSSG} + \text{NADPH} + \text{H}^+ \rightarrow 2\ \text{GSH} + \text{NADP}^+$$

These enzymes systems work together to form a cooperative antioxidant defense system. Hydrogen peroxide can inactivate the function of superoxide dismutases; the actions of catalase and glutathione peroxidase, by detoxifying cellular hydrogen peroxide, help to preserve superoxide dismutase function (50). Superoxide free radicals inhibit catalase and glutathione peroxidase, and the superoxide dismutases can protect the function of their complementary antioxidant enzymes (50).

Nonenzymatic antioxidants include lipid-soluble molecules and water-soluble molecules. The solubilities determine their intracellular location and sites of action. Their role as protectors against oxidant attack depends on their ability to undergo oxidation without compromising cellular function. Lipid-soluble antioxidant molecules are found in cell and organelle membranes. The major lipid soluble antioxidant is vitamin E (alpha-tocopherol), which protects against oxidant-induced membrane injury (53). This fat-soluble vitamin is incorporated into the lipid layer of cell membrane and functions as an intramembranous scavenger of oxygen radicals. Vitamin E is capable of breaking the domino effect of chain reaction lipid peroxidation, most likely due to the stability of the alpha tocopherol radical (* alphaTH) and because this radical does not react further with polyunsaturated lipid substrates (54). B-carotene, another lipid-soluble antioxidant, may scavenge superoxide and peroxyl free radicals under normoxic conditions; however, under hyperoxic conditions, it may have a pro-oxidant effect (55). Preliminary evidence suggests that bilirubin, formed from the catabolism of hemoglobin, may exhibit antioxidant function (56).

Water-soluble nonenzymatic antioxidants such as vitamin C are found in intracellular and extracellular spaces. Vitamin C may function cooperatively with vitamin E in breaking lipid peroxidation chain reactions, by assisting the recycling of the alpha-tocopherol radical to its reduced active form (54). In addition, vitamin C has a direct scavenging action for superoxide and hydroxyl radical. However, vitamin C is not considered a major antioxidant since it has potential pro-oxidant properties (50).

Glutathione in its reduced form (GSH) also functions as a water-soluble antioxidant that can interact directly with oxygen-derived free radicals (57). It is the most important antioxidant because of its abundance and its regulated production in all cells. Ceruloplasmin, a copper containing alpha-2-globulin, is thought to function as an antioxidant in the alveolar lining fluid with a limited capacity to scavenge oxygen free radicals directly (58). Other water-soluble compounds with potential antioxidant properties include uric acid, thiols, and taurine (56).

## NORMAL LUNG STRUCTURE

### Airways

The airways connect the outside environment (atmosphere) with the terminal respiratory or gas-exchanging units. The conducting airways are not merely rigid tubes for the passage of air, but are structures with secretory capabilities, which can dilate and contract passively in response to influences such as lung inflation and can actively respond to a variety of neurohumoral and chemical stimuli (59). There are three major groups of intrapulmonary airways: cartilaginous bronchi, membranous (noncartilaginous) bronchioles, and gas exchange ducts. There are several orders of respiratory bronchioles, the last of which leads into the first two to five orders of alveolar ducts (59).

The airways, from the trachea to the respiratory bronchioles, are covered with an epithelial lining that rests on a thin basement membrane overlying a loose network of tissue (lamina propria) containing fibers, cells, a plexus of capillaries, and unmyelinated nerves (59). The cells lining the airways are pseudostratified columnar epithelium. In the large airways, the epithelium is ciliated and columnar; the thickness of the lining decreases as the airways become smaller, so that the lining in the terminal bronchioles consists of a single layer of almost cuboidal ciliated epithelial cells. Cells in the respiratory bronchioles are flattened epithelial cells (59). The chief difference between the respiratory bronchioles and the alveolar ducts is that the alveolar ducts are completely alveolarized and do not contain ciliated respiratory epithelium.

At least eight types of cells are identified in the surface epithelium of the airways (59).

1. Ciliated epithelial cells: The dominant cells in the epithelial layer serve a protective function against injury.
2. Serous secretory cells: Normally present in the proximal airways.
3. Mucus-secreting or goblet cells.
4. Clara cells: Nonciliated cells with secretory capabilities that contain enzymes capable of detoxifying inhaled toxic substances, have a progenitor function after epithelial injury, and may differentiate into ciliated cells and brush cells (59).
5. Basal cells: Found in the epithelium as far as the bronchioles, can differentiate as needed to replace superficial ciliated and mucous cells.
6. Brush cells: Rare cells whose function remains unknown, contain microvilli, and may have a role in liquid absorption.
7. Intermediate cells: Poorly defined layer above the basal cells, are derived from basal cells, and can differentiate into ciliated cells or epithelium mucus-secreting cells.
8. Kultchitsky's (argyrophil) cells: Endocrine-like cells that are included in the amine and amine-precursor, uptake, and decarboxylation (APUD) series.

Bronchial glands, located in the submucosa beneath the lamina propria, are especially numerous in the medium-sized bronchi, less frequent in the smaller bronchi, and absent in the bronchioles. The submucosal bronchial glands contain many cell types: serous cells, mucous cells, collecting duct cells, clear cells, and myoepithelial cells. Innvervation of the bronchial glands is by the cholinergic nerves (60). Irritants initiate a reflex via the parasympathetic nerves that results in coughing and the discharge of the contents of the submucosal glands (59).

Lymphocytes have been observed in the tracheobronchial epithelium and can be recovered from bronchoalveolar lavage. Mast cells have also been identified within the bronchial mucosa and connective tissues.

### Pulmonary Parenchyma: Alveolar Structure

The alveolar walls consist of alveolar epithelium and its basement membrane, the capillary endothelium and its basement membrane, the surfactant lining, and the pulmonary interstitium. The alveolar epithelium consists of a continuous layer of cells of two principal cell types (59). Type I alveolar cells (squamous pneumocytes) make up 93% of the alveolar surface; these cells have broad, thin cytoplasmic extensions and are very susceptible to injury from blood or airborne agents. Type II alveolar cells (granular pneumocytes) have a cuboidal shape and are more numerous than type I cells, although they occupy only 7% of the alveolar surface. These cells secrete surfactant and they are the progenitor cells of the alveolar epithelium. The hallmarks of type II cells are the microvilli and the osmiophilic bodies seen on electron microscopic examination (59).

The basement membrane is composed of type IV collagen, laminin (a glycoprotein), and other macromolecules, including proteoglycans. The pulmonary interstitium is composed of connective tissue components (type I and II collagen, elastin, fibronectin, and other matrix components such as proteoglycans and glycoproteins), mesenchymal cells (fibroblasts, pericytes, and rare smooth muscle cells), and inflammatory and immune effector cells (macrophages, monocytes, and lymphocytes), with the pulmonary capillaries interwoven through the interstitium (59). The fibroblasts and the matrix of the interstitium provide the structural framework that supports the alveoli and defines the mechanical properties of the lung.

## INFLAMMATORY CELLS

In general, the histologic features of inflammation consist of the recruitment of inflammatory cells and mediators, the escape of inflammatory cells from the blood into the extravascular spaces, and alterations in blood flow and the caliber of small blood vessels accompanied by an increase in vascular permeability. Table 5 lists the resident or constituent cells and the cells that may be recruited to the airways or lungs during inflammation.

### Alveolar (Pulmonary) Macrophages

Alveolar macrophages are the predominant inflammatory cell type in the normal lung and are found both on the alveolar surface and within the pulmonary interstitium; there are 50–100 macrophages per alveolus (61,62). As an effector cell in pulmonary defense, the macrophage serves as the first line of cellular defense against inhaled particulate materials reaching the lung. Macrophages defend the lung by ingesting and degrading foreign materials, transporting particles out of the lung, and detoxifying inhaled substances. Serving the respiratory defender role, alveolar macrophages remove macromolecular debris (normal macromolecular components, effete or damaged and defense molecules that complex with their natural substrates, such as alpha-1-antitrypsin–neutrophil elastase complexes) (61).

The pulmonary macrophages are active in phagocytosis and intracellular killing of microbial organisms. Alveolar macrophages can function as an

TABLE 5 Airways and Lung Inflammation

| |
|---|
| Resident or constituent cells of airways and lungs |
| Pulmonary (alveolar) macrophages |
| Mast cells |
| Fibroblasts |
| Endothelial cells |
| Airway and alveolar epithelial cells |
| Cells recruited to airways/lungs during inflammation |
| Neutrophils |
| Eosinophils |
| Monocytes |
| T lymphocytes, helper T cells |

accessory cell in immune responses and can recruit as well as activate other inflammatory cells. They also play a role in processing of antigens, enhancing the immunologic activation of lymphocytes, and initating and/or modulating pulmonary inflammatory reactions (61,63). The ability of the alveolar macrophage to recruit and activate other inflammatory cells contributes to its role in pulmonary host defense as well as its potential for mediating lung injury (Fig. 5). This array of powerful secretory products allows the alveolar macrophage its ability to inflict significant injury to the

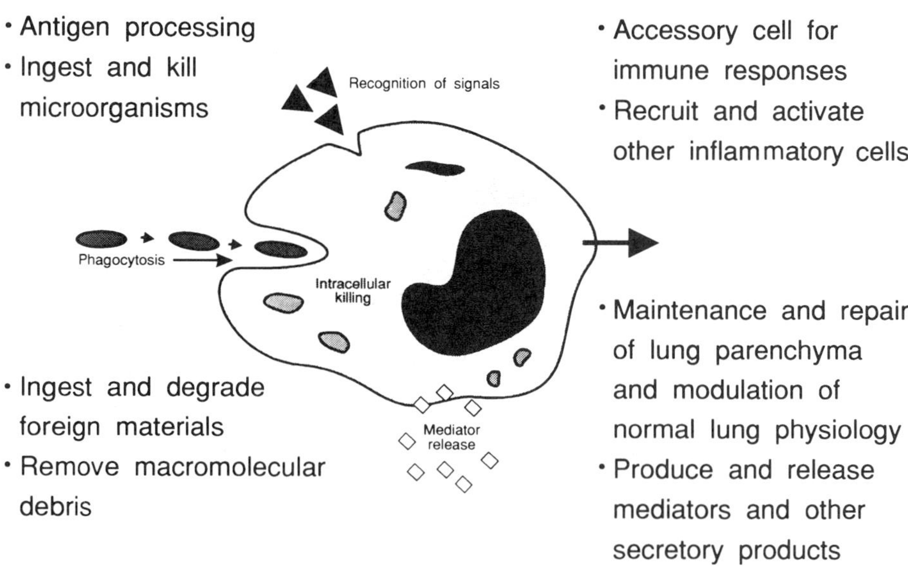


FIGURE 5 Functions of the alveolar macrophage.

normal lung. Some of the defined secretory products of the human alveolar macrophages are listed in Table 6.

Originating from stem cell precursors in the bone marrow, alveolar macrophages reach the lung through the blood as circulating monocytes (59). Transformation of blood monocytes to alveolar macrophages takes place within a few hours after arrival in the lungs and entry into the pulmonary interstitium. Once in the lung, alveolar macrophages are long-lived, with a lifespan of months or perhaps years (61).

The alveolar macrophages have receptors for IgG (Fc receptors), IgE, IgA, and complement, CR1 (C3b and C3bi receptors) and CR3 (C3bi receptors) present on the cell surfaces (61). There are no IgM receptors on the surface of alveolar macrophages, but they can bind IgM immune complexes through C3b. A variety of other receptors have been identified on alveolar macrophages including colony-stimulating factor (GM-CSF), tumor necrosis factor (TNF), platelet-activating factor (PAF), histamine, and interleukin 2 (61). These inflammatory cells are capable of interacting with a variety of cells and can secrete a number of substances that both induce and regulate inflammation. Some of these are proteases, antiproteases, lysosomal enzymes, oxidants, antioxidant, cytokines, bioactive lipids, growth factors, and other miscellaneous enzymes. For example, plasmin activator, a substance produced by the alveolar macrophage, works in concert with macrophage elastase to produce damage to host tissues (64). The conversion of plasminogen to plasmin aids in tissue destruction by stripping away the proteoglycans and fibrin and unmasking target collagen and elastin fibers, as well as generating fibrin split products from fibrin that alter vascular permeability (65).

Circulating monocytes, precursors of the alveolar macrophage, contain a serine elastase that is antigenically and biochemically related to neutrophil elastase (66) and can attack elastin and fibronectin (67). This elastase is found in large amounts on the cell surface of the monocytes, where it is available to cause damage as monocytes move through the connective tissue (66). The change of the elastase from a serine protease to a metalloenzyme elastase is one of the features that marks the differentiation of monocytes into macrophages (68). The alveolar macrophage elastase is secreted into the extracellular environment but is not stored in the cell or localized on its surface (69). This elastase is resistant to inhibition by alpha-1 antiproteinase (70).

Macrophages can contribute to lung injury through a variety of mechanisms, including the production of oxidizing agents, bioactive lipids, proteases, and cytokines. Oxidizing agents from the alveolar macrophages (superoxide anion, hydrogen peroxide, and the hydroxyl radical) can be secreted by the alveolar macrophages (61,71). Although these oxidants can damage lung tissue, the alveolar macrophages also secrete glutathione peroxidase, an antioxidant (68). Other products of the alveolar macrophages are bioactive lipids, prostaglandins and leukotrienes (e.g., LT B4, a chemoattractant for neutrophils), which provide the alveolar macrophage with a mechanism for amplifying the inflammatory response in the lung (72).

The macrophage products that are potentially important in the development of fibrosis are fibronectin and alveolar macrophage-derived growth factor (AMDGF). Fibronectin mediates normal adhesion of fibroblasts to the collagenous framework (73) and stimulates directed migration and recruitment of fibroblasts. AMDGF acts as a progression factor that stimulates fibroblasts to produce their own growth factor (74).

Alveolar macrophages interact with complement by synthesizing and secreting complement components, binding activated complement, and

TABLE 6 Secretory Products of Alveolar Macrophages

| | |
|---|---|
| *Oxidants* | *Antioxidant* |
| Superoxide anion | Glutathione |
| Hydrogen peroxide | |
| Hydroxyl radical | |
| *Proteases* | *Antiproteases* |
| Collagenase | Alpha-1-antitrypsin |
| Plasminogen activator | Alpha-2-macroglobulin |
| Elastase | Tissue inhibitor of metalloproteinases |
| Gelatinase | |
| Cathepsin L | |
| *Cytokines* | *Miscellaneous enzymes* |
| Interleukins 1α and 1β | Lysozyme |
| Tumor necrosis factor α | β-Glucuronidase |
| Interleukin 6 | Acid hydrolases |
| Interleukin 8 | Angiotensin-converting enzyme |
| Interferon gamma | |
| Transforming growth factor β | |
| Granulocyte–macrophage colony-stimulating factor | |
| Macrophage colony-stimulating factor | |
| Macrophage inflammatory protein 1 | |
| *Bioactive lipids* | *Polypeptide growth factors* |
| Cyclo-oxygenase metabolites | Platelet-derived growth factor |
| Lipoxygenase metabolites | AM insulin-derived growth factor 1 |
| Platelet-activating factor | Fibronectin |
| | Basic fibroblast growth factor |

*Source*: Modified from Ref. 61.

degrading complement through the action of proteases (75). Complement receptors on alveolar macrophages bind complement-coated particles and act synergistically with receptors for the Fc portion of IgG to facilitate particle ingestion.

Macrophages participate in complex interactions with lymphocytes. Lymphocyte mediators attract macrophages to sites of inflammation and enhance macrophage secretion of neutral proteases and oxygen radicals. Lymphokines augment the release of alpha-2-macroglobulin, prostaglandins, and interferon (76).

Interleukin 1 (IL-1) produced by macrophages is chemotactic for blood T lymphocytes and acts as a maturational signal, preparing T lymphocytes to respond to antigens or other secondary signals. IL-8, another cytokine secretory product of the alveolar macrophage, attracts and activates neutrophils, but not monocytes (61). Both IL-8 and $LTB_4$ are not released by resting alveolar macrophages but are released in large amounts after activation (61).

## Neutrophils

Neutrophils are sparse in the normal lung, with only 1 neutrophil per 100 alveoli. The pulmonary vasculature serves as a reservoir from which neutrophils can be rapidly mobilized (77). Chemotactic factors produced by alveolar macrophages (e.g., $LTB_4$), the complement cascade (e.g., $C5_a$), or bacteria can recruit neutrophils into the airways and the lung parenchyma. These chemotactic factors bind to specific receptors on the external surface of the neutrophils; this binding is associated with the influx of calcium into the cell, a reorganization of cytoskeletal proteins of the actin system, and directs the locomotion of the neutrophils (78). The chemotactic factors also increase the adhesive properties of the neutrophils and endothelial cells. The neutrophils migrate between endothelial cells of the capillaries into the interstitium and the alveolar spaces.

Once neutrophils are in the tissues they do not recirculate. Since they have little protein synthetic capacity, they are short-lived and die in a matter of hours to 1–2 days. The turnover of neutrophils can be increased (up to 10-fold) in the presence of infection or inflammation (79).

To appreciate the role of the neutrophil in lung injury, it is important to understand its role in the defense against micro-organisms and particulate matter. Particulates or micro-organisms with appropriate surface configurations interact with receptors on the neutrophil membrane to initiate phagocytosis, an active process in which cytoskeletal proteins of the actin system cause pseudopodia to form around the intruder (80). The phagocytic action of neutrophils is most effective with opsonization of the micro-organisms or the particulate matter. The major opsonins are in two of the IgG subclasses ($IgG_1$ and $IgG_3$).

During phagocytosis, cytoplasmic granules fuse with the membrane of the phagocytic vacuole and secrete hydrolytic enzymes. These have a protective role, if directed toward invading micro-organisms, but can be destructive if directed toward the tissues of the host. When host tissue is coated with immunoglobulin, injury to the host can occur when neutrophils try to phagocytize this combination (81). As the neutrophil attempts phagocytosis, an incomplete phagocytoic vacuole can be formed and the weaponry of the phagocyte can damage the host tissues rather than the invading micro-organisms (81). This response has been referred to as "frustrated phagocytosis" (82). Another situation of "frustrated phagocytosis" is in patients with cystic fibrosis (CF), in whom there is defective opsonining anti-*Pseudomonas* antibodies. Neutrophils in these patients cannot successfully accomplish phagocytosis of microcolonies of *Pseudomonas aeruginosa*, with resulting persistence of the micro-organisms.

Intracellular killing within neutrophils is accomplished by a variety of mechanisms such as oxygen radicals, cationic proteins, proteases, and lysosomal enzymes. The inflammatory process can be amplified by neutrophil proteases released during the phagocytic process; these proteases may cleave complement that can serve as chemoattractants for neutrophils (83).

There are two major types of neutrophil granules: primary or azurophil granules and the secondary or specific granules. The azurophilic granules are related to lysosomes, and contain a variety of acid hydrolases (beta-glucuronidase, beta-glycerophosphatase, alpha-mannosidase, cathepsin B, cathepsin D, N-acetyl-beta-glucosaminidase), proteases (cathepsin G, proteinase 3, collagenase), and several microbicidal components (myeloperoxidase, lysozyme, defensins, and bactericidal/permeability-increasing protein [BPI]) (83). These primary granules fuse with the phagosomes and do not generally release their contents extracellularly; however, "leakage" can occur. Antiproteinase screen offers defense against this "leakage." The specific granules contain lysozyme, lactoferrin, vitamin B-binding proteins, and cytochrome b (83). Table 7 gives a more detailed list of the contents of the neutrophil granules.

Neutrophil proteases have the potential for injuring elements of the extracellular matrix of the lungs such as collagen, elastin, and proteoglycan, if not inactivated when there is an excess unbalanced by the antiprotease protective mechanisms such as alpha-1-antitrypsin. The serine proteases (elastase and cathepsin G) found in the azurophilic granules and two metalloproteases (collagenase and gelatinase) found in the specific granules are the neutrophil enzymes with the most potential for tissue injury. Neutrophil elastase can cleave core proteins of protoglycan molecules in con-

TABLE 7 Contents of Neutrophil Granules

| | Primary granule | Secondary granule |
|---|---|---|
| Proteases | Elastase | |
| Neutral serine proteinases | Cathepsin G | |
| Metalloproteinases | Proteinase 3 | Collagenase |
| | | Gelatinase |
| Acid hydrolases | N-acetyl-β-glucosaminidase | |
| | Cathepsin B | |
| | Cathepsin D | |
| | β-Glucuronidase | |
| | β-Glycerophosphatase | |
| | α-Mannosidase | |
| Microbicidal enzymes | Myeloperoxidase | Lysozyme |
| | Lysozyme | |
| Other | Bactericidal/permeability-increasing protein | Lactoferrin |
| | Defensins | Vitamin $B_{12}$-binding proteins |
| | | Histaminase |
| | | Cytochrome b |
| | | fMet–Leu–Phe receptors |
| | | Laminin receptors |
| | | CR3 receptors |
| | | Plasminogen activator |
| | | Protein kinase C inhibitor |
| | | Complement activator |

*Source*: Modified from Abramson Ref. 83.

nective tissue and ground substance (84), and can attack host tissue proteins, glycoproteins, elastin (85), and collagen (type III and type IV) (86). Type III collagen is the major supporting component of the connective tissue and blood vessels in the lung. Type IV collagen is also important in maintaining the integrity of the epithelial and endothelial basement membranes. Fibronectin, the major cell adhesion molecule, which is a structural macromolecule, is also susceptible to neutrophil elastase (87). Elastase can hydrolyze plasma proteins, immunoglobulins, clotting factors, and complement components (88).

## Eosinophils

Eosinophils, derived from the bone marrow from a precursor stem cell, are regulated by lymphokines from T lymphocytes such as macrophage-colony stimulating factor (GM-CSF) and interleukins 5 (IL-5) and 3 (IL-3) (89–91). The life cycle of the eosinophil includes bone marrow, blood, and tissue phases. Eosinophils usually circulate for about 8 hr and then migrate into tissues; once in the tissues, the eosinophils usually live only for several days. GM-CSF has been shown to prolong the survival of human eosinophils in vitro (92,93). The migration of eosinophils into tissues is regulated by chemotactic factors, including those related to mast cells (ECF-A, $LTB_4$, and histamine), complement products, and lymphocyte–monocyte-derived products.

Receptors on the surface of eosinophils include IgG (Fc), IgA, IgE, and complement (C3 fragments) (94–96). Kay has studied the properties of the human eosinophil using monoclonal antibodies and flow cytometry to investigate the expression of receptors on normal-density and low-density eosinophils (94). There are three types of Fcγ receptors: Fcγ RI/CD 64, Fcγ RII/Cw 32, and Fcγ RIII/CD 16. The eosinophil expresses only Fcγ RII/CD w32 (94). The lack of expression of CD 16 is one major difference between eosinophils and neutrophils; this difference serves as a basis for differentiating these two cells by immunofluorescence. Monocytes bear both the Fcγ RII and Fcγ RIII receptors. Leukocyte adhesion glycoproteins, the integrins, are a family of three receptors (LFA-1, CR 3, and p150, 95). Each receptor has a alpha chain associated with a common beta chain (94). The leukocyte adhesion glycoproteins, LFA-1 alpha (CD 11a), CR3- alpha (CD 11b), and p150,95 alpha (CD 11c) and the common beta chain (CD 18), were expressed on the eosinophil and the neutrophil. Both eosinophils of low density and those of normal density did not differ in receptor expression (94).

Complement receptor (CR3) is the receptor for C3bi and has binding sites for other molecules (97). The p150,95 receptor binds C3bi and other ligands (98). LFA-1 acts with the intracellular adhesion molecule (ICAM-1) on other cells to facilitate intercellular adhesion (99).

Previous studies suggested that lower-density eosinophils are activated in terms of metabolic activity and IgG Fc and complement receptor expression (100–102). Many of these previous studies characterized IgG Fc and complement receptors on eosinophils using the rosette technique, which is a relatively imprecise method for the determination of receptor expression (94).

T-cell-derived products not only play a role in the maturation of the eosinophil but also affect the mature cell; GM-CSF and IL-5 activate mature eosinophils in regard to cytotoxicity and oxidative metabolism (93,103). IL-5 also causes hyperadherence of human eosinophils, but not neutrophils, through mechanisms dependent on CD 11/18 adhesion glycoproteins (104). The ligand for one of these adhesion glycoproteins (LFA-1) is ICAM-1 (105). Many other factors may influence the recruitment of eosinophils. The recruitment and activation of eosinophils are strongly inhibited by corticosteroids (106). Platelet-activating factor (PAF) is a potent eosinophil chemoattractant; however, it has a greater effect on neutrophil locomotion (107). The precise mechanisms responsible for local tissue eosinophilia are still largely unexplained.

The major components of the eosinophil include cell surface receptors for immunoglobulins and complement; lysophospholipase or Charcot–Leyden crystal protein, within the cell membrane and in the crystalloid free granules; and cationic proteins localized to specific granules (96). There are also enzymes able to generate PAF and leukotriene $C_4$ (96).

The eosinophil is characterized by distinctive granules with an affinity for staining with acid dyes such as eosin and by its unique electron microscopic appearance. Several types of granules are present within the eosinophil: distinctive specific or secondary granules with an electron-dense core (crystalline lattice structure) and an electron radiolucent matrix; primary granules that are round, uniformly electron-dense; and small granules containing acid phosphatase and arylsulfatase (96). Recent evidence has described another crystalloid-free granule that stains with an antibody to the Charcot-Leyden crystal protein (108). The granule-associated proteins of human eosinophils are outlined in Table 8. The most studied of the large crystalloid granules is the major basic protein (MBP), which is unique to the eosinophil and forms the electron-dense crystal-like core of the granule (96). There are three other cationic proteins contained in the large granules: eosinophil peroxidase (EPO), eosinophil-derived neurotoxin (EDN), and eosinophil cationic protein (ECP). EPO can stimulate histamine release from mast cells (EFN). The small granules of eosinophils contain arylsulfatase B and acid phosphatase. It has been shown that slow-reacting substance of anaphylaxis (SRS-A) is not inactivated by arylsulfatase, as was once proposed. Eosinophils also contain histaminase, which can degrade histamine released from mast cells. Phospholipase D, also found in eosinophils, cleaves platelet-activating factor. Lysophospholipase (membrane-associated enzyme of eosinophils) forms Charcot-Leyden crystals, which are found in the sputum of many asthmatic persons.

Eosinophils produce leukotrienes through metabolism of arachidonic acid; the predominant leukotriene produced by the eosinophils is LTC4, which induces bronchoconstriction, airway edema, and mucus production.

In the presence of eosinophilia, eosinophils may be activated with a change in morphology (vacuolization and alteration in the granules). Blood eosinophilia has been associated with the late-phase asthmatic response; there is an inverse correlation between the blood eosinophil counts and the degree of nonspecific bronchial hyperreactivity as measured by methacholine $PC_{20}$ (109). The number of hypodense eosinophils is elevated in patients with late-phase responses and better reflects the severity of asthma than does the total eosinophil count (110).

### Lymphocytes

Lymphocytes are found in the lung in the lymph nodes, lymphoid aggregates, bronchus-associated lymphoid tissue (BALT), and free in the lung parenchyma (alveoli or interstitium) (59,111). In the lung, the lymph nodes are located in the peribronchial region and are a part of the intrathoracic system of lymph nodes. Lymphoid aggregates predominate in the peripheral airways and contain a large number of plasmocytes. BALT has no identifiable germinal structure and contains more B lymphocytes than T lymphocytes. Free lymphocytes in lung parenchyma in normal subjects make up 7–10% of the inflammatory and immune effector cells present in BAL fluids (63). In normal individuals, the lymphocyte subpopulations within the lung parenchyma are similar to that of the peripheral blood: approximately 73% ± 5% are T lymphocytes, with only 6% activated (112). The activated T lymphocytes secrete lymphokines that regulate the traffic and function of other inflammatory and immune effector cells. Of the T cells, about 46% are T-helper cells and 25% are T-suppressor cells. Approximately 7% ± 1% of the alveolar lymphocytes are B lymphocytes, and only 0.1–0.3% of these actively secrete immunoglobulins (113).

### Mast Cells

Mast cells can be found in the airway lumen, bronchial epithelium, bronchial submucosa, and in the lung parenchyma. There are two types of human mast cells: tryptase-positive or T-mast cells, and mast cells that are

TABLE 8 Properties of Eosinophil Granule-Associated Proteins

| Name | Site | Activities |
| --- | --- | --- |
| Major basic protein | Core | Histamine release from basophils |
| Eosinophil cationic protein | Matrix | Neurotoxin potent<br>Helminthotoxin causes histamine release |
| Eosinophil-derived neurotoxin | Matrix | Neurotoxin |
| Eosinophil peroxidase | Matrix | Kills micro-organisms<br>Inactivates leukotriene damage to respiratory epithelium |

*Source*: Modified from Ref. 96.

both tryptase- and chymase-positive known as TC mast cells (114). Most bronchial mast cells contain tryptase as their major neutral protease and resemble mucosal rather than connective tissue type of mast cells found in rodents. The current evidence suggests that the early allergic asthmatic reaction is predominantly mast-cell-mediated, but the evidence that mast cells play a significant role in the late-phase response in asthma is debatable (89).

## LUNG INJURY IN ASTHMA

Over the last decade increasing evidence has demonstrated the role of airway inflammation as one of the major pathogenic mechanisms in asthma. In the past, most studies supporting the role of inflammation in asthma involved pulmonary function studies measuring changes in airway caliber in response to bronchial provocation by a variety of stimuli and the demonstration of chemical mediators produced by inflammatory cells. The allergen provocation model in humans (115) and animals (116) demonstrated increased bronchial responsiveness in relation to the late asthmatic reaction (LAR) that was associated in animals with histologic evidence of airway inflammation (117).

The airways are the major site of injury in asthma. Until recently, the pathologic evidence for inflammation in asthma was obtained from patients who died from asthma. The characteristic features reported in deaths from status asthmaticus included:

1. Mucus plugging of segmental bronchi and bronchioles
2. Epithelial cell damage
3. Mucous gland hyperplasia
4. Edema of submucosa
5. Inflammatory cell infiltration
6. Bronchial smooth muscle hypertrophy
7. Basement membrane

The basement membrane in patients with asthma has now been shown to be normal, with the appearance of thickening due to a dense deposition of collagen fibrils beneath the basement membrane (118). Infiltration of inflammatory cells was found in both the mucus plugs and in the airway mucosa (119–121). Infiltration of eosinophils and deposition of eosinophil products in and around the bronchial epithelium has been observed to be a prominent feature in patients with bronchial asthma (122). The histologic changes in the airways such as goblet cell hyperplasia, mucus plugging, and increase collagen deposition beneath the epithelial basement membrane were found to be similar in two children dying from status asthmaticus and two children who had open lung biopsies during remission of their asthma (123). The major difference noted was an increased number of submucosal eosinophils and more extensive denudation of epithelium in children with fatal asthma.

Through the use of fiberoptic bronchoscopy for BAL and bronchial biopsies in asthma, it has been possible to demonstrate that some of the inflammatory and structural changes observed in patients who died of asthma were also a feature of living patients with asthma (89). Laitinen et al. (124) demonstrated damage of airway epithelium in mild to moderate asthma, with ciliated cells being the most damaged cells. Ciliated cells were found to be swollen and interspaces widened on plain microscopic examination; on electron microscopic evaluation, vacuolization of the endoplasmic reticulum and loss of cilia were observed (124). Beasley et al. (125) compared ultrastructural examination of bronchial biopsies and BAL fluid from patients with mild asthma and found extensive deposition of collagen beneath the epithelial basement membrane, mast cells in various stages of degranulation, and mucosal infiltration by eosinophils with evidence of activation. A high degree of correlation between the number of epithelial cells in the lavage fluid and the degree of airway responsiveness to inhaled histamine was found in this study. Injury to the airway epithelium can lead to increased exposure of submucosal cells to allergen penetration and other inflammatory stimuli and can alter mucociliary clearance, contributing to airway obstruction from accumulation of airway secretions and mucus plugging. Disruption of the surface epithelium of airways and its tight junctions may lead to events of recruitment and activation of other inflammatory cells that can sustain the injury (126). Epithelial damage can also result in the loss of metalloendopeptidase that degrades tachykinins (127) and epithelial-derived relaxing factor (128).

Other resident cells of the airway, such as the sensory nerves, can play a significant role in the modulation of the inflammatory responses of the airways. Loss of this modulation can result in exaggerated inflammatory reactions to multiple inhaled irritants and other stimuli (129). Chemicals, dusts, and other irritants to the airways can cause release of mediators (neuropeptides) from sensory nerves, which then result in a constellation of responses called neurogenic inflammation (129). The effects of this type of inflammation include increased vascular permeability (130,131), neutrophil adhesion (131), mucus secretion (132), smooth muscle contraction (133), cholinergic neurotransmission (134), and cough (135,136). An enzyme, neutral endopeptidase, is present in airway epithelium, smooth muscle cells, and glands, as well as endothelium of postcapillary venules that can inactivate neuropeptides, serving as a autocrine regulator of neutropeptide action (129). Viral respiratory infections exaggerate neurogenic inflammatory responses of airway smooth muscle (137,138). Similar findings have been reported after inhalation of cigarette smoke (139). Human neutral endopeptidase has been cloned (140) and might be useful in the treatment of diseases in which there is release of sensory neuropeptides (129).

The inflammation in asthma shares features common to other types of inflammation: recruitment of inflammatory cells, increase in vascular congestion, and increase in tissue volume (edema). However, there are some unique features of inflammation in atopic patients with asthma: mast cell redistribution/activation, eosinophil recruitment/infiltration, fibroblast proliferation with subepithelial collagen deposition, selective T-helper cell activation, and mucus hypersecretion. Many cells and their products are involved in the inflammatory response in the airways in asthma and have the potential for airway injury: eosinophils, lymphocytes, mononuclear phagocytes, mast cells/basophils, neutrophils, and platelets (141). In patients with bronchial asthma, as in other inflammatory disorders of the airways, there are alterations in the epithelium and the epithelium is thought to contribute and modulate the inflammatory process. The bronchial epithelial cells may also play an active role in the defense of injury to the airways (141).

Strong evidence suggests that eosinophils are important proinflammatory cells in the pathogensis of asthma and asthma has been referred to as *chronic eosinophilic desquamative bronchitis* (89). The mechanism(s) for recruitment of eosinophils, in preference to the neutrophil, to the airway of asthmatic subjects is not completely understood. Eosinophils are very prominent cells in the histologic sections of patients dying from asthma (120,121). Mattoli et al. (142) examined the cellular and biochemical characteristics of patients with symptomatic nonallergic asthma and found increased number of epithelial cells, eosinophils, mast cells, and activated T lymphocytes, as well as an increased number of neutrophils. The biochemical analysis of BAL fluid in these patients revealed increased albumin, fibronectin, IL-1b, IL-6, and GMCSF (142). Using in situ hybridization techniques, mRNA for IL-5 has been identified in biopsies from patients with allergic asthma (143).

Gleich et al. have implicated the eosinophil as a potentially harmful inflammatory cell in asthma, contributing to the pathogenesis of asthma (109). Histopathologic changes induced by MBP, an eosinophil product, include shedding of the bronchial epithelium (109). Elevated levels of MBP have been found in the sputum of patients hospitalized for asthma (144). MBP has also been demonstrated by immunofluorescent studies to be localized in the respiratory epithelium in patients dying of asthma (109). Beasley et al. (125) found eosinophils in the lamina propria of patients with mild asthma and demonstrated morphologic features of activation in these cells. Wardlaw et al. demonstrated significant elevations in the marker of eosinophils and concentration of MBP in BAL fluid (145). The studies by Wardlaw et al. (145) and Lam et al. (146) suggest that bronchial hyperresponsiveness was associated with increased amounts of eosinophils and their products. Increased eosinophils and eosinophil products such as MBP have also been observed in BAL fluid during allergen-induced late-phase reactions (147,148).

The role of the T lymphocyte in the regulation and expression of the inflammatory reaction in asthma is an area of current interest and active investigation. T-cell-derived lymphokines, interleukins 4 and 5 (IL-4, IL-5), and gamma interferon are involved in the regulation of the production of IgE (149). Lymphokines are also important in the control of eosinophil production by the bone marrow (IL-5 and GMCSF) and in the regulation of mast cell differentiation (IL-3). Other lymphokines have chemotactic activity for neutrophils, eosinophils, basophils, and monocytes, and can activate and degranulate these effector cells (89,141).

T lymphocytes also play a role in the regulation of specific immune responses. Histiologic documentation of increased lymphocytes in patients with asthma has been found both in postmortem examination of the airways of patients dying with asthma (120,121) and increased "atypical intraepithelial lymphocytes" in the ultrastructural examination of bronchial biopsies from living subjects with mild asthma (118,150). Evidence of increased numbers of activated (IL-2R$^+$) T lymphocytes has been reported by Azzawi et al. with the analysis of the cellular infiltrate in atopic patients with asthma and controls, using monoclonal antibodies and immunocytochemical techniques (151). Natural killer activity, a nonspecific indicator of lymphocyte activation, has also been observed in the peripheral blood of patients with asthma (152). In patients with corticosteroid-responsive asthma and in normal controls, T lymphocytes can be inhibited by optimal concentrations of methylprednisolone in vitro (153).

Patients with chronic asthma whose disease is relatively refractory to corticosteroids have been found to have a relative decrease in the number of circulating T-suppressor (CD8$^+$) T lymphocytes (154). These patients had an abnormality of T-cell growth in vitro and their cell proliferation was not inhibited by optimal concentrations of methyl prednisolone (153). A defect in concanavalin-A-induced suppressor cell function has been reported in patients with asthma (155–158). Successful immunotherapy was associated with an increase in the relative number of T-suppressor (CD8$^+$) T cells (159).

Other evidence that T cells may be involved in the pathogenesis of asthma are the studies on status asthmaticus (acute severe asthma, ASA).

Corrigan et al. (160) demonstrated significant elevations of three surface proteins associated with T lymphocyte activation: the IL 2 receptor (IL-2 R), class II histocompatibility antigen (HLA-DR), and a late activation antigen (VLA-1) in ASA and compared their expression in control normals, patients with mild asthma, and patients with chronic obstructive pulmonary disease (COPD). The T lymphocytes were exclusively $CD4^+$ T-helper–inducer phenotype. The $CD8^+$ cells were devoid of IL-2R and VLA-1 in the asthmatic subjects and controls, and the expression of HLA-DR on these cells was not increased above that of controls (160). The percentage of $IL2R^+$ lymphocytes tended to decrease as patients improved clinically.

It is not possible at this time to define the precise role of all the infiltating inflammatory cells and the specific changes that occur in the resident cells of the airways and lungs in patients with asthma. The interaction of the complex cascade of events in airway injury and inflammation is being actively investigated. One hypothesis proposed for allergic asthma is an inappropriate response to antigen (89), in which the resident inflammatory cells of the airways become misdirected after exposure to an antigen. Another hypothesis suggests that the primary defect is in the epithelial cell, exposing the submucosal cells to increased antigen penetration and other inflammatory stimuli (89). The factors responsible for the persistence of the inflammatory response as well as the heterogeneity of asthma and the associated pathologic changes are not clearly understood.

## LUNG INJURY AND VIRAL INFECTIONS

Viral infections are an important cause of inflammatory disease of the respiratory tract. There is a high attack rate of viral pathogens during the first few years of life, when the alveoli of the lung are still developing during the early postnatal years and may be more vulnerable to injury. In contrast, the basic formation of the cartilaginous airways is complete at birth and additional divisions do not occur. Respiratory sequelae from inflammatory diseases of the airways, the pulmonary interstitium, or alveoli can be associated with variable abnormalities (clinical, physiological, histologic, and radiographic). The respiratory sequelae to inflammation can be classified by site of initial injury, type of causative agent, anatomical location of sequelae, and the nature of the sequelae (Table 9). The respiratory sequelae of inflammation vary in severity and frequency of occurrence due to various host factors (age, immunologic status, nutritional status, and genetics) and exposure to environmental agents that may cause additional airway or lung injury (e.g., passive cigarette smoking). Several disorders of the respiratory tract such as bronchiolitis, asthma, cystic fi-

TABLE 9 Classification of Respiratory Sequelae of Inflammation

| Site of Injury |
|---|
| *Airway* |
| Lower airways |
| Upper airways |
| *Lung* |
| Pulmonary parenchyma |
| Pulmonary interstitium |
| Causative agent |
| Viral respiratory agents (known or suspected) |
| Anatomical location of sequelae |
| Bronchi |
| Bronchioles |
| Pulmonary interstitum |
| Pulmonary parenchyma |
| Nature of respiratory sequelae |
| *Physiological* |
| Pulmonary function abnormalities |
| Hyperreactive airway disease |
| Clinically symptomatic |
| Abnormalities on pulmonary function studies only |
| *Roentgenographic* |
| Hyperlucent unilateral lung |
| Pulmonary fibrosis |
| Atelectasis |
| *Pathologic (Histologic)* |
| Bronchiolitis obliterans |
| Bronchiectasis |
| Interstitial lung disease (with or without fibrosis) |
| Diffuse alveolar damage |

brosis, and bronchopulmonary dysplasia share common features: inflammatory responses in the host play a role in the pathogenesis, respiratory sequelae to inflammation can occur, and the exacerbations can be related to viral respiratory tract infections and injury from viral infections may be associated with additional respiratory injury.

Epidemiologic studies suggest that viral lower respiratory tract infections in early childhood are associated with sequelae such as bronchial hyperreactivity and obstruction of the peripheral airways that may persist for variable periods of time. Studies of respiratory viruses and their relationship to airway hyperresponsiveness have also aided our understanding of airway hyperreactivity and asthma. Table 10 lists the major viral agents

TABLE 10 Major Viral Agents Associated with Respiratory Sequelae

| |
|---|
| DNA viruses |
| Adenovirus |
| Herpes virus |
| Cytomegalovirus |
| Epstein-Barr virus |
| Herpes simplex virus |
| Varicella zoster virus |
| RNA Viruses |
| Orthomyxovirus: influenza A and B |
| Paramyxovirus |
| Measles virus |
| Parainfluenza 1, 2, 3, 4 |
| Respiratory syncytial virus |
| Picornavirus |
| Coronavirus |
| Enterovirus |
| Coxsackie A |
| Echo |
| Rhinovirus |
| Coronavirus |

associated with respiratory sequelae. The course and frequency of respiratory sequelae may differ in the host impaired by congenital or acquired immunodeficiency or compromised from use of immunosuppressive agents. Although the major respiratory viruses affect the immunologically compromised host as well as the host with normal immune defenses, one important cause of viral respiratory infections in the immunologically impaired hosts is cytomegalovirus.

Adenoviruses are a complex group of viruses with several antigenic variants that produce a surface infection of respiratory mucous membranes with multiplication of virus in the mucosa. Necrotizing airway inflammation can occur as a sequela to adenovirus infection with necrosis to respiratory ciliated epithelium. The walls of the bronchi and bronchioles can become thickened due to inflammatory infiltrates or fibrosis. Destructive changes can also occur in the airways and pulmonary interstitium as a sequela to inflammation. Adenovirus types 1, 3, 4, 7, and 21 can cause severe and often fatal pneumonia, with a higher incidence of chronic lung disease in the survivors (161,162).

The common cold is the most commonly encountered viral respiratory infection in humans and may be due to various viral agents. Depending on age and exposure, causative viral agents include respiratory syncytial virus (RSV), adenovirus, parainfluenza viruses, influenza virus, coronaviruses, rhinoviruses, and other viruses (enteroviruses, measles viruses, and varicella).

Bronchiolitis can be associated with several respiratory viruses such as RSV, adenovirus, parainfluenza viruses, Influenza A and B viruses, measles, and rhinovirus. The RSV accounts for the majority of the cases of bronchiolitis, especially during epidemics. Bronchiolitis due to adenovirus is often severe and is associated with an increased incidence of respiratory sequelae, including bronchiolitis obliterans. In some series, up to 60% of children recovering from adenovirus respiratory infections develop chronic respiratory disease, characterized by recurrent infections and/or chronic reactive airway disease (163). Bronchiolitis obliterans can also follow infection with the influenza virus and measles virus. Animal studies have documented respiratory cell-mediated cytotoxicity in hamsters with parainfluenza virus type III infection (164). Dixon et al. (165) demonstrated in dogs the effect of respiratory infection on histamine-induced changes in lung mechanisms and irritant receptor discharge.

The pathologic changes of bronchiolitis involve damage to the bronchiolar epithelium with destruction of cilia, altering clearance mechanisms and leading to obstruction of the airways by the cellular debris and increased secretions. Several studies have reported recurrent wheezing following bronchiolitis. Even children with a single episode of RSV bronchiolitis in infancy were more predisposed to recurrent episodes of reactive airway disease (166). Gurwitz et al. (167) found that 57% of the children had bronchial hyperreactivity (as demonstrated by methacholine challenge) and 29% had a history of asthma or frequent wheezing in a 9–10 year follow-up of children after hospitalization for one episode of bronchiolitis.

Viral infections can act as antigens and stimulate virus-specific IgE antibody production, with the release of mediators of the immediate hypersensitivity reaction such as histamine and leukotrienes. Welliver et al. (168) were the first to show evidence that respiratory viruses can act as antigens and stimulate virus-specific IgE by demonstrating cell-bound IgE in exfoliated respiratory epithelium from infants and young children with RSV lower respiratory tract infections. These investigators found 75% RSV-specific IgE in the children with bronchiolitis during the acute phase of the respiratory illness. Three weeks later, nearly 100% of these infants and children with bronchiolitis or asthma had IgE bound to epithelial cells, in contrast to only 25% of those with upper respiratory tract infections or pneumonia without wheezing. In a subsequent report, Welliver et al. (169) quantitated the titers of IgE-specific RSV antibodies in this group of children and found that titers were higher in those with bronchiolitis or pneumonia with wheezing, in comparison to those with upper respiratory tract infections (URI) or pneumonia without wheezing. In a follow-up study of 38 infants with bronchiolitis under 6 months of age, Welliver et al. (170) monitored them from the onset of their initial episode of RSV bronchiolitis and found that 70% of the infants with higher titers of IgE-specific antibody had further documented wheezing, in comparison to 20% without RSV-specific IgE. Welliver et al. also found similar virus-specific IgE antibody response to parainfluenza virus infections in some children with croup and/or wheezing; nasal secretions contained greater amounts of histamine when airway obstruction accompanied clinical illness (171). Pre-existing airway hyperreactivity was found to be an important contributing factor in the development of wheezing or bronchiolitis at the time of parainfluenza respiratory infections (172).

Mechanisms other than the stimulation of virus-specific IgE can lead to airway hyperresponsiveness and include (172) airway injury with enhancement of airway cholinergic sensitivity, damage to airway epithelium with loss of epithelium-relaxing factor, damage to airway epithelium with loss of neutral endopeptidase, enzyme degradation of substance P, reduction in beta-adrenergic function, enhancement of basophil histamine release, and potentiation of the late-phase asthmatic response.

It is well documented that viral respiratory infections can precipitate wheezing in children known to have asthma (173–175). Viral respiratory infections can also trigger airway hyperresponsiveness in children with no previous history of asthma; the duration of airway hyperresponsiveness can also be beyond the time of the actual presence of the respiratory infection (176).

## NEONATAL LUNG INJURY

Bronchopulmonary dysplasia (BPD) is a respiratory disorder that is initiated by acute lung injury during the first 2 weeks of life; it is characterized by inflammation and results in chronic disease of the airways and lung parenchyma with a spectrum of respiratory sequelae related to unresolved lung injury. There is no universally accepted definition of this disorder and the diagnostic criteria vary. Hazinski (177) refers to BPD as a syndrome characterized by the triad of oxygen dependence, radiographic abnormalities, and respiratory symptoms in infants that persist beyond 28 days of postnatal life. O'Brodovich and Mellins specify the diagnostic criteria for BPD as (178) a respiratory disorder initiated by acute lung injury during the first 2 weeks of life; postnatal age of $> 28$ days; and significant clinical (tachypnea, retractions), radiologic (hyperinflation or cystic areas with fibrotic strands), and blood gas abnormalities (a $PaO_2 < 60$ mmHg or $pCO_2$ of 45 mmHg in ambient air at sea level). BPD was originally described by Northway et al. (179) in a group of premature infants with hyaline membrane disease (respiratory distress syndrome; RDS) that followed an atypical course. Currently, BPD includes pulmonary sequelae of RDS and other forms of neonatal acute lung injury (e.g., mechanical ventilation for recurrent apnea or poor respiratory effort due to prematurity and severe meconium aspiration). A follow-up study of survivors of BPD (mean, 8.4 years) showed persistent respiratory symptoms and pulmonary function abnormalities (180).

The incidence is higher in low-birth-weight infants, with a mean among premature infants of approximately 20% and a range of 2.4–68% (177). BPD occurs more frequently in surviving infants who weighed $<$ 1000 g (181). Avery et al. (182) reviewed 1,625 infants with birth weights of 700–1500 g in eight neonatal intensive care units (NICUs) and reported an incidence of BPD of 21–48%, with the incidence highly dependent on birth weight. Certain populations have a higher incidence of BPD. There is an increased incidence of HLA-A2 antigen in infants who develop BPD (183). There is also a higher frequency of BPD in infants with a family history of atopic diseases (184).

The causes of BPD include interacting factors of injury (from hyperoxia, barotrauma from mechanical ventilation with lung stretch, inflammation), growth factors and factors involved in injury repair, and immaturity of the lung (177). Other modifying factors include nutritional status, fluid overload, patent ductus arteriosus, genetic predisposition, and infection. The time of the lung injury is critical, with early injury leading to a greater disruption of structural integrity (177).

Although barotrauma alone has been incriminated in some cases of BPD, it is usually the combination of diffuse alveolar damage (DAD) from oxygen toxicity and barotrauma from the pressures used in mechanical ventilation or the effect of lung stretch that results in the lung injury. With longer exposure to hyperoxia there are detrimental effects including recruitment of neutrophils to the lung, necrosis of bronchiolar epithelium and type I alveolar cells with hyperplasia of type II alveolar cells, and the proliferation of fibroblasts in the lung interstitium. It is difficult to define the level of oxygen that is hyperoxic for the immature lung, since even 21% oxygen is relatively hyperoxic for the premature infant whose intrauterine oxygen tension is less than 40 mmHg. Oxygen-induced lung injury depends not only on the forced inspiratory oxygen ($FIO_2$) but also on the imbalance between oxidant production and oxidant destruction within specific lung cells (177). Although hyperoxia can affect all lung cells, the endothelial cell is especially vulnerable to injury; acute oxygen toxicity is associated with altered microvascular permeability and the development of acute pulmonary edema and acute necrotizing tracheobronchitis.

Evidence that inflammation is a factor in BPD is based on early histologic findings and on studies of tracheal effluent samples showing activated macrophages, elevated neutrophils, neutrophil elastase, and lipid inflammatory mediators such as the leukotrienes (185–188). Bronchoalveolar lavage fluid from infants who ultimately developed BPD had elevated levels of neutrophil–elastase and reduced or inactive antiprotease defenses (189–191). Ogden examined serial BAL fluid in infants with respiratory distress syndrome, infants with BPD, and normal controls; these studies suggested that pulmonary inflammation was associated with a prolonged neutrophil influx; an imbalance between neutrophil elastase and alpha-1-proteinase inhibitor may contribute to the lung damage and the development of chronic lung disease in infants with BPD (190). It has also been shown that growth factors and cytokines are produced at the site of inflammation and have potent vasoactive and mitogenic effects (191,192).

## LUNG INJURY FROM ENVIRONMENTAL IRRITANTS

The environment is a source for potential injury to the airways and lungs from a variety of agents that cause indoor pollution such as nitrous dioxide, ozone, wood smoke, and cigarette smoking. Only the latter will be discussed in any detail. Exposure to particulates and toxic gases has been associated with suppression of pulmonary host defenses. The majority of studies have evaluated the effects of tobacco smoke on pulmonary defenses (193). After exposure to tobacco smoke, alveolar macrophages have decreased phagocytosis and bactericidal activities. In animal studies the effect of wood smoke on alveolar macrophages appear to alter surface phenomena such as adherence and phagocytosis (194). The correlation of the animal studies with the effect of wood smoke on the pulmonary host defense mechanisms of children is not known.

### Nitrous Dioxide

There has been increasing concern over indoor exposure of children to nitrous dioxide ($NO_2$), both repeated short-term peak exposure and continued low exposure (195). Nitrous dioxide ($NO_2$) can be produced by the oxidation of nitrous oxide, when natural gas is used as a fuel for stoves and is burned in the atmosphere. In Great Britain, a group of school children living in homes with gas stoves were found to have higher rates of lower respiratory tract disease than those living in households with electric stoves. Homes with gas stoves had seven times higher concentrations of $NO_2$ than the households with electric stoves (196). Other studies in the United States reported $NO_2$ concentrations four times greater in kitchens with gas stoves than in households with electric stoves (197). In a study by Speizer et al., children under 2 years of age from households with gas stoves had a greater history of respiratory illness than those from homes with electric stoves; $NO_2$ concentrations were four to seven times higher in the homes with gas stoves (198).

## Cigarette Smoking

The effects of active cigarette smoking have been extensively studied in adults. Active smoking has been associated with both acute and chronic airflow obstruction, bronchial hyperreactivity (199,200), and alterations in pulmonary host defense mechanisms such as mucociliary clearance functions and activities of alveolar macrophages and neutrophils. Lavage studies from smokers show increased numbers of activated cells (macrophages and neutrophils), which actively secret proteases and oxidants (201).

Studies on the effect of cigarette smoke on the immune system in adults or in animal models of passive smoking demonstrate that nonspecific host defenses are depressed in the respiratory tract due to increased epithelial permeability (202) and impaired mucociliary transport (203,204). Inflammatory cell infiltrates have also been found in the interstitium and peribronchial areas (205,206). Cellular immunity is also adversely affected, with reduced number and activity of the natural killer cells (207,208). Smoking may decrease the elastase inhibitory capabilities of alpha-1 antitrypsin by inactivating it (209) and decreasing the synthesis of new elastin (210). Active cigarette smoking is also associated with increased levels of total IgE (211–213). The increase in IgE may represent increased sensitization to specific antigens that penetrate the damaged respiratory mucosa of smokers or a nonspecific activation of IgE production by tobacco and its by-products (214).

Although adolescents may sustain lung injury from active smoking, most of the airway and lung injury to pediatric patients probably results from exposure to passive smoking. Passive smoking is defined as the exposure of nonsmokers to the products of tobacco combustion in the environment. About 30% of adult Americans are active smokers (215). Although there are no definitive data regarding the number of children involuntarily exposed to tobacco smoking, a recent survey by the American Academy of Pediatrics estimated that 53–76% of homes in the United States contain at least one smoker (216). Thus, approximately 30 million American children may be chronically exposed to passive cigarette smoke. Within the exposed population, the degree of the exposure varies considerably due to a variety of factors: the number of cigarettes smoked indoors, the proximity of exposure, the type of ventilation during the indoor exposure, and the amount of time the child spends in the indoor environment (214).

There are two major components of environmental tobacco smoke: mainstream smoke and sidestream smoke. Mainstream smoke refers to the smoke drawn through the tobacco product, filtered by the smoker's lungs, and then exhaled by the smoker into the environment. Sidestream smoke is emitted from the burning end of the cigarette between puffs and enters the environment directly (217). In the average room during cigarette smoking, sidestream smoke comprises about 85% of the environmental smoke (217). Over 3,800 compounds have been identified in tobacco smoke; both mainstream and sidestream smoke contain measurable amounts of gaseous and particulate matter, many of which are known toxins (218). Table 11 shows that smoking in enclosed rooms can produce carbon monoxide levels greater than the national air quality standard of 9 ppm; even one smoker in an average home can significantly elevate indoor levels of suspended particulate matter (219). The amount of suspended particulates can rise as high as 700 μg/m³ in the presence of smokers (220). The particulates from passive cigarette smoke are very small, ranging from 0.1 to 1.0 μm in

TABLE 11 Selected Constituents of Environmental Tobacco Smoke (per Cigarette): Mainstream and Sidestream/Mainstream Ratio (SS/MS)

| Constituents | MS | SS/MS Ratio |
|---|---|---|
| Gases | | |
| Carbon monoxide | 10–23 mg | 2.5–4.7 |
| Carbon dioxide | 20–40 mg | 8–11 |
| Hydrogen cyanide | 400–500 μg | 0.1–0.25 |
| Ammonia | 50–130 μg | 40–170 |
| Acetic acid | 330–810 μg | 1.9–3.6 |
| Formic acid | 210–490 μg | 1.4–1.6 |
| Benzene | 12–48 μg | 10 |
| Dimethylnitrosamine | 10–40 ng | 20–100 |
| Nitrosopyrrolidine | 6–30 ng | 6–30 |
| Particulates | | |
| Total particulate | 15–40 mg | 1.3–1.9 |
| Tar | 5–40 mg | 2.1–3.4 |
| Nicotine | 1–2.5 mg | 2.6–3.3 |
| Phenol | 60–140 μg | 1.6–3.0 |
| Aniline | 360 ng | 30 |
| Benzo(a)pyrene | 20–40 ng | 2.5–3.5 |
| Benz(a)anthracene | 20–70 ng | 2–4 |
| 2-Naphthylamine | 1.7 ng | 30 |
| 4-Aminobiphenyl | 4–6 ng | 31 |

diameter, and up to 40% of those inhaled are deposited in the pulmonary compartment (221).

It is difficult to document and quantitate the exposure to passive smoking, since many of the previously used markers (i.e., carboxyhemoglobin and thiocyanate) were insensitive indicators of exposure to smoke. The short half-life (4 hr) of carboxyhemoglobin limits its usefulness in assessing chronic smoke exposure (222). Nicotine is a very sensitive and specific marker of smoke exposure, but has wide fluctuations in blood and urine levels in those exposed due to its short elimination half-life (1–2 hr) and its rapid and extensive tissue uptake (219). Cotinine, the major metabolite of nicotine, is a specific marker for tobacco, which has a long elimination half-life and can be quantitated at low levels in blood, urine, or saliva (223). The half-life of cotinine for infants is 37–160 hr, in contrast to 15–40 hr in adults (223). Several studies have shown a good correlation between urinary cotinine levels and the level of exposure to environmental tobacco smoke in all age groups (224–228).

Numerous studies of varying methodology (prospective [229–242], cross-sectional [243–246], and case–control [247–249]) from different geographic areas have evaluated the effect of parental smoking on the frequency and severity of acute respiratory illnesses in children; these studies have consistently demonstrated an increased frequency of lower respiratory tract illnesses and acute exacerbations of asthma in children of smokers compared to children of nonsmokers. The positive association of passive smoking to increased lower respiratory tract illnesses is more related to maternal smoking and stronger in infants and younger children. In general, the effect is dose related. The mechanisms for this association and the long-term consequences of the increased frequency of lower respiratory tract illnesses in infants and early childhood are not known.

A number of studies have investigated the relationship between parental smoking and chronic respiratory symptoms in children, such as cough and wheezing (236,240,250–258). Numerous studies, differing in methodology and geographic location, have documented increased frequency of cough and wheezing in young children exposed to chronic passive smoking in the environment. Children with a personal or family history of atopy appear to be particularly at risk from the adverse effects of smoking. The mechanism by which passive smoking is associated with these chronic respiratory symptoms remains unknown.

Many well-controlled studies have found small reductions in pulmonary function, decreased rates of lung growth, and increased nonspecific bronchial reactivity in children chronically exposed to parental smoking (195,246,259–262). These effects appear to be more pronounced in children with underlying reactive airway disease. Although the mechanisms for such adverse effects of passive smoking are not clearly defined, several possibilities include a direct toxic prenatal and/or postnatal effect on developing lung tissue with subsequent decreased growth and function; an increased incidence of respiratory infections in early life causing either direct damage to the lungs or a tendency to future reactive airways; and a smoke-induced chronic inflammatory state leading to alterations in pulmonary function and bronchial responsiveness (214).

Other studies demonstrating the effect of parents smoking on children include two large longitudinal studies assessing the impact of passive smoking on the long-term growth of children's lung function (263,264). Tager et al. (263) evaluated a cohort of 1,156 children (5–9 years of age) for 7 years and found that the expected increase in forced expiratory volume in 1 sec ($FEV_1$) over a 1, 2, and 5 year period was reduced by 10.7, 9.5, and 7.0%, respectively, in those children whose mothers smoked ($p = 0.015$). This study controlled for previous level of $FEV_1$ and change in height. The results in this study were independent of socioeconomic status. Another prospective study by Berkey et al. (264) of 7,834 children 6–10 years of age found similar adverse results from exposure to maternal smoking. In this latter study, after adjusting for socioeconomic status, maternal smoking was associated with a significant ($p = 0.05$) reduction in the $FEV_1$ growth rate, leading to a projected cumulative deficit of about 3% by young adulthood (264).

Two studies found no effect of parental smoking on the pulmonary functions of children (265,266). Differences in results of these two studies and previous studies probably relate to the degree of exposure to environmental tobacco smoke.

Murray and Morrison (267,268) evaluated over 200 asthmatic children between the ages of 7 and 17 and found a 13% reduction in $FEV_1$ and a 23% reduction of forced expiratory flow ($FEF_{25-75}\%$) associated with maternal, but not paternal, smoking ($p = < 0.005$). A consistent dose–response effect was also demonstrated in these studies (2). O'Connor et al. (259), using cold air inhalation challenge, also demonstrated increased nonspecific bronchoresponsiveness associated with maternal smoking in asthmatic children.

The long-term significance of lung function, particularly in those children without underlying asthma, remains uncertain; however, pulmonary mechanics seem also to be affected by smoke exposure at older ages as documented in acute exposure studies in adults.

## REFERENCES


1. Parsons PE, Worthan GS, Henson PM. Injury from inflammatory cells. In: Crystal RG, West JB, et al. (eds.), *The Lung: Scientific Foundations*, Raven Press, New York, 1991, pp. 1981–1992.
2. Larsen GL. Inflammation and cellular defences. In: Chernick V, Mellins R (eds.), *Basic Mechanisms of Pediatric Respiratory Disease: Cellular and Integrative*, BC Decker Inc, Philadelphia, 1991, pp. 347–360.
3. Barrett AJ. An introduction to proteases. In: Barrett AJ, Salvesen G (eds.), *Protease Inhibitors*, Elsevier, New York, 1986, pp. 1–22.
4. Barrett AJ, McDonald JK. *Mammalian Proteases*, Academic Press, New York, 1986.
5. Hubbard RC, Brantly ML, Crystal RG. Proteases. In: Crystal RG, West JB, et al. (eds.), *The Lung: Scientific Foundations*, Raven Press, New York, 1991, pp. 1763–1773.
6. Travis J, Salvesen GS. Human plasma proteinase inhibitors. *Annu Rev Biochem* 52:655–709, 1983.
7. Bruce MC, Poncz L, Klinger JD, et al. Biochemical and pathologic evidence for proteolytic destruction of lung connective tissue in cystic fibrosis. *Am Rev Respir Dis* 132:529–535, 1985.
8. Martodam RR, Baugh RJ, Twumasi DY, et al. A rapid procedure for the large scale purification of elastase and cathepsin G from human sputum. *Exp Biochem* 9:15–31, 1979.
9. Jackson AH, Hill SL, Afford SC, et al. Sputum sol-phase proteins and elastase activity in patients with cystic fibrosis. *Eur J Respir Dis* 65:114–124, 1984.
10. Stockley RA. Proteolytic enzymes, their inhibitors and lung diseases. *Clin Sci* 64:119–126, 1983.
11. Stockley RA, Hill SL, Morrison HM, et al. Elastolytic activity of sputum and its relation to purulence and to lung function in patients with bronchiectasis. *Thorax* 39:408–413, 1984.
12. Berger M, Sorensen RU, Tosi MF, et al. Complement receptor expression on neutrophils at an inflammatory site, the *Pseudomonas*-infected lung in cystic fibrosis. *J Clin Invest* 84:1304–1313, 1989.
13. Hubbard RC, Crystal RG. Antiproteases. In: Crystal RG, West JB, et al. (eds.), *The Lung: Scientific Foundations*, Raven Press, New York, 1991, pp. 1775–1787.
14. Knight CG. The characterization of enzyme inhibition. In: Barrett AJ, Salvesen G (eds.), *Protease Inhibitors*, Elsevier, New York, 1986, pp. 23–51.
15. Bieth JB. *In vivo* significance of kinetic constants of protein proteinase inhibitors. *Chem Med* 32:387–397, 1984.
16. Gadek JE, Fells GA, Zimmerman RL, et al. Antielastases of the human alveolar structures—implications for the proteases–antiprotease theory of emphysema. *J Clin Invest* 68:889–898, 1981.
17. Wewers MD, Casolaro MA, Crystal RG. Comparison of alpha-1 antitrypsin levels and antineutrophil elastase capacity of blood and lung in a patient

with the alpha-1 antitrypsin phenotype null-null before and during alpha-1 antitrypsin augmentation therapy. *Am Rev Respir Dis* 135:539–543, 1987.

18. Courtney M, Buchwalder A, Tessier LH, et al. High-level production of biologically active human alpha-1 antitrypsin in *Escherichia coli*. *Proc Natl Acad Sci USA* 81:669–673, 1984.
19. Rosenberg S, Barr PJ, Najarian RC, et al. Synthesis in yeast of a functional oxidation-resistant mutant of human alpha-1 antitrypsin. *Nature* 312:77–80, 1984.
20. Travis J, Owen M, George P, et al. Isolation and properties of recombinant DNA produced variants of human alpha-1 proteinase inhibitor. *J Biol Chem* 260:4384–4389, 1985.
21. Thompson RC, Ohlsson K. Isolation, properties, and complete amino acid sequence of human secretory leukocyte protease inhibitor, a potent inhibitor of leukocyte elastase. *Proc Natl Acad Sci USA* 83:6692–6696, 1986.
22. Halliwell B. Oxidants and human disease: some new concepts. *FASEB* 1:358–364, 1987.
23. Brunori M, Rotilio G. Biochemistry of oxygen radical species. *Methods Enzymol* 105:22–35, 1984.
24. Hazinski T, Kennedy KA. Pulmonary oxygen toxicity. In: Hilman BC, et al. (eds.), *Pediatric Respiratory Disease: Diagnosis and Treatment*, WB Saunders, Philadelphia, 1992.
25. Fisher AB. Intracellular production of oxygen-derived free radicals. In: Halliwell B (ed.), *Oxygen Radicals and Tissue Injury*, Upjohn Symposium, Bethesda. FASEB, 9–19, 1987.
26. Tate RM, Vanbenthuysen KM, Shasby DM, et al. Oxygen-radical-mediated permeability edema and vasoconstriction in isolated perfused rabbit lungs. *Am Rev Respir Dis* 126:802–806, 1982.
27. Elliott SJ, Schilling WP. Carmustine augments the effects of tert-butyl hydroperoxide in calcium signalling in cultured pulmonary artery endothelial cells. *J Biol Chem* 265:103–107, 1990.
28. Starke PE, Oliver CN, Stadtman ER. Modification of hepatic proteins in rats exposed to high oxygen concentration. *FASEB J* 1:36–39, 1987.
29. Deneke SM, Gershoff SN, Fanburg BL. Potentiation of oxygen toxicity in rats by dietary protein or amino acid deficiency. *J Appl Physiol* 54:147–151, 1983.
30. Reiter R, Burk RF. Effect of oxygen tension on the generation of alkanes and malondialdehyde by peroxidizing rat liver microsomes. *Biochem Pharmacol* 36:925–929, 1987.
31. Minchin RF, Boyd MR. Localization of metabolic activation and deactivation systems in the lung: significance to the pulmonary toxicity of xenobiotics. *Annu Rev Pharmacol Toxicol* 23:217–238, 1983.
32. Tate RM, Morris HG, Schroeder WR, et al. Oxygen metabolites stimulate thromboxane production and vasoconstriction in isolated saline-perfused rabbit lungs. *J Clin Invest* 74:608–613, 1984.
33. Freeman BA, Crapo JD. Biology of disease: free radicals and tissue injury. *Lab Invest* 47:412–426, 1982.

34. Saugstad OD. Oxygen radicals and pulmonary damage. *Pediatr Pulmonol* 1(3):167–177, 1985.
35. Ward PA, Till GO, Kunhel R, et al. Evidence for role of hydroxyl radical in complement and neutrophil-dependent tissue injury. *J Clin Invest* 72:789–801, 1983.
36. Johnson KJ, Ward PA. Role of oxygen metabolites in immune complex injury of lung. *J Immunol* 126:2365–2369, 1981.
37. Weiss SJ, Ward PA. Immune complex-induced generation of oxygen metabolites by human neutrophils. *J Immunol* 129:309–313, 1982.
38. Ward PA. Role of toxic oxygen products from phagocytic cells in tissue injury. *Adv Shock Res* 10:27–34, 1983.
39. Hammerschmidt DE, Weaver LJ, Hudson LD, et al. Association of complement activation and elevated plasma C5a with adult respiratory distress syndrome. *Lancet* 1:947–949, 1980.
40. Hammerschmidt DE, Jacob HS. The stimulated granulocyte as a source of toxic oxygen compounds in tissue injury. In: Autor AP (ed.), *Pathology of Oxygen*, Academic Press, New York, 1982, pp. 59–73.
41. Turrens JF, Freeman BA, Crapo JD. Hyperoxia increases $H_2O_2$ release by lung mitochondria and microsomes. *Arch Biochem Biophys* 217:411–421, 1982.
42. Forman HJ, Nelson J, Fisher AB. Rat alveolar macrophages require NADPH for superoxide production in the respiratory burst. Effect of NADPH depletion by paraquat. *J Biol Chem* 255:9879–9883, 1980.
43. Granger DN, Hollwarth MA, Parks DA. Ischemia reperfusion injury: role of oxygen derived radicals. *Acta Physiol Scand* 126:Suppl 548:47–63, 1986.
44. Kalyanaraman B. Free radicals from catecholamine hormones, neuromelanins, and neurotoxins. In: Miguel J, Quintanilha AT, Weber H (eds.), *Handbook of Free Radicals and Antioxidants in Biomedicine*, CRC Press, Boca Raton, FL, 1989, pp. 147–159.
45. Halliwell B, Gutteridge JMC. *Free Radicals in Biology and Medicine*. Clarendon Press, Oxford, 1985.
46. Fridovich I. Superoxide dismutases. *Annu Rev Biochem* 44:147–159, 1975.
47. Halliwell B, Gutteridge JMC. The importance of free radicals and catalytic metal ions in human disease. *Mol Aspects Med* 8:89–193, 1985.
48. Jamieson D, Chance B, Cadenas E, et al. The relation of free radical production to hyperoxia. *Annu Rev Physiol* 48:703–719, 1986.
49. Kellogg EW, Fridovich I. Liposome oxidation and erythrocyte lysis by enzymatically generated superoxide and hydrogen peroxide. *J Biol Chem* 252:6721–6728, 1977.
50. Sosenko IRS, Frank L. Oxidants and antioxidants. In: Chernick V, Mellins R (eds.), *Basic Mechanisms of Pediatric Respiratory Disease: Cellular and Integrative*, BC Decker, Inc., Philadelphia, 1991, pp. 315–327.
51. Heffner JE, Repine JE. Antioxidants and the lung. In: Crystal RG, West JB, et al. (eds.), *The Lung: Scientific Foundations*. Raven Press, New York, 1991, pp. 1811–1820.

52. Karlsson K, Marklund SL. Plasma clearance of human extracellular superoxide dismutase C in rabbits. *J Clin Invest* 82:762–766, 1988.
53. Burton GW, Ingold KV. Autooxidation of biological molecules. 1. The antioxidant activity of vitamin E and related chain-breaking phenolic antioxidants *in vitro*. *J Am Chem Soc* 103:6472–6477, 1981.
54. McCay PB. Vitamin E: interactions with free radicals and ascorbate. *Annu Rev Nutr* 5:323–340, 1985.
55. Burton GW, Ingold KU. Beta-carotene: an unusual type of lipid antioxidant. *Science* 224:569–573, 1984.
56. Heffner JE, Repine JE. Pulmonary strategies of antioxidant defense. *Am Rev Respir Dis* 140:531–554, 1989.
57. Ketterer B. Detoxication reactions of glutathione and glutathione transferases. *Xenobiotica* 16:957–973, 1986.
58. Gutteridge JMC, Stocks J. Ceruloplasmin: physiological and pathological perspectives. *CRC Crit Rev Clin Lab Sci* 14:257–329, 1981.
59. Murray JF. In: *The Normal Lung: The Basis for Diagnosis and Treatment of Pulmonary Disease*, W.B. Saunders, Philadelphia, 1986.
60. Meyrick B, Reid L. Ultrastructure of cells in the human bronchial submucosal glands. *J Anat* 107:281–299, 1970.
61. Crystal RG. Alveolar macrophages In: Crystal RG, West JB, et al. (eds.), *The Lung: Scientific Foundations*, Raven Press, New York, 1991, pp. 527–538.
62. Crapo JD, Barry BE, Gehr P, et al. Cell member and characteristics of the normal human lung. *Am Rev Respir Dis* 125:332–337, 1982.
63. Murphy S, Florman AL. Lung defenses against infection. A clinical correlation. *Pediatrics* 72:1–15, 1983.
64. Werb Z, Banda MJ, Jones PA. Degradation of connective tissue matrices by macrophages. I. Proteolysis of elastin, glycoproteins, and collagen by proteinases isolated from macrophages. *J Exp Med* 152:1340–1357, 1980.
65. Chapman HA, Stone OL, Vavrin Z. Degradation of fibrin and elastin by intact human alveolar macrophages *in vitro*. *J Clin Invest* 73:806–815, 1984.
66. Senior RM, Campbell EJ, Landis JA, et al. Elastase of U-937 monocyte-like cells. Comparisons with elastases derived from human monocytes and neutrophils and murine macrophage-like cells. *J Clin Invest* 69:384–393, 1982.
67. Lavi G, Zucker-Franklin D, Franklin EC. Elastase-type proteases on the surface of human blood monocytes: possible role in amyloid formation. *J Immunol* 125:175–180, 1980.
68. Janoff A. Elastases and emphysema. *Am Rev Respir Dis* 132:417–433, 1985.
69. Werb Z, Gordon S. Elastase secretion by stimulated macrophages. *J Exp Med* 142:361–377, 1975.
70. Banda MJ, Werb Z. Normal macrophage elastase. Purification and characterization as a metalloproteinase. *Biochem J* 193:589–605, 1981.
71. Joseph M, Tonnel AB, Capron A, et al. Enzyme release and superoxide anion production by human alveolar macrophages stimulated with immunoglobulin E. *Clin Exp Immunol* 40:416–422, 1980.

72. Martin TR, Altman LC, Albert RK, et al. Leukotriene $B_4$ production by the human alveolar macrophage: a potential mechanism for amplifying inflammation in the lung. *Am Rev Respir Dis* 129:106–111, 1984.
73. Bitterman PB, Rennard SI, Hunninghake GW, et al. Human alveolar macrophage growth factor for fibroblasts: regulation and partial characterization. *J Clin Invest* 70:806–822, 1982.
74. Rennard SI, Hunninghake GW, Bitterman PB, et al. Production of fibronectin by human alveolar macrophage: mechanisms for the recruitment of fibroblasts to sites of tissue injury in interstitial lung disease. *Proc Natl Acad Sci USA* 78:7147–7151, 1981.
75. Littman BH, Ruddy S. Production of the second component of complement by human monocytes: stimulation by antigen-activated lymphocytes on the lymphokines. *J Exp Med* 145:1344, 1977.
76. Nathen CF, Murray HW, Cohn ZA. The macrophage as an effector cell. *N Engl J Med* 303:622, 1980.
77. Damiano VV, Cohen AB, Tsang A, et al. A morphologic study of the influx of neutrophils into dog lung alveoli after lavage with sterile saline. *Am J Pathol* 100:349–364, 1980.
78. Reynolds HY. Lung inflammation: role of endogenous chemotactic factors in attracting polymorphonuclear granulocytes. *Am Rev Respir Dis* 127:S16–S25, 1983.
79. Cohen AB, Rossi M. Neutrophils in normal lungs. *Am Rev Respir Dis* 127:S3–S9, 1983.
80. Hensen PM. The immunological release of constituents from neutrophil leukocytes. *J Immunol* 107:1525–1527, 1971.
81. Hammerschmidt DE. The stimulated granulocyte as an effector of immune injury (or, the fickle phagocyte: friend or foe?). *J Miss State Med Assoc* 22:280–284, 1981.
82. Hammerschmidt DE. Leukocytes in lung injury. *Chest* 83:16S–19S, 1983.
83. Abramson SL, Malech H, Gallen JI. Neutrophils. In: Crystal RG, West JB, et al. (eds.), *The Lung: Scientific Foundations*, Raven Press, New York, 1991, pp. 553–563.
84. Kaiser H, Greenwald RA, Feinstein G, et al. Degradation of cartilage proteoglycan by human leukocyte granule neutral proteases. *J Clin Invest* 57:625–632, 1976.
85. Janoff A, Scherer J. Mediators of inflammation in leukocyte lysosomes. IX. Elastinolytic activity in granules of human polymorphonuclear leukocytes. *J Exp Med* 128:1137–1155, 1968.
86. Mainardi CL, Hasty DL, Sayer JM, et al. Specific cleavage of human type III collagen by human polymorphonuclear leukocyte elastase. *J Biol Chem* 255:12006–12010, 1980.
87. McDonald JA, Keley DG. Degradation of fibronectin by human leukocyte elastase. Release of biologically active fragments. *J Biol Chem* 255:8848–8858, 1980.
88. Havemann K, Gramse M. Physiology and pathophysiology of neutral proteinases of human granulocytes. *Adv Exp Med* 167:1–20, 1984.

89. Kay AB. Asthma and inflammation. *J Allergy Clin Immunol* 87(5):893–911, 1991.
90. Warren DJ, Moore MAS. Synergism among interleukin 1, interleukin 3, and interleukin 5 in the production of eosinophils from primitive hemopoietic stem cells. *J Immunol* 140:94–99, 1988.
91. Clutterbuck EJ, Hirst EMA, Sanderson CJ. Human interleukin-5 (IL-5) regulates the production of eosinophils in human bone marrow cultures: comparison and interaction with IL-1, IL-3, IL-6 and GMCSF. *Blood* 73:1504–1512, 1989.
92. Lopez AF, Williamson J, Gamble JR, et al. Recombinant human granulocyte/macrophage colony-stimulating factor stimulates *in vitro* mature neutrophil and eosinophil function, surface receptor expression and survival. *J Clin Invest* 78:1220–1228, 1986.
93. Lopez AF, Sanderson CJ, Gamble JR, et al. Recombinant human interleukin-5 is a selective activator of human eosinophil function. *J Exp Med* 167:219–224, 1988.
94. Kay AB. Modulation of eosinophil function *in vitro*. *Clin Exp Allergy* 20(Suppl. 4):31–34, 1990.
95. Hartnell A, Moqbel R, Walsh GM, et al. Fc-gamma and CD11/CD18 receptor expression on normal density and low density human eosinophils. *Immunology* 69:264–270, 1990.
96. Gleich GJ, Adolphson CR. Eosinophils. In: Crystal RG, West JB, et al. (eds.), *The Lung: Scientific Foundations*, Raven Press, New York, 1991, pp. 581–590.
97. Ross GD, Cain JA, Lachmann PJ. Membrane complement receptor type three (CR3) has lectin-like properties analogous to bovine conglutinin and functions as a receptor for zymosan and rabbit erythocytes as well as a receptor for iC3b. *J Immunol* 134:3307–3315, 1985.
98. Myones BL, Diazell JG, Hogg N, et al. Neutrophil and monocyte cell surface p150,95 has iC3b-receptor (CR4) activity resembling CR3. *J Clin Invest* 82:640–651, 1988.
99. Dustin ML, Rothlein R, Bhan AK, et al. Induction by IL-1 and interferon-gamma: tissue distribution, biochemistry and function of a natural adherence molecule (ICAM-1). *J Immunol* 137:245–254, 1986.
100. Bass DA, Grover WH, Lewis JC, et al. Comparison of eosinophils from normals and patients with eosinophilia. *J Clin Invest* 66:1558–1564, 1980.
101. Pincus SH, Schooley WR, DiNapoli M, et al. Metabolic heterogeneity of eosinophils from normal and hypereosinophilic patients. *Blood* 58:1175–1181, 1981.
102. Winqvist I, Olofsson T, Majpersson A, et al. Altered density, metabolism and surface receptors of eosinophils in eosinophilia. *Immunology* 47:531–539, 1982.
103. Yamaguchi Y, Hayashi Y, Sugama Y, et al. Highly purified murine interleukin-5 (IL-5) stimulates eosinophil function and prolongs *in vitro* survival: IL-5 is an eosinophil chemotactic factor. *J Exp Med* 167:1737–1742, 1988.
104. Walsh GM, Hartnell A, Wardlaw AM, et al. IL-5 enhances the *in vitro*

adhesion of human eosinophils but not neutrophils, in a leukocyte integrin (CD11/18)-dependent manner. *Immunology* 71:258–265, 1990.
105. Rothlein R, Dustin ML, Marlin SD, et al. A human intercellular adhesion molecule (ICAM-1) distinct from LFA-1. *J Immunol* 137:1270–1274, 1986.
106. McFadden ER Jr. Corticosteroids and cromolyn sodium in modulators of airway inflammation. *Chest* 94:181–184, 1988.
107. Wardlaw AJ, Moqbel R, Cromwell O, et al. Platelet activating factor. A potent chemotactic and chemokinetic factor for human eosinophils. *J Clin Invest* 78:1701–1706, 1986.
108. Dvorak AM, Letourneau L, Login GR, et al. Ultrastructural localization of the Charcot-Leyden crystal protein (lysophospholipase) to a distinct crystalloid-free granule population in mature human eosinophils. *Blood* 72:150–158, 1988.
109. Filley WV, Holley KE, Kephart GM, et al. Identification by immunofluorescence of the eosinophil granule major basic protein in lung tissues of patients with bronchial asthma. *Lancet* 2:11–16, 1982.
110. Frick WE, Sedgwick JB, Busse WW. The appearance of hypodense eosinophils in antigen-dependent late phase asthma. *Am Rev Respir Dis* 139:1401–1406, 1989.
111. Gee JBL, Smith GJW. Lung cells and disease. *Basics RD* 9:42, 1981.
112. Hunninghake GW, Fulmer JD, Young RC, et al. Localization of the immune response in sarcoidosis. *Am Rev Respir Dis* 120:49, 1979.
113. Lawrence EC, Martin RR, Blaese RM, et al. Increased bronchoalveolar IgG-secreting cells in interstitial lung disease. *N Engl J Med* 302:1186, 1980.
114. Irani A-M, Schwartz LB. Mast cell heterogeneity. *Clin Exp Allergy* 19:143–155, 1989.
115. Cartier A, Thomson NC, Frith PA, et al. Allergen-induced increase in bronchial responsiveness to histamine: relationship to the late asthmatic response and change in airway caliber. *J Allergy Clin Immunol* 70:170–177, 1982.
116. Chung KF, Becker AB, Lazarus SC, et al. Antigen-induced airway hyperresponsiveness and pulmonary inflammation in allergic dogs. *J Appl Physiol* 58:1347–1353, 1985.
117. Hutson PA, Church MK, Clay TP, et al. Early and late-phase bronchoconstriction after allergen challenge of nonanesthetized guinea pigs. I. The association of disordered airway physiology to leukocyte infiltration. *Am Rev Respir Dis* 137:548–557, 1988.
118. Roche WR, Beasley R, Williams JH, et al. Subepithelial fibrosis in the bronchi of asthmatics. *Lancet* 1:520–524, 1989.
119. Houston JC, De Navasquez S, Trounce JR. A clinical and pathological study of fatal cases of status asthmaticus. *Thorax* 8:207–213, 1953.
120. Dunnill MS. The pathology of asthma with special reference to changes in the bronchial mucosa. *J Clin Pathol* 13:27–33, 1960.
121. Dunnill MS, Massarella GR, Anderson JA. A comparison of the quantitative anatomy of the bronchi in normal subjects, in status asthmaticus, in chronic bronchitis, and in emphysema. *Thorax* 24:176–179, 1969.
122. Filley WV, Holley KE, Kephart GM, et al. Identification by immunoflu-

orescence of eosinophil granule major basic protein in lung tissues of patients with bronchial asthma. *Lancet* 2:11–16, 1982.
123. Cutz F, Levison H, Cooper DM. Ultrastructure of airways in children with asthma. *Histopathology* 2:407–421, 1978.
124. Laitinen LA, Heino M, Laitinen A, et al. Damage of the airway epithelium and bronchial reactivity in patients with asthma. *Am Rev Respir Dis* 131:599–606, 1985.
125. Beasley R, Roche WR, Roberts JA, et al. Cellular events in the bronchi in mild asthma and after bronchial provocation. *Am Rev Respir Dis* 139:806–817, 1989.
126. Hulbert WM, McLean T, Hogg JC. The effect of acute airway inflammation on bronchial reactivity in guinea pigs. *Am Rev Respir Dis* 132:7–11, 1985.
127. Borson DB, Brokaw JJ, Sekizawa K, et al. Neutral endopeptidase and neurogenic inflammation in rats with respiratory infections. *J Appl Physiol* 66: 2653–2658, 1989.
128. Vanhoutte PM. Epithelium-derived relaxing factor(s) and bronchial reactivity. *J Allergy Clin Immunol* 83:855–861, 1989.
129. Nadel JA. Mechanisms of inflammation and potential role in the pathogenesis of asthma. *Allergy Proc* 12(2):85–88, 1991.
130. Saria A, Lundberg JM, Skofitsch G, et al. Vascular protein leakage in various tissues induced by substance P, capsaicin, bradykinin, serotinin, histamine, and by antigen challenge. *Naunyn Schmiedebergs Arch Pharmacol* 324:212–218, 1983.
131. Umerno E, Nadel JA, Huang HT, et al. Inhibition of neutral endopepidase potentiates neurogenic inflammation in the rat trachea. *J Appl Physiol* 66: 2647–2652, 1989.
132. Borson DH, Corrales R, Varsano S, et al. Enkephalinase inhibitors potentiate substance P-induced secretion of "$SO_4$-macromolecules from ferret trachea. *Exp Lung Res* 12:21–36, 1987.
133. Lundberg JM, Martling C-R, Saria A. Substance P and capsaicin-induced contraction of human bronchi. *Acta Physiol Scand* 19:49–53, 1983.
134. Tanaka DT, Grunstein MM. Mechanisms of substance-P induced contraction of rabbit airway smooth muscle. *J Appl Physiol* 57:1551–1557, 1984.
135. Kohrogi H, Graf PD, Sekizawa K, et al. Neutral endopeptidase inhibitors potentiate substance P- and capsaicin-induced cough in awake guinea pigs. *J Clin Invest* 82:2063–2068, 1988.
136. Kohrogi H, Nadel JA, Malfroy B, et al. Recombinant human enkephalinase (neutral endopeptidase) prevents cough induced by tachykinins in awake guinea pigs. *J Clin Invest* 84:781–786, 1989.
137. Jacoby DB, Tamaoki J, Borson DB, et al. Influenza infection causes airway hyperresponsiveness by decreasing enkephalinase. *J Appl Physiol* 64:2653–2658, 1988.
138. Dusser DJ, Jacoby DB, Djokic TD, et al. Virus induced airway hyperresponsiveness to tachykinins: role of neutral endopeptidase. *J Appl Physiol* 67:1504–1511, 1989.
139. Dusser DJ, Djokic TD, Borson DB, et al. Cigarette smoke induces bron-

choconstrictor hyperresponsiveness to substance P and inactivates airway neutral endopeptidase in the guinea pig. Possible role of free radicals. *J Clin Invest* 84:900–906, 1989.
140. Malfroy B, Kuang WJ, Seeburg PH, et al. Molecular cloning and amino acid sequence of human enkephalinase (neutral endopeptidase). *FLBS Lett* 229:206–210, 1988.
141. Kay AB, Durham SR. T-lymphocytes, allergy and asthma. *Clin Exp Allergy* 21(suppl 1):17–21, 1991.
142. Mattoli S, Mattoso VL, Soloperto M, et al. Cellular and biochemical characteristics of bronchoalveolar lavage fluid in symptomatic nonallergic asthma. *J Allergy Clin Immunol* 87:794–802, 1991.
143. Hamid Q, Azzawi M, Moqbel R, et al. Expression of mRNA for interleukin 5 in mucosal bronchial biopsies from asthma. In: *Proceedings of 1990 Meeting of the Collegium Internationale Allergologieuum*, Basel, Karger, 1990.
144. Dor J, Ackerman SJ, Gleich G. Charcot-Leyden crystal protein and eosinophil granule major basic protein in sputum of patients with respiratory disease. *Am Rev Respir Dis* 130:1072–1077, 1984.
145. Wardlaw AJ, Dunnette S, Gleich GJ, et al. Eosinophils and mast cells in bronchoalveolar lavage in mild asthma: relationship to bronchial hyperreactivity. *Am Rev Respir Dis* 137:62–69, 1988.
146. Lam S, LeRiche J, Phillips D, et al. Cellular and protein changes in bronchial lavage fluid after late asthmatic reaction in patients with red cedar asthma. *J Allergy Clin Immunol* 80:44–50, 1987.
147. Diaz P, Gonzalez MC, Galleguillos FR, et al. Leukocytes and mediators in bronchoalveolar lavage during allergen-induced late-phase asthmatic reactions. *Am Rev Respir Dis* 139:1383–1389, 1989.
148. de Monchy JG, Kauffman HF, Venge P, et al. Bronchoalveolar eosinophils during allergen-induced late asthmatic reactions. *Am Rev Respir Dis* 131:373–376, 1985.
149. Leung DYM, Geha RS. Regulation of the human IgE antibody response. *Int Rev Immunol* 2:75–91, 1987.
150. Jeffery PK, Nelson FC, Wardlaw AJ, et al. Quantitative analysis of bronchial biopsies in asthma. *Am Rev Respir Dis* 135:A316, 1987.
151. Azzawi M, Bradley B, Jeffery PK, et al. Identification of activated T-lymphocytes and eosinophils in bronchial biopsies in stable atopic asthma. *Am Rev Respir Dis* 142:1407–1413, 1990.
152. Timonen T, Stenius-Aarnala B. Natural killer cell activity in asthma. *Clin Exp Immunol* 59:85–90, 1985.
153. Pozansky MC, Gordon ACH, Douglas JG. Resistance to methylprednisolone in cultures of blood mononuclear cells from glucocorticoid-resistance asthmatic patients. *Clin Sci* 67:639–645, 1984.
154. Pozansky MC, Gordon ACH, Grant IWB, et al. A cellular abnormality in glucocorticoid resistant asthma. *Clin Exp Immunol* 61:135–142, 1985.
155. Haper TB, Gaumer HR, Waring W, et al. A comparison of cell-mediated immunity and suppressor T cell function in asthmatic and normal children. *Clin Allergy* 10:555–563, 1980.

156. Rola-Pleszcynski M, Blanchard R. Suppressor cell function in respiratory allergy. *Int Arch Allergy Appl Immunol* 64:361–370, 1981.
157. Rivlin J, Kuperman O, Freier S, et al. Suppressor T-lymphocyte activity in wheezy children with and without treatment by hyposensitization. *Clin Allergy* 11:353–356, 1981.
158. Hwang KC, Fikrig SM, Friedman HM, et al. Deficient concanavalin A-induced suppressor-cell activity in patients with bronchial asthma, allergic rhinitis, and atopic dermatitis. *Clin Allergy* 15:67–72, 1985.
159. Rocklin RE, Sheffer AL, Greineder DR, et al. Generation of antigen-specific suppressor cells during allergy desensitization. *N Engl J Med* 310:1349–1352, 1984.
160. Corrigan CJ, Hartnell A, Kay AB. T-lymphocyte activation in acute severe asthma. *Lancet* 1:1129–1132, 1988.
161. James AG, Lang WR, Liang AY, et al. Adenovirus type 21 bronchopneumonia in infants and young children. *J Pediatr* 95:530–533, 1979.
162. Similä S, Linna O, Lanning P, et al. Chronic lung damage caused by adenovirus type 7: a ten-year follow-up study. *Chest* 80(2):127–131, 1981.
163. Rooney JC, Williams HE. The relationship between proved viral bronchiolitis and subsequent wheezing. *J Pediatr* 79:744, 1971.
164. Henderson FW. Pulmonary cell-mediated cytotoxicity in hamsters with parainfluenza virus type 3 pneumonia. *Am Rev Respir Dis* 120:41, 1979.
165. Dixon M, Jackson DM, Richards IM. The effect of a respiratory tract infection on histamine-induced changes in lung mechanism and irritant receptor discharge in dogs. *Am Rev Respir Dis* 120:843, 1979.
166. Eisen A, Bacal HL. The relationship of acute viral bronchiolitis to bronchial asthma. *Pediatrics* 31:859, 1963.
167. Gurwitz D, Mindorff C, et al. Increased incidence of bronchial reactivity in children with a history of bronchiolitis. *J Pediatr* 98:551, 1981.
168. Kattan M, Levison H, Bryan AC. Lung mechanics in asymptomatic children after bronchiolitis. *Am Rev Respir Dis* (Suppl) 227:357, 1976.
169. Welliver RC, Kaul TN, Ogra PL. The appearance of cell-bound IgE in respiratory-tract epithelium after respiratory-syncytial-virus infection. *N Engl J Med* 303(21):1198–1202, 1980.
170. Welliver RC, Wong DT, Sun M, et al. The development of respiratory syncytial virus-specific IgE and the release of histamine in nasopharyngeal secretions after infection. *N Engl J Med* 305(15):841–846, 1981.
171. Welliver RC, Wong DT, Sun M, et al. Parainfluenza virus bronchiolitis. Epidemiology and pathogenesis. *Am J Dis Child* 140(1):34–40, 1986.
172. Welliver RC, Wong DT, Middleton E Jr, et al. Role of parainfluenza virus-specific IgE in pathogenesis of croup and wheezing subsequent to infection. *J Pediatr* 101(6):889–896, 1982.
173. Busse WW. Viral infections and allergic disease. *Clin Exp Allergy* 21(1):68–71, 1991.
174. Minor TE, Dick EC, DeMeo AN, et al. Viruses as precipitants of asthmatic attacks in children. *JAMA* 227:292–298, 1974.

175. McIntosh K. Respiratory syncytial virus infections in infants and children: Diagnosis and treatment. *Pediatr Rev* 9(6):191–196, 1987.
176. Empey DW, Laitinen LA, Jacops L, et al. Mechanisms of bronchial hyperreactivity in normal subjects after upper respiratory tract infections. *Am Rev Respir Dis* 113:131–139, 1976.
177. Hazinski TA. Bronchopulmonary dysplasia. In: Chernick V (ed.), *Kendig's Disorders of Respiratory Tract in Children*, 5th ed., W.B. Saunders, Philadelphia, 1990, pp. 300–320.
178. O'Brodovich HM, Mellins RB. Bronchopulmonary dysplasia—unresolved neonatal acute lung injury. *Am Rev Respir Dis* 132:694–709, 1985.
179. Northway WH Jr, Rosan RC, Porter DY. Pulmonary disease following respiratory therapy of hyaline membrane disease. *N Engl J Med* 267:357–368, 1967.
180. Smyth JA, Tabachnik E, Duncan WJ, et al. Pulmonary function and bronchial hyperreactivity in long-term survivors of bronchopulmonary dysplasia. *Pediatrics* 68:336, 1981.
181. Saigal S, Rosenbaum P, Stoskopf B, et al. Outcome in infants 501 to 1000 gm birth weight delivered to residents of the McMaster Health Region. *J Pediatr* 105:969–976, 1984.
182. Avery ME, Tooley WH, Keller MPH, et al. Is chronic lung disease in low birth weight infants preventable? A survey of eight centers. *Pediatrics* 79(1): 26–30, 1987.
183. Clark DA, Pincus LG, Oliphant M, et al. HLA-A2 and chronic lung disease in neonates. *JAMA* 248:1868–1869, 1982.
184. Nickerson BG, Taussig LM. Family history of asthma in infants with bronchopulmonary dysplasia. *Pediatrics* 65:1140–1144, 1980.
185. Irving LB, Jordana M, O'Brodovich HM, et al. Alveolar macrophage activation in BPD. *Am Rev Respir Dis* 133:A207, 1986.
186. Stenmark KR, Eyzaguirre M, Remigio L, et al. Recovery of PAF and leukotrienes from infants with severe BD: clinical improvement with cromolyn treatment. *Am Rev Respir Dis* 131:A236, 1985.
187. Merrit TA, Cochrane CG, Holcomb K, et al. Elastase and α1-proteinase inhibitor activity in tracheal aspirates during respiratory distress syndrome: role of inflammation in the pathogenesis of BPD. *J Clin Invest* 72:656–666, 1983.
188. Burnett D, Chamba A, Hill SL, et al. Neutrophils from subjects with chronic obstructive lung disease show enhanced chemotaxis and extracellular proteolysis. *Lancet* 2:1043, 1987.
189. Clement A, Chadelat K, Sardet A, et al. Alveolar macrophage status in bronchopulmonary dysplasia. *Pediatr Res* 23:470, 1988.
190. Ogden BE, Murphy SA, Saunders GC, et al. Neonatal lung neutrophils and elastase/proteinase inhibitor imbalance. *Am Rev Respir Dis* 130:817–821, 1984.
191. Johnson DE, Lock JE, Elde RP, Thompson TR. Pulmonary neuroendocrine cells in hyaline membrane disease and bronchopulmonary dysplasia. *Pediatr Res* 16:446, 1986.

192. Johnson MD, Gray ME, Carpenter GR, et al. Ontogeny of epidermal growth factor receptor/kinase and of lipocortin-1 in the ovine lung. *Pediatr Res* 25:535, 1989.
193. Harris JD, Swenson EW, Johnson JE III. Human alveolar macrophages. Comparison of phagocytic ability, glucose utilization and ultrastructure in smokers and nonsmokers. *J Clin Invest* 49:2086–2096, 1970.
194. Fick RB, Paul ES, Merrill WW, et al. Alterations in the antibacterial properties of rabbit pulmonary macrophages exposed to wood smoke. *Am Rev Respir Dis* 129:76–81, 1984.
195. Hasselblad V, Humble CG, Graham MC, et al. Indoor environment determinants of lung function in children. *Am Rev Respir Dis* 123:479–485, 1981.
196. Melia RJW, Florey C Du V, Altman DS, et al. Association between gas cooking and respiratory disease in children. *Br Med J* 2:149, 1977.
197. Wade WA, Cote WA, Yocum JE. A study of indoor air quality. *J Air Pollut Control Assoc* 25:933, 1975.
198. Speizer FE, Ferris B, Bishop YMM, et al. Respiratory disease rates and pulmonary function in children associated with $NO_2$ exposure. *Am Rev Respir Dis* 121:3, 1980.
199. Chiang ST, Wang BC. Acute effects of cigarette smoking on pulmonary function. *Am Rev Respir Dis* 101:860–868, 1970.
200. Gerrard JW, Cockcroft DW, Mink JT, et al. Increased nonspecific bronchial reactivity in cigarette smokers with normal lung function. *Am Rev Respir Dis* 122:577–581, 1980.
201. Hunninghake GW, Crystal RG. Cigarette smoking and lung destruction: accumulation of neutrophils in the lungs of cigarette smokers. *Am Rev Respir Dis* 128:833–838, 1983.
202. Hulbert WC, Walker DC, Jackson A, et al. Airway permeability to horseradish peroxidase in guinea pigs: the repair phase after injury by cigarette smoke. *Am Rev Respir Dis* 123:320–326, 1981.
203. Wanner A. Clinical aspects of mucociliary transport. *Am Rev Respir Dis* 116:73–125, 1977.
204. Park SS, Kikkawa Y, Goldring IP, et al. An animal model of cigarette smoking in beagle dogs: correlative evaluation of effects on pulmonary function, defense, and morphology. *Am Rev Respir Dis* 115:971–979, 1977.
205. Ludwig PW, Schwartz BA, Hoidal JR, et al. Cigarette smoking causes accumulation of polymorphonuclear leukocytes in alveolar septum. *Am Rev Respir Dis* 131:828–830, 1985.
206. Stecenko A, McNicol K, Sauder R. Effect of passive smoking on the lungs of young lambs. *Pediatr Res* 20:853–858, 1986.
207. Sopori ML, Gairola CC, DeLucia AJ, et al. Immune responsiveness of monkeys exposed chronically to cigarette smoke. *Clin Immunol Immunopathol* 36:338–344, 1985.
208. Tollerud DJ, Clark JW, Brown LM, et al. Association of cigarette smoking with decreased numbers of circulating natural killer cells. *Am Rev Respir Dis* 139:194–198, 1989.

209. Janoff A, Carp H, Lee DK, et al. Cigarette smoke inhalation decreases alpha-1-antitrypsin activity in rat lung. *Science* 206:1313–1314, 1979.
210. Osmon M, Jerome OC, Roffman S, et al. Cigarette smoke impairs elastin resynthesis in lungs of hamsters with elastase-induced emphysema. *Am Rev Respir Dis* 640–643, 1985.
211. Gerrard JW, Heiner DC, Ko CG, et al. Immunoglobulin levels in smokers and non-smokers. *Ann Allergy* 44:261–262, 1980.
212. Burrows B, Halonen M, Barbee RA, et al. The relationship of serum immunoglobulin E to cigarette smoking. *Am Rev Respir Dis* 124:523–525, 1981.
213. Warren CPW, Holford-Strevens V, Wong C, et al. The relationship between smoking and total IgE levels. *J Allergy Clin Immunol* 69:370–375, 1982.
214. Van Wye JE. Passive smoking. In: Hilman BC, et al. (eds.), *Pediatric Respiratory Disease: Diagnosis and Treatment*, W.B. Saunders, Philadelphia, 1992.
215. Weiss ST. Passive smoking and lung cancer: what is the risk? *Am Rev Respir Dis* 133:1–3, 1986.
216. American Academy of Pediatrics, Committee on Environmental Hazards. Passive smoking: a hazard to children. *Pediatrics* 77:755–757, 1986.
217. Fielding JE, Phenow KJ. Health effects of involuntary smoking. *N Engl J Med* 319:1452–1460, 1988.
218. National Research Council, Committee on Passive Smoking. *Environmental Tobacco Smoke; Measuring Exposures and Assessing Health Effects*. Washington, D.C., National Academy Press, 1986.
219. U.S. Department of Health and Human Services. *The Health Consequences of Involuntary Smoking: A Report of the Surgeon General*. DHEW publication DHHS-CDC-87-8398. Washington, D.C., Government Printing Office, 1986.
220. Repace JL, Lowrey AH. Indoor air pollution, tobacco smoke, and public health. *Science* 208:464–472, 1980.
221. Stober W. Lung dynamics and uptake of smoke constituents by nonsmokers: a survey. *Prev Med* 13:589–601, 1984.
222. Weiss ST, Tager IB, Schenker M, et al. The health effects of involuntary smoking. *Am Rev Respir Dis* 128:933–942, 1983.
223. Pattishall EN, Strope GL, Etzel RA, et al. Serum cotinine as a measure of tobacco smoke exposure in children. *Am J Dis Child* 139:1101–1104, 1985.
224. Wald NJ, Boreham J, Bailey A, et al. Urinary cotinine as marker of breathing other people's tobacco smoke. *Lancet* 1:230–234, 1984.
225. Matsukura S, Taminato T, Kitano N. Effects of environmental tobacco smoke on urinary continine excretion in nonsmokers: evidence for passive smoking. *N Engl J Med* 311:828–832, 1984.
226. Greenberg RA, Haley NJ, Etzel RA, et al. Measuring the exposure of infants to tobacco smoke: nicotine and cotinine in urine and saliva. *N Engl J Med* 310:1075–1078, 1984.
227. Labrecque M, Marcoux S, Weber JP, et al. Feeding and urine cotinine values in babies whose mothers smoke. *Pediatrics* 83:93–97, 1989.
228. Greenberg RA, Bauman KE, Glover LH, et al. Ecology of passive smoking by young infants. *J Pediatr* 114:774–780, 1989.

229. Harlap S, Davies AM. Infant admissions to hospital and maternal smoking. *Lancet* 1:529–532, 1974.
230. Colley JRT, Holland WW, Corkhill RT. Influence of passive smoking and parental phlegm on pneumonia and bronchitis in early childhood. *Lancet* 2:1031–1034, 1974.
231. Leeder SR, Corkhill RT, Irwig LM, et al. Influence of family factors on the incidence of lower respiratory illness during the first year of life. *Br J Prev Soc Med* 30:203–212, 1976.
232. Rantakallio P. Relationship of maternal smoking to morbidity and mortality of the child up to the age of five. *Acta Paediatr Scand* 67:621–631, 1978.
233. Fergusson DM, Horwood LJ, Shannon FT. Parental smoking and respiratory illness in infancy. *Arch Dis Child* 55:358–361, 1980.
234. Fergusson DM, Horwood LJ, Shannon FT. Parental smoking and lower respiratory illness in the first three years of life. *J Epidemiol Commun Health* 35:180–184, 1981.
235. Fergusson DM, Hons BA, Horwood LJ. Parental smoking and respiratory illness during early childhood: a six-year longitudinal study. *Pediatr Pulmonol* 1:99–106, 1985.
236. Ware JH, Dockery DW, Spiro A. Passive smoking, gas cooking, and respiratory health of children living in six cities. *Am Rev Respir Dis* 129:366–374, 1984.
237. Pedreira FA, Guandolo VL, Feroli EJ, et al. Involuntary smoking and incidence of respiratory illness during the first year of life. *Pediatrics* 75:594–597, 1985.
238. Chen Y, Li W, Yu S. Influence of passive smoking on admissions for respiratory illness in early childhood. *Br Med J* 293:303–306, 1986.
239. Chen Y, Li W, Yu S, et al. Chang-Ning epidemiological study of children's health: passive smoking and children's respiratory diseases. *Int J Epidemiol* 17:348–355, 1988.
240. Somerville SM, Rona RJ, Chinn S. Passive smoking and respiratory conditions in primary school children. *J Epidemiol Commun Health* 42:105–110, 1988.
241. Groothuis JR, Gutierrez KM, Lauer BA. Respiratory syncytial virus infection in children with bronchopulmonary dysplasia. *Pediatrics* 82:199–203, 1988.
242. Wissow LS, Warshow M. Passive smoking exacerbates seasonal variation in acute visits for asthma. *Am J Dis Child* 142:401, 1988.
243. Evans D, Levison MJ, Feldman CH, et al. The impact of passive smoking on emergency room visits of urban children with asthma. *Am Rev Respir Dis* 135:567–572, 1987.
244. Ekwo EE, Weinberger MM, Lachenbruch PA, et al. Relationship of parental smoking and gas cooking to respiratory disease in children. *Chest* 84:662–668, 1983.
245. Schenker MB, Samet JM, Speizer FE. Risk factors for childhood respiratory disease: the effect of host factors and home environmental exposures. *Am Rev Respir Dis* 128:1038–1043, 1983.

246. Burchfiel CM, Higgins MW, Keller JB, et al. Passive smoking in childhood: respiratory conditions and pulmonary function in Techumseh, Michigan. *Am Rev Respir Dis* 133:966–973, 1986.
247. Pullan CR, Hey EN. Wheezing, asthma, and pulmonary dysfunction 10 years after infection with respiratory syncytial virus in infancy. *Br Med J* 284:1665–1669, 1982.
248. McConnochie KM, Roghmann KJ. Parental smoking, presence of older siblings, and family history of asthma increase risk of bronchiolitis. *Am J Dis Child* 140:806–812, 1986.
249. Hayes EB, Hurwitz ES, Schonberger LB. Respiratory syncytial virus outbreak on American Samoa. *Am J Dis Child* 143:316–321, 1989.
250. Charlton A. Children's coughs related to parental smoking. *Br Med J* 288:1647–1649, 1984.
251. Andrae S, Axelson O, Bjorksten B, et al. Symptoms of bronchial hyperreactivity and asthma in relation to environmental factors. *Arch Dis Child* 63:473–478, 1988.
252. Tsimoyianis GV, Jacobson MS, Feldman JG. Reduction in pulmonary function and increased frequency of cough associated with passive smoking in teenage athletes. *Pediatrics* 80:32–36, 1987.
253. Geller-Bernstein G, Kenett R, Weisglass L. Atopic babies with wheezy bronchitis. *Allergy* 42:85–91, 1987.
254. Cogswell JJ, Mitchell EB, Alexander J. Parental smoking, breast feeding, and respiratory infection in development of allergic diseases. *Arch Dis Child* 62:338–344, 1987.
255. Murray AB, Morrison BJ. Passive smoking increases the frequency of asthma in children who have had atopic dermatitis. *J Allergy Clin Immunol* 83:195, 1989.
256. McConnochie KM, Roghmann KJ. Breast feeding and maternal smoking as predictors of wheezing in children ages 6 to 10 years. *Pediatr Pulmonol* 2:260–268, 1986.
257. Neuspiel DR, Rush D, Butler NR, et al. Parental smoking and post-infancy wheezing in children: a prospective cohort study. *Am J Public Health* 79:168–171, 1989.
258. Weiss ST, Tager IB, Speizer FE, et al. Persistent wheeze: its relation to respiratory illness, cigarette smoking, and level of pulmonary function in a population sample of children. *Am Rev Respir Dis* 122:697–707, 1980.
259. O'Connor GT, Weiss ST, Tager IB, et al. The effect of passive smoking on pulmonary function and nonspecific bronchial responsiveness in a population-based sample of children and young adults. *Am Rev Respir Dis* 135:800–804, 1987.
260. Vedal S, Schenker MB, Samet JM, et al. Risk factors for childhood respiratory disease: analysis of pulmonary function. *Am Rev Respir Dis* 130:187–192, 1984.
261. Spinaci S, Arossa W, Burgiani M, et al. The effects of air pollution on the respiratory health of children: a cross-sectional study. *Pediatr Pulmonol* 1:262–266, 1985.

262. Tager IB, Weiss ST, Rosher B, et al. Effect of parental cigarette smoking on pulmonary functions of children. *Am J Epidemiol* 110:15–26, 1979.
263. Tager IB, Weiss ST, Munoz A, et al. Longitudinal study of the effects of maternal smoking on pulmonary function in children. *N Engl J Med* 309:699–703, 1983.
264. Berkey CS, Ware JH, Dockery DW, et al. Indoor air pollution and pulmonary function growth in preadolescent children. *Am J Epidemiol* 123:250–260, 1986.
265. Dodge R. The effects of indoor pollution on Arizona children. *Arch Environ Health* 37:151–155, 1982.
266. Lebowitz MD, Armet DB, Knudson R. The effect of passive smoking on pulmonary function in children. *Environ Int* 8:371–373, 1982.
267. Murray AB, Morrison BJ. The effect of cigarette smoke from the mother on bronchial responsiveness and severity of symptoms in children with asthma. *J Allergy Clin Immunol* 77:575–581, 1986.
268. Murray AB, Morrison BJ. Passive smoking and the seasonal difference of severity of asthma in children. *Chest* 94:701–708, 1988.

7

# Increasing Asthma Morbidity and Mortality

R. MICHAEL SLY

*Children's National Medical Center*
*and The George Washington University*
*School of Medicine and Health Sciences*
*Washington, D.C.*



Reversibility of airway obstruction has long been regarded as part of the definition of asthma (1). Fatal asthma is so unusual that it calls for investigation. Progressive increases in rates of death from asthma demand the intense scrutiny they have received in the past few years.

## HISTORICAL PERSPECTIVE

As early as the 2nd century AD, Aretaeus the Cappadocian observed that airway obstruction due to asthma could progress to the point of causing suffocation (2). In the 12th century Moses Maimonides (3) asserted that

> . . . should the rules of management [of asthma] go unheeded and one's desires and habits be followed indiscriminately, the gap between onset [of episodes] will grow shorter, and the duration and intensity gradually increase until a peak is reached which may well end in death. . . (3)

The rules have changed since the 12th century, but asthma still can be fatal, sometimes even when patients have heeded the rules as we understand them.

In the 18th century Millar observed that severe asthma was most frequent in "the lower class of people" and identified severe, chronic asthma as a risk factor for death (4). In the following century Henry Hyde Salter agreed that prognosis depended on the duration and frequency of acute episodes of asthma (5).

Nevertheless, death from asthma was so rare that many able clinicians doubted that asthma could be fatal. Laennec declared that anyone with asthma could look forward to a long life (6), and Sir William Osler asserted that "the asthmatic pants into old age" (7).

In 1963 Alexander drew attention to the increased frequency in deaths from asthma in the United States from 1930 to 1952 followed by a sudden decline in deaths (8). Rates of death from asthma increased from 2.5: 100,000 general population in 1937 to 4.5 by 1951 and 1952 (9). Annual deaths from asthma peaked at 6943 in 1952. Rates of death then decreased to 3.6:100,000 by 1955 and 2.8 by 1959. Alexander commented that during the earlier period of increasing asthma mortality, fatal asthma had been associated often with respiratory infection (8). He thought that the introduction of antibiotics might have resulted in increased prominence of viral pneumonia and increased frequency of fatal asthma and that the subsequent decrease in rates of death might have been due to increasingly widespread use of adrenal corticosteroids for the treatment of asthma.

## EPIDEMIC ASTHMA

A progressive increase in mortality from asthma in England and Wales began in 1960. Mortality rates increased from 2.60:100,000 general population in 1960 to 4.35 in 1965 and 4.24 in 1966 (10). The increase in mortality was greatest among children 10–14 years of age, for whom the rate increased from 0.33 in 1959 to 2.46 in 1966. Increases were least in those below 5 years of age and beyond 55 years of age. Total annual deaths from asthma peaked at 2080 in 1965, and numbers of deaths fell in all age groups after March, 1967.

Correlation of numbers of deaths with numbers of prescriptions and sales of pressurized bronchodilator aerosols suggested the possibility of an adverse effect of metered dose inhalers, but total sales did not decrease until 1967, 1 year after the initial decrease in deaths (11). Data from 174 deaths at 5–34 years of age during one 6 month period disclosed that 84% of the fatalities occurred in subjects who had been using β-agonist inhalers (12).

Isoprenaline-Forte, a preparation of isoproterenol in a pressurized canister that delivered 400 μg for each actuation instead of the usual 80 μg, accounted for 30% of the nebulizer sales in England and Wales during the epidemic. It was implicated by the observation that no increase in mortality from asthma had occurred at that time in the United States or Canada, where Isoprenaline-Forte had never been marketed. No increases in mortality occurred in the Netherlands and Belgium where it was not marketed until 1966, and even then there were relatively few sales there (13). However, there was an increase in mortality in Japan, although Isoprenaline-Forte was not marketed there either.

Publication of articles drawing attention to the increasing mortality from asthma in England and Wales did not begin to appear in the medical literature until August, 1965. This was probably somewhat late to have any major impact on mortality that year although that was the year in which the epidemic peaked. It is possible, however, that information about it had been disseminated orally somewhat earlier. Manufacturers did not modify instructions for patients until 1968, after the mortality rates had already decreased. Bronchodilator aerosol sales were not limited to prescriptions until December, 1968 (11).

Similar increases in mortality from asthma began in Australia in 1964 (14). There mortality decreased after 1966 and had returned to the pre-epidemic baseline by 1968. Throughout this period there was a progressive increase in sales of pressurized bronchodilator aerosols, including isoproterenol, metaproterenol, and isoproterenol as Isoprenaline-Forte (14). Thus, these data do not implicate overuse of bronchodilator aerosols as a cause of increased mortality in Australia.

Some deaths did occur after overuse of bronchodilator inhalers (15), and some may have followed overreliance on inhalers that had previously afforded relief of symptoms in patients who delayed seeking further help until it was too late. The available data do not implicate overuse of metered dose inhalers as a major cause of the increased mortality from asthma in 1961 to 1968.

## RECENT INCREASES IN MORTALITY

After the peak of 6943 deaths from asthma in the United States in 1952, numbers of deaths decreased, reaching a low of 1674 deaths in 1977 (Fig. 1). Data from the National Center for Health Statistics indicate that there have been progressive increases since then, however, to 4597 deaths in 1988, the most recent year for which complete data are available (16).

To understand these data it is necessary to understand the impact of the Ninth Revision of the International Classification of Diseases, which took effect in 1979. This revision discontinued a linkage between asthma and two other conditions that are sometimes associated, bronchitis and emphysema. Previously, deaths had been ascribed to bronchitis when both bronchitis and asthma were mentioned on the death certificate, but since 1979 they have been coded as due to asthma. Coding of two highly stratified random samples of deaths from 1976 according to both the eighth and ninth revisions estimated that implementation of the ninth revision increased assignment of deaths to asthma by 35.44% (17,18).

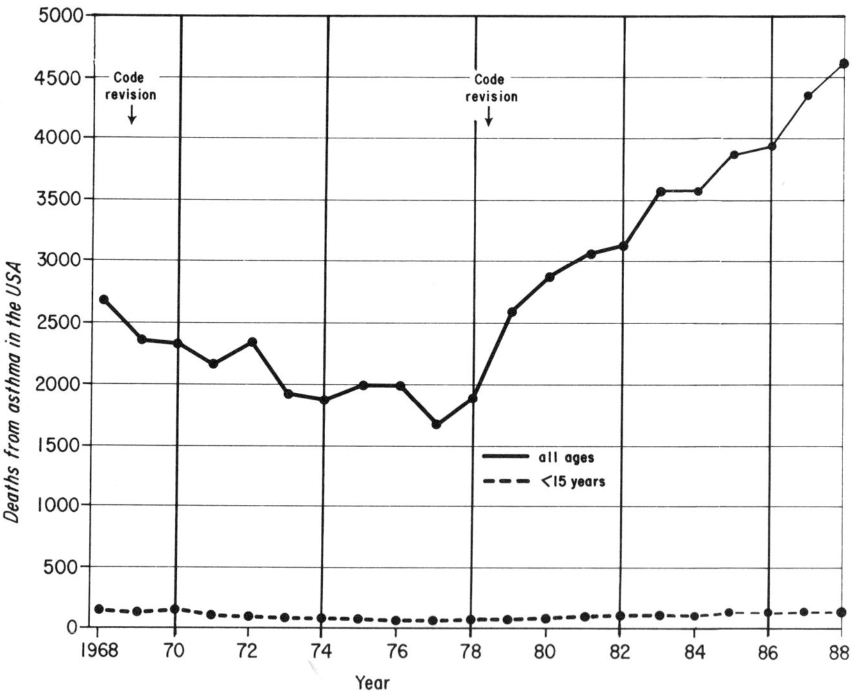


FIGURE 1 Deaths for asthma in the United States by year. (Modified from Ref. 18.)

The 39% increase in deaths from asthma in 1979 was well within the 95% confidence interval, indicating that the increase that year could have been due entirely to the revision of the International Classification of Diseases (ICD). Increases that have continued since then cannot be accounted for in that way, however (Fig. 1).

Rates of death from asthma have also increased from a low of 0.8: 100,000 general population in 1977 and 1978 to 1.2 in 1979 and 1.9 in 1988.

Rates of death from asthma have increased progressively with age from a low of 0.1:100,000 general population at 1–4 years of age in 1988 to 0.3 at 5–14 years of age, 0.4 at 15–24 years of age, 0.5 at 25–34 years, 1.0 at 35–44, 1.8 at 45–54, 3.6 at 55–64, 6.1 at 65–74, 10.4 at 75–84 and 14.6 at 85 or older (16). Because most deaths from asthma occur in persons beyond 55 years of age, aging of the population could account in part for increases in numbers and rates of death (19).

Age-adjusted rates of death correct for aging of the population by indicating the rates that would have existed if the age-specific rates for the particular year had prevailed in a population with the same age distribution as that of the United States in 1940. Age-adjusted rates of death from asthma have increased from 0.6:100,000 in 1977 to 0.9 in 1979 (the year of adoption of the ninth revision of the ICD) and 1.4 in 1988 (Fig. 2) (16,20).

Rates of death from asthma have been much higher among blacks than whites and have been increasing more rapidly among blacks (Fig. 3). Age-adjusted rates of death among whites increased from 0.5:100,000 in 1977 to 1.1 in 1988, while those for blacks increased from 1.5 in 1977 and 1978 to 3.5 in 1988 (16,20). On the other hand, rates of death from asthma for

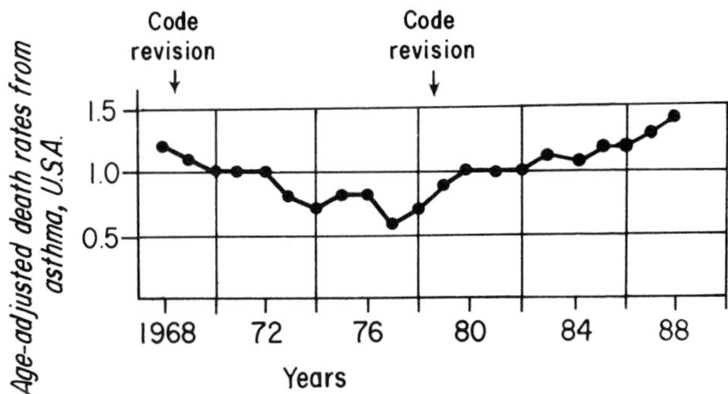


FIGURE 2 Age-adjusted death rates from asthma (per 100,000 general population) in the United States by year. (Modified from Ref. 19.)

Native Americans, Japanese, Chinese, and Filipinos residing in the United States have been lower than those for whites (20).

Although deaths from asthma have been more rare in children than adults, deaths in children less than 15 years of age increased in the United States from a low of 54 in 1977 to a peak of 125 in 1985 and have decreased slightly to 119 in 1988 (Fig. 4) (16,21). The increase in rate of death from asthma from 0.1:100,000 in 1979 to 0.4 by 1986 in children 10–14 years of age has been the greatest proportionate increase for any age group.

Rates of death from asthma have been higher among boys than girls but higher among women than men (16,18,21).

Disparities related to race have been even greater among children than adults. Among white children 10–14 years of age rates of death from asthma increased from 0.1:100,000 in 1979 to 0.3 in 1986 while those for black children increased from 0.3 to 1.2 (19,21). Among white adolescents 15–19 years of age rates increased from 0.2:100,000 in 1979 to 0.3 in 1986; for blacks, the increase was 0.7 to 1.4 in 1986.

Rates of death from asthma have been much lower in the United States than in many other countries, where there have also been recent increases in mortality (Fig. 5) (20). Rates have been increasing in Canada, England and Wales, and Australia, and rates increased sharply in New Zealand until reaching a peak at 8.1:100,000 in 1980. Since then rates have been decreasing in New Zealand.

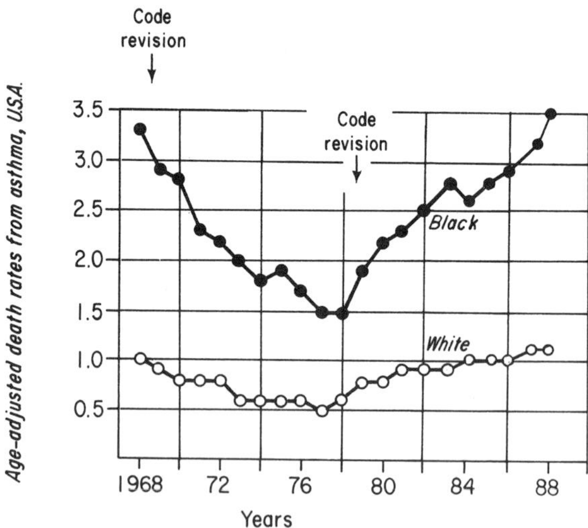


FIGURE 3 Age-adjusted asthma death rates per 100,000 general population in the United States by year for blacks and whites. (Modified from Ref. 19.)

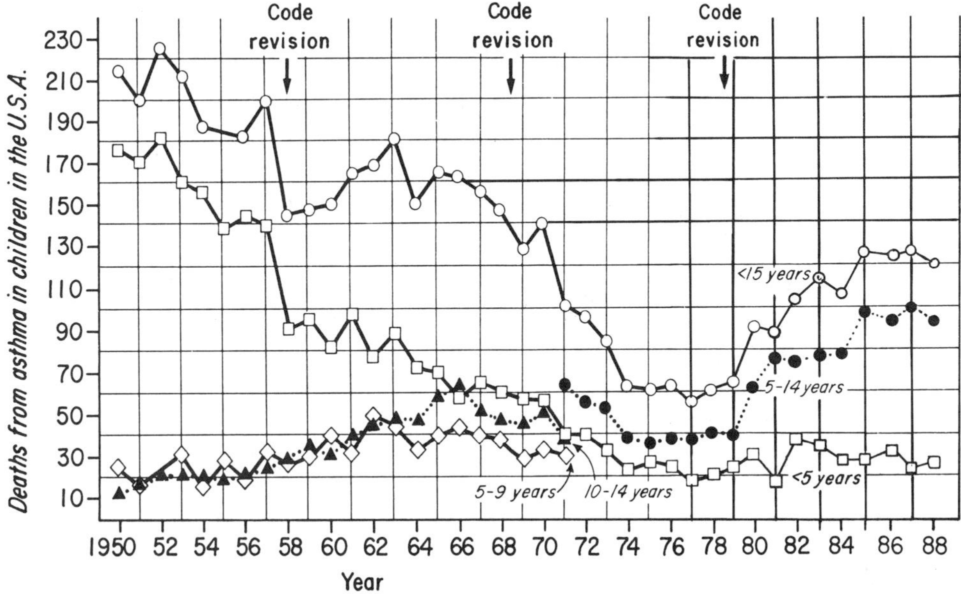


FIGURE 4 Deaths from asthma in children by year and by age group, United States, 1950–1988. (Modified from Sly RM. *Pediatric Allergy, 3rd ed*, New Hyde Park, NY, Medical Examination, 1984, used with permission.)

## ACCURACY OF CERTIFICATION OF DEATHS AS DUE TO ASTHMA

Reliability of these data depends heavily upon accuracy of certification of death as due to asthma. Reviews of circumstances surrounding death when asthma has been mentioned anywhere on the death certificate have disclosed frequent inaccuracies of certification, often due to confusion with chronic bronchitis or emphysema (22–25). Deaths of persons more than 70 years of age have accounted for most inaccuracies of certification. Certification of deaths as due to asthma has been reported accurate in 90% of cases at 15–44 years of age (23) and in 94% of children less than 15 years of age (26).

Postmortem examinations have been done in approximately 50% of deaths from asthma of persons 5–34 years of age in the United States from 1979 to 1984 (20), but in fewer than 20% of the deaths in all age groups. Results of such examinations often have not been considered in assigning the cause of death on the death certificate. Clinical information may be more important than pathologic findings in determining the cause of death

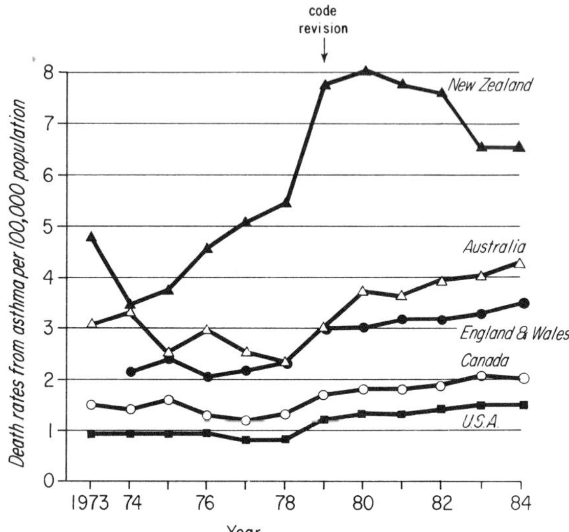


FIGURE 5 Asthma death rates per 100,000 general population by year in New Zealand, Australia, England and Wales, Canada, and the United States. (Modified from Ref. 18.)

in such a patient, although findings at the time of autopsy usually are consistent with asthma whether or not asthma was the cause of death (27,28).

## PATHOLOGIC FINDINGS

Postmortem examination of asthmatic children and adults who have died from status asthmaticus usually have disclosed extreme hyperinflation and filling of the airways with viscid, mucoid secretions (27,29,30). There are often areas of atelectasis. The mucous plugs contain desquamated epithelial cells, eosinophils, and sometimes Charcot-Leyden crystals. Eosinophilic infiltration of the mucosa and submucosa, focal denudation of the mucosa, and hyperplasia of goblet cells, mucous glands, and airway muscle are characteristic (27,29,31). There is apparent thickening of the basement membrane due to an increase in collagen beneath the basement membrane. Loss of cilia and of ciliated epithelial cells probably has impaired mucociliary clearance markedly (27,32).

Lung biopsy of asymptomatic asthmatic patients can disclose similar but less extensive changes (27,32).

Both the major basic protein of eosinophil granules and eosinophil peroxidase can cause damage and desquamation of bronchial epithelial cells (33). Immunofluorescent studies of lung specimens from a child who had died from asthma have disclosed deposition of major basic protein at the base of an area of a bronchus denuded of epithelium and in association with eosinophil degranulation in areas of epithelial desquamation (33). These observations suggest an important role for the eosinophil and its products in the epithelial destruction often associated with fatal asthma. However, epithelial desquamation may also occur in such patients without evidence of degranulation of eosinophils (33).

Postmortem examination of children who have died from asthma has failed to disclose mucoid obstruction of airways occasionally (34). This might be accounted for by sudden, extreme airway obstruction due to bronchoconstriction in a patient with heightened airway reactivity. Sudden, extreme increases in airway obstruction followed by cardiac arrest have occurred in occasional patients hospitalized for asthma who have survived only as a result of immediate, aggressive intervention (34). Those asthmatic patients subject to sudden, severe respiratory crises such as these often have large circadian variations in peak expiratory flow rate of more than 50% (35). Variation in peak expiratory flow rate has been found to correlate with nonspecific airway reactivity (36).

The bronchial hyperresponsiveness typical of asthma may be due in part to increased thickness of the airway walls, which can result in occlusion of the lumen after less smooth muscle contraction than in nonasthmatic subjects. Postmortem examination of the airways of asthmatic patients has shown increased thickness of the walls of membranous and cartilaginous airways due to increased thickness of the epithelium and submucosa as well as the muscle (37). These changes are probably due to chronic inflammation, including vascular congestion, exudation, connective tissue deposition, epithelial metaplasia, and muscular hyperplasia and hypertrophy.

## LOCATIONS OF DEATHS

Increases in rates of death from asthma have occurred in every state since 1979 (20). Evaluations of variables associated with fatal asthma are most conclusive when limited to impact on deaths at 5–34 years of age, because of the high accuracy of certification of death as due to asthma in this age group (23,26). Rates of death from asthma at 5–34 years of age have increased in all regions of the United States for both blacks and for whites (38). Rates have been highest for blacks in the North Central region and

Northeast, and the disparity between rates for blacks and whites has been greatest there.

Much of the increase in these two regions has been due to increases in mortality rates in Cook County, Illinois, and in New York City. In 1985 Cook County and New York City accounted for 21.1% of the deaths from asthma at 5–34 years of age, but only 6.8% of the U.S. population in that age group resided there (39).

Examination of asthma mortality at less than 35 years of age from 1982 to 1987 has identified certain neighborhoods in New York City with excessive mortality rates: neighborhoods characterized independently by extreme poverty and black or Hispanic populations (40).

Over all age groups, rates of death from asthma for residents in metropolitan statistical areas and New England county metropolitan areas increased from 1.23:100,000 general population in 1980 to 1.50 in 1984, while that in nonmetropolitan areas increased from 1.42 to 1.55 (20). Metropolitan rates increased for both blacks and whites. The percentage of deaths from asthma at 5–34 years of age that occurred among metropolitan residents varied from 70 to 78% during 1979 to 1984 in whites and from 79 to 88% for blacks (20). In 1980 81% of our black population and 73% of whites lived in standard metropolitan statistical areas.

The problem has not been failure to reach a hospital. Data from the 40 states where the place of death was indicated on the death certificate from 1979 through 1984 disclose that 70% of blacks who died from asthma at 5–34 years of age and 77% of whites died at hospitals, either as inpatients or at emergency rooms (Fig. 6) (38). Forty-six percent of black children and adolescents less than 20 years of age and 47% of white children and adolescents who died from asthma died at hospitals (21). Of course these data do not indicate how many were already moribund when they reached the hospital, but they contrast strikingly with data from the 2 year national study of asthma mortality in New Zealand. Only 15% of 271 deaths from asthma at less than 70 years of age occurred at hospitals in New Zealand, and there was no death in anyone who had survived at least 30 min after reaching the hospital, which is long enough for the intensive treatment available there to take effect (24,41). These observations raise serious questions about the adequacy of management of asthma at many hospitals in the United States.

Data from the National Hospital Discharge Survey indicate increases in rates of discharge from hospitals after admission for treatment of asthma at 5–34 years of age from 100:100,000 general population in 1979 to 128 in 1982 and 125 in 1986 (Fig. 7) (38). The rate for whites changed from 78:100,000 in 1979 to 95 by 1986; that for blacks increased from 180 in

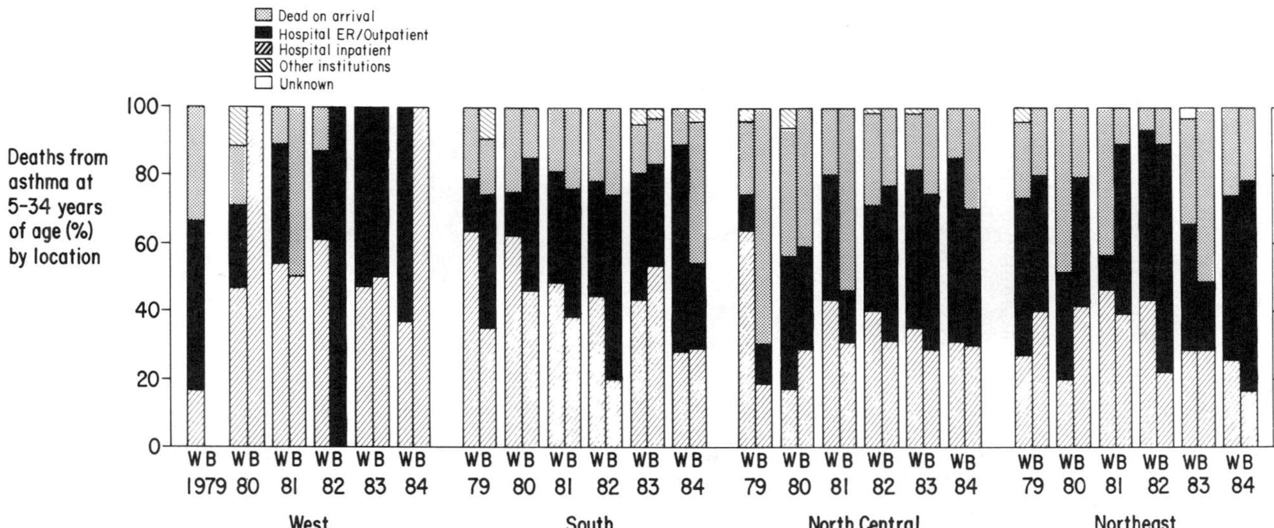


FIGURE 6 Percentage of deaths from asthma in whites (W) and blacks (B) 5–34 years of age that occurred while hospital inpatients, in hospital emergency rooms or outpatient departments, those dead on arrival, those who died at other institutions, and those for whom death certificates did not indicate the place of death by region and year. Data exclude 10 states and the District of Columbia, where death certificates did not indicate these details. (From Ref. 38.)

1979 to 310 in 1982 before decreasing to 264 by 1986. Rates for both blacks and whites increased significantly across time.

Asthmatic patients have been reaching hospitals for treatment at increasing rates, but it is possible that they have not been receiving the necessary expert care. Analysis of deaths from asthma at 5–34 years of age in 1980 in nine regions of the United States disclosed variations in mortality rates from 0.105:100,000 in the East North Central states to 0.271 in the Mountain states for whites and from 0.637 in the South Atlantic states to 1.343 in the Middle Atlantic states for blacks (Table 1). After an adjustment for regional area was made, multiple linear regression indicated a positive relationship between asthma mortality and medical specialist density, although this was statistically significant only for whites (42). The more medical specialists in the region, the higher the mortality from asthma! Of course analysis of such data by relatively large regions may be misleading because of local geographic conditions including distance that may limit

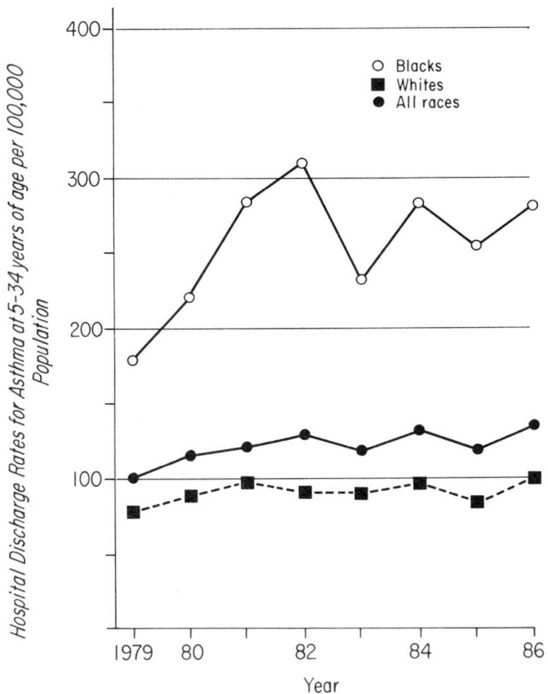


FIGURE 7 Hospital discharge rates following admission for treatment of asthma, United States, at 5–34 years of age by year. (Data from National Hospital Discharge Survey.)

access to care, but barriers other than distance may be even more important. Such associations in smaller regions would not be reliable because of the low rates of death from asthma.

A decreased prevalence of asthma in Briançon, France, at an elevation of 1350 m has been associated with a decreased prevalence of positive allergy skin tests to house dust mites (43). This suggests that decreased temperatures and decreased humidity at high geographic elevations may inhibit proliferation of mites and result in a lower prevalence of asthma. However, geographic elevation has had no discernible effect on asthma mortality rates in the United States, possibly because of the mobility of our population and importance of causes of asthma other than mites (44).

## POSSIBLE CAUSES OF INCREASING MORTALITY

### Prevalence

An increase in prevalence of asthma might account for an increase in mortality rates. Comparisons of rates of prevalence of asthma across time are complicated by differences in methodology and slight differences in

TABLE 1 Rates of Death from Asthma per 100,000 General Population and 95% Confidence Intervals for Blacks and Whites 5–34 Years of Age by Geographic Region and Division, 1980

| | Blacks | | | Whites | | |
|---|---|---|---|---|---|---|
| Region and division | Deaths | Death rate | [95% CI][a] | Deaths | Death rate | [95% CI] |
| West | | 0.905 | [0.468, 1.584] | | 0.263 | [0.192, 0.352] |
| Pacific | 10 | 0.862 | [0.414, 1.586] | 32 | 0.259 | [0.175, 0.370] |
| Mountain | 2 | 1.211 | [0.147, 4.372] | 14 | 0.271 | [0.148, 0.455] |
| North Central | | 1.179 | [0.822, 1.639] | | 0.108 | [0.072, 0.157] |
| West North Central | 5 | 1.102 | [0.357, 2.57] | 9 | 0.116 | [0.053, 0.220] |
| East North Central | 31 | 1.192 | [0.805, 1.705] | 19 | 0.105 | [0.063, 0.164] |
| Northeast | | 1.313 | [0.915, 1.83] | | 0.180 | [0.125, 0.250] |
| Middle Atlantic | 32 | 1.343 | [0.907, 1.920] | 26 | 0.181 | [0.118, 0.266] |
| New England | 3 | 1.066 | [0.220, 3.11] | 10 | 0.176 | [0.084, 0.324] |
| South | | 0.659 | [0.489, .870] | | 0.149 | [0.109, 0.200] |
| West South Central | 14 | 0.693 | [0.378, 1.164] | 13 | 0.139 | [0.074, 0.238] |
| East South Central | 11 | 0.677 | [0.338, 1.21] | 8 | 0.138 | [0.059, 0.272] |
| South Atlantic | 28 | 0.637 | [0.424, .924] | 22 | 0.161 | [0.101, 0.243] |

[a] 95% C.I. based on Poisson distribution of deaths.
*Source*: Ref. 42.

definitions of asthma, but successive surveys by the National Center for Health Statistics have indicated changes in prevalence of asthma among children 6–11 years of age (Table 2) (45). Prevalence increased from 5.3% in 1963–1965 and 4.8% in 1971–1974 to 7.6% in 1976–1980. Asthma was defined as a current history of asthma diagnosed by a physician at some time in the past and/or frequent trouble with wheezing during the past 12 months, excluding colds or the flu. Among black adolescents 12–17 years old there was a significant increase in prevalence from 4.6% in 1971–1974 to 10.1% in 1976–1980, but interpretation of these data is complicated by a significant decrease in 1971–1974 from 7.0% in 1966–1969. These surveys disclosed no significant changes in prevalence among whites 12–17 years of age, for whom rates in the successive surveys were 5.8%, 6.3%, and 5.9% (45).

More recent data from annual Health Interview Surveys have indicated an increase in prevalence of asthma of 60% from 1979–1989 for children and adolescents less than 18 years of age and an increase of 71% for adults 18–44 years old (Fig. 8). Large though these increases are, they are not sufficient to account fully for the increases in mortality rates with rates of mortality at 10–14 years of age that have quadrupled (21).

It is not clear why there should have been an increase in prevalence of asthma, but certain environmental variables have been identified as risk factors. Data from the Child Health Supplement to the 1981 National Health Interview Survey indicated a prevalence of 4.4% among black children less than 18 years of age and a prevalence of 2.5% among white children (46). More than 80% of the children with asthma at 6–17 years of age had had the onset of asthma at less than 6 years of age, including 71% of the white children and 90% of the blacks (46). Onset had been during the first year for 35% of both whites and blacks but during the second year for 9% of whites and 26% of blacks and during the third year

TABLE 2 Cumulative Prevalence of Asthma (%) at 6–11 Years of Age

| Survey | Total | White | Black |
|---|---|---|---|
| HES II, 1963–1965 | 5.3 | 5.2 | 5.5 |
| NHANES I, 1971–1974 | 4.8 | 4.7 | 5.1 |
| NHANES II, 1976–1980 | 7.6* | 7.2* | 9.6 |

* $p < 0.01$ compared with NHANES I.
HES, Health Examination Survey; NHANES, National Health and Nutrition Examination Survey.
*Source*: Ref. 45.

for 10% of whites and 23% of blacks. Higher rates of onset of asthma during only the second and third years for black children suggests an adverse impact on them of environmental variables.

Increased rates of asthma were associated with poverty, maternal smoking, large family size, small home size, low birth weight, and maternal age less than 20 years at the child's birth (46). After these other risk factors were controlled for, race and poverty were no longer significant risk factors. Thus, socioeconomic factors that cause crowding and possibly increased exposure to house dust mite allergens and to respiratory infectious agents may increase the risk of asthma.

Maternal smoking during pregnancy at the rate of at least 1/2 pack per day was a risk factor for asthma, and it was assumed that smoking usually continued after birth of the child (47).

Analysis of data from the Second National Health and Nutrition Examination Survey of 1976–1980 also identified certain risk factors for asthma (48). For children 6 months–11 years of age the prevalence of asthma was 3.0% for white children and 7.2% among blacks and prevalence of frequent wheezing during the previous 12 months "apart from colds and flu" was 6.2% among whites and 9.3% among blacks. As disclosed by other surveys, prevalence was higher among boys than girls. Other risk factors for asthma or frequent wheezing were low family income, living in a central city, low birth weight, young maternal age, premature birth, not having been breast fed, and increasing body mass index, triceps skinfold thickness, and total food energy intake (48). After adjusting for these other variables, black children were still at increased risk for asthma.

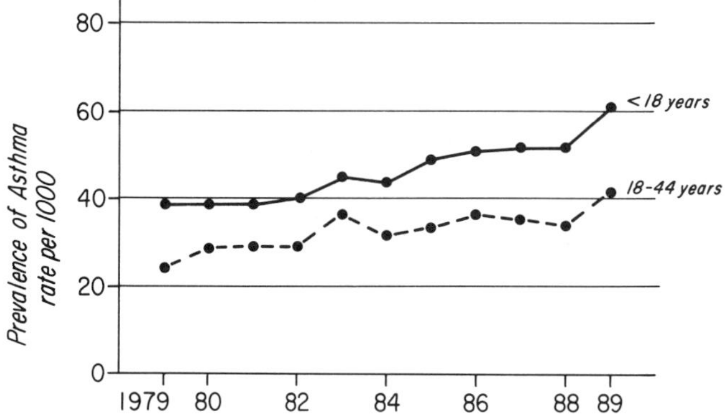


FIGURE 8 Prevalence of current asthma per 1,000 general population by year. (Data from National Health Interview Surveys).

## Effects of Treatment

Increasing mortality from asthma during a decade when there has been increasingly widespread use of inhaled β-agonists and slow-release theophylline in the United States has suggested possible drug toxicity. Administration of theophylline to fat rats in relatively high dosages can enhance the toxic effect of parenteral isoproterenol or terbutaline, increasing the frequency of fatal cardiac arrhythmias, an effect potentiated by adrenal corticosteroids (49). The clinical relevance of these observations is uncertain, but treatment of acute asthma in children and adolescents with intravenous isoproterenol has been associated with increased serum concentrations of the cardiac-specific creatine phosphokinase MB isoenzyme (50). Postmortem examination of an adolescent who died after developing a cardiac arrhythmia while receiving intravenous isoproterenol has disclosed focal myocardial necrosis (51). It is clear that inhalation of β-agonists is far safer than intravenous infusion.

On the other hand, review of the 271 deaths from asthma in the 2 year national survey in New Zealand in 1981–1983 disclosed only nine deaths for which excessive use of a β-agonist might have been a contributing factor (24). Excessive drug therapy was implicated in only 2 of the 16 children less than 15 years of age in this group (26). One had used the entire contents of a β-agonist inhaler within 2 days, but used it only three times during the 3 hr before death. The other may have received four or five slow-release theophylline tablets within 8 hr but was thought to have died from severe asthma.

Data from New Zealand are of special interest because of the very high rates of death from asthma there, where rates peaked at 8.1:100,000 in 1980 (20). However, New Zealand mortality rates have been decreasing since then (Fig. 5). In 1980 New Zealand sales of β-agonist inhalers and corticosteroid inhalers increased by 60% each over the previous year, theophylline sales increased by 100%, and cromolyn sales increased by 33% (52). Sales have continued to increase since then, suggesting that the previously higher mortality rates from asthma were due to undertreatment rather than overtreatment. The per capita rate of β-agonist inhaler sales in New Zealand in 1980 was four times that in the United States (53).

Another difference between treatment of asthma in New Zealand and the United States has been the availability of fenoterol in New Zealand. Inhalation of fenoterol can cause more tachycardia and more extreme hypokalemia than albuterol or terbutaline at dosages that elicit comparable bronchodilation (54). Case–control studies have established that use of fenoterol has doubled the risk of death from asthma in New Zealand compared with use of albuterol (55). Much of the high rate of deaths from asthma in New Zealand may have been due to the popularity of fenoterol there.

Some deaths from asthma have been due to inadequate treatment by emergency technicians, who often have been neither trained nor equipped for administration of epinephrine by injection and are not prepared for administration of β-agonists by inhalation. These deficiencies of care delivered by emergency personnel emphasize the importance of prescribing injectable epinephrine for use when the patient is unable to communicate with emergency personnel or unable to inhale a β-agonist effectively.

Prompt, effective treatment is essential. When provisions for responses to emergency calls in Paris were revised to provide for immediate dispatching of an ambulance with a physician whenever the caller mentioned asthma, average delays in treatment were reduced from an average of 28 min to 10 min, and there was a sixfold reduction in rates of mortality among patients who called for emergency care of asthma (56).

## Risk Factors

A case–control study of 44 deaths from asthma in New Zealand disclosed an association of fatal asthma with poorer medical care than that received by other asthmatic patients matched for age, sex, and race (57). Community control subjects were selected at random from patients who had consulted generalists for treatment of asthma at the same time as when the deaths had occurred, and a random sample of hospital control subjects was selected from patients discharged from the hospitals after admission for asthma. Medical care scores were below average nearly three times as often among those who died as compared with the community controls. Medical care was evaluated with a 12-item medical management score (Table 3).

There had been no measurement of pulmonary function nearly three times as often among those who died as among the community controls (Table 4). Noncompliance with recommendations for medical management was far more frequent among those who died than among the controls.

Those who died were 16 times as likely to have been admitted to a hospital for treatment of asthma during the previous year than the community controls and 8.5 times as likely to have required an emergency room visit (Table 5). Seven of those who died had had previous respiratory arrests, and 20 of the 44 had had life-threatening episodes of asthma, defined as disturbance of consciousness or "appreciable hypercapnia" due to asthma. None of the community controls had had either.

The only significant risk factors detected by comparison with the hospital controls were previous life-threatening episodes and psychosocial problems

TABLE 3 Sound Medical Management During Previous 12 Months

| |
|---|
| How to use inhaler demonstrated |
| Use of peak flow meter at home |
| Physician and patient agree about drugs in regular use |
| Continuity of care by physician |
| Referral for consultation for severe asthma |
| Adequate communication between primary care physician and consultant |
| Pulmonary function measured within past year |
| Pulmonary function measured at each visit |
| Patient advised what to do for unusually severe episode of asthma |
| When to increase β-agonist |
| When to start corticosteriods (for subjects with severe asthma) |
| Where to get help |

*Source*: Ref. 57.

that might have impaired perception of worsening asthma or compliance. These included alcoholism, personality disorder, depression, recent bereavement, and recent unemployment (57).

A case–control study of 21 deaths from asthma 1 month–6 years after discharge from a residential treatment center for asthma in the United States has also implicated psychosocial dysfunction as an important risk factor (58). Those who had died were matched for age, sex, race, and severity of illness with surviving asthmatic children 7–14 years of age at the time of admission to the residential treatment facility. Histories of hypoxic seizures, use of inhaled beclomethasone, and reductions of corticosteroid dosage by more than 50% during hospitalization were significantly more frequent among those who died, but identified those who died only when associated with psychological difficulty (Table 6). Factors that did not differentiate those who died from controls included inhaler abuse (recognized in 11 who died and in 9 controls), nocturnal asthma, corticosteroid dependence, and adrenal suppression as measured by serum cortisol concentrations.

Most deaths from asthma have occurred in patients with severe asthma, although inadequacies of management suggest that most deaths have been preventable. Some deaths have occurred in patients considered to have only mild asthma. Forty-four of 163 deaths from asthma in Victoria, Australia, in 1986–1987 occurred in patients 5–39 years of age (59). Twelve of these 44 deaths occurred in patients with only mild asthma, many of whom could participate in strenuous activity. Another 13 had had only moderate asthma. Twenty-nine of the deaths in this age group occurred within 20 min of the onset of symptoms or, in a few cases, after sudden

TABLE 4 Medical Management and Relative Risk of Death from Asthma with 95% Confidence Limits

| Risk Factor | Hospital control subjects (39 matched pairs) | Community control subjects (44 matched pairs) |
|---|---|---|
| Below-average medical care score | 1.9 (0.7,5.1) | 2.9* (1.2,8.0) |
| Pulmonary function not measured in past year | 1.1 (0.4,3.1) | 2.7* (1.1,7.6) |
| Three or more types of asthma drug prescribed in past year | 1.7 (0.6,5.1) | 3.0* (1.04, 10.5) |
| Three or more types of asthma drug taken in past year | 1.0 (0.4, 2.3) | 2.4 (0.96,6.9) |
| Noncompliance with medical treatment | 1.4 (0.6,3.8) | ∞** (5.2, ∞) |

* $p < 0.05$.
** $p < 0.01$, compared with relative risk of 1.0.
*Source*: Ref. 57.

TABLE 5 Indicators of Severity and Relative Risk of Death from Asthma with 95% Confidence Limits

| Indicator | Hospital control subjects (39 matched pairs) | Community control subjects (44 matched pairs) |
|---|---|---|
| Hospitalized for asthma in past year | 0.8 (0.3,2.1) | 16.0* (2.5,665.7) |
| Emergency room visit for asthma in past year | 1.1 (0.4,2.9) | 8.5* (2.0,75.9) |
| Previous respiratory arrest | 5.0 (0.6,237.1) | ∞* (1.4, ∞) |
| Previous life-threatening asthma | 3.8** (1.2,15.5) | ∞* (4.9, ∞) |
| Psychosocial problem | 3.5** (1.04, 13.7) | |

Relative risk is ratio of discordant pairs.
* $p < 0.01$, compared with relative risk of 1.0.
** $p < 0.05$, compared with relative risk of 1.0.
*Source*: Ref. 57.

TABLE 6 Physiological and Psychological Variables Differentiating Children and Adolescents Who Died of Asthma from Matched Control Subjects

| Variable | No. of patients | | |
|---|---|---|---|
| | Deaths | Control subjects | p[a] |
| Physiological | | | |
| History of seizures associated with episodes of asthma | 9 | 1 | 0.01 |
| Inhaled beclomethasone dipropionate | 13 | 6 | 0.05 |
| Prednisone decreased >50% of initial dosage during hospitalization | 13 | 5 | 0.01 |
| More symptoms of asthma during week before discharge compared to 4 weeks before discharge | 8 | 2 | 0.05 |
| Psychological | | | |
| Disregard of perceived asthma symptoms | 7 | 2 | 0.06 |
| Self-care in hospital not appropriate for age | 15 | 5 | 0.01 |
| Patient–staff conflict | 15 | 6 | 0.01 |
| Parent–staff conflict | 15 | 6 | 0.01 |
| Patient–parent conflict | 12 | 5 | 0.05 |
| Maniplative use of asthma | 19 | 12 | 0.01 |
| Emotional disturbance | 18 | 9 | 0.01 |
| Depressive symptoms | 16 | 9 | 0.05 |
| History of emotional/behavior reactions to separation or loss | 15 | 6 | 0.01 |
| Family dysfunction (parental psychopathology, intense marital conflict, alcoholism, inability to cope with financial difficulties) | 17 | 11 | 0.05 |

[a] p value from chi-square for differences in probabilities.
*Source*: Ref. 58.

worsening after stabilization or improvement in response to initial treatment. Nineteen deaths occurred at 5–19 years of age; 10 in children and adolescents with mild asthma, and 15 within 20 min of the onset of symptoms. Such rapid progression of symptoms mandates prompt attention to symptoms even when apparently mild initially and preparation of patients to manage their own treatment initially and to seek assistance immediately when there is any question about the adequacy of their response to treatment.

The possibility of rapid progression of symptoms also indicates the importance of preventing symptoms by adequate long-term management of asthma. Yet, a study of asthmatic schoolchildren in Baltimore disclosed that 24% of the white children and 44% of the blacks relied upon emergency rooms as their source of primary care for asthma (60). Although emergency rooms should be excellent sources of care for acute asthma, their personnel cannot provide the intensive evaluation and comprehensive management necessary for optimal long-term management of asthma.

### Failure of Diagnosis

Adequate management of asthma is possible only after accurate diagnosis. Study of 147 deaths in England in which asthma was mentioned anywhere on the death certificate disclosed that in 4 of the 89 deaths due to asthma the diagnosis had not been made before death and in five others asthma had not been recognized during the final episode (61).

Failures of diagnosis are common. Study of 179 7-year-old schoolchildren who had had at least one episode of wheezing since entry to school in England disclosed that asthma had been diagnosed in only 21, although only 14 of the schoolchildren had not been examined by a physician (62). Thirty-one of the children had had more than 12 episodes of wheezing during the previous year, but only 11 of them had been diagnosed as having asthma. One-third of these 31 children with very frequent symptoms had received no bronchodilator therapy, and two-thirds of the 179 children with some symptoms had received no bronchodilator. Absenteeism fell 10-fold in the 31 with frequent symptoms after treatment with cromolyn or beclomethasone was begun (62).

In patients known to have asthma, underestimation of the severity of airway obstruction by patients, their families, and their physicians often has been implicated as having contributed to death. More frequent objective evaluation of pulmonary function should facilitate recognition of airway obstruction that requires treatment (63).

## RECOMMENDATIONS

Alleviation of socioeconomic inequities may be necessary for us to make a major impact on morbidity and mortality from asthma. Improvements in access to medical care and adequate prenatal care through provision of adequate medical insurance should be helpful.

Patients at high risk of death from asthma should be warned of that risk, and all asthmatic patients should be aware of the possibility of a fatal episode. Those at high risk require especially close monitoring and should receive psychotherapy when appropriate for psychological dysfunction.

Physicians should provide patients with written suggestions for emergency management for the patient to present to emergency personnel who may be unfamiliar with the optimal treatment of acute asthma and certainly will be less familiar with the patient than his or her regular physician.

Any severely asthmatic patient also needs a written crisis plan to guide his or her own management of severe episodes. This plan should indicate when and how to increase treatment and where to get further help when necessary. A Medic-Alert bracelet or emblem may be helpful to emergency personnel confronted with a patient who may be unable to communicate with them.

Most deaths from asthma are avoidable. Although reasons for recent increases in mortality from asthma remain obscure, better education of patients, health care providers, and the public should reverse this alarming trend.

## REFERENCES

1. Glaser J. Differential diagnosis of bronchial asthma in infancy and childhood. *Ann Allergy* 4:409–424, 1946.
2. Adams F, ed (translated by Adams F). *The Extant Works of Aretaeus the Cappadocian*, London, Sydenham Society, 1856.
3. Maimonides M. Treatise on asthma. In: Muntner S (ed.), *Treatise on Asthma*, Philadelphia, JB Lippincott, 1963.
4. Millar J. *Observations on the Asthma and Whooping Cough*, London, T Cabel, 1769.
5. Salter HH. *On Asthma, Its Pathology and Treatment*, London, Churchill, 1860.
6. Laennec RTH (translated by Forbes J). *A Treatise on the Diseases of the Chest and Mediate Auscultation*, 3rd ed, London, Thomas and Underwood, 1829.
7. Osler W. *The Principles and Practice of Medicine*, Edinburgh and London, Young J Pentland, 1892:498.
8. Alexander HL. A historical account of death from asthma. *J Allergy* 34:305–313, 1963.
9. US Dept Health, Education, and Welfare. Vital statistics of the United States, 1950–60.
10. Speizer FE, Doll R, Heaf P. Observations on recent increase in mortality from asthma. *Br Med J* 1:335–339, 1968.
11. Inman WHW, Adelstein AM. Rise and fall of asthma mortality in England and Wales in relation to use of pressurized aerosols. *Lancet* 2:279–285, 1969.
12. Speizer FE, Doll R, Heaf P, Strang LB. Investigation into use of drugs preceding death from asthma. *Br Med J* 1:339–343, 1968.
13. Stolley PD. Asthma mortality. Why the United States was spared an epidemic of deaths due to asthma. *Am Rev Respir Dis* 105:883–890, 1972.
14. Gandevia B. Pressurized sympathomimetic aerosols and their lack of relationship to asthma mortality in Australia. *Med J Aust* 1:273–277, 1973.

15. Speizer FE. Historical perspectives: the epidemic of asthma deaths in the United Kingdom in the 1960s. *J Allergy Clin Immunol* 80:368–372, 1987.
16. U.S. Department of Health and Human Services. Advance report of final mortality statistics, 1988. NCHS Monthly Vital Statistics Report 1990; 39(7).
17. Klebba AJ, Scott JH. Estimates of selected comparability ratios based on dual coding of 1976 death certificates by the eighth and ninth revisions of the International Classification of Diseases. DHEW Pub. (PHS) 80-1120, vol 28, no 11(suppl) Feb 29, 1980.
18. Sly RM. Increases in deaths from asthma. *Ann Allergy* 53:20–25, 1984.
19. Sly RM. Mortality from asthma. *N Engl Reg Allergy Proc* 7:425–434, 1986.
20. Sly RM. Mortality from asthma, 1979–1984. *J Allergy Clin Immunol* 82:705–717, 1988.
21. Sly RM. Mortality from asthma in children 1979–1984. *Ann Allergy* 60:433–443, 1988.
22. Ormerod LP, Stableforth DE. Asthma mortality in Birmingham, 1975–7; 53 deaths. *Br Med J* 280:687–690, 1980.
23. British Thoracic Society. Accuracy of death certificates in bronchial asthma. *Thorax* 39:505–509, 1984.
24. Sears MR, Rea HH, Beaglehole R, et al. Asthma mortality in New Zealand: a two-year national study. *NZ Med J* 98:271–275, 1985.
25. Barger LW, Vollmer WM, Felt RW, Buist AS. Further investigation into the recent increase in asthma death rates: a review of 41 asthma deaths in Oregon in 1982. *Ann Allergy* 60:31–39, 1988.
26. Sears MR, Rea HH, Fenwick J, et al. Deaths from asthma in New Zealand. *Arch Dis Child* 61:6–10, 1986.
27. Cutz E, Levison H, Cooper DM. Ultrastructure of airways in children with asthma. *Histopathology* 2:407–421, 1978.
28. Gleich GJ, Motojima S, Frigas E, et al. The eosinophilic leukocyte and the pathology of fatal bronchial asthma: evidence for pathologic heterogeneity. *J Allergy Clin Immunol* 80:412–415, 1987.
29. Buranakul B, Washington J, Hilman B, et al. Causes of death during acute asthma in children. *Am J Dis Child* 128:343–350, 1974.
30. Nguyen MT, Patterson K, Sly RM. Causes of death from asthma in children. *Ann Allergy* 55:448–453, 1985.
31. Hossain S. Quantitative measurement of bronchial muscle in men with asthma. *Am Rev Respir Dis* 107:99–109, 1973.
32. Laitinen LA, Heino M, Laitinen A, et al. Damage of the airway epithelium and bronchial reactivity in patients with asthma. *Am Rev Respir Dis* 131:599–606, 1985.
33. Gleich GJ, Flavahan NA, Fujisawa T, et al. The eosinophil as a mediator of damage to respiratory epithelium: a model for bronchial hyperreactivity. *J Allergy Clin Immunol* 81:776–781, 1988.
34. Wood DW, Lecks HJ. Deaths due to childhood asthma. Are they preventable? *Clin Pediatr* 8:677–687, 1976.
35. Hetzel MR, Clark TJH, Branthwaite MA. Asthma: analysis of sudden deaths and ventilatory arrests in hospital. *Br Med J* 1:808–811, 1977.

36. Ryan G, Latimer KM, Dolovich J, et al. Bronchial responsiveness to histamine: relationship to diurnal variation of peak flow rate, improvement after bronchodilator, and airway calibre. *Thorax* 37:423–429, 1982.
37. James AL, Pare PD, Hogg JC. The mechanics of airway narrowing in asthma. *Am Rev Respir Dis* 139:242–246, 1989.
38. Sly RM, O'Donnell R. Regional distribution of deaths from asthma. *Ann Allergy* 62:347–354, 1989.
39. Weiss KB, Wagener DK. Changing patterns of asthma mortality. Identifying target populations at high risk. *JAMA* 264:1683–1687, 1990.
40. Weiss KB, Carr W, Zeitel L. Geographic variations in asthma hospitalizations and deaths in New York City (abstract). *J Allergy Clin Immunol* 85:195, 1990.
41. Rea HH, Sears MR, Beaglehole R, et al. Lessons from the national asthma mortality study: circumstances surrounding death. *NZ Med J* 100:10–13, 1987.
42. Sly RM, O'Donnell R. Association of asthma mortality with medical specialist density. *Ann Allergy* 68:340–344, 1992.
43. Charpin D, Kleisbauer J-P, Lanteaume A, et al. Asthma and allergy to house-dust mites in populations living in high altitudes. *Chest* 93:758–761, 1988.
44. Sly RM, O'Donnell R. Lack of effect of geographic elevation on mortality from asthma. *Ann Allergy* 63:495–497, 1989.
45. Gergen PJ, Mullally DI, Evans RE III. National survey of prevalence of asthma among children in the United States, 1976 to 1980. *Pediatrics* 81:1–7, 1988.
46. Weitzman M, Gortmaker S, Sobol A. Racial, social, and environmental risks for childhood asthma. *Am J Dis Child* 144:1189–1194, 1990.
47. Weitzman M, Gortmaker S, Walker DK, Sobol A. Maternal smoking and childhood asthma. *Pediatrics* 85:505–511, 1990.
48. Schwartz J, Gold D, Dockery DW, et al. Predictors of asthma and persistent wheeze in a national sample of children in the United States. *Am Rev Respir Dis* 142:555–562, 1990.
49. Nicklas RA, Whitehurst VE, Donohoe RF, et al. Concomitant use of beta-adrenergic agonists and methylxanthines. *J Allergy Clin Immunol* 73:20–24, 1984.
50. Maguire JF, Geha RS, Umetsu DT. Myocardial specific creatine phosphokinase isoenzyme elevation in children with asthma treated with intravenous isoproterenol. *J Allergy Clin Immunol* 78:631–636, 1986.
51. Kurland G, Williams J, Lewiston NJ. Fatal myocardial toxicity during continuous infusion intravenous isoproterenol therapy of asthma. *J Allergy Clin Immunol* 63:407–411, 1979.
52. Keating G, Mitchell EA, Jackson R, et al. Trends in sales of drugs for asthma in New Zealand, Australia, and the United Kingdom, 1975–81. *Br Med J* 289:348–351, 1984.
53. Sly RM. Effects of treatment on mortality from asthma. *Ann Allergy* 56:207–212, 1986.
54. Wong CS, Pavord ID, Williams J, et al. Bronchodilator, cardiovascular, and hypokalaemic effects of fenoterol, salbutamol, and terbutaline in asthma. *Lancet* 336:1396–1399, 1990.

55. Grainger J, Woodman K, Pearce N, et al. Prescribed fenoterol and death from asthma in New Zealand, 1981–7: a further case–control study. *Thorax* 46:105–111, 1991.
56. Barriot P, Riou B. Prevention of fatal asthma. *Chest* 92:460–466, 1987.
57. Rea HH, Scragg R, Jackson R, et al. A case–control study of deaths from asthma. *Thorax* 41:833–839, 1986.
58. Strunk RC, Mrazek DA, Fuhrmann GSW, et al. Physiologic and psychological characteristics associated with deaths due to asthma in childhood. *JAMA* 254:1193–1198, 1985.
59. Robertson CF, Rubinfeld AR, Bowes G. Deaths from asthma in Victoria: a 12-month survey. *Med J Aust* 152:511–517, 1990.
60. Mak H, Johnston P, Abbey H, et al. Prevalence of asthma and health service utilization of asthmatic children in an inner city. *J Allergy Clin Immunol* 70:367–372, 1982.
61. Hills EA, Somner AR, Stewart CJ, et al. Accuracy of death certificates in bronchial asthma. *Thorax* 39:505–509, 1984.
62. Speight ANP, Lee DA, Hey EN. Underdiagnosis and undertreatment of asthma in childhood. *Br Med J* 286:1253–1256, 1983.
63. Williams AJ, Church SE. A near fatal asthma attack in a patient unaware of deteriorating lung function. *Eur J Respir Dis* 71:259–262, 1987.

# 8

# Relationship of Viral and Bacterial Infections to Bronchial Hyperreactivity

**KETAN K. SHETH and WILLIAM W. BUSSE**

*University of Wisconsin Medical School*
*Madison, Wisconsin*

Respiratory infections have a very important influence on asthma and possibly the development of airway hyperresponsiveness. For many patients with asthma, especially children, respiratory infections provoke wheezing. Less well established is the possibility that respiratory infections are a pivotal event in the onset of asthma. The relationship of respiratory infections and asthma has focused on two major issues: the epidemiology of respiratory infections and asthma, and the mechanisms of virus-induced asthma. This chapter will focus on these issues and use respiratory syncytial virus (RSV) bronchiolitis as a clinical model for the mechanisms of viral-induced airway hyperresponsiveness.

## VIRAL RESPIRATORY INFECTIONS EXACERBATE ASTHMA

For decades clinicians "knew" that respiratory infections provoked asthma in many of their patients. Initial attention was focused upon bacteria as the causative agents. However, prospective studies conclusively indicated that viral, not bacterial, respiratory infections triggered asthma. For example, McIntosh and co-workers (1) selected 32 young children, aged 1–5 years of age, and prospectively evaluated exacerbations of wheezing with respiratory tract infections. Of the 139 asthma attacks experienced by these children, 58 episodes (42%) occurred during a viral respiratory infection, of which RSV was the most frequent. Although bacteria such as *Haemophilus influenzae, Streptococcus pneumoniae*, β-hemolytic *Streptococcus*, and *Staphylococcus aureus* were also cultured, their presence did not correlate with an asthma attack.

A prospective outpatient study from the University of Wisconsin evaluated 16 children, aged 3–11 years,with histories of 4 or more asthma attacks associated with respiratory illnesses during the previous year (2). Detailed clinical records profiled each child's asthma severity, which was further substantiated with biweekly examinations. During an asthma exacerbation, or apparent upper respiratory tract infection (URI), additional bacterial and viral cultures were collected and asthma symptoms carefully quantitated.

The 16 children experienced 61 episodes of asthma; 42 occurred in conjunction with a symptomatic respiratory infection and 24 were confirmed by culture and/or serum hemagglutination titers to be viral. In this study, rhinovirus was the most frequently isolated virus in association with wheezing. Some patients had episodes of asymptomatic viral infection, but asthma was not worsened. Only one episode of wheezing coincided with a bacterial infection.

Horn et al. (3) also found that RSV was an important pathogen for children who wheezed with respiratory infections. Furthermore, they noted that the development of constitutional symptoms was important for a flare of asthma to occur, and that patients at increased risk for wheezing with viral respiratory infections were young children, more often boys than girls, with a history of allergic diseases or positive skin tests, and airway hyperresponsiveness in response to an exercise challenge. Wheezing was more likely to occur with the cold if the children were symptomatic with malaise, mucus production, or cough. Some asymptomatic patients had respiratory viruses recovered on routine culture, but experienced no increase in wheezing. Taken together, these observations indicate that wheezing with a cold is dependent not only on the presence of respiratory viruses but also on the development of constitutional symptoms.

In a large study of pediatric outpatients at the University of North Carolina, 6,165 patients were evaluated for lower respiratory illnesses during which 1,851 (30%) had wheezing (4). Wheezing with a respiratory illness was more common in children less than 2 years old. Yet 19% of patients over 9 years of age wheezed with respiratory infections. RSV, parainfluenza, adenovirus, and *Mycoplasma pneumoniae* accounted for over 80% of the isolates in children with wheezing.

In contrast, the relationship between respiratory infections and episodes of wheezing is not as striking in adults. When both children and adults were evaluated, respiratory viruses were more frequently identified during episodes of asthma in children under 10 years of age than in adults (5). Eight adult subjects evaluated by Minor et al. (5) had only three documented viral infections with increased wheezing. Although an explanation for such findings is not clear, it is likely that asthma flares are more difficult to sharply delineate, and the pattern of wheezing often appears chronic rather than episodic in adults. Similarly, when Hudgel and co-workers (6) evaluated 19 adult asthmatic patients over a 15 month period, 76 episodes of asthma were recorded but only 8 could be documented with a viral URI. Although clinically apparent viral respiratory infections precipitate asthma in adults, the relative frequency appears less than in children.

Not all subjects are susceptible to wheezing with respiratory infections, nor are all respiratory viruses, or strains of one virus, capable of provoking asthma. Half of a normal adult volunteer population experimentally infected with rhinovirus by Halperin et al. (7) had positive cultures from their lower respiratory tract at bronchoscopy; neither spirometry nor bronchoprovocation with histamine changed during the respiratory illness. When the same investigators inoculated asthma volunteers with rhinovirus, only 4 of the 21 infected asthmatic patients had a 10% or greater decrease in forced expiratory volume in 1 sec ($FEV_1$) and a concomitant increase in airway sensitivity to inhaled histamine (8). Although the investigators interpreted their findings to show that experimental rhinovirus infections aggravate airway reactivity in a minority of adult patients with asthma, an exacerbation of wheezing with other viral pathogens is more likely to play an important role in this relationship. This frequency of wheezing during URIs is not unusual for adults (5,6). Moreover, it is important to recall that symptomatic respiratory infections, not merely the recovery of viruses from the airway, are more inclined to incite asthma in both children and adults (2). Thus, the effect that a viral respiratory infection has on lung function will be dictated by many factors including the patient's age, underlying airway hyperreactivity, the particular respiratory virus, and the development of significant symptoms (rhinorrhea, malaise, etc.).

## ROLE OF BACTERIAL RESPIRATORY INFECTIONS AS PRECIPITANTS OF ASTHMA

To determine the contribution of bacterial infections to wheezing, Berman et al. (9) performed transtracheal aspirations during an "infectious" flare of asthma in 27 adult patients. Bacteria was cultured from airway aspirates, but differences in the number of colonies found in asthmatic patients and asymptomatic control subjects was not significant, and the recovery of bacteria did not correlate with clinical illness.

However, it is premature to conclude that bacteria are unimportant to asthma. There is renewed interest in the role of bacterial sinusitis and wheezing (10–12). Most commonly, asthma and sinusitis are found in nonallergic adults with nasal polyps. Moreover, Rachelefsky and co-workers (11) found that children can experience similar flares of wheezing with sinusitis. Forty-eight children with asthma and radiographic evidence of sinusitis were treated for sinus disease. After antibiotic treatment, 67% had normal pulmonary functions compared with 0% prior to treatment. Moreover, when antibiotic therapy led to resolution of their sinusitis, nearly 80% of the treated children were able to discontinue use of bronchodilators because their asthma was obviously better controlled. Zimmerman and coworkers (13) confirmed the high prevalence of abnormalities found by sinus x-ray in children with lower respiratory tract symptoms of cough or wheeze

(31%) compared to controls (0%), but were unable to support the hypothesis that sinusitis was a factor in the aggravation of asthma and increased need for medication. Although these observations are intriguing, additional insight is needed to understand how sinusitis exacerbates asthma. Thus, sinus infections are common in asthmatic patients, and the site of the respiratory infection (sinuses vs. airway) may dictate the contribution of bacterial illness to asthma. The mechanism(s) by which sinusitis influences asthmatic symptoms are likely to be different from that of viral respiratory infections. It is conceivable that sinusitis and asthma may coexist as complications of the same respiratory infection.

## ROLE OF RESPIRATORY INFECTIONS AND DEVELOPMENT OF ASTHMA

In comparison to the question of whether viral respiratory infections exacerbate asthma, the issue becomes more complex when the role of respiratory illnesses is examined "in the causation and perpetuation of airways hyperresponsiveness and, by implication, recurrent, chronic wheeze-associated respiratory illnesses including asthma" (14). Although a significant body of information suggests an association between respiratory tract illness in early life and later development of airway dysfunction, this relationship cannot be definitively established and underscores the complexity of factors surrounding the development of bronchial reactivity and asthma (15).

Eisen and Bacal (16) found that children hospitalized for bronchiolitis prior to age 2 had an increased risk for asthma. Rooney and Williams (17) also evaluated retrospectively the records of infants hospitalized for bronchiolitis at 18 months or younger; allergic manifestations and a family history of asthma were more frequent in children who eventually experienced one or more episodes of wheezing. Finally, McConnochie and Roghmann (18) identified 77 patients who had bronchiolitis at 25 months or younger and compared their outcome to children without a history of bronchiolitis. When these children were evaluated approximately 7 years later, only upper respiratory allergy, bronchiolitis, and passive smoking exposure were found to be independent predictors of wheezing following bronchiolitis.

It is therefore apparent that final conclusions on the relationship between respiratory infections in infancy and later asthma must consider a host of influences, including parental smoking, air pollution, underlying airway reactivity, and gender. A more difficult issue to resolve is the relationship between respiratory infections and the genesis of airway hyperresponsiveness.

## LONG-TERM SEQUELAE OF ACUTE BRONCHIOLITIS IN INFANCY

To evaluate the potential effect of bronchiolitis on airway responsiveness, Sims and co-workers (19) identified 25 8-year-old children who had had RSV infections and quantitated bronchial "lability" by exercise tests. Fifty-one percent had recurrent wheeze by history compared with 3% of a control group. Although the fall in the peak flow to exercise was greater in children who had bronchiolitis compared to controls, airway reactivity to exercise was not different between children with or without subsequent episodes of wheezing. Since other variables confounded their study, Sims and colleagues could not prove that respiratory infections led to the later development of asthma.

Zweiman et al. (20) evaluated 35 children 5 years after hospitalization for acute bronchiolitis; 50% continued to have asthma, although often of diminished intensity. Children most likely to be "persistent wheezers" were offspring of parents with atopic illnesses. Other efforts have been made to ascertain if lower respiratory tract viral infections in early life cause persistent pulmonary function abnormalities. Pullan and Hey (21) retrospectively identified 130 children admitted to hospitals during the first year of life with RSV lower respiratory tract infection and evaluated them 10 years later. Forty-two percent of the hospitalized children had had further episodes of wheezing, while only 19% of control subjects experienced similar airway symptoms. However, few patients (6.2% vs. 4.5% of controls) had troublesome respiratory symptoms by 10 years of age. Furthermore, although a threefold increase in bronchial reactivity was found in the children with bronchiolitis, atopy was not increased. Analogous conclusions were reached by Weiss and co-workers (22) when they assessed the outcome of an antecedent acute respiratory illness on airway responsiveness and atopy in young adults.

Sly and Hibbat (23) prospectively evaluated 48 infants who had RSV infections in the first year of life. During the 5 year follow-up, 92% (cumulative prevalence) reported symptoms suggestive of asthma; however, the number reporting asthma symptoms each year declined over the 5 year interval. Although 67% of these patients had a positive bronchoprovocation response to histamine at the 5 year follow-up, there was no correlation between bronchial responsiveness to histamine, family history of atopy, or clinical asthma. Thus, the authors concluded that while the majority of children who have RSV infections in the first year will report symptoms suggestive of asthma, no correlation is possible between clinical history, histamine challenge, and family history of allergic disease.

Mok and Simpson (24) evaluated 200 children 7 years after hospitalization for acute lower respiratory tract infection. One hundred of these children had documented RSV infections; 47% had recurrent wheezing vs. 17% of matched controls. Lung function was significantly lower in the hospitalized infants vs controls ($FEV_1$ 91.3% vs. 95% of predicted values, $p < 0.005$). Their results suggest that children who had been hospitalized with RSV bronchiolitis have increased respiratory symptoms, asthma, and bronchial hyperreactivity compared to controls at 7 years of age. To assess bronchial reactivity in children who had bronchiolitis, Gurwitz et al. (25) studied 48 children 10 years after hospitalization using methacholine bronchoprovocation; 57% had bronchial hyperreactivity but only 14 children still had asthma, which was mild.

It has been hypothesized that the occurrence of wheezing in infancy may be an "infectious challenge test" to unmask previously dysfunctional lungs. The possibility has also been raised that a predisposition to wheezing in infancy depends more on intrinsic airway structure or bronchial responsiveness than atopy (26). Furthermore, the respiratory tract outcome could depend on the interaction of lung function and other variables including airway responsiveness, tendency towards allergic disease, and environmental factors such as allergens, smoking, or pollution. To clarify the relationship between premorbid lung function and wheezing with respiratory illnesses, Martinez and colleagues (27) conducted a prospective study of respiratory illness in infancy and childhood. They enrolled 1,246 healthy, normal infants for study. Of these, 124 had lung function values determined *prior* to any lower respiratory infection. Included in these measurements were patterns of tidal expiratory patterns, specifically the ratio of time to peak tidal expiratory flow ($T_{me}$) divided by total expiratory time ($T_E$), or the $T_{me}/T_E$ ratio. Morris and Lane (28) had previously shown that decreasing $T_{me}/T_E$ ratios correlated with lower lung function in patients with progressive chronic obstructive lung disease.

Thirty-six infants developed a lower respiratory infection and 24 wheezed with at least 1 of these infections. There was no difference in preinfection lung function between those infants who did not have a lower respiratory infection and those with an infection but no wheezing (Table 1). In contrast, infants who wheezed with the initial respiratory infection had diminished $T_{me}/T_E$ values and reduced expiratory system conductance when measured *prior* to wheezing with the infection. These data suggest that alterations in lung function are compatible with reduced airway conductance and predict wheezing with respiratory infections in infants. Thus, it appears that a given child's response to infection is determined by not only the infection but also the pre-existing lung function.

TABLE 1 Pulmonary Function and LRI Outcome

| Index | No LRI | LRI (no wheeze) | (Wheeze) | p Value |
|---|---|---|---|---|
| $T_{me}/T_E$ | 31.2 ± 9.2 (88) | 31.4 ± 8.5 (12) | 25.4 ± 6.9* (24) | 0.01 |
| $G_{RS}$(liter/sec/cm $H_2O$) | 0.035 ± 0.009(30) | 0.036 ± 0.010(6) | 0.028 ± 0.006**(11) | 0.04 |
| FRC(ml) | 103.2 ± 16.7 (71) | 102.5 ± 15.6 (8) | 97.1 ± 20.8 (15) | 0.63 |
| $\dot{V}_{max}$(ml/sec) | 131.2 ± 47.9 (77) | 119.1 ± 44.0 (11) | 118.6 ± 51.2 (21) | 0.5 |

Values are given as mean ± SD. The number of subjects is shown in parentheses. All values are age or length adjusted.
*p <0.01 for comparison with the no-LRI group.
**p <0.05 for comparison with the no-LRI group.
*Source*: Ref. 27.

In a 3 year follow-up of the initial cohort (27), Martinez et al. (29) examined the relationship between initial lung function and *both* the incidence of new onset wheezing in second and third year of life and recurrent wheezing in infants who wheezed during the first year of life. Infants who wheezed during the first year of life had lower levels of respiratory conductance, maximal flow at end-expiration, initial airway conductance, and functional residual capacity. Infants who first wheezed in the second and third year of life or had only 1 wheezing illness in 3 years also had lower levels of maximal flows at end expiration. Collectively, these studies suggest that "critically narrower peripheral airways may be an important predisposing factor for recurrent obstructive airway episodes during the first 3 years of life" (29).

Taussig et al. (30) also noted that lower levels of lung function predispose to wheezing with lower respiratory infection, as opposed to the infection per se. The precise nature of this predisposition remains to be defined but may lie in airway geometry, airway–parenchyma interaction, or mucosal and smooth muscle response. Furthermore, this pulmonary–structural predisposition may be enhanced by an exaggerated IgE response to viral infection (31,32), resulting in more inflammation and severe wheezing. Since the majority of infants who wheeze with lower respiratory infections do not continue to do so throughout life (33), it is likely that pulmonary function abnormalities that promote wheezing with viral infections are modified with the growth and development of the lung. Long-term outcome may be more closely linked to the persistence of continued airway damage or bronchospasm associated with the development of atopy and true clinical asthma (26).

## RESPIRATORY SYNCYTIAL VIRUS

### RSV Bronchiolitis as a Model for Respiratory Infections and Asthma

Bronchiolitis caused by RSV provides an excellent model to study respiratory infections and the pathogenesis of asthma. It is the most important respiratory pathogen of infancy and early childhood as well as causing the most severe disease in the first several months of life. It infects almost all children in the first years of life and accounts for sizable outbreaks of infection each year, while continuing to cause symptomatic infections throughout life. Each year 95,000 children in the United States are hospitalized with lower respiratory tract RSV infection and more than 4,500 die (34).

## Epidemiology and Clinical Characteristics

In 1956 Morris and colleagues isolated a new virus that they called chimpanzee coryza agent (CCA) from a colony of chimpanzees who developed colds with coryza (35). In 1957, Chanock (36) isolated a similar agent from an infant who had bronchopneumonia and another infant who had laryngotracheobronchitis. Subsequently, these viruses were grouped together into a category called RSV.

It is in the family of paramyxoviridae, in the genus *Pneumovirus*. It is an enveloped, medium-sized virus of 120–300 nm. Its major antigenic specificity is provided by the fusion envelope proteins, (F1 and F2), which play an important role in the infectivity and spread of the virus. Another protein, the G protein, is responsible for viral absorption during infection. Both the F and G proteins are the focus of efforts to develop a vaccine against RSV infection.

There are two subtypes of RSV: A and B, distinguished by antigenic differences in the G protein (34). Infants produce different antibody responses to each subtype. Recent observations appear to substantiate the important differences between the subtypes. To examine the effect of RSV subtype on clinical manifestation of disease, McConnochie et al. (37) reviewed 157 children who had RSV infections from 1985 through 1987 in Rochester, New York. Ninety-five of the children had subtype A while 62 had subtype B. No significant difference emerged between the two subtypes with regard to bronchiolitis or wheezing. However, subtype A provoked significantly worse retractions, rales, tachypnea, acidosis, and hypercarbia. Moreover, the incidence of apnea was five times higher and mechanical ventilation eight times greater in children infected with subtype A. This suggests that the subtype may have a crucial role in the severity of illness associated with RSV infections.

These infections can be further classified into upper and lower respiratory tract illnesses. Symptoms of upper respiratory tract RSV illnesses include cough, otitis media, tracheobronchitis, and croup. Lower respiratory tract manifestations include pneumonia, in which the patient has rales with or without wheezing, and bronchiolitis, in which the patient has wheezing and hyperinflation on chest x-ray. The clinical pattern of RSV infections usually begins with a prodrome of rhinitis followed in several days by fever and cough. Progression to rales, wheezes, hypoxemia, and pulmonary infiltrates may occur. In some infants, apnea may ensue. Early in the infection there is an increase in the total white blood cell count with a concomitant increase in the percentage of polymorphonuclear leukocytes (PMNs) and immature neutrophil forms. Subsequently, the total white blood cell count decreases with a predominance of lymphocytes.

The virus is usually shed from day 2 until day 10 of the illness. Spread of RSV is usually by a large droplets or infected secretions, with nasal secretions being infectious for up to 6 hr. Inoculation of RSV is usually through the eyes or nose. Consequently, prevention of nosocomial RSV infection has been shown with the use of eye/nose goggles (38) and gown–glove isolation in health care workers (39). In a family setting, RSV is often introduced by an older sibling who has a "mild" cold. Moreover, the intrafamilial spread is related to increasing number of family members (40).

The risk of infection and reinfection with respiratory syncytial virus is significant. Glezen et al. (41) found that 118 of 119 children evaluated during the first 5 years of life developed a primary RSV infection by 24 months of age. Moreover, the risk of reinfection was also significant in the first 2 years of life. A significant risk of primary infection occurs in children who attend day care. Ninety-eight percent of children in day care were infected during the first exposure to RSV. In outbreaks during 2 subsequent years, the reinfection rate was 74% and 65%, respectively (4).

### Pathogenesis

The illness with RSV infections is dependent upon virus and host characteristics. First, RSV has a greater tropism for bronchial epithelium in the terminal airways than in the upper respiratory tract. Second, in infants the terminal bronchioles have a small diameter and easily obstruct. Furthermore, peribronchial infiltrates of lymphocytes, macrophages, and plasma cells lead to edema, mucus secretion, and epithelial necrosis that occlude airway lumens to produce hyperinflation and atelectasis (42). However, the severity of RSV infection cannot be attributed only to occlusion of small airways (43), and immunologic factors appear important in determining the severity of RSV illness.

### Antibody-Mediated Immunity

The initial IgM antibody response to RSV begins within several days of infection and lasts for 1–2 weeks; IgG antibodies subsequently appear with peak levels at 4 weeks and then disappear by 2 months after infection. IgG antibody in nasopharyngeal secretion mediates antibody-dependent cellular cytotoxicity (ADCC) to suggest that it is necessary for recovery. The IgA response is more variable and first appears in the nasopharyngeal secretions at about the same time that the virus disappears from the respiratory tract; these observations suggest that IgA is principally involved in terminating the viral shedding (44). Nasal IgA development in adult volunteers appears to correlate better with immunity than serum IgA levels.

It had been hypothesized that due to the lack of a specific secretory IgA during the first nasal challenge with RSV, transplacentally acquired IgG could diffuse into the lumen of the infant airway during an acute viral infection and result in the formation of immune complexes with the virus (45). These immune complexes, in turn, could mediate an arthus-like reaction in the lung or initiate the invasion of granulocytes, resulting in pneumonia (46). Furthermore, phagocytosis of RSV antibody immune complexes have been shown to stimulate the oxidative and arachidonic acid metabolism in neutrophils (47). Production of inflammatory mediators and mediators of airway destruction in the respiratory tract of children could contribute to the development of more serious forms of disease at the time of primary RSV infection.

More recent data appear to point to a minor role for immune complexes in the pathogenesis of RSV infections. Infants who have the highest titers of transplacentally acquired RSV specific IgG appeared to develop less severe disease than those infants with low titers of such antibodies (48). Furthermore, Hemming et al. (49) have recently shown that treatment with intravenous immunoglobulin of a high titer against RSV does not appear to worsen the disease, suggesting a minimal role of antibodies in the pathogenesis. Toms et al. (50) evaluated the serum antibodies to the fusion and large glycoprotein G of respiratory syncytial virus in 57 infants infected with the virus. They found that neither IgG nor IgM responses correlated with the clinical assessment of the severity of infection in the infants. Moreover, IgM responses were weakly correlated with reduced secretion of infectious virus in the upper respiratory tract. Taken together this suggests that "antibody to RSV in the IgG, IgM and IgA isotypes provides incomplete protection against reinfection and potentially has some role in eradication of infection but such antibody does not appear to contribute to the pathogenesis of disease" (43).

### RSV-Specific IgE Antibody Responses

The development of virus-specific IgE antibody in the respiratory tract appears to be related to the appearance of more severe disease. Welliver et al. (31) tested 79 infants (less than 12 months old) with documented RSV infection for the presence of IgE-specific antibody to the infecting virus (Fig. 1). The clinical patterns of illness were classified into four groups: upper respiratory tract illness, pneumonia without wheezing, pneumonia and wheezing, and wheezing (bronchiolitis). Nasal secretions from each patient were measured for IgE-specific antibody to RSV and histamine. When RSV-IgE antibody titers were compared with the patient's

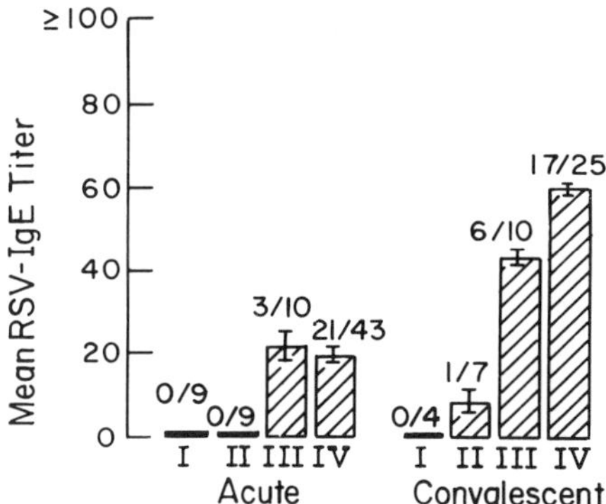


FIGURE 1 The RSV IgE response analyzed according to illness group. The fractions represent the number of patients positive for RSV IgE per number tested. Bars represent arithmetic mean for the RSV IgE titer (± 1 SE). Group I had upper respiratory tract disease only, group II pneumonia without wheezing, group III pneumonia with wheezing, and group IV bronchiolitis without pneumonia. The acute phase represents the first 7 days after the onset of illness, and the convalescent phase the 14–90th day after the onset of illness. (From Ref. 31.)

clinical illness, a striking and intriguing association appeared. IgE titers to RSV were highest in patients with lower respiratory tract illness and evidence of airway obstruction. Furthermore, patients with the highest RSV-IgE titers also had the lowest arterial $pO_2$ values, signifying worse disease.

Similarly, parainfluenza virus (PV)-specific IgE responses were examined in individuals with upper respiratory illness alone or bronchiolitis. Welliver et al. (51) found PV-specific IgE antibody in 8 of 12 with bronchiolitis but only 1 of 10 with upper respiratory disease alone. These studies indicate that respiratory viruses stimulate IgE-specific antibody responses and that the intensity of the response is associated lower airway obstructive disease.

A biological role for virus-specific IgE is strengthened by the presence of chemical mediators in respiratory tract secretions. The frequency and mean concentrations by which histamine was detected were greater in children with bronchiolitis (lower airway disease) than subjects without wheezing (Table 2). Although these observations imply that histamine is a marker for the type and severity of illness from RSV, the correlations were weaker than those noted with IgE-specific antibody titers.

Volovitz et al. (52) measured leukotriene $C_4$ ($LTC_4$) in nasopharyngeal secretions of 73 infants with either RSV bronchiolitis or upper respiratory tract infection alone. $LTC_4$ was detected twice as frequently in patients

TABLE 2 Histamine Content of Nasopharyngeal Secretions Following RSV Infection

| Illness | No. with histamine/ no. tested (%) | Histamine content (ng/mg protein in fluid) (mean ± SE) |
|---|---|---|
| Upper respiratory infection alone | 1/2 (50) | 1.1 ± 1.0 |
| Pneumonia, no wheezing | 2/10 (20) | 0.6 ± 0.01 |
| Bronchiolitis | 27/37 (73) | 2.8 ± 0.2 |

*Source*: Ref. 31.

with bronchiolitis as those with upper airway disease alone; moreover, the concentration of $LTC_4$ was six times higher in those with bronchiolitis (Table 3). Furthermore, the quantity of $LTC_4$ measured directly correlated with the magnitude of RSV-IgE response in nasal secretions. Further studies by Volovitz (53) (Fig. 2) compared groups of children with or without wheezing during respiratory illness and matched healthy controls. The concentration of $LTC_4$ in wheezing children with viral shedding (1520 ± 228 pg/0.1 ml) was consistently elevated compared with children who wheezed without viral shedding (709 ± 147 pg/0.1 ml). Little $LTC_4$ was measured in healthy children. Their data suggest not only that respiratory viruses are a stimuli for release of mediators of inflammation, but also that viral-induced bronchospasm may be related to direct cell-virus interactions or the release of pharmacologically active mediators in the respiratory tract through virus-IgE interactions. Skoner et al. (54) found elevated plasma histamine and prostaglandin metabolites in infants with acute bronchiolitis (Table 4). Again, a correlation was noted between plasma elevations of these mediators and disease severity. Since plasma measurements in a

TABLE 3 $LTC_4$ Release in Nasopharyngeal Secretions of Infants and Children with RSV Infection

| Diagnosis | No. with $LTC_4$/ no. tested (%) | Group mean $LTC_4$ concentration (pg/0.1 ml fluid) |
|---|---|---|
| Upper respiratory infection alone | 7/21 (33) | 224 ± 114* |
| Bronchiolitis | 29/43 (67) | 1271 ± 239* |

*p <0.02
*Source*: Ref. 52.

TABLE 4 Plasma Histamine (pg/ml) and 13,14-Dihydro-15-Keto-$PGF_{2a}$ (pg/ml) Levels Before and After Initial Therapy for Acute Bronchiolitis

| Mediator | Group I (n = 9) | Group II (n = 14) | Group III (n = 12) | Group IV (n = 9) |
|---|---|---|---|---|
| Histamine | 1,923 ± 980 | 1,035 ± 240* | 9,210 ± 5,242 | 360 ± 125 |
| PG metabolite | 1,033 ± 419** | 1,613 ± 527** | 27 ± 7 | 68 ± 25 |

Group I, acute bronchiolitis before therapy; group II, acute bronchiolitis 15 min–48 hr after therapy; group III, nonwheezing infants 6 months after bronchiolitis; group IV, nonwheezing infants 18 months after bronchiolitis.

*$p < 0.05$ compared to 18 month value.

**$p < 0.025$ compared to 6 and 18 month values

*Source*: Ref. 54.

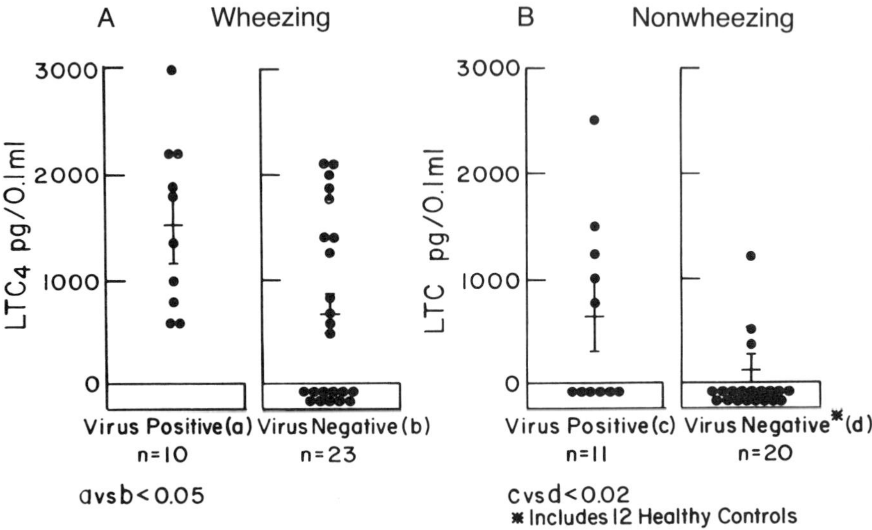


FIGURE 2 Effect of viral infection on $LTC_4$ concentration in children (A) with and (B) without wheezing. Significantly higher concentrations of $LTC_4$ were found in both wheezing and nonwheezing infants infected with virus. (From Ref. 53.)

comparative control group indicated that the histamine and prostaglandin elevations were not a mere reflection of general illness, a role for these mediators is suggested in the clinical characteristics of bronchiolitis.

### Virus-Specific IgE Concentrations Predict Future Wheezing Episodes

To evaluate further the significance of virus-specific IgE antibody, Welliver et al. (55) prospectively monitored 38 infants for 48 months after an initial episode of bronchiolitis. Only 20% of infants with undetectable titers of RSV IgE had subsequent episodes of documented wheezing (Table 5). In contrast, 70% of those children with high RSV IgE antibody titers experienced wheezing. To explain their observation, the authors questioned whether RSV infection in early age identifies individuals with airways congenitally prone to obstruction. As a consequence, the investigators concluded:

> Results, which suggest that the number of wheezing episodes experienced after RSV bronchiolitis can be predicted on the basis of a genetically determined phenomenon (overproduction of IgE), are more consistent with the concept that the increased frequency of lower respiratory tract illnesses, airway hyperreactivity, and small airway dys-

TABLE 5 Risk of Subsequent Wheezing after RSV Bronchiolitis Analyzed by Peak RSV IgE Titer in Nasopharyngeal Secretions

| RSV IgE titer in secretions | Subjects with titer | Documented subsequent wheezing episode No. (%) | p |
|---|---|---|---|
| Undetectable | 15 | 3 (20) | |
| 1–6 | 13 | 6 (46) | <0.025 |
| > 6 | 10 | 7 (70) | <0.025 |

p values are compared with undetectable levels.
*Source*: Ref. 55.

function observed in children examined years after an episode of bronchiolitis are also genetically determined.

Furthermore, recent data suggest that Ribavirin treatment may effect RSV-specific antibody production. Rosner et al. (56) recently studied 48 patients with RSV who were treated with Ribavirin. They found that treated subjects had lower RSV-specific IgE and IgA in convalescent serum than controls, suggesting that treatment with Ribavirin inhibits IgE and IgA response with subsequent diminution in release of inflammatory mediators thus, perhaps, lessening the risk of future wheezing.

### T-Cell-Mediated Hypersensitivity

Immunoregulatory defects in the T-cell-mediated response to RSV infection may also play a role in the pathogenesis of the disease. Welliver (57) examined the peripheral blood T lymphocyte subpopulations in 72 children with upper respiratory infection, pneumonia without wheezing, or bronchiolitis due to RSV infection. They used monoclonal antibodies to membrane antigens to determine the T-lymphocyte subpopulations: T-helper ($T_4$) and T-suppressor ($T_8$). There was no difference in the percentage of peripheral blood mononuclear cells that were $T_4$ positive at the time of acute infection or in convalescent serum between the three groups. There was also no difference in the three groups at the time of acute infection in $T_8$-positive cells. An interesting finding was that the percentage of $T_8$-positive cells in the convalescent serum of patients with bronchiolitis was significantly lower than in those patients with an upper respiratory infection alone or pneumonia without wheezing. Furthermore, an inverse correlation was found between the number of $T_8$-positive cells and peak RSV-IgE titers in nasal secretions. Their data suggest "that a defect in suppressor cell numbers and function in patients with bronchiolitis due to RSV may explain both the exaggerated lymphoproliferative responses to RSV antigen as well as the overproduction of RSV-IgE" (57). Moreover, improved suppressor cell function may result in milder subsequent infections because of improved regulation of RSV-specific IgE.

## MECHANISMS OF VIRUS-INDUCED AIRWAY HYPERRESPONSIVENESS

A number of mechanisms have been identified to explain how viral respiratory infections enhance airway responsiveness or provoke an attack of asthma (Table 6). As each of these mechanisms is reviewed, it should become apparent that no single, unifying cause has yet to be established, but rather that the virus effects are multiple, interrelated, and interactive.

### Effect on Hyperresponsiveness and Late-Phase Asthma

To evaluate the effects of respiratory infection on airway responsiveness, Lemanske et al. (58) experimentally infected subjects with rhinovirus and determined its action on a nonallergic stimulus of airway contraction, histamine, and an IgE-dependent activator, antigen. The patients were evaluated on three separate occasions: at baseline, during acute infection, and recovery. Each study period was separated by approximately 4 weeks with the following determinations made at each testing. First, airway response to inhaled histamine was determined and provided an index of airway reactivity. Second, both the immediate and late-phase asthmatic responses (LAR) to inhaled antigen were evaluated. Thus, the effect of a rhinovirus infection on nonspecific airway responsiveness and response to antigen could be compared.

TABLE 6 Mechanisms of Virus-Induced Asthma

| |
|---|
| Sensitization of rapidly adapting afferent vagus sensory fibers |
| Damage to airway epithelium |
|   Loss of relaxing factor |
|   Inactivation of enkephalinase, substance P degrading enzyme |
| Beta-adrenergic blockade |
| Production of virus-specifc IgE antibody |
| Development of late asthmatic reactions to inhaled antigen |
| Enhanced leukocyte inflammatory function |

**Effect on Airway Response to Histamine and Antigen**

All 10 patients had a rhinovirus respiratory infection at time of study as ascertained by either virus recovery from nasal washings and/or a rise in hemagglutination titer, or both. During the acute rhinovirus respiratory infection, airway responsiveness to histamine increased significantly over baseline values (Fig. 3). Likewise, the acute airway reactivity to inhaled antigen increased. The change in airway responsiveness to histamine and antigen was similar, suggesting that the respiratory infection effects on the immediate responsive to antigen related to alterations in nonspecific bronchial reactivity.

The airways' response to inhaled antigen is not necessarily limited to immediate bronchoconstriction. Many individuals experience immediate bronchoconstriction and a recurrence of airway obstruction 4–8 hr after inhalation of antigen, the LAR. The LAR is characterized by a number

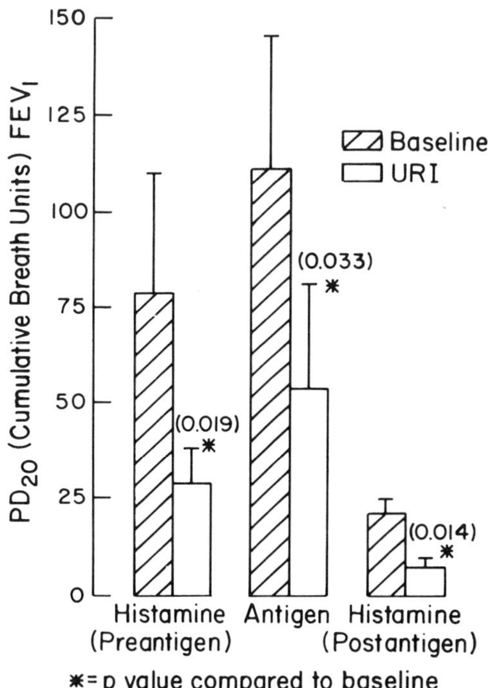


FIGURE 3 The effect of acute rhinovirus respiratory infection on airway reactivity to histamine and antigen along with reactivity to histamine following antigen challenge. Values are mean ± SEM, n = 10. (From Ref. 58.)

of features (59): diminished responsiveness to bronchodilator, increased airway reactivity, and the presence of bronchial inflammation. These features of LAR resemble chronic asthma and are the component of an airways' response to inhaled antigen most likely to yield insight into the pathogenesis of this disease. For these reasons, the effect of the viral respiratory illness on the late-phase asthmatic response to inhaled antigen was also determined. Prior to rhinovirus inoculation, only 1 of the 10 patients had an LAR to inhaled antigen (Fig. 4). However, during the acute respiratory infection, 8 of 10 patients experienced late-phase airway obstruction. Furthermore, when evaluated during the recovery period (4 weeks after rhinovirus inoculation), 5 of the 7 patients available for testing still had late airway obstructive responses to inhaled antigen. These observations indicate that rhinovirus respiratory infection not only increased airway responsiveness but also changed the pattern of the airway response to inhaled antigen.

The recovery pattern of airway responsiveness following the viral respiratory infection as also evaluated. Although increased airway responsiveness was still detected 4 weeks after rhinovirus inoculation, there was a trend toward recovery to both inhaled histamine and the immediate response to antigen. However, as already discussed, the increased frequency of late-phase asthmatic reactions to antigen was still noted 4 weeks after viral infection. These observations suggest that the viral respiratory infection has a greater, and possibly more lasting, effect on factors that participate in the development of LARs.

### Possible Mechanisms

Virus-associated airway hyperresponsiveness is a multifactorial process involving a complex interplay of IgE-dependent reactions, epithelial damage, autonomic nervous system dysfunction, and enhanced inflammation (60). In addition, individual patient features, such as inborn lung function and a family history of atopy, may also contribute to the outcome in specific patients (26).

To begin to unravel the mechanisms by which a respiratory viral infection increases the potential for late-phase asthma, it is helpful to examine those steps involved in the airways' response to antigen. From this analysis a number of sites emerge as being potentially susceptible to respiratory virus effects and may eventually influence the development of late-phase asthma (Fig. 5). Of the identified influences, interest has focused on factors which could cause, or accentuate, airway inflammation: mediator release and function of inflammatory cells.

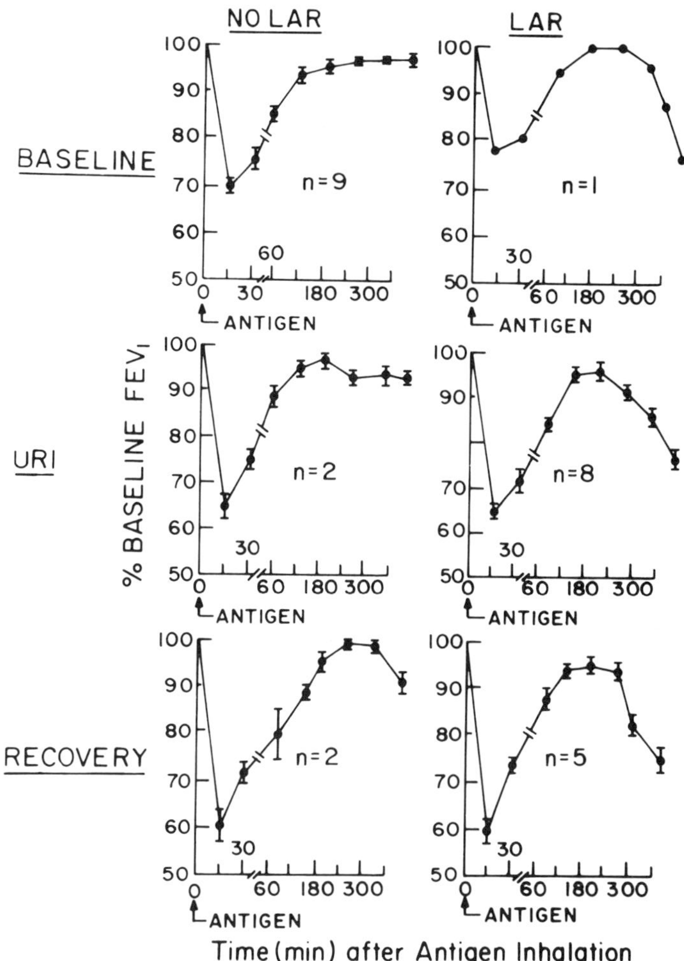


FIGURE 4 The pattern of airway response to inhaled ragweed antigen in patients before, during, and after an acute rhinovirus infection. (From Ref. 58.)

## Effect on the Inflammatory Response and Late-Phase Asthmatic Responses

In IgE-mediated reactions, the tissue response, whether the skin, nose, or airway, is influenced by IgE sensitization of mast cells and basophils, release of bronchospastic and inflammatory mediators from sensitized cells, and the response of the target organ, which, in asthma, is bronchial smooth muscle. Welliver and colleagues (31,32) have evidence that respiratory

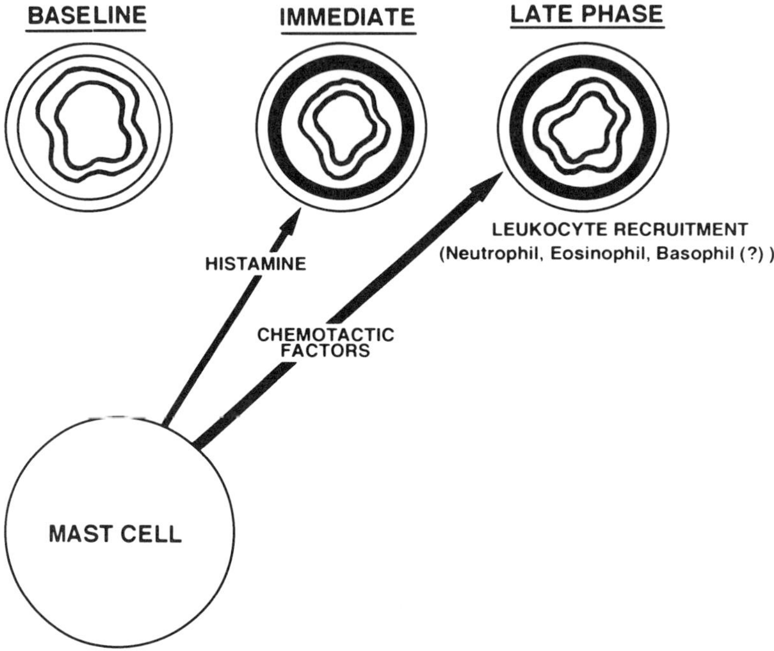


FIGURE 5 Mechanisms by which rhinovirus infection promotes the development of late-phase asthma. During the "baseline" period of the respiratory infection, airway reactivity is increased. Changes in mast cell mediator or the cells recruited to the airway may determine the likelihood of a late-phase reaction. (From Busse WW, Calhoun WJ. Infections. In: Barnes PJ, Rodger IW, Thomson NC (eds.), *Asthma: Basic Mechanisms and Clinical Management*, Harcourt Brace Jovanovich, London.

viruses stimulate the production virus-specific IgE. However, there are no available data to suggest that the concentration of IgE antibody necessarily determines either the intensity or likelihood of a late reaction (58,59).

To evaluate the effects of respiratory viruses on another facet of the immediate hypersensitivity response, mediator release, basophil histamine secretion was determined. For these studies, isolated human white cells were obtained, incubated in vitro with live respiratory virus, challenged with antigen, and histamine release was measured. We, and others, have found increased IgE-dependent basophil histamine release following an in vitro incubation with live respiratory viruses (61,62). There is evidence that enhanced basophil histamine release occurs, in part, as interferon is produced during the virus–leukocyte incubation and then acts on sensitized basophils. On the other hand, Chonmaitree et al. (63) incubated leukocytes from healthy, nonallergic donors with different strains of inactivated respiratory viruses and found that respiratory viruses could augment IgE-mediated histamine release with or without interferon present. They concluded that although interferon may play a role in virus-induced hypersensitivity reactions, other mechanisms were probably also involved.

In the studies that showed increased airway reactivity to histamine and the development of late-phase asthma during a rhinovirus infection (58), basophil histamine release was also enhanced. Although this association does not indicate a cause and effect relationship between enhanced leukocyte secretion and changes in airway reactivity and the development of an LAR, it does imply that the in vivo viral infection had effects upon human basophil function similar to that found with in vitro exposure to respiratory viruses. Furthermore, T-cell depletion, prior to virus incubation, appears to decrease basophil histamine release (64), suggesting an integral role for T Cells in the virus–leukocyte interaction.

Since the role of basophils in allergic disease and asthma is not fully established, it is difficult to ascertain the relevance of in vitro and in vivo studies with basophils. Nonetheless, recent investigations at Johns Hopkins Hospital may help to clarify the contribution of basophils in allergic diseases.

To evaluate nasal responses to inhaled antigen, Naclerio and his colleagues (65) found that nasal histamine concentrations increased during both the immediate and late-phase nasal response to inhaled antigen. Prostaglandin $D_2$ ($PGD_2$) was also measured and found elevated only during the acute-phase reaction. Because histamine is found in both the mast cell and basophil whereas $PGD_2$ is limited to the mast cell, the rise in histamine during late-phase nasal response was attributed to the basophil. Although the basophil has not been established as a participant in late-phase airway obstructive reaction, the changes in basophil function during respiratory viral infections may be relevant to the development of a late asthmatic reaction.

Late-phase reactions also involve leukocyte recruitment. When Lett-Brown and colleagues (66) incubated leukocytes with a parainfluenza virus and then measured leukocyte chemotaxis to a C5 peptide component of complement or a leukocyte-derived chemotactic factor, only basophils demonstrated enhanced chemotaxis. Furthermore, if interferon was substituted for virus, basophil migration was likewise enhanced. When looked at collectively, these observations are a further example that basophil function may be particularly susceptible to effects of respiratory viruses, with an end result being the promotion of this cell's inflammatory potential and hence greater contribution to the allergic reaction.

### Effect on Polymorphonuclear Leukocyte Function

Since other cells (i.e., neutrophils and eosinophils) are also associated with airway inflammation and late-phase asthmatic reactions, we have begun to examine the effect of respiratory viruses on their function. Isolated neutrophils were incubated in vitro with influenza virus and then activated to generate superoxide. Superoxide generation was increased when neutrophils had been incubated with influenza virus (67). Since superoxide is toxic to pulmonary tissues and may cause bronchial injury (68), it is possible that respiratory virus enhancement of the inflammatory function of leukocytes promotes airway injury and the likelihood of increased responsiveness.

To integrate these findings into an understanding of the development of late-phase asthma, we hypothesize the following series of events. During initiation of the allergic response in the airway, inflammatory cells (neutrophils, eosinophils, and possibly basophils) are recruited to the airway and, when activated, release inflammatory mediators. The amount of inflammatory mediators released will determine the intensity of the response and possibly whether a late-phase reaction occurs. If this same allergic reaction occurs during a viral respiratory infection, leukocytes recruited to the airway are "primed" and, when activated, produce a greater inflammatory response. Thus, because the cells recruited to the lung during the respiratory illness are activated leukocytes, the likelihood for airway injury and the development of a late asthmatic reaction increases (Fig. 5).

## OTHER MECHANISMS

### Alterations in Autonomic Nervous System Function

Airway smooth muscle function is regulated by the autonomic nervous system. Beta-adrenergic receptors on bronchial smooth muscle are activated by catecholamines and reduce bronchial smooth muscle tone. In addition, beta-adrenergic receptors on leukocytes modulate their inflammatory response and mediator release. Nearly three decades ago, Szentivanyi (69) proposed that diminished beta-adrenergic function was found in patients with asthma and that autonomic nervous system imbalance contributed to the bronchial hyperresponsiveness and bronchoconstriction in asthma. He further suggested that viral infections exacerbate "beta-blockade" to increase further the underlying airway abnormalities in asthma.

The existence of diminished beta-adrenergic function has been proposed to explain airway hyperresponsiveness and the lack of complete bronchodilation with the administration of catecholamines in patients with asthma. Although evidence for "beta-blockade" exists in asthma, the precise role of altered autonomic nervous system function has yet to be fully established.

Isolated human leukocytes can be used as an in vitro model to evaluate beta-adrenergic function in asthma with suppression of lysosomal enzyme release being the test response. Leukocytes isolated from patients during viral respiratory infection (70), or following incubation with respiratory viruses (71), had diminished beta-adrenergic function. These observations indicated that respiratory viruses can alter the beta-adrenergic function of circulating human leukocytes. Even though airway smooth muscle beta-adrenergic function may not be altered by respiratory viruses, the virus-associated autonomic nervous system dysfunction can affect regulation of the leukocyte-dependent inflammation. Since catecholamines normally inhibit leukocyte inflammatory responses, virus alteration of beta-adrenergic function may increase cellular secretion of inflammatory mediators. The consequence of virus-associated changes in leukocyte regulatory responses could translate to increased tissue inflammation.

Viral upper respiratory infections also enhance airway cholinergic sensitivity. In a study of 16 nonasthmatic patients, Empey et al. (72) documented a significant increase in airway sensitivity to inhaled histamine. Since the enhanced response to inhaled histamine was blocked by atropine, the authors speculated that airway injury by respiratory viruses sensitized rapidly adapting sensory fibers of the vagus nerve to promote reflex bronchospasm. These observations indicate that respiratory viruses may not have to change directly the function of airway smooth muscle to promote bronchial hyperreactivity but can accomplish this alteration by "indirect" methods (73).

To localize and characterize further the effect of a respiratory virus on cholinergic function, Fryer and Jacoby (74) evaluated parainfluenza action on cholinergic receptor binding. In membrane preparations from guinea pig lung, parainfluenza virus incubation decreased cholinergic agonist binding. Although not conclusive, their observations suggest that the virus effect is on the $M_2$ receptor of the lung. Because "$M_2$ receptors modulate vagally induced bronchoconstriction in the lungs, the investigators postulate that the virus-induced decrease in agonist affinity for $M_2$ receptors is responsible for the increase in vagally mediated bronchoconstriction observed in animals and man with viral respiratory infections" (74).

### Damage to Airway Epithelium

Damage to airway epithelium can also contribute to airway hyperreactivity (75). In addition to serving as a protective barrier to the diffusion of antigens and noxious substances, bronchial epithelium actively produces substances that modulate airway responsitivity and smooth muscle tone (76). Since some respiratory viruses directly injure airway epithelium, the consequences of this damage have been examined.

In studies with parainfluenza-3-infected guinea pigs, Saban et al. (77) detected enhanced isolated airway contractility to the neuropeptide substance P. In addition, Jacoby and co-workers (78) found that isolated ferret trachea, which had been incubated with influenza virus, had epithelial desquamation, increased contractility to substance P, and reduced activity of enkephalinase, an epithelial-derived enzyme that degrades substance P. Based on these findings, Jacoby et al. (78) proposed that the influenza virus infection altered enkephalinase activity such that the substance P-induced contraction was enhanced.

Moreover, damage to epithelium may lead to the loss of epithelium-derived relaxing factor(s) (79). These factor(s) include inhibitory cyclo-oxygenase metabolites of arachidonic acid (80) that may reduce cholinergic neurotransmitter release (81). In this fashion, virus-associated damage to airway epithelium would further alter control of airway caliber and reactivity without directly affecting smooth muscle physiology.

The role of neuropeptides in airway inflammation has been further elucidated by McDonald (82), who demonstrated that naturally occurring viral infections caused rat tracheas to become more susceptible to neurogenic inflammation that arose from direct stimulation of vagal sensory nerves or by injection of capsaicin or substance P. The enhanced susceptibility to inflammation occurred even in the absence of virus-induced changes in the airway such as increased vascular permeability, adherence of neutrophils to blood vessel walls, or influx of neutrophils into tracheal mucosa. Moreover, the increased susceptibility to neurogenic inflammation outlasted the brief pathologic changes observed with acute infection. Taken collectively, the described changes in airway epithelium could promote airway responsiveness. Evidence that increased airway reactivity enhances the likelihood for late asthmatic reactions has yet to be established.

### Viral Effects on the Cellular Immune Response

To appreciate more fully the effects of a viral respiratory infection on airway function, it is essential to consider the complex interaction of respiratory viruses with the cellular immune system. To initiate an immune response, viruses must first attach to a target cell. Evidence now indicates that this attachment occurs through a specific cell surface receptors (83) called the T-cell receptor (TCR). Following cellular processing, which may involve intracellular alteration of the virus, viral antigen peptides may be expressed on the cell surface bound to molecules encoded by the major histocompatibility complex (MHC). T lymphocytes are activated by binding of their TCR to this newly expressed antigen–MHC complex on antigen-presenting cells such as macrophages. After binding, proliferation and differentiation occur into the two types of functional T cells: helper cells (CD4) and killer cells (CD8).

### Cellular Adhesion Molecules

Before specific binding occurs, however, T lymphocytes bind to other cells by means of surface adhesion molecules (84). Recent studies have augmented our understanding of cellular adhesion molecules, which participate in cell–cell interaction, regulate cell migration, and act as receptors for antigens, including certain viruses. Such interactions have potential importance for viral infections, the development of inflammation, airway hyperresponsiveness, and asthma.

Three families of adhesion molecules have been identified: the immunoglobulin superfamily, which includes antigen-specific receptors of T and B lymphocytes; the integrin family, which are important in the regulation of cellular adhesion and migration; and the selectin family, which participate in lymphocyte and neutrophil activation with vascular endothelium (85). The T-cell surface adhesion molecules that interact with target cells have been identified with monoclonal antibodies and are termed lymphocyte function-related antigens (LFA-1, LFA-2 [CD2], LFA-3). The ligand for LFA-1 is ICAM-1 (intercellular cell adhesion molecule). While LFA-1 is expressed only on leukocytes, ICAM-1 is expressed on a wide variety of cells including endothelial cells, fibroblasts, epithelial cells, lymphocytes, and monocytes (86). The LFA-1/ICAM-1 interaction is important for regulating inflammation, with inflammatory mediators such as $\gamma$-interferons, interleukin-1, and tumor necrosis factor causing strong induction of ICAM-1.

### ICAM-1 Rhinovirus Receptor

The major human rhinovirus receptor has been identified as ICAM-1 (84,87). Virus binding to ICAM-1 may stimulate production of cytokines that may induce ICAM-1 production on neighboring cells to enhance further adhesion and spread of infection. The host cell response promoted via ICAM-1/rhinovirus interaction increases mucus secretions and sneezing, providing another mechanism to increase infectivity (85,86). Although preliminary, these findings promise to have important implications for future study and for our understanding of the pathogenesis of virus-induced airway hyperresponsitivity.

Viral infections may alter the regulation of IgE synthesis by modifying the combined actions of T-helper and T-suppressor lymphocytes (88). To evaluate the effect of viral infection on IgE synthesis, Lin and associates (89) studied children allergic to house dust following a community-acquired influenza A illness. Twelve of their study patients experienced attacks of asthma in association with the influenza illness. When compared to subjects who did not wheeze during the influenza infection, patients with increased asthma symptoms had alterations in their T-helper/T-suppressor lymphocyte ratio and increases in specific house dust antibody. Thus, Lin and associates (89) postulated that virus infection-associated changes in the T-helper/T-suppressor cell ratio may result in an increased lymphoproliferative response to antigen, which, in turn, can contribute to increased symptoms of asthma.

## SUMMARY

The mechanisms involved in the development of airway hyperresponsiveness, airway obstruction, and recurrent wheezing with viral respiratory infections have yet to be fully appreciated. Nonetheless, current evidence indicates that viruses, or products of virus-infected cells, influence the inflammatory property and potential of many cells. Precisely how these virus effects translate into increased airway injury, responsiveness, and obstruction will require further work. As the mechanisms of these interactions are established, our understanding of asthma's pathogenesis and treatment will improve.

## ACKNOWLEDGMENT

This work was supported in part by NIH grants HL 44098 and AI 26609.

## REFERENCES

1. McIntosh K, Ellis EF, Hoffman LS, Lybass TG, Eller JJ, Fulginiti VA. The association of viral and bacterial respiratory infections with exacerbations of wheezing in young asthmatic children. *J Pediatr* 83:578–590, 1973.
2. Minor TE, Dick EC, DeMeo AN, Ouellette JJ, Cohen M, Reed CE. Viruses as precipitants of asthmatic attacks in children. *JAMA* 227:292–298, 1974.
3. Horn MEC, Gregg I. Role of viral infection and host factors in acute episodes of asthma and chronic bronchitis. *Chest* 63:44–47, 1973.
4. Henderson FW, Clyde WA, Collier AM, et al. The etiology and epidemiologic spectrum of bronchiolitis in pediatric practice. *J Pediatr* 95:183, 1979.
5. Minor TE, Dick EC, Baker JW, Ouellette JJ, Cohen M, Reed CE. Rhinovirus and influenza A infections as precipitants of asthma. *Am Rev Respir Dis* 113:149–153, 1976.

6. Hudgel DW, Lanston E Jr, Selner JC, McIntosh K. Viral and bacterial infections in adults with chronic asthma. *Am Rev Respir Dis* 120:393–397, 1979.
7. Halperin SA, Eggleston PA, Hendley JO, Suratt PM, Gröschel DHM, Gwaltney JM Jr. Pathogenesis of lower respiratory tract symptoms in experimental rhinovirus infection. *Am Rev Respir Dis* 128:806–810, 1983.
8. Halperin SA, Eggleston PA, Beasley P, Suratt P, Hendley JO, Gröschel DHM, Gwaltney JM Jr. Exacerbations of asthma in adults during experimental rhinovirus infection. *Am Rev Respir Dis* 132:976–980, 1985.
9. Berman SZ, Mathison DA, Stevenson DD, Tan EM, Vaughan JH. Transtracheal aspiration studies in asthmatic patients in relapse with "infective" asthma and in subjects without respiratory disease. *J Allergy Clin Immunol* 56:206–214, 1975.
10. Slavin RG, Cannon RF, Friedman WH, et al. Sinusitis and bronchial asthma. *J Allergy Clin Immunol* 66:250–254, 1980.
11. Rachelefsky GS, Katz RM, Siegel SC. Chronic sinus disease associated with reactive airway disease in children. *Pediatrics* 73:526–529, 1984.
12. Friedman R, Ackerman M, Wald E, Casselbrandt M, Friday G, Frieman P. Asthma and bacterial sinusitis in children. *J Allergy Clin Immunol* 74:185–189, 1984.
13. Zimmerman B, Stringer D, Feanny S, Resiman J, Hak H, Rashad N, deBenedicts F, McLaughlin J, Levison H. Prevalence of abnormalities found by sinus x-rays in childhood asthma: lack of relation to severity of asthma. *J Allergy Clin Immunol* 80:268–273, 1987.
14. Tager IB. Epidemiology of respiratory infections in the development of airway hyperreactivity. *Semin Respir Med* 11:297–305, 1990.
15. Samet JM, Tager IB, Speizer FE. The relationship between respiratory illness in childhood and chronic air-flow obstruction in adulthood. *Am Rev Respir Dis* 127:508–523, 1983.
16. Eisen AH, Bacal HL. The relationship of acute bronchiolitis to bronchial asthma—a 4-to-14 year follow-up. *Pediatrics* 31:859–861, 1963.
17. Rooney JC, Williams HE. The relationship between proven viral bronchiolitis and subsequent wheezing. *J Pediatr* 79:744–747, 1971.
18. McConnochie KM, Roghmann KJ. Bronchiolitis as a possible cause of wheezing in childhood. *Pediatrics* 74:1–10, 1984.
19. Sims DG, Downham MAPS, Gardner PS. Study of 8-year-old children with a history of respiratory syncytial virus bronchiolitis in infancy. *Br Med J* 1:11–14, 1978.
20. Zweiman B, Schoenwetter WF, Pappano JE, et al. Patterns of allergic respiratory disease in children with a past history of bronchiolitis. *J Allergy* 48:283–286, 1971.
21. Pullan CR, Hey EN: Wheezing, asthma, and pulmonary dysfunction 10 years after infection with respiratory syncytial virus in infancy. *Br Med J* 284:1665–1669, 1982.
22. Weiss ST, Tager IB, Munoz A, Speizer FE. The relationship of respiratory infections in early childhood to the occurrence of increased levels of bronchial responsiveness and atopy. *Am Rev Respir Dis* 131:573–578, 1985.

23. Sly P, Hibbert M. Childhood asthma following hospitalization with acute viral bronchiolitis in infancy. *Pediatr Pulmonol* 7:153–158, 1989.
24. Mok JY, Simpson H. Outcome of acute lower respiratory tract infection in infants: preliminary report of seven-year follow-up study. *Br Med J* 285:333–337, 1982.
25. Gurwitz D, Mindorff C, Levison H. Increased incidence of bronchial reactivity in children with a history of bronchiolitis. *J Pediatr* 98:551–555, 1981.
26. Morgan WJ. Viral respiratory infection in infancy: provocation or propagation? *Semin Respir Med* 11:306–313, 1990.
27. Martinez FD, Morgan WJ, Wright AL, Holberg CJ, Taussig LM, Group Health Medical Associates Personnel. Diminished lung function as a predisposing factor for wheezing respiratory illnesses in infants. *N Engl J Med* 319:1112–1117, 1988.
28. Morris MJ, Lane DJ. Tidal expiratory flow patterns in air-flow obstruction. *Thorax* 36:135–142, 1981.
29. Martinez FD, Morgan WJ, Wright AL, Holberg C, Taussig LM. Initial airway function is a risk factor for recurrent wheezing respiratory illnesses during the first three years of life. *Am Rev Respir Dis* 143:312–316, 1991.
30. Taussig LM, Harris TR, Lebowitz MD. Lung function in infants and young children: functional residual capacity, tidal volume, and respiratory rate. *Am Rev Respir Dis* 116:233–239, 1977.
31. Welliver RC, Wong DT, Sun M, Middleton E Jr, Vaughan RS, Ogra PL. The development of respiratory syncytial virus specific IgE and the release of histamine in nasopharyngeal secretions after infection. *N Engl J Med* 305:841–846, 1981.
32. Welliver RC, Wong DT, Middleton E Jr, Sun M, McCarthy RN, Ogra PL. Role of parainfluenza virus-specific IgE in pathogenesis of croup and wheezing subsequent to infection. *J Pediatr* 101:889–896, 1982.
33. Voter KZ, Henry MM, Stewart PW, Henderson FW. Lower respiratory illness in early childhood and lung function and bronchial reactivity in adolescent males. *Am Rev Respir Dis* 137:302–307, 1988.
34. Hall CB, McBride JT. Respiratory syncytial virus—from chimps with colds to conundrums and cures. *N Engl J Med* 325:57–58, 1991.
35. Morris JA, Bount RE, Savage RE. Recovery of cytopathogenic agent from chimpanzees with coryza. *Proc Soc Exp Biol Med* 92:544–549, 1956.
36. Chanock R, Roizman B, Myers R. Recovery from infants with respiratory illness of a virus related to chimpanzee coryza agent (CCA): I: isolation, properties and characterization. *Am J Hyg* 66:281–290, 1957.
37. McConnochie KM, Hall CB, Wash EE, et al. Variation in severity of respiratory syncytial virus infections with subtype. *J Pediatr* 117:52–62, 1990.
38. Gala CL, Hall CB, Schnabel KC, et al. The use of eye–nose goggles to control nosocomial respiratory syncytial virus infection. *JAMA* 256:2706–2708, 1986.
39. Leclair JM, Freeman J, Sullivan BF, et al. Prevention of nosocomial respiratory syncytial virus infections through compliance with glove and gown isolation precautions. *N Engl J Med* 317:329–334, 1987.

40. Monto AS, Lim SK. The Tecumseh study of respiratory illness. III. Incidence and periodicity of respiratory syncytial virus and mycoplasma pneumonia infections. *Am J Epidemiol* 94:290–301, 1971.
41. Glezen WP, Taber LH, Frank AL, et al. Risk of primary infection and reinfection with respiratory syncytial virus. *Am J Dis Child* 140:543–566, 1986.
42. Hall CB. Respiratory syncytial virus. In: Feigen RD, Cherry JD (eds.), *Textbook of Pediatric Infectious Diseases*, WB Saunders, Philadelphia, 1987, pp. 1653–1676.
43. Welliver RC. Detection, pathogenesis and therapy of respiratory syncytial virus infections. *Clin Microbiol Rev* 1:27–39, 1988.
44. McIntosh K, Maters HB, Orr I, et al. The immunologic response to infection with respiratory syncytial virus in infants. *J Infect Dis* 138:24–32, 1978.
45. Nadal D, Ogra PL. Development of local immunity: role in mechanisms of protection against or pathogenesis of respiratory syncytial viral infections. *Lung* Suppl:379–387, 1990.
46. Bienenstock J. *Immunology of the Lung and Upper Respiratory Tract*. McGraw-Hill, New York, 1984.
47. Faden H, Kaul TN, Ogra PL. Activation of oxidative and arachidonic acid metabolism in neutrophils by respiratory syncytial virus antibody complexes: possible role in disease. *J Infect Dis* 148:110–116, 1983.
48. Glezen WP, Paredas A, Allison JE, Taber LH, Frank AL. Risk of respiratory syncytial virus infection for infants from low-income families in relationship to age, sex, ethnic group and maternal antibody level. *J Pediatr* 98:708–715, 1982.
49. Hemming VG, Rodriguez W, Kim HW. Intravenous immunoglobulin treatment of respiratory syncytial virus infections in infants and young children. *Antimicrob Agents Chemother* 31:1882–1886, 1987.
50. Toms GL, Webb MSC, Milner PD, Milner AD, Routledge EG, Scott R, Stokes GM, Swarbrick A, Taylor CE. IgG and IgM antibodies to viral glycoprotein in respiratory syncytial virus infections of graded severity. *Arch Dis Child* 64:1661–1665, 1989.
51. Welliver RC, Wong DT, Sun M, McCarthy N. Parainfluenza virus bronchiolitis. Epidemiology and pathogenesis. *Am J Dis Child* 140:34–40, 1986.
52. Volovitz B, Welliver RC, DeCastro G, Krystofik DA, Ogra PL. The release of leukotriene in the respiratory tract during infection with respiratory syncytial virus: role in obstructive airway disease. *Pediatr Res* 24:504–507, 1988.
53. Volovitz B, Faden H, Ogra PL. Release of leukotriene $C_4$ in respiratory tract during acute viral infection. *J Pediatr* 112:218–222, 1988.
54. Skoner DP, Fireman P, Caliguiri L, Davis H. Plasma elevations of histamine and prostaglandin metabolite in acute bronchiolitis. *Am Rev Respir Dis* 142:359–364, 1990.

syncytial virus-specific IgE response for recurrent wheezing following bronchiolitis. *J Pediatr* 109:766–780, 1986.

56. Rosner IK, Welliver RC, Edelson PJ. Effect of Ribavirin therapy on respi-

ratory syncytial virus-specific IgE and IgA responses after infection. *J Infect Dis* 155:1043–1046, 1987.
57. Welliver RC, Kaul TN, Sun M, et al. Defective regulation of immune responses in respiratory syncytial virus infection. *J Immunol* 133:1925–1936, 1984.
58. Lemanske RF Jr, Dick EC, Swenson CA, Vrtis RF, Busse WW. Rhinovirus upper respiratory infection increases airway reactivity in late asthmatic reactions. *J Clin Invest* 83:1–10, 1989.
59. Lemanske RF Jr, Kaliner MA. Late-phase allergic reactions. In: Middleton E Jr, Reed CE, Ellis EF, Adkinson NF Jr, Yunginger JW (eds.), *Allergy: Principles and Practice*, St. Louis, C.V. Mosby, 1988, pp 224–246.
60. Frick WE, Busse WW. Respiratory infections: their role in airway responsiveness and pathogenesis of asthma. *Clin Chest Med* 9:539–549, 1988.
61. Ida S, Hooks JJ, Siraganian RP, Notkens AL. Enhancement of IgE-mediated histamine release from human basophil by viruses: role of interferon. *J Exp Med* 145:892–896, 1979.
62. Busse WW, Swenson CA, Borden EC, Treuhauft MW, Dick EC. The effect of influenza A virus on leukocyte histamine release. *J Allergy Clin Immunol* 71:382–388, 1983.
63. Chonmaitree T, Lett-Brown MA, Tsong Y, Goldman AS, Baron S. Role of interferon in leukocyte histamine release caused by common respiratory viruses. *J Infect Dis* 157:127–132, 1988.
64. Huftel MA, Swenson CA, Borcherding WR, et al. Enhanced basophil histamine release (HR) following *in vitro* incubation with live influenza A virus is attenuated by T-cell depletion. *J Allergy Clin Immunol* 87:211A, 1991.
65. Naclerio RM, Proud D, Togias AG, Adkinson NF Jr, Meyers DA, Kasey-Sobotka A, Plaut M, Norman PS, Lichtenstein LM. Inflammatory mediators in late antigen-induced rhinitis. *N Engl J Med* 313:65–70, 1985.
66. Lett-Brown MA, Aelvoet M, Hooks JJ, Georgiades JA, Thueson DO, Grant JA. Enhancement of basophil chemotaxis *in vitro* by virus-induced interferon. *J Clin Invest* 67:547–552, 1981.
67. Busse WW, Vrtis RF, Steiner R, Dick EC. *In vitro* incubation with influenza virus primes human polymorphonuclear leukocyte generation of superoxide. *Am J Respir Cell Mol Bio* 4:347–354, 1991.
68. Cross CE, Halliwell B, Borish ET, Pryor WA, Ames BN, Saul RL, McCord JM, Harman D. Oxygen radicals and human disease. *Ann Intern Med* 107:526–545, 1987.
69. Szentivanyi A. The beta-adrenergic theory of atopic abnormality in asthma. *J Allergy* 42:203–223, 1968.
70. Busse WW. Decreased granulocyte response to isoproterenol in asthma during upper respiratory infections. *Am Rev Respir Dis* 115:783–791, 1977.
71. Busse WW, Anderson CL, Dick EC, Warshauer D. Reduced granulocyte response to isoproterenol, histamine, prostaglandin E, after *in vitro* incubation with rhinovirus 16. *Am Rev Respir Dis* 122:641–646, 1980.
72. Empey DW, Laitinen LA, Jacobs L, Gold WM, Nadel JA. Mechanisms of

bronchial hyperreactivity in normal subjects after upper respiratory tract infection. *Am Rev Respir Dis* 133:131–139, 1976.

73. deJongste JC, Kerrebijn, KF. Is bronchial hyperresponsiveness in humans a smooth muscle abnormality? *Prog Clin Biol Res* 263:255–265, 1988.
74. Fryer Ad, El-Fakahany EE, Jacoby DB. Parainfluenza virus type 1 reduces the affinity of agonists for muscarinic receptors in guinea-pig lung and heart. *Eur J Pharmacol* 181:51–58, 1990.
75. Laitinen LA, Heino M, Laitinen A, Kava T, Haahtela T. Damage of the airway epithelium and bronchial reactivity in patients with asthma. *Am Rev Respir Dis* 131:599–606, 1985.
76. Nadel JA. Role of airway epithelial cells in the defense of airways. *Prog Clin Biol Res* 263:331–339, 1988.
77. Saban R, Dick EC, Fishleder RJ, Buckner CK. Enhancement by parainfluenza 3 infection of contractile responses to substance P and capsaicin in airway smooth muscle from the guinea pig. *Am Rev Respir Dis* 136:586–591, 1987.
78. Jacoby DB, Tamaoki J, Bornson DB, Nadal JA. Influenza infection causes airway hyperresponsiveness by decreasing enkephalinase. *J Appl Physiol* 64:2653–2658, 1988.
79. Vanhoutte PM. Epithelium-derived relaxing factor(s) and bronchial reactivity. *J Allergy Clin Immunol* 83:855–861, 1989.
80. Butler GB, Adler KB, Evans JN, Morgan DW, Szarek JL. Modulation of rabbit airway smooth muscle response by respiratory epithelium. *Am Rev Respir Dis* 135:1099–1104, 1987.
81. Barnett K, Jacoby DB, Nadel JA, Lazarus SC. The effects of epithelial cell supernatant on contraction of isolated canine tracheal smooth muscle. *Am Rev Respir Dis* 138:780–783, 1988.
82. McDonald DM. Respiratory tract infections increase susceptibility to neurogenic inflammation in the rat trachea. *Am Rev Respir Dis* 137:1432–1440, 1988.
83. White JM, Littman, DR. Viral receptors of the immunoglobulin superfamily cell. *Cell* 56:725–728, 1988.
84. Bierer BE, Burakoff SJ. T cell adhesion molecules. *FASEB J* 2:2584–2590, 1988.
85. Springer TA. Adhesion receptors of the immune system. *Nature* 346:425–434, 1990.
86. Staunton DE, Merluzzi VJ, Rothlein R, Barton R, Marlin SC, Springer TA. A cell adhesion molecule, ICAM-1, is the major surface receptor for rhinoviruses. *Cell* 56:849–853, 1989.
87. Greve JM, Davis G, Meyer AM, Forte CP, Yost SC, Marlor CW, Kamark ME, McClelland A. The major human rhinovirus receptor is ICAM-1. *Cell* 56:839–847, 1989.
88. Roitt IM, Brostoff J, Male DK. *Immunology*, 2nd ed, Gower Medical Publishing, London, 1989, pp 19.3–19.6.
89. Lin CY, Kuo YC, Liu WT, Lin CC. Immunomodulation of influenza virus infection in the precipitating asthma attack. *Chest* 93:1234–1238, 1988.

# 9

# Wheezing in Infants and Young Children

**JOHN JOSEPH REISMAN, GERARD J. CANNY, and HENRY LEVISON**

*The Hospital for Sick Children and University of Toronto Toronto, Ontario, Canada*

## INTRODUCTION

Wheezing, a term commonly used by parents and physicians, has had numerous definitions (1–3). Consistent with the present generally accepted definitions, we define wheezing as a prolonged musical, adventitial lung sound of varying intensity that can be heard with and sometimes without a stethoscope (1,2). Although usually expiratory, wheezes can be both expiratory and inspiratory. Wheezing can be caused by a wide variety of medical conditions, but before the approach to the evaluation of the wheezing infant is discussed, it is crucial to consider the anatomical and physiological aspects of wheezing and how they relate to the unique aspects of the anatomy and physiology of the infant's respiratory tract.

## ANATOMICAL AND PHYSIOLOGICAL CONSIDERATIONS

Wheezing results from partial obstruction of the airway and may be caused by single or multiple points of narrowing within the airway. There can be multiple sites of obstruction, but because a critical airflow velocity is required to generate sound, the site of obstruction is usually in the larger bronchi. A similar obstruction in smaller airways may not lead to wheezing as the flow of air is too slow to generate the sound. Small airway obstruction can, however, result in wheezing by a different mechanism; wheezing may originate from larger bronchi even when the disease is confined to the small airways, because there can be dynamic compression of the large airways by positive pleural pressure being generated to overcome the added resistance caused by the small airway disease (3).

In the past, work with model airways revealed that airway wall vibrations occur when the expiratory effort exceeds that required to generate a maximum flow in the airway. Electronic analysis of a variety of respiratory sounds suggests a predominant origin from turbulent flow from within central airways (4,5). Normal inspiratory breath sounds likely result from a jet mechanism of sound production from below the larynx. Expiratory sounds include a component of sound generated by airstream convergence at airway bifurcations (4,5). The generation of sound is complicated because flow turbulence depends on the diameter of the airway and on characteristics of the gas flowing through the airway, including the density, the viscosity, and the linear velocity. In addition, it is important to note that the sounds are propagated differently depending on the density of the underlying lung tissue. Sounds travel more slowly through atelectatic lung than through well-inflated lung. Wheezing is a particular airway sound that is described as being musical and continuous, lasting more than 200 msec in duration. The oscillation frequency causing the sound depends on airflow velocity and the mass and elasticity of the airway wall. A fixed obstruction in a large-caliber airway results in monophonic-type wheezing, whereas diffuse airway obstruction results in musical noises of various pitches called polyphonic wheezing (4). Recent technical advances will provide us with new knowledge concerning acoustics of the lung. Detailed images of respiratory sounds provided by respirosonography may enhance our understanding of the processes involved in generating the sounds we hear with our stethoscopes (6).

It is worthwhile considering unique aspects of the anatomy and physiology of the infant's respiratory tract to understand the reasons for the increased severity of respiratory symptoms in infants and their increased likelihood of developing respiratory failure.

### Increased Peripheral Airway Resistance

The peripheral airways resistance in infants and young children is significantly greater than that in adults (7–9), and as a result, small airway disease in infants and young children has a greater impact on increasing total resistance.

### Decreased Elastic Recoil Pressure and Early Airway Closure

Relative lack of elastic recoil in the infant lung may lead to early airway closure even during tidal breathing in normal infants (7). This can result in decreased ventilation and ventilation-perfusion mismatching. In disease states resulting in airway inflammation, the combination of relatively small peripheral airways and diminished elastic recoil results in airway closure even at high lung volumes and a more significant impact on gas exchange.

### Deficient Collateral Channels of Ventilation

The infant lung is deficient in both the pores of Kohn, which are interalveolar channels, and the canals of Lambert, which are bronchoalveolar connections (10). As a result, disease states causing small airways obstruction are more likely to lead to areas of atelectasis owing to the deficiency in collateral ventilation.

## MECHANICAL CONSIDERATIONS

Several factors put an infant's respiratory system at a mechanical disadvantage compared to that of an older child or adult. The rib cage is very compliant in the infant; in addition, the diaphragm inserts horizontally rather than obliquely, as it does in the adult (11,12). Anyone who has examined children with airway obstruction realizes how dramatic retraction of the rib cage can be. A diaphragm that inserts horizontally leads to a decreased efficiency of contraction as well as a greater tendency to cause inward motion of the rib cage (11,12). If diaphragmatic contraction results in indrawing and inward motion of the rib cage, less force is available to move air into the lungs and do the work of breathing. For a given respiratory requirement, there is a substantial increase in the work of breathing. An additional important consideration is that the infant diaphragm is less well equipped to cope with an increased workload as there are fewer fatigue-resistant muscle fibers compared to the adult diaphragm (13).

In addition to the increased compliance of the rib cage, the trachea and major bronchi are more compliant in the infant and young child. The combination of compliant upper airways with relatively increased peripheral airway resistance leads to upper airway compression when positive pleural pressures are generated in expiration to overcome small airway obstruction.

## EVALUATION OF THE WHEEZY INFANT

### History

Table 1 includes a list of the most frequently seen causes of wheezing in infancy. The first and most important task in evaluation of a wheezy infant is development of a thorough history. One must determine if the problem is acute or if there are elements of chronicity. A first-time episode of wheezing associated with signs of an upper respiratory tract infection and occurring in the late fall, winter, or early spring may suggest a diagnosis of bronchiolitis.

TABLE 1 Causes of Wheeze/Cough in Infants and Young Children

| Common | Uncommon | Rare |
|---|---|---|
| Asthma | Bronchopulmonary dysplasia | Left ventricular failure |
| Bronchiolitis | Foreign body | Vascular anomalies |
| Recurrent aspiration | Cystic fibrosis | Mediastinal masses |
| | | Bronchiolitis obliterans |
| | | Immune deficiency states |
| | | Tracheobronchial anomalies |

A history of wheeze, cough, or shortness of breath that follows viral infections, physical activity, exposure to cigarette smoke, cold air, dust, or animals suggests hyperreactive airways may be the underlying problem. Seasonal variation in the incidence of wheeze may be an associated feature. A family history of asthma or atopic disorders such as eczema is very helpful. Inquiries should be made as to the existence of smokers and pets in the home and the method of house heating. Other factors to be considered are the rapidity of onset of previous respiratory difficulties, the need for hospital admission, intensive care unit admission, and need for ventilatory support. A medication history should be recorded with attention to drug dosage, mode of administration, and response, especially with respect to bronchodilators. There may be a relevant family history of asthma, ezcema, and allergy.

Infants and toddlers are at risks for inhalation of a wide variety of foreign bodies, and this possibility should always be inquired into. Careful attention should be paid to the feeding history. Recurrent regurgitation or choking with feeds indicates that aspiration may be the problem.

A history of bulky stools and failure to thrive should alert the clinician to the possibility of cystic fibrosis as the underlying cause of the wheeze. It must be remembered, however, that failure to thrive is not always seen, and chronic respiratory disease of other etiologies can cause growth failure.

Prematurity and a history of the respiratory disease syndrome requiring mechanical ventilatory support may lead one to consider a diagnosis of bronchopulmonary dysplasia.

As always, with disorders of the respiratory system, a history of cardiac disease may be relevant.

The history is also important in helping establish that the respiratory noises the parents are describing are indeed wheezes. Inspiratory noises and stridor are likely to be associated with such conditions as laryngotracheomalacia, and in such cases, the parents may remark that the symptoms disappear when the infant hyperextends his or her neck.

## Physical Examination

A thorough physical examination is indicated in the evaluation of the wheezing infant. General inspection and first impressions are particularly important. A determination as to whether the child looks chronically ill should be made. Cyanosis and clubbing indicate the possibility of cystic fibrosis, suppurative lung disease, or cardiac disease. Standardized growth curves should be used to plot height and weight. Poor growth parameters and failure to thrive also point to the presence of chronic disease.

Evidence of atopic disease may be seen on the head and neck examination. These include allergic shiners, tranverse nasal creases (allergic gape), Dennie's sign (lines radiating from the lower aspect of the palpebral fissure), or boggy erythematous nasal mucosae. Observation of the child may show evidence of mouth breathing or an "allergic salute," an upward rubbing motion of the nose with the hand. Examination of the posterior pharynx may show a cobblestone pattern due to hypertrophic lymphoid follicles caused by postnasal drip.

The respiratory and cardiac examinations are obviously important. Inspection of the chest may reveal hyperinflation indicative of obstructive airway disease. Cough, wheeze, and a prolonged expiratory phase of respiration are typical of asthma but are also seen in any condition causing lower airway obstruction. A search should be made for unilateral or asymmetrical wheezes, which can signify aspiration of debris or a foreign body, or the presence of significant mucus plugging. Crackles are found with pneumonia, bronchiectasis, pulmonary congestion, and fibrotic lung disease. They are indicative of pathology in the terminal airways and alveoli. Cardiac examination may reveal pathological heart murmurs, cardiomegaly, and other signs of cardiac disease. The presence of stridor suggests an upper airway problem. The abdominal, dermatological, and neurological examination may help uncover an underlying disease process. As with all diagnostic dilemmas, the physical examination may yield no clues whatsoever as to what is going on.

## Laboratory Investigations

In the majority of cases, the physician will have a good idea of which investigations are needed after a careful history and physical examination have been performed.

For infants and young children who have a history of wheezing, and who have never had previous radiological investigations, we generally obtain a posterior-anterior and lateral chest radiograph. If a foreign body is suspected or if there is evidence of emphysema secondary to airway obstruction, then inspiratory and expiratory films should be performed. If there is any question of foreign body aspiration, rigid bronchoscopy is indicated (14).

If, on the basis of the history, one considers that gastroesophageal reflux or aspiration secondary to swallowing problems is the likely cause of the child's respiratory difficulty, then a barium swallow with careful attention to the mechanics of swallowing is indicated.

Anatomical abnormalities and abnormal masses may need further radiological investigations, including ultrasound, computed-tomography (CT) scanning, and magnetic resonance imaging. Depending on the results of these investigations, one may then need to consider bronchoscopy of biopsy.

Serological tests are occasionally helpful in the evaluation of the wheezing child. A complete blood count and differential may reveal an eosinophilia indicative of allergic disease. An increased white blood cell count might indicate the presence of an active infectious process, and an elevated erythrocyte sedimentation rate points to active infection or inflammation. Neutropenia may be associated with some of the immune deficiency states. A tuberculin test (5-TU) should be performed in any child with chronic respiratory symptoms of an unexplained etiology.

If failure to thrive is associated with the wheezing, or if there is malabsorption or any other reason to suspect cystic fibrosis, then a sweat chloride test (performed by pilocarpine iontophoresis) should be done.

Immunoglobulin and IgG subclass determinations are important if an immune deficiency state is suspected, based on a history of chronic infections, failure to thrive, or unexplained bronchiectasis (15,16).

Depending on the findings of the history and physical examination, and the age of the child, allergy skin testing may be useful; an atopic profile may thus be identified.

Physicians are at a disadvantage in looking after infants and young children with wheezing as there is not the array of pulmonary function tests available to characterize the degree of airway obstruction and bronchial hyperresponsiveness that there is for children over the age of 5 years. Infant pulmonary function testing can be performed in certain centers and has been used in evaluating infants and young children with a variety of pulmonary disorders. England has reviewed the different infant pulmonary function tests available, with a focus on the mechanics and rationale of these tests (17). A variety of techniques are available. Measurements of functional residual capacity, dynamic compliance, and respiratory resistance can be obtained using an infant body plethysmograph (18). However, few centers possess such equipment, the skilled personnel, and time necessary for such evaluations. For evaluating infants with obstructive lung disease, two methods have been developed that enable the forced expiratory flow-volume relationship to be examined. Motoyama described a technique of forced deflation that can generate a maximal expiratory flow-volume curve. However, it requires endotracheal intubation as well as deep sedation and muscle relaxation and, thus, would be practical only in an intensive care unit setting (19). The rapid thoracoabdominal compression technique was described by Wohl originally and has been modified by others (20,21). With this method, forced expiratory flows are produced using an inflatable jacket that compresses the thorax and abdomen at the end-inspiratory phase of tidal breathing. This technique can be used in an outpatient setting, but does require that the infant be sedated with an agent such as chloral hydrate. Commercial equipment packages are available to carry out this technique, but our feeling at this time is that there are still concerns with the technique and controversial issues concerning the achievement of flow limitation. The practice of infant pulmonary function testing should probably still be carried out in a research setting by investigators with a solid understanding of pulmonary mechanics and an ability to properly understand and interpret the results.

## DIAGNOSTIC ENTITIES

### Asthma in Early Life

Asthma is the most common chronic disorder of childhood in industrialized nations (22). Although it is rarely a cause of mortality, it is a major cause of school absenteeism, hospitalization, and health care cost (22–28). It is likely that asthma morbidity is associated with underdiagnosis, undertreatment, poor education, and inadequate supervision. Estimates of asthma prevalence vary widely, for a variety of reasons. The variation may be due to genetic environmental, or cultural factors or to the fact that different definitions and methods are used in screening populations. A review of the literature reveals that the estimates of asthma prevalence in infants and young children under 2 years of age range from 5 to 10% (29,30). A recent review of the experience of the Emergency Room of The Hospital for Sick Children, Toronto, Canada, demonstrated that over a 16-month period there were 3358 visits by 1864 different asthmatic patients for treatment of acute asthma (31). The male-to-female ratio of our study population was 1.9:1, and the mean age was 5.6 years. Study of the age distribution of these patients revealed that 6% were infants less than 1 year of age, and 47% of the visits were made by individuals between 1 and 4 years of age. Other research has shown that as many as 50% of childhood asthmatics develop symptoms prior to their first birthday (32). Despite significant medical advances in the treatment of acute asthma and the maintenance therapy of the stable asthmatic, morbidity from asthma seems to be on the increase, especially in preschool children (22,33).

Asthma is a chronic illness characterized by increased airway responsiveness to various stimuli. This responsiveness manifests itself as a widespread narrowing that may reverse on its own or in response to therapy. The airway obstruction is produced by a combination of airway smooth muscle spasm, inflammatory edema of the mucosa lining the airway, and mucus plugging. Pathologically, on a microscopic level, changes are most marked in the peripheral airway and include smooth muscle hypertrophy, goblet cell metaplasia, basement membrane thickening and increased collagen deposition beneath the basement membrane, inflammatory cell infiltration, and epithelial cell shedding (34). However, for patients only mildly or intermittently affected by their asthma, the lining of the respiratory tree may appear entirely normal (35).

## Etiological Considerations

The cause of asthma is not understood completely, but there is agreement that the characteristic feature is bronchial hyperreactivity. In studies performed on older children, up to 90% of the subjects with frequent episodes of wheezing in the previous year demonstrated reactivity to methacholine/histamine, particularly when there was concurrent evidence of atopy (36). In young infants, recent studies have demonstrated that bronchial hyperreactivity is detectable shortly after birth, and it has been postulated that this reactivity may result from interaction between genetic, atopic, and environmental factors (37). It has been known for some time that disorders such as asthma, eczema, and allergic rhinitis seem to run in some families and are at least partly hereditary in nature. It has been determined that the risk of having a child with asthma is greater when one or both parents have asthma than when neither parent is affected (38,39). A familial component is also felt to be relevant to the development of increased responsiveness to methacholine and histamine, regardless of the presence or absence of atopy (40). Young and co-workers found that histamine-induced responsiveness may be present shortly after birth in normal, asymptomatic infants, and that the responsiveness correlated with a family history of asthma and parental smoking, but not with markers of atopy (41).

Atopy, the increased tendency to form IgE antibodies on exposure to common environmental antigens, is present in most patients with asthma. The atopic predisposition is also partly hereditary, and recent data suggest a possible autosomal dominant pattern of inheritance linked to a gene locus on chromosome 11 (42). It has been postulated that exposure to and the development of antibodies to allergens such as house dust mites, animal dander, grasses, and pollens in the early years may influence the development of asthma (43).

The respiratory viruses, including rhinovirus, respiratory syncytial virus (RSV), influenza, and parainfluenza viruses, are the most common trigger of wheeze in young children with asthma (44). In addition, infections with pertussis, croup, bronchiolitis, and *Chlamydia* pneumonia may lead to the development of asthma and airway hyperreactivity. Significant bronchiolitis infection has been associated with the development of lung function abnormalities, increased airway hyperreactivity, and an increased chance of having asthma later in childhood. It may have an even greater tendency to do so in families with a strong atopy history. It is not known whether the RSV causes these problems directly, or whether the infections occur in infants with a genetic predisposition to develop airway hyperreactivity. Martinez and co-workers have found, using infant pulmonary function testing techniques, that the risk of wheezing during respiratory infections in early childhood was higher in infants with diminished lung function detected earlier in life (45). It may be that the infants who are more likely to wheeze later in life are born with narrower peripheral airways.

The importance of parental smoking in the development of asthma is worth consideration. Maternal smoking has been shown to increase symptom severity in children with asthma, and the effect seems more pronounced in males and older children with asthma (46). The effect of intrauterine exposure to cigarette smoke has also been studied (47). The exposure has been noted to result in increased cord blood IgE levels, increased airway responsiveness at birth, and an increased risk of developing asthma and atopy in the early childhood years. The combination of maternal smoking in a household with a child with eczema is more likely to result in the child developing asthma than if the mother is not a smoker (48).

Other factors that may impact on the development of asthma in childhood are living in areas with higher levels of air pollution and socioeconomic factors such as low family income, low birthweight, and young maternal age. Finally, it remains controversial as to whether breast feeding protects against the development of atopic disease.

## DIAGNOSIS AND EVALUATION OF ASTHMA IN INFANCY AND EARLY CHILDHOOD

Within the Chest Division of The Hospital for Sick Children, Toronto, Canada, we generally agree that any child, regardless of age, with three or more episodes of wheezing and/or dyspnea is considered asthmatic until proven otherwise. A history of episodic illness triggered by the usual factors and improvement of symptoms after taking antiasthma medications help confirm the diagnosis. It should be remembered, however, that not all asthmatic children present with wheeze. About 5% of childhood asthmatics present with a chronic or recurrent cough as the only symptom (49). Attention should be paid to the pattern of symptoms, their frequency, severity, and diurnal and seasonal variation. A search should be made for precipitating or aggravating factors, including the relationship to viral upper respiratory tract infections, weather change, allergen and irritant exposure, and physical activity. Inquiries should be made into the home environment and presence of dust and cigarette smoke. Other factors that may influence the child's asthma are the method of home heating and cooking, the presence of rugs and feather bedding in the bedroom, and the existence of cats and dogs in the home.

In taking the history and doing the physical examination, the physician should pay careful attention to the growth and development of the asthmatic child, and stigmata of failure to thrive and chronic illness should be looked for so that other, less common causes of wheezing, such as those listed in Table 1, can be ruled out. Table 2 summarizes clinical features of other conditions that can cause wheeze in early childhood. Other than a chest radiograph for those presenting with wheeze for the first time, or those with asymmetrical lung findings, laboratory investigations can usually be kept to a minimum. As many young children with asthma are atopic,

TABLE 2 Clinical Features Suggestive of an Alternative Diagnosis to Asthma

| |
|---|
| History |
| Symptoms presenting in neonatal period |
| Requirement of ventilation in neonatal period |
| Wheeze associated with feeding/vomiting |
| Sudden onset of cough/choking |
| Steatorrhea |
| Stridor |
| Physical examination |
| Failure to thrive |
| Heart murmur |
| Clubbing |
| Unilateral signs |
| Investigations |
| No reversibility of airflow obstruction with bronchodilator |
| Focal, persistent, or atypical chest radiographic findings |

one must consider performing skin testing to identify allergens that may be aggravating asthma symptoms identified in the clinical assessment. We utilize the skin prick test, not intradermal testing, because the latter has been associated with a greater number of false-positive test results (50). The skin testing extracts should be selected on the basis of what allergens are common and by the patient's history. In our experience, the most important allergens to consider are dust mites (*Dermatophagoides pteronyssinus, D. farinae*), cats, dogs, horses, pollens, and molds. Saline testing to exclude dermatographia and histamine testing to exclude anergy or recent anti-histamine ingestion controls are also part of our test panel. The radioallergosorbent test (RAST) can be used if it is feared that skin testing could cause anaphylaxis. We do not routinely use RAST testing our clinic setting. We do not usually perform skin testing in children under 3 years of age. The younger the child, the more difficult it is to perform these tests; however, if offending allergens can be identified, advice on avoidance and environmental control can be given.

Occasionally, the history and physical evaluation do not give the clinician as much information as would be liked, and in such cases, a diary card can be given to the parents. The parent records the frequency and severity of symptoms over a period of time and then returns the card to the physician. This allows for a better assessment of disease impact and response to therapy.

## MANAGEMENT OF ASTHMA IN INFANCY AND EARLY CHILDHOOD

Once the diagnosis of asthma has been made and the impact of the illness established, a treatment strategy can be devised. The following are our goals in managing young children with asthma:

1. To maximally control symptoms with the minimal number of medications
2. To reduce the frequency and severity of acute attacks
3. To educate the child and family about asthma and its management
4. To minimize the need to keep the child home from day care, nursery school, or kindergarten
5. To allow the child to grow and develop normally
6. To limit medication side effects

Three broad categories of therapy need to be considered when devising a comprehensive management plan. These are patient and family education and supervision, environmental control, and pharmacological therapy. The issue of family education is too often dealt with superficially, but there is no question that an informed parent is more likely able to cope with an asthmatic infant. Poor parental understanding may be a contributing factor in the requirement for emergency room visits and hospitalizations, and thus, education programs might well impact on asthma morbidity. Parents who attend the Chest and Asthma Clinic at our institution receive a detailed educational program accompanied by a clearly written handbook that explains the nature and mechanisms of asthma, factors that lead to exacerbations, how to recognize and appreciate the severity of an asthma attack, and information about asthma medications, routes of delivery, and possible side effects. As a component of the educational process, we feel it is important to have a member of the education team observe a parent administer the medication using the correct technique.

Environmental control can help reduce exposure to various common irritants and allergens. Harmful factors that can often be avoided include secondhand cigarette smoke, smoke and fumes from gas or wood stoves, pet dogs and cats if they seem to aggravate symptoms, and house dust. Many young children are sensitive to the house dust mite and may benefit from antidust measures applied to their sleeping quarters. Such measures include keeping pets out of the bedroom and, certainly, off of the bed, removing carpets, stuffed animals, and fluffy toys from the bedroom, and frequent cleaning with damp cloths. Mattresses and pillows should be of nonallergenic material (no feathers!) and should be enclosed in zippered vinyl mattress and pillow covers. Washing bedding with water at least 60°C can help eliminate the dust mite. Many households tend to overuse vaporizers and humidifiers, and this should be discouraged as mites thrive in warm, moist conditions. In humid summers, air conditioning can reduce humidity levels and thus decrease mite numbers. For those children who are exquisitely sensitive to dust and dust mites, a trial with antimite chemicals such as benzylbenzoate may be worthwhile (51).

During the spring and fall, seasonal pollens can be partially avoided by keeping windows and doors closed as much as possible and relying on window or central air conditioners for ventilation. As soon as children are old enough to play outdoors, it becomes more difficult to avoid pollens. Many parents seem obsessed with a notion that avoidance of various foods such as dairy products will lead to improvement of their young child's symptoms. It is generally agreed that food allergy plays a minimal role in causing exacerbations of childhood asthma, and exclusion diets should not be utilized as a form of therapy unless there are clear indications that a child has sensitivity to a certain food (52). The most common food sensitivities include milk, eggs, and peanuts. Parents of children who have experienced anaphylactic reactions to foods such as peanuts must be educated in the importance of avoiding such triggers and instructed in the use of and provided with a form of emergency-use subcutaneous epinephrine. Our clinic does not believe in the use of allergy hyposensitization shots in general, and certainly not for infants and young children.

Treating young asthmatics provides the clinician with a considerable challenge for a variety of reasons. It is generally harder to administer medications to infants, and there is a relative deficiency of data concerning the dosage and therapeutic benefit of many antiasthma medications for this age group. Our clinic prefers to utilize the inhalational route of medication delivery. This can be accomplished with the use of either a compressed air nebulizer or a spacer device with a mask attachment (53). We have been attempting to use the latter route more frequently because with practice it seems to be very effective. Previous research has questioned whether children under the age of 18 months benefit from beta-2 agonists; however, recent studies of infants with acute asthma at our institution have shown that there can be a beneficial response to nebulized albuterol (54,55). For treatment of infants with very mild and infrequent asthma, a trial of an oral beta-2 agonist given on an intermittent basis may be all that is required. If this is felt to be inadequate, a beta-2 agonist should be administered by the inhaled route. The addition of inhaled ipratropium bromide can provide additional bronchodilation if required. Although there are clinicians who prescribe theophylline for infants and young children with asthma, our clinic tends not to because there are considerable difficulties with side effects. Children with persistent symptoms require regular maintenance treatment with a prophylactic anti-inflammatory agent such as inhaled cromolyn sodium or oral ketotifen. If symptoms persist despite the use of the above prophylactic agents, a trial of inhaled corticosteroid medication is indicated. As with other inhaled medication, these agents can be administered with a spacer device and mask attachment. In general, once we have achieved control of symptoms using beta-2 agonists, we use them to control symptoms on an as-needed basis and just administer the prophylactic agent regularly. When using inhaled corticosteroids, we attempt to use low dosages (200–400 μg/day) because dosages in this range are less likely to cause adrenal suppression (56). If necessary, we increase the dose, but an occasional severely affected patient may require alternate-day oral prednisone to achieve adequate control.

## BRONCHIOLITIS

Acute viral bronchiolitis is an important cause of wheezing in infants and young children. It occurs in children under the age of 24 months and accounts for 50–70% of lower respiratory illness in infancy. The most common cause is the respiratory syncytial virus (RSV); however, the illness can also result from infection with parainfluenza, influenza, and adenovirus (57). The seasonal incidence of bronchiolitis ranges from late fall to spring. From a pathological point of view, there are several detectable changes. Obstruction at the bronchiolar level occurs secondary to submucosal edema, peribronchial cellular infiltrates, mucus plugging, and intraluminal cellular debris. This leads to patchy obstruction and gas trapping distal to the obstruction. A patchy interstitial pneumonia may also accompany the above changes. Physiologically, the obstruction leads to gas exchange interference, with hypoxia being the first detectable change in the blood gas profile.

The role of RSV viral infection and other viral infections in the etiology of recurrent wheeze and asthma has been discussed in the previous section on asthma, but it is important to remember that some series show as many as 50% infants with bronchiolitis will go on to have recurrent episodes of wheezing later in life. Bronchiolitis due to infection with types 3, 7, and 21 adenovirus has been associated with the development of a severe form of chronic lung disease known as bronchiolitis obliterans. Native Canadian Indians and Polynesians in New Zealand seem to be particularly prone to infection with adenovirus. In addition to bronchiolitis obliterans, the hyperlucent lung syndrome (Swyer-James syndrome) can develop.

## Clinical Manifestations

Viral bronchiolitis usual presents with a prodrome typical of a viral upper respiratory tract infection. Within a few days (or less if the infection is more severe), symptoms of lower respiratory tract infection develop. The fever is usually low grade (38°C); however, the infants are usually irritable, ill looking, dyspneic, and have a reduced appetite. The parents may remark that the child is wheezing or has a wheezy cough.

Physical examination reveals a variety of physical findings, depending on the severity of the illness, and bronchiolitis may result in mild to severe respiratory distress. The respiratory rate usually ranges from 50 to 80 breaths/min. There may be flaring of the alae nasi, and subcostal and intercostal indrawing is present in moderately to severely affected infants. Severely infected patients may present with apneic spells, and sudden death has been reported in infants with bronchiolitis. Examination of the chest may reveal evidence of hyperinflation with an increase in anterior-posterior diameter and hyperresonance on percussion. On auscultation, it is usually possible to detect both diffuse crackles and wheezes. On abdominal examination, both the liver and spleen may be palpable owing to the hyperinflated lungs causing depression of the diaphragm. Cardiac examination should be directed at looking for evidence of extreme tachycardia (>200 beats/min), which, combined with periodic breathing, signals impending respiratory failure. Evidence of dehydration may be present and is likely due to increased insensible losses associated with fever and tachypnea and decreased fluid intake.

### Laboratory Investigations

The chest radiograph usually shows evidence of hyperinflation. Peribronchial thickening is often noted and appears as irregular linear shadows and increased thickness of airways seen end-on. Patchy areas of atelectasis may be evident. Viral cultures reveal a pathogenic agent in up to 70% of children with bronchiolitis (58). More rapid detection can be accomplished with the aid of immunofluorescence techniques. In a recent study completed in the Emergency Room of The Hospital for Sick Children, 24 of 34 nasopharyngeal swabs examined for the presence of virus were positive: 21 for RSV, one for paramyxovirus, one for parainfluenza virus, and one for influenza A (59). To assess the effect on gas exchange in the acute phase of the illness in moderately to severely affected infants, arterial blood gases should be performed. Hypoxemia is invariably present. In more severely affected infants, carbon dioxide retention occurs. In recent years, transcutaneous oxygen saturation monitoring has been very useful in following the status of patients with bronchiolitis (50).

Most infants recover from bronchiolitis, although there is a mortality rate of probably less than 1%. Therapy for acute bronchiolitis includes supportive measures such as supplementary oxygen. The role of bronchodilating agents, including sympathomimetic agents, theophylline, and anticholinergic agents, and the role of corticosteroids remain controversial. In a recent study of 40 infants at The Hospital for Sick Chlidren, Toronto, we found that children with acute bronchiolitis demonstrated significantly greater improvement when they received nebulized albuterol than when they received a placebo (59). Infants with severe bronchiolitis, congenital heart disease, chronic lung disease (e.g., bronchopulmonary dysplasia), or immunodeficiency, and who are less than 6 weeks of age are at risk of developing severe sequelae from RSV infection and should be considered for Ribavirin antiviral therapy (60). Systemic steroids do not appear to be efficacious in bronchiolitis.

## ASPIRATION SYNDROMES

As outlined in Table 1, aspiration is an important cause of recurrent wheezing in infants and young children. Recurrent aspiration can mimic asthma or recurrent respiratory tract infections. The usual material aspirated most commonly includes milk and other gastric contents and foodstuffs. The aspiration results in an inflammatory reaction of the airways and alveoli. If the problem is persistent, there can be the development of chronic intestitial lung disease with pulmonary fibrosis and bronchiolitis obliterans. Table 3 outlines a variety of causes of recurrent aspiration.

### Swallowing Incoordination

Difficulties associated with swallowing are a common cause of recurrent aspiration in infancy. This is usually associated with bouts of coughing and choking associated with feeding, and rattly breathing. Nasal escape of milk and other foods may also be noted. In infants with neurological damage, persistent drooling may indicate difficulties with coordination of the swallowing mechanism. Transient swallowing difficulties associated with neuromuscular immaturity have been described. Symptoms usually improve as the infant matures over the first year of life.

TABLE 3 Aspiration in Infancy

| |
|---|
| Swallowing dysfunction |
| Central nervous system dysfunction, e.g., perinatal damage |
| Neuromuscular immaturity |
| Central nervous system depression caused by drugs, toxins, and poisons |
| Familial dysautonomia |
| Structural lesions of mouth, tongue, nasopharynx, jaw |
| Regurgitation |
| Gastroesophageal reflux |
| Hiatus hernia |
| Esophageal obstruction due to |
| Atresia |
| Stricture |
| Stenosis |
| Vascular ring |
| Achalasia |
| Esophageal dysmotility |
| Pharyngeal and esophageal damage due to burns |
| Abnormal communication |
| Tracheoesophageal fistula |
| Laryngotracheoesophageal cleft |
| Bronchobiliary fistula |
| Bronchojejunal fistula |
| Bronchogastrointestinal fistula |

### Regurgitation

Esophageal or pharyngeal overfilling with spillover into the larynx results in material being aspirated into the respiratory tree. Vomiting and regurgitation of partially digested or undigested foodstuffs are characteristic. If the vomiting occurs between meals, it is more suggestive of esophageal reflux. Reflux without vomiting or choking can occur during sleep. Gagging and vomiting occurring at the time of food ingestion suggest the presence of esophageal obstruction. Reflux can result in cough and wheeze even if material is not aspirated into the respiratory tree; acid coming in contact with the mucosa of the lower esophagus irritates vagal receptors, which in turn can result in bronchoconstricting vagal efferent signals.

### Abnormal Communication

Conditions such as tracheoesophageal fistula (TEF), including the H-type fistula, which makes up approximately 2–5% of TEFs, are a less common cause of aspiration of material into the tracheobronchial tree. Fluid consumption can result in sudden bouts of coughing, choking, and cyanosis. Jejunal and biliary communications have also been described.

### Evaluation of Aspiration

After the history and physical examination have led one to consider aspiration as a potential problem, a chest radiograph should be performed. Recurrent aspiration may present, with patchy or diffuse areas of atelectasis and overinflation (3). Advanced disease may be associated with fibrosis and bronchiectasis. Infants tend to aspirate in the supine position. This leads to disease involving the dependent portions of the lung, primarily the right upper lobe and, sometimes, the right lower lobe. Right upper lobe changes include streaky densities and loss of volume. The minor fissure may appear to be shifted upward. The middle lobe is usually spared in all but severe aspiration cases. The left lung is not affected as frequently as the right. On the left side, changes tend to involve the medial segments of the lung (3). In children aspirating while upright, changes occur in the lower lobes.

The chest radiograph can confirm a physician's suspicion that a child is aspirating. The barium swallow under fluroscopic control may allow the diagnosis to be established. Aspiration due to gastroesophageal reflux may be more difficult to confirm, as often the barium swallow is not helpful. Other investigations that may play a role include a radionucleide milk scan in which the ultimate fate of radiolabeled milk is followed (not particularly useful in the experience of the respirologists at this institution), esophagoscopy with biopsy, and 24-hr pH probe monitoring. The latter investigation is the most sensitive test in looking for reflux but may not be performed in some institutions. Analysis of tracheal or bronchial secretions obtained bronchoscopically for fat-laden macrophages confirms aspiration, but their absence does not rule out the diagnosis.

## Foreign Body Aspiration

Toddlers and young children may aspirate foreign bodies of all possible descriptions into their airways. A witnessed episode of choking after food ingestion or after putting a toy in the mouth helps make the diagnosis, which can be harder to make in the event the episode was unwitnessed or did not result in acute symptoms. Kim and co-workers reviewed a large series of foreign body ingestions at The Hospital for Sick Children, Toronto (61). Boys were twice as likely to aspirate foreign bodies as girls were. Sixty-five percent of all cases occurred in children between 6 months and 3 years of age. Peanuts made up 50% of the foreign matter inhaled, and in general, foreign material was most often vegetable. However, parents should be warned that pieces of frankfurter, which are frequently used as "finger" foods, can find their way into the upper airway and should be finely chopped if served to young children. Kim et al. found a history of aspiration in about 85% of the patients (61). There is frequently a history of sudden onset of wheezing and respiratory difficulties in a child who was previously healthy. There may not be a classic history of a choking episode, so a high index of suspicion is necessary. Esophageal foreign bodies most commonly cause dysphagia, but can cause wheezing and cough by compressing the trachea.

Clues for physicians include asymmetry of air entry, unilateral wheezing, and unilateral hyperinflation. Tachypnea, cough, stridor, and mediastinal shift may be present. The diagnosis is frequently difficult to make, and whereas 65% of the time the diagnosis was made within 1 week, in 17% of the cases the diagnosis was not made until at least 1 month later (61). The respiratory difficulty can be mistakenly diagnosed as asthma or respiratory tract infection, as cough and fever can be associated. When material is aspirated more distally into the respiratory tree, recurrent pneumonia may be mistakenly diagnosed.

Radiological investigations include a posterior-anterior and lateral chest radiograph, and care should be taken to show the entire region from the mouth to below the diaphragm. Opaque foreign bodies or a lucent outline of nonradiopaque material may be visible. Evidence of hyperinflation with contralateral mediastinal shift and paradoxical diaphragmatic motion on fluoroscopy or sequential films should be sought. Inspiratory and expiratory films may help determine the presence of air trapping. A tracheal foreign body such as a coin is usually seen head-on in the lateral view, whereas a similar esophageal foreign body will appear head-on in the posterior-anterior view. Any suspicion of foreign body aspiration must be investigated using rigid bronchoscopy (14). With regard to the ultimate location of aspirated foreign bodies, the right mainstem bronchus and bronchus intermedius are involved in approximately 50% of cases, with the left main bronchus being the site in about 30% (61).

## CYSTIC FIBROSIS

Cystic fibrosis (CF) classically presents as failure to thrive, malabsorption, and chronic cough, but the first presenting symptom in a patient with CF may be wheezing. We have recently reviewed the incidence of wheezing in patients with CF in the CF clinic population followed at The Hospital for Sick Children, Toronto (62). It was found that 25% of infants who were diagnosed as having CF before 2 years of age had physician-documented wheezing during the first 2 years of life. Interestingly, wheezing had resolved in 50% of the infants by age 2 years and in 75% by age 4 years. Pulmonary function test abnormalities were more evident at 7 and 13 years in the group that wheezed, as compared to the group that did not. A sweat chloride test should be performed if CF is a possible diagnosis in the infant with chronic respiratory problems.

## BRONCHOPULMONARY DYSPLASIA

A history of prematurity with requirement for oxygen and mechanical ventilation in the neonatal period should lead one to consider bronchopulmonary dysplasia (BPD) as the possible cause of wheezing. Many infants with BPD go on to have recurrent wheezing and respiratory difficulty and benefit from antiasthmatic therapy as they have bronchial hyperreactivity (63,64). Radiological evidence includes patchy areas of atelectasis, hyperinflation, and fibrosis on the chest radiograph.

## VASCULAR RINGS

Aortic arch abnormalities can result in the formation of vascular rings or structures that compress the trachea and cause airway obstruction. Embryologically, there is either persistence of a vessel that should regress or abnormal regression of a vessel. The most common of these anomalies include a double aortic arch, right aortic arch with a ductus arteriosus or ligamentum arteriosus, anomalous innominate artery, and the pulmonary sling (3,65).

Although stridor is the most likely symptom, wheeze, recurrent infection, dysphagia, and apnea have been described. As with other causes of tracheal obstruction such as laryngotracheomalacia, the patient may tend to rest with the next hyperextended. Neck flexion may reproduce symptoms noted by the parents. Reflex apnea may also occur in this condition.

Radiological investigations can contribute to making the diagnosis. A right-sided aortic arch can be detected on a plain film, as can tracheal shift or compression. Pulmonary slings can result in asymmetrical areas of hyperinflation due to compression of the right mainstem bronchus. The barium swallow can be a particularly useful investigation and may show a persistent indentation. The location of the indentation may point to a particular diagnosis (65). Before repair can be carried out, more complete anatomical detail can be characterized with echocardiography and/or angiography. Surgical repair may not completely abolish symptoms as the trachea can remain persistently abnormal at the site of the original compression.

## CARDIOGENIC WHEEZE

A variety of cardiac conditions can result in bronchial obstruction and wheezing. Most commonly, this is due to a large left-to-right cardiovascular shunt such as that seen with a large ventricular septal defect or patent ductus arteriosus (66,67). The problems arise when a distended pulmonary artery and/or an enlarged left atrium compresses large airways. Cardiomegaly due to a variety of causes can result in bronchial compression. If the bronchial compression is complete, atelectasis can result, whereas if the blockage is incomplete, an emphysematous picture may be evident. If there is complete obstruction of a mainstem bronchus (more commonly the left), complete atelectasis of the lung may result. The most common sites of compression are the left main bronchus, the left upper lobe bronchus, and the bronchus to the right middle lobe. Factors that favor cardiac problems manifesting themselves this way in the first year or life include the high pulmonary artery pressures present and the lack of stiffness in the airway cartilage.

With respect to cardiac disease, wheezing may result from causes other than airway compression. Left ventricular failure can result in distention of the pulmonary vascular bed, as can obstructed pulmonary veins. The resulting bronchiolar wall edema causes increased peripheral resistance and can lead to wheezing and other respiratory difficulties. If there is a cardiac murmur or cardiomegaly on the radiograph, cardiac consultation should be obtained, and other investigations, such as electrocardiography, echocardiography and angiography, may be indicated. It should be noted that murmurs and cardiomegaly may not be evident in certain conditions, such as obstructed pulmonary veins, and an index of suspicion and experience will be required to make the proper diagnosis.

## MEDIASTINAL MASSES AND PULMONARY MASS LESIONS

Chronic cough or wheezing can occasionally be caused by airway compression due to a mass lesion in the mediastinum (4,68). This may be detected as an abnormal mass on a plain posterior-anterior and lateral chest radiograph. Filler and co-workers have previously reviewed the presentation of a variety of these lesions at our institution (69). Neurogenic tumors in the posterior mediastinum made up about one-third of the lesions, with the most common anterior or middle mediastinal masses being lymphomatous. The location and distribution of these lesions can be seen in Table 4. The history may reveal a gradual or more sudden onset of symptoms. The physical examination may provide evidence of cervical or other lymphadenopathy, stridor, and/or wheeze or may reveal no abnormality. Depending on the illness, there may be manifestations of systemic disease. Once it has been determined that there is a lesion on plain chest films, investigation by such modalities as barium swallow, ultrasound, and CT scanning can be arranged. Most often surgical and/or oncological consul-

TABLE 4 Mass Lesions of the Mediastinum

| | |
|---|---|
| Superior | Anterior |
| Cystic hygroma | Thymoma |
| Thymic tumor | Teratoma |
| Hemangioma | Cystic hygroma |
| Teratoma | Pericardial cyst |
| Mediastinal abscess | Thyroid lesion |
| | Lymphoma |
| | Morgagni hernia |
| Middle | Posterior |
| Lymphoma | Neurogenic tumor |
| Great vessel anomalies | Enterogenic cyst |
| Bronchogenic cyst | Neurenteric anomaly |
| Enlarged and/or infected lymph nodes | Bronchogenic cyst |
| Angiomatous lesion | Esophageal lesion |
| | Bochdalek hernia |

tations will be required to evaluate and treat the conditions listed. When evaluating mediastinal adenopathy, one should not neglect tuberculin skin testing. Complete blood counts, bone marrow aspiration, and tests of vanillylmandelic acid, homovanillic acid, and epinephrine metabolites may be indicated. Bronchoscopy can be helpful in locating the site of airway compression. With solid lesions, the final diagnosis is not usually made until a thoracotomy and biopsy have been completed.

## ABNORMALITIES OF THE LARYNX, TRACHEA, AND BRONCHI

Abnormalities of the tracheobronchial tree can result in a wide variety of respiratory tract symptoms, including chronic cough, stridor, wheeze, cyanosis, and dyspnea (70). Laryngeal lesions classically cause inspiratory stridor, although inspiratory and expiratory wheezing can also result. Lesions may be congenital or acquired. Laryngeal stenosis and laryngeal webs can result in stridor that is both inspiratory and expiratory. Laryngoceles are rare cystic lesions that are in communication with the laryngeal ventricles. Depending on their size and location, they can cause obstruction of the larynx and even present as a neck mass anterior to the sternocleidomastoid muscles of the neck. Hoarseness or absence of voice, recurrent infection, and the variety of respiratory symptoms listed above can result from such lesions. Acquired laryngeal problems include traumatic dislocation of the cricoarytenoid joint, acquired subglottic stenosis, and angioneurotic edema.

Tracheal narrowing and stenosis may be congenital or acquired. Congenital lesions include such rare anomalies as tracheal webs. Stenosis of the trachea can be short segment, and reparable, or long segment, which is by and large irreparable. Tracheoesophageal fistulae may also lead to tracheal stenosis at the site of communication. Subglottic and tracheal stenosis can be acquired from the trauma of repeated intubation sometimes necessary for premature infants with respiratory distress syndrome. The trachea can also be narrowed owing to cartilage deficiencies, as in tracheomalacia, or as a component of a more diffuse laryngotracheobronchomalacia. In such situations, the trachea may be of normal caliber until compressed by positive intrathoracic pressure that can develop when the infant has a superimposed infection causing peripheral airway disease. Anomalous vessels may also cause tracheal compression.

Some congenital bronchial lesions can lead to wheeze and a variety of respiratory symptoms. Bronchi may be narrow owing to agenesis, atresia, or stenosis. Webs have been described in bronchi. As with the trachea, there can be compression of the bronchi by enlarged or anomalous vessels, and bronchi can also be affected by cartilage anomalies.

Making the diagnosis of the laryngotracheobronchial abnormalities can be difficult on plain films of the chest. The barium swallow may reveal esophageal anomalies that can give a clue as to the diagnosis. Ultimately, laryngoscopy and bronchoscopy allow the diagnosis to be established. With such investigation, the site of the lesion can be detected. Occasionally, a pulsatile compressing vessel can be identified if an anomalous vascular lesion is the cause of the problem, and in classic tracheomalacia, the trachea can be seen to be abnormally floppy and collapse on expiration.

## CONCLUSION

Wheezing is a common complaint in the infant and young child. Although asthma is by far the most common cause, a multitude of other possibilities need to be considered in different clinical situations. Usually, the diagnosis can be established after a thorough history and physical examination have been performed. Radiological investigations and occasionally bronchoscopic examination will allow the diagnosis to be established in cases that are more diagnostically challenging.

## REFERENCES

1. Mikami R, Murao M, Cugell DW, Chretian J, et al. International Symposium on lung sounds. Synopsis of proceedings. *Chest* 92:342, 1987.
2. Pasterkamp H, Montgomery M, Wiebicke W. Nomenclature used by health care professionals to describe breath sounds in asthma. *Chest* 92:346, 1987.
3. Levison H, Tabachnik, Newth CJL. Wheezing in infancy, croup and epiglottitis. *Cur. Concepts Pediatr* 12(3):1–65, 1982.
4. Pasterkamp H. The history and physical examination. In: Kendig and Chernick (eds), *Disorders of the Respiratory Tract in Children*, 5th ed., WB Saunders, Philadelphia, 1990.
5. Pasterkamp H, Wiebicke W, Fenton R. Subjective assessment vs computer analysis of wheezing in asthma. *Chest* 91:376, 1987.
6. Pasterkamp H, Carson C, Daien D, Oh Y. Digital respirosonography. New images of lung sounds. *Chest* 96:1405, 1989.
7. Bryan AC, Mansell Al, Levison H. Development of mechanical properties of the respiratory system. In: Hodson WA (ed.), *Development of the Lung*, Vol 6, Marcel Dekker, New York, 1977.
8. Hogg JC, Williams J, Richardson JB et al. Age as a factor in the distribution of lower airway conductance and in the pathologic anatomy of obstructive lung disease. *N Engl J Med* 282:1283, 1970.
9. Wohl MEB. Lung mechanics in the developing human infant. In: Chernick V, Mellins RB (eds.), *Basic Mechanisms of Pediatric Respiratory Disease*, BC Decker, Philadelphia, 1991.

10. Macklin CC. Alveolar pores and their significance in the human lung. *Arch Pathol* 21:202, 1936.
11. Muller NL, Bryan AC. Chest wall mechanics and respiratory muscles in infants. *Pediatr Clin North Am* 26:503, 1979.
12. Bryan AC, Wohl MEB. Respiratory mechanics in children. In Fishman AP (ed): *Handbook of Physiology*, Section 3: The Respiratory System. American Physiological Society, Bethesda, MD, 1986.
13. Keens TG, Bryan AC, Levison H, et al. Developmental pattern of muscle fiber types in human ventilatory muscles. *J Appl Physiol* 44:909, 1978.
14. Cotton E, Yasuda K. Foreign body aspiration. *Pediatr Clin North Am* 31:937, 1984.
15. Bjorkander J, Bake B, Hanson L. Bronchitis in patients with hypogammaglobulinemia and other immunodeficiencies. *Eur J Respir Dis* 63 (Suppl 118):97, 1982.
16. Umetsu DT, Ambrosino DM, Quinti I, et al. Recurrent sinopulmonary infection and impaired antibody response to bacterial capsular polysaccharide antigen in children with IgG subclass deficiency. *N Engl J Med* 313:1247, 1985.
17. England SJ. Current techniques for assessing pulmonary function in the newborn and infant: Advantages and limitations. *Pediatr Pulmonol* 5:48, 1988.
18. Stocks J, Levy NM, Godfrey S. A new apparatus for the accurate measurement of airway resistance in infancy. *J Appl Physiol* 43:155, 1977.
19. Motoyama EK. Pulmonary mechanics during early postnatal years. *Pediatr Res* 11:220, 1977.
20. Adler S, Wohl ME. Flow-volume relationship at low lung volumes in healthy term newborns. *Pediatrics* 61:636, 1978.
21. Taussig LM, Landau LI, Godfrey S, Arad I. Determinants of forced expiratory flows in newborn infants. *J Appl Physiol* 53:1220, 1982.
22. Weiss KB, Wagener DK. Changing patterns of asthma mortality: Identifying target populations at risk. *JAMA* 264:1683, 1990.
23. Speight, ANP, Lee DA, Hey EN. Underdiagnosis and undertreatment of asthma in childhood. *Br Med J* 286:1253, 1983.
24. Clifford RD, Radford M, Howell JB, Holgate ST. Prevalence of respiratory symptoms among 7 and 11 year old school children and association with asthma. *Arch Dis Child* 64:1118, 1989.
25. Hill RA, Standen PJ, Tattersfield AE. Asthma, wheezing and school absence in primary schools. *Arch Dis Child* 64:246, 1989.
26. Storr J, Barrell E, Lenney W. Asthma in primary schools. *Br Med J* 295:251, 1987.
27. Gergen PJ, Weiss KG. Changing patterns of asthma hospitalization among children: 1979–1987, *JAMA* 264:1688, 1990.
28. Marion RJ, Creer TL, Reynolds RVC. Direct and indirect costs associated with childhood asthma. *Ann Allergy* 54:31, 1985.
29. Williams H, McNicol KN. Prevalence, natural history and relationship of wheeze, bronchitis and asthma in children: An epidemiologic study. *Br Med J* 4:321, 1969.

30. Dees SC. Asthma in infants and young children. *JAMA* 175:365, 1961.
31. Canny GJ, Reisman J, Healy R, et al. Acute asthma: Observations regarding the management of a pediatric emergency room. *Pediatrics* 83:507, 1989.
32. Selander P. Asthmatic symptoms in the first year of life. *Acta Pediatr* 49:265, 1960.
33. Mao Y. Canadian pediatric asthma: Morbidity, mortality and hospitalization data. In: *Treatment of Pediatric Asthma: A Canadian Concensus*. (MEDICINE Publishing Foundation Symposium. Series 29). MES Medical Education Services, Toronto, 1991, pp. 9–17.
34. Cutz E, Levison H, Cooper DM. Ultra structure in airways in children with asthma. *Histopathology* 2:407, 1978.
35. Lozewicz S, Wells C, Gomez E, et al. Morphological integrity of the bronchial epithelium in mild asthma. *Thorax* 45:12, 1990.
36. Clough JB, Williams JD, Holgate ST. Effect of atopy on the natural history of symptoms, peak expiratory flow, and bronchial responsiveness in 7- and 8-year old children with cough and wheeze. *Am Rev Respir Dis* 143:755, 1991.
37. Le Souef PN, Geelhoed GC, Turner DJ, Morgan SEG, Laundau LI. Response of normal infants to inhaled histamine. *Am Rev Respir Dis* 139:62, 1989.
38. Davis JB, Bulpitt, CJ. Atopy and wheeze in children according to parental atopy and family size. *Thorax* 36:185, 1981.
39. Horwood LJ, Ferguson DM, Hens BA, Shannon FT. Social and familial factors in the development of early childhood asthma. *Pediatrics* 75:859, 1985.
40. Hopp RJ, Bewtra AK, Nair N, Townley R. Bronchial reactivity patterns in nonasthmatic parents of patients. *Ann Allergy* 61:184, 1988.
41. Young S, Le Souef PN, Geelhoed G, et al. The influence of a family history of asthma and parental smoking on airway responsiveness in early infancy. *N Engl J Med* 324:1168, 1991.
42. Cookson WOCM, Sharp PA, Faux JA, Hopkin JM. Linkage between immunoglobulin E responses underlying asthma and rhinitis and chromosome 11q. *Lancet* 1:1292, 1989.
43. Sporik R, Holgate SJ, Platts-Mills TAE, Cogswell JJ. Exposure to house dust mite allergen (Der p1) and the development of asthma in childhood: A prospective study. *N Engl J Med* 323:502, 1990.
44. Busse WW. Respiratory infections: their role in airway responsiveness and the pathogenesis of asthma. *J Allergy Clin Immunol* 85:671, 1990.
45. Martinez FD, Morgan WJ, Wright AL, Holberg C, Taussig LM. Initial airway function is a risk factor for recurrent wheezing respiratory illnesses during the first 3 years of life. *Am Rev Respir Dis* 143:312, 1991.
46. Murray AB, Morrison BJ. The effect of cigarette smoke from the mother on bronchial responsiveness and severity of symptoms in children with asthma. *J Allergy Clin Immunol* 76:575, 1986.
47. Magnusson CG. Maternal smoking influences cord serum IgE and IgD levels and increases the risk for subsequent infant allergy. *J Allergy Clin Immunol* 78:898, 1986.
48. Murray AB, Morrison BJ. It is children with atopic determatitis who develop

asthma more frequently if the mother smokes. *J Allergy Clin Immunol* 86:732, 1990.

49. Reisman JJ, Canny GJ, Levison H. The approach to chronic cough in childhood. *Ann Allergy* 61:163, 1988.
50. Bousquet J. In vivo methods for study of allergy skin tests, technique and interpretation. In: Middleton E, Reed CE, et al. (eds), *Allergy, Principles and Practice*, 3rd ed. CV Mosby, St. Louis, 1988, pp. 419–436.
51. Platts-Mills TAE. Allergen avoidance at home: What really works? *J Respir Dis* 10:53, 1989.
52. Bock AL, Lee WY, Remingio LK, May CD. Studies of hypersensitivity reactions to foods in infants and children. *J Allergy Clin Immunol* 62:327, 1978.
53. O'Callaghan C, Milner AD, Swarbrick A. Spacer device with facemask attachment for giving bronchodilators to infants with asthma. *Br Med J* 198:160, 1989.
54. Bentur L, Kerem E, Canny GJ, et al. Response of acute asthma to beta 2 agonist in children less than than two years of age. *Ann Allergy* 65:122, 1990.
55. Bentur L, Canny, GJ, Shields MD, et al. A controlled trial of nebulized albuterol in children under the age of 2 years with acute asthma. *Pediatrics* 89(1):133, 1992.
56. Varsano I, Volovitz B, Malik H, Amir Y. Safety of 1 year of treatment with budesonide in young children with asthma. *J Allergy Clin Immunol* 85:914, 1990.
57. Denny FW, Collier AM, Henderson FW, et al. The epidemiology of bronchiolitis. *Pediatr Res* 11:235, 1977.
58. Wohl ME, Chernick V. Bronchiolitis. *Am Rev Respir Dis* 118:759, 1978.
59. Schuh S, Canny G, Reisman JJ, et al. Nebulized albuterol in acute bronchiolitis. *J Pediatr* 117:633, 1990.
60. Taber LH, Knight V, Gilbert BE, et al. Ribavirin aerosol treatment of bronchiolitis associated with respiratory syncytial virus infection in infants. *Pediatrics* 72:613, 1983.
61. Kim GI, Brummitt MW, Humphrey A, et al. Foreign body in the airway: A review of 202 cases. *Laryngoscope* 83:347, 1973.
62. Kerem E, Reisman J, Corey M, et al. Wheezing in cystic fibrosis patients: Clinical course, pulmonary function and survival analysis. *Pediatrics* (submitted for publication).
63. O'Brodovich HM, Mellins RB. Bronchopulmonary dysplasia. *Am Rev Respir Dis* 132:694, 1985.
64. Smyth JA, Tabachnik E, Duncan WJ, et al. Pulmonary function and bronchial hyperreactivity in long-term survivors of bronchopulmonary dysplasia. *Pediatrics* 68:336, 1981.
65. Keith HH. Vascular rings and tracheobronchial compression in infants. *Pediatr Ann* 6:8, 1977.
66. Moss AJ, McDonald LV. Cardiac disease in the wheezing child. *Chest* 71 (Suppl 2):187, 1977.

67. Snashall PD, Fan Chung K. Airway obstruction and bronchial hyperresponsiveness in left ventricular failure and mitral stenosis. *Am Rev Respir Dis* 144:945, 1991.
68. Eigen H. The clinical evaluation of chronic cough. *Pediatr Clin North Am* 29:67, 1982.
69. Filler RM, Simpson JS, Ein SH. Mediastinal masses in infants and children. *Pediatr Clin North Am* 26:677, 1979.
70. Holinger PH. Congenital anomalies of the tracheobronchial tree. *Postgrad Med* 36:454, 1964.

# 10

## Treatment of Wheezing Infants

**HERMAN J. NEIJENS and JOHAN C. DE JONGSTE**

*University Hospital Rotterdam/*
*Sophia Children's Hospital*
*Rotterdam, The Netherlands*

## STRATEGIES FOR TREATMENT

Asthma usually begins in the first years of life, and it is likely that the underlying pathophysiological processes in the airways have their origin in early childhood. Treatment in young children should be directed against the development of these processes. Over recent years a significant improvement occurred in our understanding of the pathophysiology of asthma. Our knowledge has grown about the regulation of cells that induce a variable but often persistent, inflammation. These cells and their mediators are able to induce changes in bronchial structures that are typical for asthma.

It has been shown that in patients with asthma endobronchial inflammation may be present even when asthmatic symptoms are mild or absent (1). Thus the activity of bronchial inflammation can only partly be assessed on the basis of symptoms and lung function variables.

Before asthmatic symptoms in young children have fully developed, it is conceivable that airway inflammation is built up gradually. However, hardly any information is available on the presence and development of this process in the first years of life.

These concepts have a number of consequences. Since airway inflammation persists when patients are free of symptoms, continuation of anti-inflammatory treatment may be indicated to prevent a recurrence of asthmatic attacks: a prophylactic approach. Markers of inflammation or cell activation obtained from bronchoalveolar lavage or blood may be a more reliable indication of the underlying disease activity than symptoms or lung function, and in the future may be used to guide therapy, as is already the case in liver and kidney diseases. However, this must be further studied before reliable markers can be used in the treatment of patients.

The drugs used in asthma therapy are classified into those with anti-inflammatory actions and bronchodilators. Anti-inflammatory action has the effect to turn down cell activation, and release of mediators and to allow the recovery of mucosal disruption, vascular leakage, and smooth muscle hypertrophy. These effects are found to be associated with a reduction in bronchial responsiveness. The clearest example of drugs with anti-inflammatory activity are corticosteroids, and probably disodium cromoglycate. The term *prophylactic therapy* is often used, but may produce confusion, since bronchodilators may also prevent symptoms but do not suppress bronchial inflammation and bronchial responsiveness.

Drugs with bronchodilating action are beta-agonists, anticholinergics, and theophylline. In the present concept of treatment, anti-inflammatory drugs are central and should be prescribed over long periods of time. Bronchodilating drugs are given additionally when bronchial obstruction is present. These drugs should be limited in their use to periods when obstruction is present.

Consensus discussions are currently being held worldwide (2–4). These aim to find an optimal and agreed scheme of the various drugs, alone or in combination, in relation to asthma symptoms and age of the patients.

These concepts may also indicate that an early start of anti-inflammatory treatment may be worthwhile, aimed at suppressing vicious circles in mechanisms from the very beginning. Some studies have even investigated the benefit of initiating therapy before symptoms occur, in children who have a high risk of asthma (5,6). Although these primary prevention studies produce remarkable indications that the occurrence of asthmatic symptoms can be influenced, additional studies are needed before an optimal approach can be established.

The objectives of treatment should be as few symptoms as possible, normal activities of daily life, undisturbed sleep, prevention of attacks, and little variability in airflow rates. Although reduction of bronchial hyperresponsiveness as a relevant aim in treatment is broadly accepted, it remains to be established.

The diagnosis of asthma may be difficult to determine in wheezy infants. Objective assessment of disease severity is a problem in young children, since lung function cannot be measured by standard techniques. If symptoms in a young child are suggestive of asthma, a trial of antiasthma medication is indicated and a prompt response may strongly support the presence of asthma.

Several causes different from asthma may be involved in the child who wheezes, although asthma is by far the most common cause. Alternative diagnoses should be considered and recognized in order to supply optimal treatment. Wheezing in infants has a number of possible causes. The most frequent ones are listed in Table 1. Signs in the medical history, recurrent infections, and poor response to asthma therapy are suggestive for a disease different from asthma. Once suspicion has been raised, appropriate diagnostic tests usually discover the abnormality.

## DRUGS USED TO TREAT INFANTILE ASTHMA

Inhaled therapy has advantages over oral therapy, but many young asthmatic patients receive oral treatment, since inhalation is often difficult in children under 5. The inhaled drugs usually administered in young children are listed in Table 2. It has been stated that infants under 1 year of age are poor responders to beta-agonists and anticholinergics (7,8). A therapeutic trial is currently the only way to identify responses to bronchodilators in an individual young child. When bronchodilators are regularly needed or attacks are not sufficiently suppressed, anti-inflammatory therapy is

TABLE 1 Possible Causes of Wheezing in Infants

| Cause | Signals | Analysis | Treatment |
|---|---|---|---|
| Asthma | Variable obstruction, hypersecretion | See this chapter | See this chapter |
| Viral bronchiolitis | Widespread crepitations, oxygen desaturation, prominent hyperinflation | (Rapid) RSV test | Oxygen<br>Ribavirin(?) |
| Gastric aspiration | Regurgitation, vomiting, nightly coughing, sometimes lung infections | X-ray esophagus, monitoring of esophageal pH | Semiupright position, solid food, prokinetic drug |
| Bronchopulmonary dysplasia | Preterm birth, oxygen and artificial ventilation, recurrent infections, "spells" | Chest x-ray | Oxygen, diuretics, corticosteroids, nebulized bronchodilators |
| Tracheal malacia | Inspiratory stridor (variable) | X-ray trachea, flexible bronchoscopy | In several cases: aortopexy |
| Anatomical abnormalities: lung (cysts, stenosis etc.) heart (L → R shunt large right atrium) | (variable) persistent obstruction, tachypnea, recurrent infections | Bronchoscopy, chest x-ray, CT/MRI scan, echocardiography, angiography, (as appropriate) | Surgical |
| Foreign body | Sudden onset, coughing, dyspnea, signs of infection | During in-/expiration, chest x-ray | Removal, rigid bronchoscopy |

TABLE 2 Bronchodilators

| Drug | Route | Dosage |
|---|---|---|
| *Beta-2-sympathicomimetics* | | |
| Salbutamol | Oral | 0.1 mg/kg, 3 times daily |
| | Metered-dose inhaler<br>Powder device | 0.1–0.4 mg, up to 8 times daily |
| | Nebulizer | 0.5–2.0 mg, up to 8 times daily |
| | Parenteral | s.c./i.m. 0.01 mg/kg<br>i.v. loading 0.005–0.01 mg/kg<br>maintenance 0.001–0.002 mg/kg/min<br>under monitoring (pulse, blood pressure) |
| Terbutaline | Oral | 0.075 mg/kg, 3 times daily |
| | Metered-dose inhaler<br>Powder device<br>(Turbuhaler) | 0.25–0.5 mg, up to 8 times daily |
| | Nebulizer | |
| | Parenteral | s.c./i.m. 0.01 mg/kg;<br>i.v. under monitoring |
| Fenoterol | Oral | 0.075 mg/kg dose, 3 dd |
| | Metered-dose inhaler<br>Powder device | 0.2–0.4 mg, up to 8 dd |
| | Nebulizer | up to 8 dd |
| Anticholinergics | | |
| Deptropine | Oral | 0.02–0.03 mg/kg, 3 times daily |
| Thiazinamium | Oral | 7 mg/kg, 3 times daily |
| | Parenteral | 0.7–1 mg/kg i.m. |
| Ipratropium bromide | Metered-dose inhaler | 0.02–0.04 mg, 1–8 times daily |
| | Nebulizer | 0.250 mg/ml, 1–4 times daily |

s.c., subcutaneously; i.m., intramuscularly; i.v., intravenously.

indicated. A proper choice of inhalation device is essential and will be discussed separately.

### Beta-Agonists

Beta-agonists are generally considered as the first choice of drugs to treat bronchial obstruction. Oral beta-agonists often have side effects, such as tremor and tachycardia. This therapy is sometimes adequate for children who wheeze incidentally, and may be given for practical reasons. However, when the response/side effects ratio is unfavorable and adequate bronchodilatation cannot be achieved, inhalation therapy provides a more satisfactory alternative with rapid relief of airway obstruction.

### Anticholinergics

Anticholinergics, administered either orally or by inhalation, often give relatively effective bronchodilation in young asthmatic children, with very few side effects. The oral preparations detropine and thiazinamium are licensed only in a limited number of countries; these are often effective in wheezy infants. However, few or no reliable controlled data are available on these drugs in young children.

A relatively large proportion of wheezy children respond to nebulized ipratropium bromide with clinical and lung function improvements (7,8). Ipratropium bromide is therefore worth trying in young children alone or in combination with a beta agonist. Ipratropium bromide can only be given by inhalation.

### Theophylline

Good evidence is available that preschool asthmatic children respond well to theophylline. Theophylline is probably mainly effective as a bronchodilator. Although additional effects such as inhibition of mediator release have been claimed, their contribution to the in vivo effect is unclear. Theophylline has a high incidence of side effects, such as tachycardia, decreased appetite, behavioral changes, and insomnia. Dangerous complications such as seizures may easily be induced from modest overdosage.

The introduction of slow-release preparations has diminished the short-term variability of theophylline serum concentrations. Theophylline can be prescribed as slow-release minipellets in capsules or in low-dosage tablets; both are convenient for young children and minipellets can be taken by babies. Slow-release preparations are especially appropriate for children who have nocturnal or early morning symptoms. However, since such symptoms may indicate poor asthma control, appropriate anti-inflammatory treatment should be considered seriously.

The metabolism of theophylline changes during the first years of life. For infants older than 6 months of age, the average dosage of theophylline required to obtain therapeutic blood levels decreases from 25 to 20 mg/kg/day from baby to toddlerhood (9). Since metabolism may vary between and within patients, it is important to monitor theophylline blood levels to obtain optimal dosing, which can be done in ambulatory patients using a dried blood spot test (10).

### Disodium Cromoglycate

Disodium cromoglycate (DSCG) inhibits the early and late asthmatic response after the inhalation of allergen dose-dependently, and prevents allergen-induced increase in bronchial hyperresponsiveness (BHR) (11). DSCG reduces bronchoconstriction due to exercise (12), to cold air (13), fog (14), and sulfur dioxide (15). Long-term treatment with DSCG may decrease BHR, but its main potency is probably to protect against a seasonal rise in BHR after challenge, such may occur during the pollen season (16).

DSCG reduces the symptoms of asthma in young children when supplied on a long-term basis. Both the efficacy and safety of DSCG have been demonstrated in children from 2 years, while data on children under 2 are limited (17–19).

Thus, it is certainly worthwhile to treat young children with frequent symptoms not easily controlled by bronchodilators on demand using DSCG for several months to assess its value. In children under 1 difficulties in administration and the usually poor results do not justify its use as a first-line drug (17).

### Inhaled Corticosteroids

The main action of corticosteroids in the treatment of asthma is considered to be suppression of the inflammatory response. Corticosteroids reduce the recruitment of leukocytes such as eosinophils and neutrophils to inflammatory sites, modulate the spectrum of mediators by direct effects upon eosinophils, T lymphocytes, macrophages, and endothelial cells, and inhibit local proliferation of mast cells (20). Furthermore, corticosteroids potentiate the beta-2-adrenoreceptor effects of catecholamines on airway smooth muscle (21), although the clinical relevance is not sure. Long-term treatment with inhaled corticosteroids significantly reduces airway inflammation and epithelial damage, as has been shown in adult patients with asthma (22).

Pretreatment with inhaled corticosteroids decreases or abolishes the late reaction after allergen challenge. The protective effect on early allergic responses and exercise-induced bronchoconstriction can be demonstrated after several weeks of therapy. Inhaled corticosteroids are the most potent reducers of BHR, but do not bring BHR into the normal range in most patients (23). This effect needs a relatively long period of treatment. After 6 months a substantial decrease in BHR can mostly be observed, although a further reduction continues to develop over the course of several years.

The main limiting factor to more general use in childhood asthma, in particular in infants, has been the worry about side effects, which so far have proved potential rather than actual. Although inhaled corticosteroids may lead to a slight dose-dependent reduction of baseline adrenal cortisol production, the clinical significance is far from clear. Some observations suggest that growth inhibition may occur using normal dosages in young children (24). Most long-term follow-up studies, however, have shown normal growth even with relative high dosages (25). More information is needed about the efficacy and side effects of inhaled corticosteroids in infants. New inhaled corticosteroids with an improved effect/side effect ratio are being introduced, which might be important, especially for infants.

Although inhaled corticosteroids are often very effective in controlling asthma, their value in infants is not extensively studied. Beclomethasone dipropionate demonstrated good efficacy in children between 1 and 5 years of age treated for at least 1 year (26). Administration to infants may be possible by a nebulizer solution, which is available in some countries.

### Ketotifen and Antihistamines

Ketotifen has been found by some studies (27) to reduce symptoms and the need for comedication in young children when supplied for several months in an adequate dosage. However, some other studies have reported negative results (28). An important condition for efficacy seems a treatment period of at least 12 weeks.

Ketotifen has strong antihistamine-1 activity with some anti-inflammatory effects in vitro and in animal experiments. The drug has no bronchodilating effect and no reduction in bronchial responsiveness could be shown (29). Several other antihistamines have claimed to have a comparable mode of action and efficacy, such as astemizole, terfenadine, and cetirizine, but have not been studied sufficiently in childhood asthma.

## MAINTENANCE THERAPY

Increasing emphasis is being laid on the importance of long-term suppression of inflammatory processes by maintenance therapy. The present consensus reports (2–4) state that prophylactic treatment should be started in patients who have moderate to severe asthma. A stepwise medication plan has been proposed by most consensus reports. Decisions can be based on efficacy, risk of side effects and applicability. The guideline of the Dutch consensus report is reported below (3).

In young children a trial of ketotifen (Zaditen) may be conducted to assess its effects, which often needs a period of at least 3 months. The advantages of ketotifen in young children are its oral administration and multiorgan effectivity (i.e., nose, skin). To avoid sedation, the daily dose may be divided in a skewed manner, for instance, 25% as the morning dose and 75% as the evening dose.

The next step in prophylactic treatment is DSCG (Intal, Lomudal). DSCG is used in young children if ketotifen has not been proved or is not considered useful and as first-line drug in many children above 4 years of age. The inhaled route is the only mode of administration, which necessitates its use as an aerosol with spacer device or a nebulizer compressor system. It often takes at least 3 weeks or more to assess the response.

If these drugs are not able to induce adequate control of symptoms, inhaled corticosteroids are certainly indicated. There has been a trend to use this drug in increasing numbers of young children over the last few years. However, more information is needed about their merits and risks in young children before inhaled corticosteroids can be advocated as first-line maintenance treatment.

## ACUTE ASTHMA

Acute dyspnea is most frequently caused by asthma, although other conditions may need to be considered, especially in infants. Information that can have relevance for therapy includes the trigger responsible for the attack, how the child has responded to therapy in previous attacks, what regular therapy the child is receiving, what additional therapy already has been given and its effects. Signs of severity should be carefully determined to allow one to choose adequate treatment:

Heart and respiratory rate
Quality of chest auscultatory findings (diminished air entry?)
Retractions
Flaring
Pulsus paradoxus
Pallor or cyanosis (sometimes difficult to detect in artificial light)
Anxiety
Restlessness

Tiredness
Exhaustion
Unconsciousness (in severe situations)

Blood gases should be measured when the attack is accompanied by one or more signs of severity. Repeated blood gas measurements can provide information on the progress of the asthma attack. Oxygen saturation followed continuously by transcutaneous oximetry has been found very useful to assess the severity of the attack, the need for and flow of oxygen supplementation, as well as the effect of antiasthma therapy.

Lung function values produce an objective measurement to assess the degree of bronchial obstruction, but cannot be registered by the standard techniques in infants. Peak flow measurements are often possible from the age of 5–6 years onwards, but measurements during acute asthma attacks are often not feasible.

Drug therapy in the case of an exacerbation can be chosen stepwise, depending on the severity, previous response to therapy, and the age of the child (Fig. 1). The initial treatment is to provide an inhaled bronchodilator. Beta-agonists are usually the first choice, although in infants anticholinergics may be even more powerful to relieve bronchial obstruction and mucus production. One or both should be tried. Whenever the effect is not sufficient, the combination of a beta-agonist plus an anticholinergic is often useful. The combination is somewhat more effective than a standard dose of either (8).

In case of difficulties with inhaling, as is often the case in young children, or with a severe attack, the deposition can be improved by using an appropriate spacer device. A nebulizer/compressor system is even more effective. Since oxygen saturation in infants with an asthmatic attack is often decreased, and may further diminish after administration of a bronchodilator, aerosols should preferably be generated with oxygen-enriched air.

Inhaled bronchodilators should be given. Even if the child has received this form of treatment before coming to the hospital, cumulative dose is often useful and safe under well-controlled conditions. Careful observation for side effects is necessary. Five to 10 min after completion of the inhalation, the degree of airway obstruction should be reassessed.

Several lines of action may then emerge. When the child improves dramatically, he or she should be observed for some time. If improvement is maintained, the child can return home. Necessary instructions should be given for adaptations in therapy, for instance, frequent inhalations of bronchodilators (every 3–4 hr) or the start of additional therapy, such as theophylline or a short course of oral prednisone.

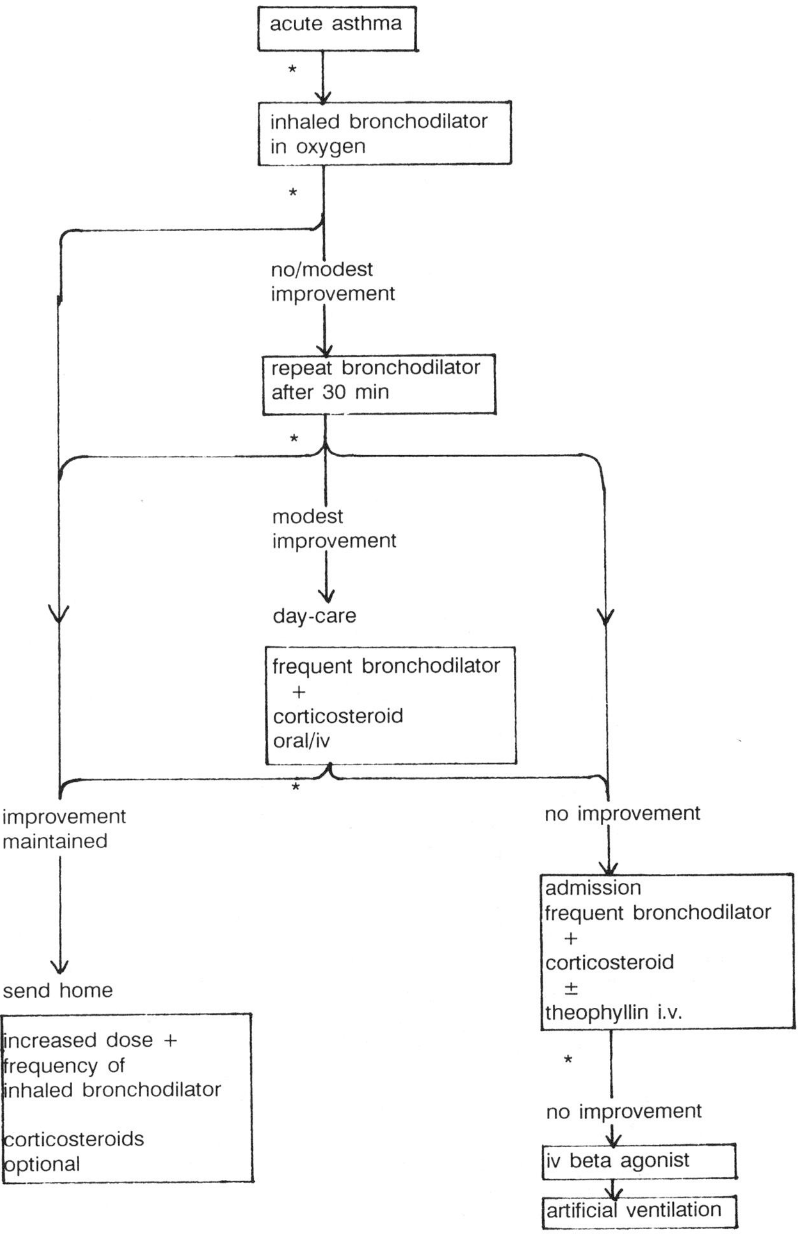


FIGURE 1 Management of asthmatic attacks. * = Assessment of severity, including oximetry. Oxygen should be given to maintain $SaO_2 > 90\%$.

When the child shows improvement but continues to have signs of obstruction or desaturation, a second inhalation of a bronchodilator after 30 min should be given. Usually the child needs to be further controlled (for instance, in the ambulatory department or on the ward) and will require frequent inhalations (every 2–4 hr), if necessary, combined with systemic corticosteroids and possibly other treatment (oxygen, theophylline).

When the child has no response to nebulized bronchodilators, he or she should be hospitalized and given systemic corticosteroids and intravenous theophylline and, if necessary, an intravenous beta-2-mimetic. Monitoring of transcutaneous oxygen saturation and heart rate are mandatory under those conditions.

The dosage of systemic corticosteroids in the case of severe attacks should be equivalent to 1–2 mg prednisolone/kg/day; the dosage of intravenous hydrocortisone is 10–20 mg/kg/day. An initial bolus dosage of 1–2 mg/kg of prednisolone is recommended.

In severe attacks, intravenous theophylline treatment can be initiated by a loading dose of 5 mg/kg, injected during at least 20 min, for those not receiving oral theophylline. When the child is receiving regular theophylline therapy, half of the loading dose can usually be given. After loading, the child should receive a continuous infusion of 0.9 mg/kg/hr, preferably monitored by serum theophylline measurements.

Many young children in respiratory difficulty will need oxygen. The need for oxygen should be carefully considered and oxygen supplied, preferably monitored by measurement of blood gasses and transcutaneous oxygen monitoring. There is no risk of respiratory depression due to oxygen treatment in acute asthma in children.

Sedatives have no place in the management of acute severe asthma because they have the risk of depressing the child and may complicate clinical decisions.

## INHALATION SYSTEMS

Correct inhalation using metered-dose inhalers is difficult or impossible for children under 5–6 years of age. In young children, a dry powder system is therefore preferable. As an alternative, spacer devices, such as an Aerochamber, Nebuhaler or Volumatic, can be used by children as young as 3 years of age, who can be encouraged to pant in and out through the one-way valve system. Below that age most of the children do not generate enough negative inspiratory pressure to open the valve. An open system may be applicable in even younger children. A coffee-cup method has been proposed, which seems to be suitable for most children over the age of 2 years. Other comparable open systems may be used as well (Fig. 2).

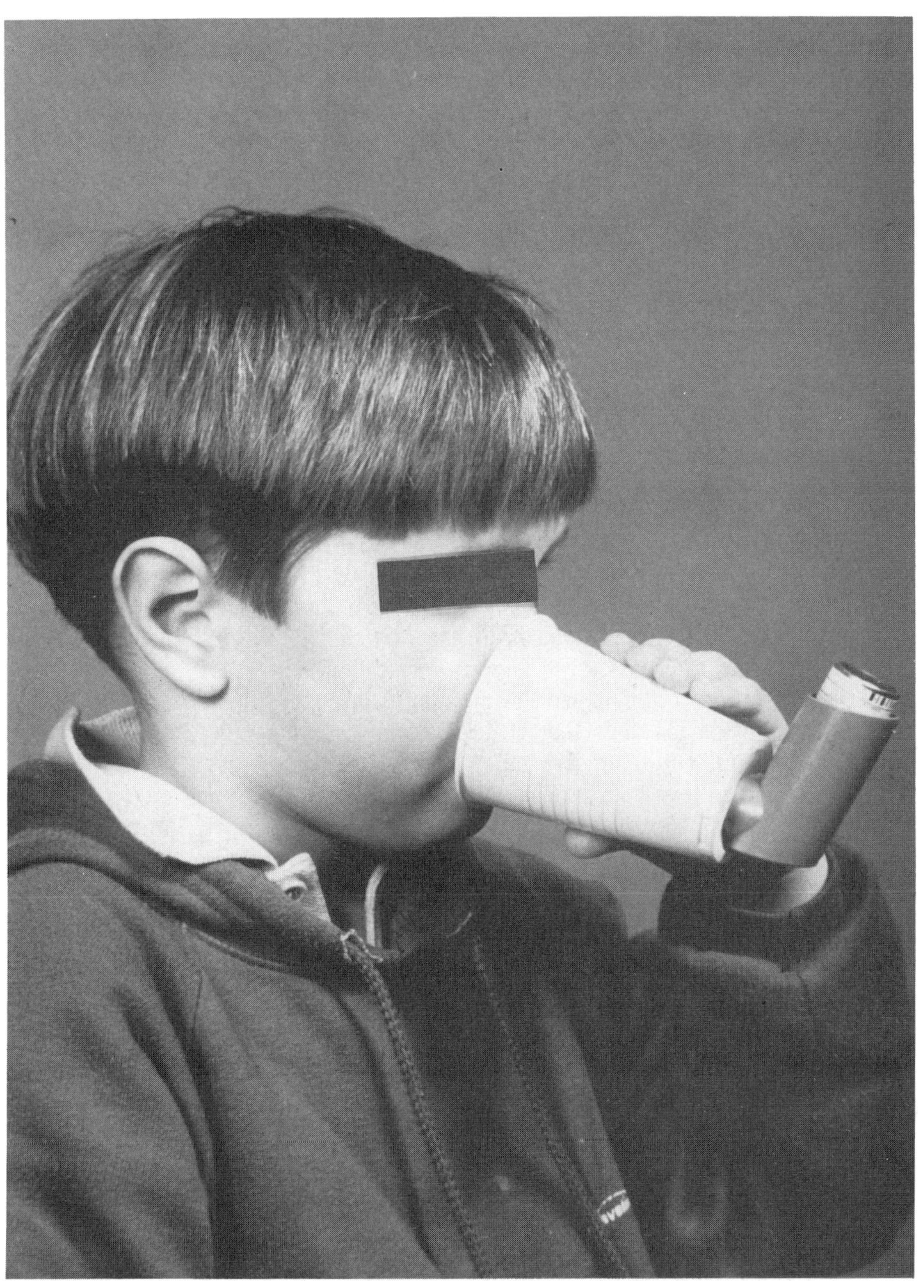

FIGURE 2 Open inhalation system for use with children.

These systems also provide a useful back-up for times when those normally able to use powder delivery systems have such severe airways obstruction that they are unable to generate adequate inspiratory flow rates. Nebulizers that produce aerosols with sufficiently small particles provide the most effective technique for delivery of aerosol to the lower airways. It may be the preferred method for very young children and patients with severe asthma.

## ADDITIONAL THERAPY

Antibiotics are indicated only in a minority of young children with asthma. Antibiotic treatment has to be considered only if a bacterial infection seems to be present. Recognition of a bacterial infection in relation to symptoms of asthma is often not easy. Although green sputum may indicate a bacterial infection, this sign is often not obvious in young children, since they tend to swallow their sputum directly after coughing. Hence, recognition of bacterial infection from sputum by straining or culture is often not available. Nose or pharyngeal swabs are not reliable.

Appropriate antibiotics are amoxycillin, cotrimoxazol, or a cephalosporin, since pneumococci, *Haemophilus influenzae*, or streptococci are usually responsible for respiratory infections in children.

Some asthmatic children often have bacterial respiratory infections. The explanation for repeated bacterial invasions is uncertain, but bronchial obstruction and compromised mucociliary clearance probably are important. Subnormal levels of serum IgG subclasses or low specific concentrations of antibody to *Haemophilus influenzae*, pneumococci, and possibly other microorganisms may explain the increased infection risk in these patients (30).

Viral respiratory infections are probably the most frequent cause of recurrent wheezing episodes, particularly in the infant. Antiviral treatment, although potentially important for asthmatic subjects, is presently not available to some extent. Ribavirin has been proposed for the treatment of respiratory syncytial virus (RSV) bronchiolitis in children who have an increased risk (31), but its value is not yet established by enough controlled studies.

## PHYSIOTHERAPY

Physiotherapy in children with asthma stimulates expectoration of sputum from the central airways and optimal use of respiratory muscles. In general, the contribution of physiotherapy has been difficult to prove.

Techniques to enhance sputum expectoration may be of value when sputum accumulates and hampers ventilation. This is, however, hardly the case in childhood asthma. It should optimally be preceded by nebulized bronchodilator drugs and saline to facilitate mobilization of sputum plugs. Vibration or clapping on the chest wall is traditionally applied and should mobilize sputum from the airway walls. It is, however, highly unlikely that this has any effect and cannot be recommended in the treatment of childhood asthma. Training in optimal respiratory maneuvers usually cannot be initiated before the age of 4.

## GASTROESOPHAGEAL REFLUX

Gastroesophageal reflux may provoke asthmatic symptoms and also recurrent respiratory infections, although this latter complication seems far less frequent. The presence of reflux should be considered in young asthmatic children with recurrent vomiting or regurgitation, acute nocturnal episodes of cough and wheezing, insufficient response to adequate asthma therapy, repeated pulmonary infiltrates, or failure to thrive.

The precise contributing role of reflux in respiratory symptoms is often difficult to determine, but it seems wise to treat reflux to observe its effect on asthmatic phenomena. The presence of asthma may potentially facilitate reflux by forced coughing, inducing high abdominal pressure, as well as by theophylline, which may relax the lower esophageal sphincter.

The monitoring of esophageal pH for 24 hr is generally considered to be the best way to diagnose the presence and degree of reflux. X-ray examination of the esophagus is often used as a screening method to detect reflux and to investigate the presence of anatomical malformations. Endoscopy and eosophageal biopsy can confirm these abnormalities more precisely. Milk scans have the option to detect reflux, as well as lung aspiration, but their reliability is limited.

Treatment by a (semi) upright position, solid food, and prokinetic drugs (Domperinome, cisapride) is often applied to diminish reflux. An $H_2$ blocker or antacidic compounds may be given for protection against acid fluid. Surgical procedures are confined to the treatment of refractory and severe reflux or anatomical abnormalities.

## AVOIDANCE OF ALLERGENS AND POLLUTANTS

One of the important risk factors for childhood asthma is allergen exposure. The type of allergen, the dose, and the age at first exposure all appear to be important, and it seems that the first 6 months of life are particularly important for sensitization (32–34). There is obviously a genetic factor, which may be associated with a gene on chromosome 11g (35), but environmental factors are found to have a role as well (36).

A very low exposure to allergens during the period of development of IgE antibodies may lead to diminished primary sensitization. This requires a careful avoidance of allergens for at least 6 months, which is difficult to perform in an optimal manner. Not enough evidence has been found to support of this approach.

Secondary allergen avoidance tries to prevent contact with relevant allergens once the patient has been sensitized and may react. Allergen avoidance studies have been variable in their success (37). This may partly be explained by the various opinions about the threshold levels of antigen exposure in susceptible subjects leading to sensitization. Platts-Mills and De Weck (38) proposed 2μm house dust mite antigen (Der p1) per g as a risk factor for mite allergen. Price et al. (39) found 0.5 μg Der p1/g dust relevant in this respect. The last group showed that measurement of antigen levels in carpets is not a good indicator of inhaled antigen, but airborne levels as measured by a sampler are more relevant. The level of airborne Der p1 was significantly higher above wool carpets than above synthetic ones or hard floors.

Murray and Fergusson (40) conducted an extremely thorough allergen avoidance trial that involved several procedures (removing all feather bedding, vacuuming procedures, removal of carpet and clothes from the child's bedroom, and removal of any other "mite-carrying" materials) and found a pronounced difference in wheezing and medication between the control and study group. It seems worthwhile to reduce house dust to a minimum, particularly in the bedroom. Measures that aim to reduce the house dust mite include replacing feather pillows and mattresses and woolen blankets by synthetic ones that can be washed frequently, placing an impermeable sheet between the undersheet and the mattress to prevent distribution of mites, removing woolen carpets, and cleaning the rooms frequently.

Children whose parents smoke, and in particular mothers who smoke, have a higher frequency of respiratory illness (41). The effect of passive smoking may be even more important in the prenatal period when the influence may affect immunologic functions (IgE increase) and perhaps lung growth (42).

Reduced ventilation leading to increased condensation and a damp home may cause greater mold colonization, associated with an increase in respiratory symptoms and an increased frequency of allergy (43,44).

Air pollution and smoking may contribute to the generation of bronchial inflammation, as well as sensitization to allergens, although their quantitative roles are far from clear. Parents of "at risk" babies should be warned of the effect of cigarette smoke and indoor pollution, and as informed about allergen avoidance.

## SUMMARY

Infants with asthma can present a very challenging problem to physicians. The disease is probably often underestimated. Proper recognition and evaluation should be the basis of adequate therapy, based on the present concepts of pathophysiology.

The therapeutic option is to control the symptoms, as well as the underlying airway inflammation to diminish the risk of symptoms. Treatment schedules in infants for maintenance therapy and for acute attacks are proposed and discussed. The relevance of additional therapeutic measures (oxygen, inhalant systems, physiotherapy, role of reflux, avoidance of allergens and pollutants) is considered.

## REFERENCES

1. Laitinen LA, Laitinen A. Mucosal inflammation and bronchial hyperreactivity. *Eur Respir J* 1:476–491, 1988.
2. Warner JO, Götz M, Landau LI, Levison H, Milner AD, Pederson S, Silverman M. Management of asthma: a consensus statement. *Arch Dis Child* 64:1065–79, 1989.
3. Van der Laag J, van Aalderen WMC, Duiverman EJ, Nagelkerke AF, van Essen-Zandvliet EEM, van Nierop JC. Astma bij kinderen consensus over lange termijn behandeling. *Dutch J Med* 135:2316–2323, 1991.
4. Warner JO, Neijens HJ, et al. Asthma: a follow-up statement from an international pediatric asthma consensus group. *Arch Dis Child*, in press.
5. Nogawa T, Shinohara D, Tagachi N, Takeuchi Y, Abe T, et al. Long-term treatment with ketotifen in infants with bronchiolitis and recurrent wheezy infants. *Shonika-Shinzyo* 50:2611–14, 1987.
6. Ikura Y, Naspitz CK, Mikawa H, Talaricofich S, Baba M, Sole D, Nishima S. Prevention of asthma by ketotifen in infants with atopic dermatitis. *Ann Allergy* 68:233–236, 1992.
7. Henry RL, Hiller EJ, Milner AD, Hodges IGC, Stokes GM. Nebulized ipratropium bromide and sodium cromoglycate in the first two years of life. *Arch Dis Child* 59:54–57, 1984.
8. Silverman M. The role of anticholinergic antimuscarinic bronchodilator therapy in children. *Lung* Suppl 304–309, 1990.
9. Neijens HJ, Duiverman EJ, Graatsma BH, Kerrebijn KF. Clinical and bronchodilating efficacy of controlled-release theophylline as a function of its serum concentrations in preschool children. *J Pediatr* 107:811–815, 1985.
10. Rattenburg JM, Tsanakas J. Acceptance of domiciliary theophylline monitoring using dried blood spots. *Arch Dis Child* 63:1449–52, 1988.
11. Mattoli S, Foresi A, Corbo GM, Valente S, Ciappi G. Effects of two doses

of cromolyn on allergen-induced late asthmatic response and increased responsiveness. *J Allergy Clin Immunol* 97:747–754, 1987.
12. Neijens HJ, Wesselius T, Kerrebijn KF. Exercise-induced bronchoconstriction as an expression of bronchial hyperreactivity. A study of its mechanisms in children. *Thorax* 517–522, 1981.
13. Murphy S. Cromolyn sodium. In: Jenne JW, Murphy S (eds.), *Drug Therapy for Asthma. Lung Biology in Health and Disease*, vol. 31. Marcel Dekker, New York/Basel, pp. 688–690.
14. Fuller RW, Collier JG. Sodium cromoglycate and atropine block the fall in $FEV_1$ but not the cough induced by hypotonic mist. *Thorax* 39:766–770, 1984.
15. Sheppard D, Nadel JA, Boushey HA. Inhibition of supher dioxide-induced bronchoconstriction by disodium cromoglycate in asthmatic subjects. *Am Rev Respir Dis* 124:257–259, 1981.
16. Van Essen-Zandvliet EEM, Kerrebijn KF. The effect of anti-asthma drugs on bronchial hyperresponsiveness. *Immunol Allergy Clin North Am* 10 (3):483–501, 1990.
17. Geller-Bernstein C, Levin S. Nebulized sodium cromoglycate in the treatment of wheezy bronchitis in infants and young children. *Respiration* 71:13–18, 1982.
18. Church MK, Warner JO. Sodium cromoglycate and related drugs. *Clin Allergy* 15:311–320, 1985.
19. Newth CJL, Newth CV, Turner JAP. Comparison of nebulized sodium cromoglycate and oral theophyllin in controlling symptoms in chronic asthma in pre-school children. A double blind study. *Aust NZ J Med* 12:232, 1982.
20. Schleimer RP. Effects of glucocorticosteroids on inflammatory cells relevant to their therapeutic applications in asthma. *Am Rev Respir Dis* 1991.
21. Shensfield GM, Hodson ME, Clark SW, Paterson JW. Interaction of corticosteroids and cathecholamines in the treatment of asthma. *Thorax* 30:430–435, 1975.
22. Lundgren R, Söderberg M, Horstedt P, Stenling R. Morphological studies of bronchial mucosal biopsies from asthmatics before and after ten years of treatment with inhaled steroids. *Eur Respir J* 1:883–889, 1988.
23. Kerrebijn KF, van Essen-Zandvliet EEM, Neijens HJ. Effect of long-term treatment with inhaled corticosteroids and beta-agonists on the bronchial responsiveness in children with asthma. *J Allergy Clin Immunol* 79:653–9, 1987.
24. McKenzie CA. Growth in asthmatic children clinical experience with inhaled fluticasone proprionate. *Proc ERS (Brussels)* 4045, 1991.
25. Selroos O. The effects of inhaled corticosteroids on the natural history of obstructive lung disease. *Eur Respir Dis* 1:354–365, 1991.
26. Freigant B. Long-term follow-up of infants and children treatment with beclomethasone aerosol by a special inhalation device. *Ann Allergy* 45:13, 1980.
27. Neijens HJ, Knol K. Oral prophylactic treatment in wheezy infants. *J Allergy Clin Prac* 1:17–23, 1988.
28. Loftus BG, Price JF. Long-term, placebo controlled trial of ketotifen in the management of preschool children with asthma. *J Allergy Clin Immunol* 79:350–5, 1987.

29. Tinkelman DG, Moss BA, Bukantz SC, Scheffer AL, Dobken JH, Chodosh S, Cohen BM, Rosenthal RR, Rappaport I, Buckley CE, Chusid EL, Deutsch AJ, Settipane GA, Burns RBP. A multicenter trial of the prophylactic effect of ketotifen, theophylline, and placebo in atopic asthma. *J Allergy Clin Immunol* 76:487–97, 1985.
30. Page R, Friday G, Stillwagon P, Skoner D, Caliquiri L, Fireman P. Asthma and selective immunoglobulin subclass deficiency: improvement of asthma after immunoglobulin replacement therapy. *J Pediatr* 112:127–31, 1988.
31. Smith D, Frankel LR, Mathers LH, Tang ATS, Arigno RC, Prober CG. A controlled trial of aerosolised ribavirin in infants receiving mechanical ventilation for severe respiratory syncytial virus infection. *N Engl J Med* 325:24–9, 1991.
32. Kjellman NM, Croner S. Cord blood IgE determination for allergy prediction—a follow-up to seven years of age in 165 children. *Ann Allergy* 53:167–71, 1984.
33. Lau S, Falkenhorst G, Weber A, et al. High mite-allergen exposure increases the risk of sensitization in atopic children and young adults. *J Allergy Clin Immunol* 84:718–25, 1989.
34. Sporik R, Holgate ST, Platts-Mills TAE, et al. Exposure to house-dust mite allergen (Der p1) and the development of asthma in childhood. A prospective study. *N Engl J Med* 323: 502–7, 1990.
35. Cookson WOCM, Faux JA, Sharp PA, Hopkin JM. Linkage between immunoglobulin E responses underlying asthma and rhinitis and chromosome 11q. *Lancet* 1:1292–4, 1989.
36. Schwartz J, Gold D, Dockery DW, Weiss ST, Speizer FE. Predictors of asthma and persistent wheeze in a national sample of children in the United States. *Am Rev Respir Dis* 142:555–562, 1990.
37. Warner JA, Warner JO. Allergen avoidance in childhood asthma. *Respir Med* 85:101–105, 1991.
38. Platts-Mills TAE, de Weck AL. House mite allergens and asthma. A worldwide problem. *J Allergy Clin Immunol* 83:416–427, 1989.
39. Price JA, Pollock I, Little SA, Longbottom JL, Warner JO. Measurement of air-borne mite antigen in the homes of asthmatic children. *Lancet* 336:895–897, 1990.
40. Murray AB, Ferguson AC. Dust-free bedrooms in the treatment of asthmatic children with house dust mite allergy: a controlled study. *Pediatrics* 7:418–422, 1983.
41. Holt PG, Turner KJ. Respiratory symptoms in the children of smokers: an overview. *Eur J Respir Dis* 65 suppl 133:109–120, 1984.
42. Tayler B, Wadsworth J. Maternal smoking during pregnancy and lower respiratory tract illness in early life. *Arch Dis Child* 62:76–79, 1987.
43. Waegemaekers M, van Wageningen N, Brunekreef B, Boley JSM. Respiratory symptoms in damp homes. *Allergy* 44:192–198, 1989.
44. Dijkstra L, Houthuys D, Brunekreef B, Akkerman I, Boley JSM. Respiratory healthy effects of the indoor environment in a population of Dutch children. *Am Rev Respir Dis* 142:1172–1178, 1990.

# 11

# Evaluation of the Child with Chronic Cough and/or Wheezing

**FRANK S. VIRANT and GAIL G. SHAPIRO**

*University of Washington School of Medicine*
*Seattle, Washington*

Asthma is a pulmonary disorder characterized by reversible airway obstruction and bronchial hyperresponsiveness. Asthma typically appears clinically as wheezing, a high-pitched expiratory sound generated by turbulent airflow, and cough. Although some wheezing is common, pediatric asthma may occur with cough as the sole presenting feature (1,2). Often these children will have a history of frequent colds that "settle in the chest," chronic bronchitis, or "recurrent pneumonia" (3). Careful scrutiny of such cases often reveals a lack of objective measurement of pulmonary function. As a result, asthma is frequently misdiagnosed and undertreated, leading to needless acute and chronic morbidity (4).

Childhood asthma exists as a spectrum of disease states. At one end is the child with overlooked "silent asthma" who never wheezes, and yet never has normal lung function. At the other end is the easily recognized child with severe asthma who constantly wheezes to a greater or lesser degree. In between are children who obviously have acute episodes of asthma from three to six times per year. Some children in this group have no obvious functional impairment between episodes, while others may demonstrate some residual airway obstruction or subtle symptoms. In a given patient, documenting the pattern of chronic asthma has important implications for the type and duration of therapy. For example, the patient with intermittent episodes frequently will do well with a bronchodilator as needed. However, when abnormal lung function is present between episodes, regular therapy designed to decrease bronchial hyperresponsiveness, for example, cromolyn sodium or corticosteroids, is crucial for adequate disease control (5–8).

When presented with a child who has chronic cough and/or wheezing, pulmonary function testing should be performed if the patient can cooperate. Frequently, abnormal air flows will confirm the diagnosis of asthma. Although normal airflow measurements do not exclude the diagnosis of asthma, they would heighten suspicion of other respiratory, cardiovascular, or central nervous system disorders as a source for the observed symptoms.

## DIFFERENTIAL DIAGNOSIS

Although most children with recurrent episodes of coughing and wheezing do have asthma, a number of other conditions must be considered (see Table 1). In the absence of associated airway infection, the appearance of symptoms early in life should raise concern about congenital problems such as laryngomalacia, tracheomalacia, laryngeal webs, tracheoesophageal fistula, tracheostenosis, bronchiostenosis, and vascular rings (surrounding the airway) (9). Foreign body aspiration must be considered when the onset of symptoms is abrupt, particularly in the child below 2 years of age (10). When this diagnosis is suspected, an expiratory chest radiograph will often

TABLE 1 Differential Diagnosis of Cough and/or Wheezing during Childhood

| |
|---|
| Upper respiratory tract |
| Foreign body |
| Mucus in the nose creating "wheeze" |
| Middle respiratory tract |
| Epiglottitis |
| Foreign body |
| Laryngomalacia/tracheomalacia |
| Laryngotracheobronchitis |
| Laryngeal webs |
| Pertussis |
| Toxic inhalation (dust, gas, talc) |
| Tacheoesophageal fistula |
| Tracheostenosis/bronchiostenosis |
| Lower respiratory tract |
| $Alpha_1$-antritrypsin deficiency |
| Asthma |
| Bronchiectasis |
| Bronchiolitis |
| Bronchopulmonary dysplasia |
| Congenital anomalies |
| Cystic fibrosis |
| Foreign body |
| Gastroestophageal reflux |
| Hypersensitivity lung diseases (molds, fibers, etc.) |
| Pulmonary eosinophilia (Loeffler's syndrome) |
| Pulmonary hemosiderosis |
| Pulmonary interstitial emphysema |
| Toxic inhalation (dust, gas, fumes) |
| Tumor |
| Cardiovascular system |
| Mitral valve prolapse |
| Vascular rings (around airways) |
| Nervous system |
| Hyperventilation syndrome |
| Swallowing mechanism dysfunction (aspiration) |

*Source*: Adapted from Siegel SC, Katz RM, Rachelefsky GS. Asthma in infancy and childhood. In: Middleton E, Ellis E, Reed C (eds.), *Allergy Principles and Practice*, CV Mosby, St. Louis, 1983; and Ellis E. Asthma in infancy and childhood. In: Middleton E, Reed C, Ellis E (eds.), *Allergy Principles and Practice*, CV Mosby, St. Louis, 1988.

demonstrate obstruction of air flow from the lung on the affected side, manifest as hyperlucency or tracheal shift.

Bronchopulmonary dysplasia and pulmonary interstitial emphysema are frequently apparent radiographically, and should be suspected in a child born prematurely who has required prolonged ventilatory support. Cystic fibrosis should be excluded with a sweat test in older infants with recurrent sinopulmonary disease, failure to thrive, or nasal polyps.

Careful physical examination should demonstrate that obstruction is not coming from the upper airway, for example from nasal mucus or choanal atresia, or from the middle respiratory tract, as with epiglottitis or laryngotracheobronchitis. Bronchiectasis should be considered in the presence of focal lower respiratory tract obstruction, particularly in the setting of recurrent pneumonitis.

In the first year of life, the distinction between asthma and bronchiolitis may be subtle (11,12). Differentiation does not significantly affect therapy. In fact, the presence of significant chronic asthma may only be apparent as the child demonstrates recurrent cough or wheezing with subsequent infection (13). The two most common viral agents implicated in asthma initiation are respiratory syncytial virus (RSV) and parainfluenza virus (14,15).

When confronted with the coughing or wheezing child, a careful history will commonly reduce the differential diagnoses to only a few considerations. A subsequent directed physical examination will often clarify the clinical picture. Once the diagnosis of asthma is apparent, appropriate laboratory evaluation can document the degree of dysfunction, and elucidate the importance of amplifying factors, for example allergy and sinus disease, which will have profound implications for therapy.

## CLINICAL EVALUATION

### Presenting History

As suggested above, a comprehensive initial history frequently should suggest a limited group of diagnoses. For example, the appearance of symptoms shortly after birth greatly increases the likelihood of a congenital abnormality as a source for symptoms. The abrupt onset of cough or wheezing in a young child, particularly associated with eating and in the absence of a current airway infection, should be considered secondary to foreign body aspiration until proven otherwise. The probability of asthma as a source for chronic symptoms is increased in the presence of several risk factors, including onset of symptoms with viral airway infection (16,17), concomitant history of allergy (18,19), or a strong family history of asthma (20,21).

Most often, asthma *will* be the source of chronic cough and/or wheezing. In this setting, a detailed history should elucidate the disease process from its onset to the present, and allow the clinician to learn what types of medication have been used to this point. In addition, the history should identify factors important in inducing acute episodes of bronchospasm and document the presence of other environmental factors such as allergens or irritants that might be responsible for exacerbating a patient's asthmatic symptoms on a chronic basis.

Although patients with asthma may present in a variety of ways, most children will have common clinical features that can be diagnosed from the history alone. Typically asthma is characterized by intermittent episodes of respiratory obstruction with symptoms most prominent on expiration. Although expiratory wheezing is most common, inspiratory symptoms may appear as asthma worsens, or wheezing may be totally absent as air flow is further limited in the presence of profound obstruction. An inspiratory wheeze can occur with moderate asthma but is not characteristic of the disease. Upper airway sources of obstruction, for example, foreign body or laryngotracheitis, should be considered, particularly if inspiratory symptoms predominate.

Coughing generally accompanies wheezing, or occasionally may be the only symptom of asthma. Asthma exacerbations, although often episodic initially, frequently progress to fewer and shorter symptom-free intervals. Symptoms are nearly always worse at night or early in the morning, and tend to improve through the day. When symptoms have historically improved after use of inhaled beta-adrenergic drugs, subcutaneous epinephrine, or oral theophylline, the diagnosis of asthma is confirmed. Although typical exacerbations over 7–10 days may improve spontaneously, lung function may remain abnormal for several weeks.

Asthmatic symptoms are frequently age-related. A younger child may have a history of recurrent bronchitis, bronchiolitis, or pneumonia, persistent coughing with colds, recurrent croup, or a "rattly chest." Although older children also may have a history of chest tightness with "colds," they often will have a history of persistent wheezing on exposure to dust, animals, or a variety of other airway irritants including cigarette smoke, wood smoke, pollution, or strenuous exercise.

Finally, the clinician should be aware of two special problems when confronted with an obvious asthmatic history: gastroesophageal reflux and chronic sinus disease. Gastroesophageal reflux (GER) should be considered in any infant with postprandial vomiting or nocturnal asthmatic symptoms (particularly cough), or in an older child with complaints of dysphagia or "heartburn" (22–24). Relevant studies may include an upper gastrointestinal radiographic series or technetium scan followed by prolonged esophageal pH monitoring. A second, more common problem, chronic sinus disease, should be considered in any child with a history of increasing nasal congestion, purulent rhinorrhea, nocturnal cough (often to the point of vomiting), or gradual chronic worsening of asthma (25,26). Generally, a modified Waters view sinus radiograph will document the presence of significant sinus involvement. Once significant GER or chronic sinusitis is documented, aggressive directed therapy will often markedly reduce the severity of chronic asthma and obviate the need for chronic systemic steroid therapy.

## Past Medical History

When a child presents with a brief current history, it is useful to ask about previous episodes of coughing or wheezing, with emphasis on any obvious precipitating or exacerbating factors. The occurrence of previous episodes increases the likelihood of asthma. Knowledge of previous exacerbating sinusitis, pneumonitis or bronchitis, would likewise increase the suspicion of a current chronic process, and also raise concerns about immunodeficiency.

In the obviously asthmatic child the past medical history should explore clinical signs of atopy including eczema, episodic urticaria, chronic middle ear effusion, and hay fever. The presence of any of these factors increases the probability of a significant allergic component to the chronic cough and/or wheeze. It is also important to ask directly about exercise as a trigger for cough, wheeze, or dyspnea. These symptoms are commonly ignored or tolerated, and are important to elicit, since exercise-induced bronchospasm (EIB) will occur in 90% of children with asthma and in 40% of allergic "nonasthmatic" children (27).

Finally, it is important to ascertain any adverse reactions to medications, especially antibiotics, beta-adrenergics, or antihistamines. These classes of medications are frequently required in the child with chronic cough or wheezing, and it is useful to know which drugs have been efficacious and well tolerated.

## Family History

Family history should focus on the immediate family, but also can include extended family members known to the informant. Prior research suggests that a unilateral family history of asthma or allergic rhinitis is associated with a 35% frequency of such conditions in the offspring, while a bilateral family history increases this incidence to 65%. In children with obvious asthma, the frequency of other family members with known asthma or suggestive symptoms is very high, regardless of whether symptoms are related to allergic triggers (28). The clinician should realize that the initial family history is often incomplete and somewhat unreliable, and the informant will frequently volunteer additional information on subsequent visits, having had the opportunity to question other family members and become more comfortable with a new physician.

The environmental history is a unique part of the evaluation of a child with chronic cough or wheezing. Careful questioning about exacerbating factors at home, school, or day care will provide important information about potential allergens that the patient is exposed to frequently. This information, coupled with identification of specific allergic factors by skin or radioallergosorbent (RAST) testing provides the basis for environmental control or avoidance therapy. Table 2 is an example of a useful environmental checklist.

## Physical Examination

In the child with chronic cough or wheezing, the physical examination should focus on overall growth and development, respiratory mechanics and chest evaluation, and signs of other allergic conditions that frequently coexist in asthmatic children.

Since asthma and asthma therapy can affect growth adversely, a child's height and weight should be measured and recorded on initial and subsequent visits. A pattern of growth retardation in the asthmatic child may be from chronic hypoxemia with severe or poorly controlled asthma, from a food elimination diet based on surmised food allergy (which may or may not be true), or from the injudicious use of systemic steroids for asthma management (29–31). Heart rate and rhythm should be documented along with blood pressure, since many frequently used asthmatic medications, for example beta-adrenergic drugs, corticosteroids, and theophylline, may have an adverse effect on the cardiovascular system.

Respiratory examination should begin with observation of breathing rate, the color of lips and nail beds, signs of obstruction including expiratory phase prolongation, and any evidence for dyspnea including intercostal retractions or the use of accessory muscles to lift the shoulders during breathing. Chronic pulmonary hyperinflation with shouldered posture often leads to an increase in anterior–posterior chest diameter and a "pseudo-rachitic" chest deformity. The clinician should always look for evidence of finger clubbing or cyanosis. When either of these signs are apparent, other chronic pulmonary diseases must be considered in the differential diagnosis, especially cystic fibrosis and bronchiolitis obliterans.

In the younger child it is best to examine the lungs first, when the patient is still somewhat cooperative. Examination of the lungs frequently reveals rhonchi or unequal breath sounds, which may clear partially on changing position or with cough. Compression of the chest during expiration may accentuate latent wheezes by increasing airflow through obstructed pas-

TABLE 2 Environmental History

Home
- Location: city, suburb, rural
- Outdoor factors: landscaping, flowering, and pollinating plants in area
- Age of home: length of time in house (months, years)

Construction
- Type: rambler, 2-story, split level, other
- Basement: finished, unfinished, earth, none
- Crawl space: presence of vapor barrier

Heating and Cooling
- Type: forced air, electric baseboard, space heater or wall furnace, radiator, fireplaces, woodstove
- With forced air: type of filter (none, fiberglas, permanent, electrostatic) and frequency of filter change
- Cooling system: central, window, evaporative

Mold and moisture
- Condensation or mildew: windows, walls, bath, basement, none
- Humidifiers: furnace, cold mist, steam (determine frequency of cleaning)
- Exhaust fans: kitchen, bathrooms

Clothes dryer
- Location: separate room, garage, kitchen, basement, porch, other
- Vent: outside, crawl space, none, other

Patient's bedroom
- Location: basement, main floor, upper floor
- Number of children sharing room
- Flooring: wood, tile or linoleum, area rug, wall-to-wall carpet
  - Rug: wool, cotton, synthetic, fiber, shag, pile, none
  - Pad: felt, rubberized felt, rubber, synthetic, unknown, none
- Windows: curtains, drapes, shades, miniblinds, none
- Beds (consider all beds in room)
  - Mattress: innerspring, foam
  - Springs: box or coil
  - Bedding: synthetic, wool, cotton, other
  - Pillow: feather, foam, synthetic, other
  - Mattress pad: cotton, synthetic
  - Spread: linty, nonlinty
- Furniture: dresser, book, bookcase, chairs, nightstand, lamps, radio, television, stereo, houseplants, books, toy box, shelves, washable toys, nonwashable toys
- Closet: clothing, shoes, toys and games, sports equipment, storage, other

Living room
- Flooring: wood, tile or linoleum, area rug, wall-to-wall carpet
  - Rug: wool, cotton, synthetic, fiber, shag, pile, none
  - Pad: felt, rubberized felt, rubber, synthetic, unknown, none

Furniture: television, upholstered chairs, upholstered sofa, love seat, toys or games, books, other
Furniture content: innerspring, foam, down, synthetic, antique, fabric, other
Throw pillows: kapok, cotton, synthetic, foam, none, other
Family room or den
Flooring: wood, tile or linoleum, area rug, wall-to-wall carpet
Rug: wool, cotton, synthetic, fiber, shag, pile, none
Pad: felt, rubberized felt, rubber, synthetic, unknown, none
Furniture: television, upholstered chairs, upholstered sofa, love seat, toys or games, books, other
Furniture content: innerspring, foam, down, synthetic, antique, fabric, other
Throw pillows: kapok, cotton, synthetic, foam, none, other
Pets
Type
Where allowed in house: entire house, patient's bedroom, family (television) room, outdoors only
Smoking
By whom: none, mother, father, other
Quantity per day
Plants
Number
Location
Other environmental factors (animals, smoke, other factors)
Babysitter's home or daycare
Other parent's or relatives' homes
School or employment
Vacation home or recreational vehicles, other
Hobbies (patients and family members)
Indoor
Outdoor

---

sages. Although wheezing usually is elicited with forced expiration, some children will show only prolongation of expiration without overt wheezing. Older children or adolescents frequently will resist forceful exhalation because they have realized that this maneuver may induce coughing and accentuate bronchospasm. Accordingly, they must frequently be exhorted to try their best, and reassured that it's "okay to cough" during the exam. Children with severe asthma often "breathe from the top of their lungs" and move too little air with each tidal breath to generate a wheeze. Careful examination should verify the lower respiratory tract as a source for wheezing apart from other sounds such as stridor, which may occur in the laryngeal area but transmit sounds to the lower airway during pulmonary auscultation. Marked pulmonary hyperinflation can cause liver displacement downward, and a shift in the point of cardiac maximal impact. Although wheezing and rhonchi make cardiac examination difficult, it is important to document heart rate or rhythm abnormalities, since chronic pulmonary obstruction and its therapy may adversely affect the cardiovascular system.

In addition to growth pattern and lower airway examination, assessment should include evaluation of the eyes, ears, nose, and skin. Significant findings will heighten the probability of an allergic component as a source for cough and wheezing, and reveal other clinical problems that may need appropriate therapy. Examination of the conjunctiva should focus on signs of edema or inflammation, including any discharge. In the child who is receiving chronic steroid therapy, a slit-lamp examination should be performed by an ophthalmologist to evaluate for any signs of early cataract formation. Ear examination should assess any evidence of chronic middle ear effusion or eustachian tube dysfunction. Nasal evaluation includes documentation of mucosal pallor or erythema, the presence and character of rhinorrhea (clear versus purulent), or other obstructive phenomena such as foreign bodies or nasal polyps. The presence of nasal polyps in a child should raise concern about cystic fibrosis or chronic sinus disease and associated aspirin sensitivity. Finally, the clinician should note any eczema, which tends to occur in flexor areas such as wrists, elbows, ankles, and knees, including any purulent component.

## LABORATORY EVALUATION

A directed history and physical examination should always be considered an initial, essential step in the evaluation of a child with chronic cough or wheezing. Guided by this initial information, the astute clinician can then choose appropriate adjunctive laboratory procedures to clarify further the causes and provide a functional assessment of disease severity. Baseline studies help to define initial therapy, and can often be used as a reference in subsequent visits for ascertaining response to initial treatment.

### Nasal Cytology

Examination of nasal secretions will often provide useful clues about causes in patients with chronic cough or wheeze (see Table 3). Children with infectious rhinitis (either bacterial or viral) generally demonstrate a predominance of neutrophils when secretions are examined microscopically. Significant eosinophilic rhinitis generally suggests an allergic component

TABLE 3 Differential Diagnosis of Rhinitis

| | Eosinophilic Allergic | Eosinophilic Nonallergic | Neutrophilic | Vasomotor |
|---|---|---|---|---|
| Clinical findings | Typically during childhood | Adulthood, often young | Any age | Adulthood, rare in children |
| | Sneezing, nasal pruritus, clear rhinorrhea | Severe obstruction; anosmia, polyps common | Purulent secretions, sinus tenderness, nocturnal cough | Congestion, minimal rhinorrhea |
| | Episodic or perennial | Perennial symptoms | Appearance most common during fall and winter | Variable presentation |
| | Triggers are often obvious (e.g., dust mites, animals, pollens) | Often aspirin sensitive; frequent asthma and sinus disease | Infection typical; can be caused by irritation (e.g., cigarette or wood smoke) | Can be hormonal (e.g., thyroid disease, pregnancy) |
| Nasal cytologic findings | Eosinophils<br>± Basophils<br>± Neutrophils | Eosinophils<br>± Basophils<br>± Neutrophils | Neutrophils often with intracellular bacteria | Generally unremarkable |

in children, although it may be a sign of NARES (nonallergic rhinitis with eosinophilia), a condition often associated with nasal polyposis and aspirin sensitivity. Thus, nasal cytologic findings should not be considered specific, but can be useful in directing further evaluation.

The first step in nasal cytologic evaluation is obtaining an adequate sample. In general, an older child can blow his or her nose into a piece of plastic wrap. If a child is too young to cooperate with this, or if the nose seems dry, a cotton swab can be placed in the nasal vault to collect secretions. An alternative technique utilizes a plastic curette (Rhinoprobe) that is gently scraped below the inferior turbinate. Samples are then transferred from plastic wrap, cotton applicator, or plastic curette onto a glass slide. After appropriate heat fixing, the secretions are prepared with Hansel's stain for examination according to the protocol outlined in Table 4.

## Radiography

During an initial acute wheezing episode, anteroposterior and lateral chest films should be obtained to help identify areas of pneumonia (32,33). If the pneumonia becomes persistent or recurrent, follow-up radiographs should be obtained to define the course of the disease process. Subsequently, a film taken during a period of well-being can confirm that the initial process has really resolved and serve as a good baseline for the future.

Particularly in the first few months of life, it is important to remember that structural abnormalities may underlie a clinical pattern of chronic wheezing with or without pneumonia. Although this is much less common than reversible airway disease, a chest x-ray can help to exclude more uncommon structural problems, for example, peribronchial lymphoid hyperplasia, vascular rings, and pulmonary sequestration.

Occasionally, with persistent cough unresponsive to intense medical management, recurrent localized pneumonitis, or poorly defined radi-

TABLE 4 Nasal Cytologic Preparation

| |
|---|
| Transfer the specimen to a glass slide, dry, and fix with heat |
| Stain for 30 sec with Hansel's stain (1:500 eosin and 1:200 methylene blue in alcohol) |
| Add distilled water to take up stain for 30 sec |
| Wash with water |
| Decolorize with methanol or 95% ethyl alcohol (do not overdecolorize) |
| Dry and examine under oil immersion |

ographic abnormalities, further studies such as computed chest tomography (with and without radiocontrast) or bronchoscopy may be necessary.

The possibility of foreign body aspiration should always be considered when a toddler or preschool child presents with abrupt onset of wheezing. Since the physical examination frequently is not helpful in this setting, appropriate radiographic studies are essential. Comparison of films taken in inspiration and expiration may demonstrate air trapping distal to the area obstructed by the foreign body. Especially when plain radiographs are unrevealing in the face of a suggestive history, fluoroscopy during respiration should be performed. In experienced hands, this technique improves sensitivity and can greatly simplify bronchoscopy and removal of the foreign body.

There is increasing evidence that sinus disease can exacerbate bronchial hyperresponsiveness and chronic asthma severity (25,26). Research suggests that aggressive therapy of wheezing children who show abnormal sinus radiographs can alleviate both upper and lower airway symptoms as sinus disease resolves. Accordingly, sinus radiographs should be performed when the history and physical examination reveal increasing asthma severity, chronic purulent rhinorrhea, or recurrent nocturnal cough. Since maxillary disease is most common, either alone or with ethmoid involvement, a Waters (occipitomental) view is often adequate. Ethmoid visibility can be enhanced with a modified Waters radiograph, in which the chin is tipped up 37 degrees instead of the usual 42 degrees, or with a Caldwell view (anteroposterior). Lateral head films are rarely needed, since sphenoid and frontal sinusitis is unusual in childhood (34,35).

In evaluating sinus radiographs, remember that maxillary and ethmoid sinuses should be pneumatized in infancy and that crying does not cause sinus clouding or opacity. Frontal and sphenoid sinuses generally are radiologically visible during the early to mid-school-age years. Therapy should be influenced by research showing that antral punctures from sinuses with chronic severe membrane thickening, clouding and opacification, or air fluid levels frequently yield bacteria. The most common organisms, frequently beta-lactamase positive, include *H. influenzae*, *S. pneumoniae*, and *M. catarrhalis* (previously *B. catarrhalis*) (36,37). When aggressive treatment fails, a coronal sinus CT scan should be performed. The scan often will reveal occult ethmoid disease or clarify the need for sinus lavage and surgical intervention.

### Gastroesophageal Reflux Tests

A young child with failure to thrive, chronic regurgitation, recurrent pneumonitis, and nocturnal spasmodic cough, should alert the clinician to the possibility of gastroesophageal reflux (GER) (24). Initially, a barium study should be obtained to assess swallowing function and disclose any structural abnormalities. Although marked reflux can frequently be seen during a barium examination, more sensitive techniques are often needed. Technetium or other radionuclide studies can be used to evaluate gastric emptying, reflux, or evidence of pulmonary aspiration. Manometry can be used to document lower esophageal sphincter pressure, which tends to be significantly decreased in persons with GER. Intraluminal pH monitoring is the most sensitive means of diagnosing GER, and also enhances specificity by allowing for correlation between reflux episodes and respiratory symptoms. A standardized examination, the Tuttle test, involves placement of a three-lumen tube, including nasogastric tube, pH probe, and manometer, in the lower esophagus. The pH is monitored during a baseline phase and after the introduction of acid into the stomach. During a subsequent 1 hr period of observation, two episodes of decreased esophageal pH to less than 4.0 define the presence of significant reflux. Sensitivity can be further enhanced with longer-term monitoring. A 24 hr tracing, for example, can be evaluated for frequency of reflux episodes, acid clearance time, and the relationship of coughing, wheezing, or cyanosis with altered esophageal pH (38).

## Pulmonary Function Tests

Pulmonary function testing is a simple, inexpensive procedure that can be done by primary care physicians as well as specialists. Evaluation during acute episodes quantifies the degree of obstruction and response to bronchodilator treatment. Subsequent studies can be used to evaluate resolution of acute episodes or assess chronic disease severity.

Objective measurement of pulmonary function is important for adequate clinical sensitivity in the management of asthma. It is not unusual, for example, to see mild or even moderate pulmonary airflow obstruction with spirometry even though the patient denies distress and sounds free of wheezes. Numerous studies further suggest that physical examination alone frequently underestimates asthma severity (39–41). Without objective lung function measurement, the clinician will be at a distinct disadvantage in determining both acute and chronic asthma therapy.

Assessment of pulmonary function on children under age 3 years is limited to resistance measurements, which are not currently practical for the ambulatory setting. By age 3–4 years many children can reproducibly perform peak expiratory flow rate (PEFR) maneuvers. PEFR is a measurement of large airway flow, and decreases greater than 10% indicate significant obstruction. Since the technique is very effort-dependent, it is important for office staff to spend a good deal of time with appropriate teaching. Used correctly in the home, PEFR meters can help patients and their parents to detect deterioration in lung function and assess response to bronchodilator therapy. At present, several types of inexpensive PEFR devices are available for $25–35.*

Most school-aged children can be taught to perform an adequate forced expiratory maneuver that will yield a valuable spirometric tracing. Proper technique involves inhalation to total lung capacity, followed by vigorous forced expiration into the spirometer over 6 sec. The subsequent curve of expiratory volume against time yields useful information on large and small airway flows, and may suggest restrictive as well as obstructive pulmonary disease. The forced expiratory volume in 1 sec ($FEV_1$), normally about 80% of vital capacity, measures initial airway emptying or large airway flow. The slope of the curve from 25 to 75% of vital capacity ($FEF_{25-75\%}$) or the maximal expiratory flow at midvital capacity (MMEF) is indicative of smaller airway flow.

Proper interpretation of a child's pulmonary function data involves comparison with air flows in normal subjects of the same age, gender, and height. Interpretation will be appropriate only if the predicted normal values have been obtained directly from children rather than a computer-generated extrapolation from adult normal values (42). If one accepts two standard deviations from the mean as within normal limits, a normal $FEV_1$ is at least 80% of predicted, and a normal $FEF_{25-75\%}$ is over 65% of predicted. Normal patients will typically have an $FEV_1$/FVC ratio of at least 80%. Although these parameters are useful, it is always important to look at the raw numbers and the trend in air flows. Realizing that bona fide obstruction should be maximal in the smaller airways, a careful review of the tracing and numbers is indicated when the data do not correlate with the clinical picture. Often scrutiny will reveal technical errors in data entry, suboptimal technique, or simply poor patient effort.

Since spirometry is very effort-dependent, the best of three forced expiratory tracings should be used as the best estimate of a patient's pulmonary function. Performance of multiple vital capacity maneuvers enables the clinician to assess patient effort and ensure quantitative consistency between trials. When patients are uncooperative or cannot appropriately perform the usual techniques, effort-independent methods such as plethysmography can be used in a hospital setting.

---

*Assess peak flowmeter (standard, low range) available from Center Laboratories, Port Washington, New York; Mini-Wright peak flowmeter (standard, low range) available from: Dura Pharmaceuticals, San Diego, California; Keller Medical Specialties, Antioch, Illinois.

## Bronchoprovocation Tests

A variety of bronchoprovocation tests can be useful when the cause of a patient's chronic cough is unclear. These techniques are particularly helpful when presented with a suggestive asthmatic history in the face of normal resting pulmonary function. Although some of these diagnostic maneuvers require expensive, sophisticated equipment, most procedures can be adapted for routine clinical use in the office setting.

Exercise tolerance testing can be used to evaluate the presence and severity of exercise-induced bronchospasm (EIB). Such an evaluation should be considered in patients with asthma or allergic rhinitis. In fact, nearly 90% of children with asthma will experience significant bronchoconstriction after vigorous activity, as will 40% of children with allergic rhinitis (43). Unrecognized, EIB can create suboptimal athletic performance, resistance to participation with school or extracurricular sports, or even a long-term sedentary lifestyle. Even a thorough history may not elicit EIB. For example, it is common for children with obvious chronic asthma to deny the need for bronchodilator treatment before or after exercise because they do not want to appear different to their peers, or prefer to think they are simply in poor physical condition. An exercise tolerance test will invariably document significant EIB in this setting. Subsequent discussion and therapy will not only enhance performance during exercise but also frequently will provide a sense of relief to the child and improved self-esteem.

Routine exercise testing requires generation of vigorous aerobic activity for 6–8 min at 80–90% of maximal myocardial oxygen consumption capacity. A variety of exercise forms can be used, including running, cycling, rowing, kayaking, or swimming. Free running appears to be the most asthmagenic form of exercise, presumably because it creates more intense water and heat loss from the airway (44,45). When free running is not practical, or when the degree of exercise and environmental variables must be standardized, a treadmill can be used (46). A positive test will generally demonstrate significant bronchoconstriction 5–15 min following the exercise tolerance test. Because of patient variability, it is prudent to monitor pulmonary function before, immediately after, and at 3, 5, 10, 15, and 20 min after exercise. Significant EIB is suggested by a decrease of more than 12% in $FEV_1$, 25% in $FEF_{25-75\%}$, or 12% in PEFR. Such decrements reflect a change greater than 2 standard deviations above the effect of exercise on the normal population (47). If bronchospasm is documented after exercise, patients should be told they may experience a "late phase" response hours later and also be instructed on appropriate therapy (48,49).

A patient with chronic cough will periodically have results from a history, physical examination, and baseline pulmonary function tests that do not provide a definitive diagnosis of asthma. In these cases, a variety of inhalation challenges can provide important information about increased nonspecific airway reactivity to help clarify the diagnosis. In general, these techniques, if performed under standardized protocol regimens, have high sensitivity and specificity. Methacholine or histamine challenges are commonly used for both diagnostic and research purposes in children and adults (50–52). In children, the specificity of methacholine challenges is somewhat decreased, presumably due to the length of the test and risk of fatigue at higher challenge concentrations (53). On the other hand, a challenge with methacholine provides excellent sensitivity approaching 95% compared with other techniques, such as cold air or distilled water inhalation (54). From a clinical perspective, this means that appropriate methacholine challenges will miss very few children with a significant asthmatic component to their chronic cough. Given the excellent predictive value of the test, methacholine results can be used to initiate antiasthma therapy promptly or reconsider the differential diagnosis rather than forcing one to rely on empiric treatment (55).

Distilled water inhalation and eucapneic hyperventilation of cold air are other valuable provocative challenges (56,57). These techniques are useful because alterations in airway heat and water content will stimulate bronchospasm in asthmatic but not normal subjects. Although well tolerated and specific in children, these procedures lack the high degree of sensitivity that the clinician needs in a diagnostic procedure. More recently, hyperosmolar saline challenge has been used in children with much greater levels of sensitivity than distilled water or cold air inhalation (58).

In principle, inhalation challenge with specific antigens can be used to identify environmental factors that produce a patient's symptoms (59,60). Although standardized protocols are available for such challenges, several problems limit widespread application. Commercially available antigens often are not identical to the patient's exposure, so one is forced to prepare material from a patient's sample, which is typically a very time- and labor-intensive process. Particularly when several antigens are in question, one has to consider the time and expense involved in being able to evaluate only one exposure at a time. Research would suggest that the specificity of inhalation challenges can be poor, creating difficulty in differentiating patients with rhinitis from those with asthma on the basis of bronchial challenge results. From a safety standpoint, an office employing specific antigen inhalation challenges must be prepared for a significant portion of positive responders having a delayed, often profound, late-phase response to the test. This secondary drop in lung function can occur from 4 to 12 hr after the initial exposure, and must be anticipated in the clinical or research setting with appropriate supervision.

Standardized protocols for bronchoprovocation use either a tidal volume breathing method or an intermittent inhalation technique (61–63). The tidal volume method has the subject breathing sequential dilutions of the continually nebulized agent, allowing 2 min of tidal volume respiration per dilution. Pulmonary function tests are typically performed 3 min after each dilution until the full range of appropriate challenge has been completed or the $FEV_1$ drops 20% or more. The intermittent technique involves patient inhalation after self-actuation of a solenoid valve Rosenthal dosimeter. The patient then takes five breaths of each concentration before performing spirometry. As with the tidal volume method, the patient continues with the test until the highest concentration is completed or until the $FEV_1$ has decreased by at least 20%. Studies would suggest that these two methodologies are comparable (64). For documentation, the provocative dose or concentration of agent capable of causing an $FEV_1$ decrease of 20% is called the $PD_{20}$ or $PC_{20}$.

The specificity of bronchoprovocation challenges in children can be greatly enhanced if the clinician considers several factors. First, testing should not be performed immediately following a viral illness, since this disease process can induce transient reactivity for up to 8 weeks. Second, younger children may often find it difficult to synchronize the use of dosimeter with inhalation appropriately. Best results in this age group are found using the tidal volume method and encouraging the child to cooperate and expend maximal effort on pulmonary function testing, particularly if the test has gone on for several minutes. Finally, a standardized chemical inhalation challenge should not be performed if the child cannot reliably perform spirometry, since specificity will be poor. Recent studies with techniques utilizing computerized sound analysis to evaluate airflow changes after challenge suggest that reproducible study of children less than 5 years of age may be possible (65). Additional research needs to be done to determine if this newer technology will have widespread application.

### Total Serum IgE Evaluation

Determination of total serum IgE can be useful in a child with evident chronic asthma. Nearly 80% of children with significant allergic asthma will have a total serum IgE level greater than 2 standard deviations from the nonallergic population's mean (66). Although one can have an elevated IgE without manifesting allergic disease, this is rare in childhood. In general, even though a viral illness may have been an initial precipitant of clinical asthma, an elevated IgE level in a child suggests that a component of the patient's pulmonary hyperresponsiveness is due to an allergic response to environmental factors. Subsequent appropriate identification of specific allergic triggers will define appropriate environmental control measures that can have a significant beneficial impact on the chronic course of the child's asthma.

Total serum IgE can be determined by a variety of methodologies. Radioimmunoassay (RIA) can be performed as a traditional competitive displacement procedure, or the more recently developed noncompetitive immunoradiometric assay (67,68). Although these techniques are very sensitive, they have the disadvantage of requiring radioactive agents. Alternative techniques that do not require radioactivity include the use of a fluorochrome or a chlorometric enzyme immunoassay. With the development of more sensitive instruments, even nephalometry or rate nephalometry can be used with reasonably good sensitivity.

### Allergen-Specific Skin Tests

Pediatric asthma is frequently exacerbated by exposure to environmental allergens. In these children, antigen-specific IgE bound to basophils and mast cells combines with antigen, resulting in the release of a variety of mediators. The chemicals released produce immediate bronchoconstriction and late-phase airway inflammation. In a given patient, the same antigen-specific IgE found in the airway can be detected in the skin.

Performed properly, allergy skin testing is a very sensitive bioassay for antigen-specific IgE. A positive skin test reaction mirrors the pathophysiological findings seen in the lung. Antigen applied to the skin reacts to specific mast-cell-bound dermal antibody, which induces mediator release. Histamine will generally create local vasodilation with wheal and flare within 10–15 min, and a variety of chemotactic factors may create a delayed inflammatory response hours later (69,70). In the asthmatic subject, these responses are analogous to the early- and late-phase bronchospasm observed after antigen inhalation.

Although true-positive skin tests indicate that a patient has antigen-specific IgE, it does not prove that exposure creates clinically significant disease. The predictive value of a positive skin test is typically enhanced if the skin reactivity is intense or when moderate reactivity occurs in conjunction with a positive provocative history.

The foundation for reliable skin testing rests on obtaining antigen extracts (ideally standardized) from a quality-controlled laboratory. Allergens should be diluted only when necessary for testing purposes and stabilized with glycerin or albumin (71). Testing materials should be appropriately refrigerated and must be monitored frequently to ensure that their shelf life has not expired.

Even with fresh, stable allergens, poor technique can result in loss of sensitivity. For example, if epicutaneous antigen application is too superficial, or intradermal testing is too deep, the expected response may be blunted. Test results may also be confusing if appropriate positive histamine and negative saline controls are not applied, or if tests are placed too closely together, allowing for the formation of overlapping wheals.

If skin test results are to reflect the presence of specific IgE, it is critical to withhold all antihistamines at least 48 hr before testing. This is particularly true for hydroxyzine (72) and terfenadine and, in some cases, astemizole may need to be restricted for up to a month (73). If a child has taken antihistamines within 24 hr, it is often appropriate to apply a histamine control before a battery of tests is applied to ensure adequate skin reactivity.

Virtually any child can be reliably skin tested. At the same time, it is important to realize that infants and young children generally will have a smaller wheal response to histamine and positive allergens, and frequently may experience more nonspecific trauma with the process of injection (74,75). In this setting, positive and negative skin test controls are crucial.

The choice of skin testing materials should be limited to pertinent allergens that could exacerbate the child's asthma, and be guided by the initial history. At the same time, a patient should not be tested with allergens that have clearly caused anaphylaxis in the past. Such testing provides no new information and could be life-threatening.

Although proper skin testing should only create dermal exposure, a patient may react to several allergens with risk of anaphylaxis. Accordingly, epinephrine, oxygen, and antihistamines must be readily available with easy access to supportive treatments such as airways, intravenous fluids, vasopressors, and corticosteroids.

### Allergen-Specific RAST Tests

As an alternative to allergen-specific skin tests, serum IgE against a specific antigen can be measured with the RAST test (76,77). In this procedure, antigens are coupled to an inert carrier such as latex or cellulose. This matrix is then incubated with patient sera. During a reaction period, any available allergen-specific IgE in the serum will react with the matrix-bound antigen. In the final step, an anti-IgE antibody is allowed to react with the antigen–antibody complexes. This final antibody is either radiolabeled or enzyme-linked so that positive reactions can be easily detected with a gamma-counter or spectrophotometer.

In general, RAST testing is less sensitive and significantly more expensive than skin testing (78). Clinical situations in which RAST testing might be preferable include a child with severe eczema who lacks sufficient normal skin area to allow appropriate skin testing, or a patient with dermatographism in whom needle application is likely to evoke a significant response independent of allergen addition.

## SUMMARY

When presented with a coughing or wheezing child, the clinician should focus on a careful comprehensive history. Key features include onset of symptoms, exacerbating factors, useful treatments, and the presence of other associated chronic symptoms. The past history should include gestational age at birth, perinatal problems including congenital anomalies, adverse reaction to medications, and any other significant chronic medical problems. Often a synthesis of these historical factors will suggest a congenital problem, foreign body, gastroesophageal reflux, or a variety of problems associated with prematurity. If not, asthma should be suspected.

An appropriate physical examination should focus on overall growth and development, respiratory mechanics including chest examination, and signs of nasal disease that could adversely influence asthma, including allergic rhinitis and chronic sinusitis. Based on the history and directed physical examination, appropriate laboratory evaluation should clarify the diagnosis and quantify disease severity. Appropriate studies might include nasal cytology, sinus and lung radiographs, gastroesophageal reflux studies, pulmonary function tests including provocative challenge, or measurement of both total and specific IgE.

A comprehensive evaluation will frequently disclose the diagnosis of asthma. Armed with objective data, the clinician should be able to create a comprehensive management plan including environmental control, pharmacotherapy for bronchoconstriction and airway hyperresponsiveness, and treatment of concomitant nasal disease. If asthma has been ruled out, the history should be carefully rescrutinized to help direct further laboratory evaluation.

## REFERENCES

1. Konig P. Hidden asthma in childhood. *Am J Dis Child* 135:1053, 1981.
2. Clotier MM, Laughlin GM. Chronic cough in children: a manifestation of airway hyperreactivity. *Pediatrics* 67:6, 1981.
3. Taussig LM, Smith SM, Blumenfeld R. Chronic bronchitis in childhood—what is it? *Pediatrics* 67:1, 1981.
4. Speight AND, Lee DA, Hey EN. Underdiagnosis and undertreatment of asthma in childhood. *Br Med J* 286:1253, 1983.

5. Eigen H, Reid JJ, Dahl R, et al. Evaluation of the addition of cromolyn sodium to bronchodilator maintenance therapy in the long-term management of asthma. *J Allergy Clin Immunol* 80:612, 1987.
6. McFadden ER Jr. Cromolyn: first-line therapy for chronic asthma? *J Respir Dis* 8:39, 1987.
7. Kaliner M. Mechanisms of glucocorticosteroid action in bronchial asthma. *J Allergy Clin Immunol* 76:321, 1985.
8. Williams MH Jr. Corticosteroids in asthma therapy: role of inhaled corticosteroids. *J Respir Dis* Suppl:S44, 1988.
9. Berdon WE, Baker DH. Vascular anomalies and the infant lungs: rings, slings and other things, *Semin Roentgenol* 7:39, 1972.
10. Weissberg D, Schwartz I. Foreign bodies in the tracheobronchial tree. *Chest* 91:730, 1987.
11. Wittig HS, Chang CH. Bronchiolitis or asthma. *Pediatr Clin North Am* 16:55, 1969.
12. Reynolds EOR. Bronchiolitis. In: Kendig EI Jr (Ed.), *Pulmonary Disorders*, W.B. Saunders, Philadelphia, 1972.
13. Busse WW. Respiratory infections: their role in airway responsiveness and pathogenesis of asthma. *J Allergy Clin Immunol* 85:671, 1990.
14. McIntosh K, Ellis EF, Hoffman LS, et al. The association of viral and bacterial respiratory infections with exacerbations of wheezing in young asthmatic children. *J Pediatr* 82:578, 1973.
15. Minor TE, Dick EC, DeMeo AN, et al. Viruses as precipitants of asthmatic attacks in children. *JAMA* 336:292, 1974.
16. Gurwitz D, Mindorff C, Levison H. Increased incidence of bronchial reactivity in children with a history of bronchiolitis. *J Pediatr* 98:551, 1981.
17. Duivermann EJ, Neijens HJ, Van Strik R, et al. Lung function and bronchial responsiveness in children who had bronchiolitis. *Pediatr Pulmonol* 3:38, 1987.
18. Fergusson DM, Horwood LJ, Shannon FT. Parental asthma, parental eczema, and asthma, and eczema in early childhood. *J Chron Dis* 36:517, 1983.
19. Davis JB, Bulpitt CJ. Atopy and wheeze in children according to parental atopy and family size. *Thorax* 35:671, 1980.
20. Horwood LJ, Fergusson DM, Hons BA, Shannon FT. Social and familial factors in the development of early childhood asthma. *Pediatrics* 75:859, 1985.
21. Sibbald B, Horn MEC, Gregg I. A family study of the genetic basis of asthma and wheezy bronchitis. *Arch Dis Child* 55:54, 1980.
22. Berquist WE, Rachelefsky GS, Kadden M, et al. Gastroesophageal reflux-associated recurrent pneumonia and chronic asthma in children. *Pediatrics* 68:29, 1981.
23. Herbst JJ. Gastroesophageal reflux and pulmonary disease. *Pediatrics* 68:132, 1981.
24. Shapiro GG, Christie D. Gastroesophageal reflux and asthma. *Clin Rev Allergy* 1:39, 1983.
25. Rachelefsky GS, Katz RM, Siegel SC. Chronic sinus disease with associated reactive airway disease in children. *Pediatrics* 73:526, 1984.

26. Slavin RG. Relationship of nasal disease and sinusitis to bronchial asthma. *Ann Allergy* 49:76, 1982.
27. Pierson WE. Exercise-induced bronchospasm in children and adolescents. *Pediatr Clin North Am* 35:1031, 1988.
28. Schwartz M. Heredity in bronchial asthma: clinical and genetic study of 191 asthma probands and 50 probands with Baker's asthma. *Acta Allergol* 5(suppl 2), 1952.
29. Ellis EF. Adverse effects of corticosteroid therapy. *J Allergy Clin Immunol* 80:515, 1987.
30. Balfour-Lynn L. Growth and childhood asthma. *Arch Dis Child* 61:1049, 1986.
31. Shohat M, Shohat T, Kedem R, et al. Childhood asthma and growth outline. *Arch Dis Child* 62:63, 1987.
32. Gilles JD, Reed MH, Simons FE. Radiographic findings in acute childhood asthma. *J Can Assoc Radiol* 29:28, 1978.
33. Eggleston PA, Ward BH, Pierson WE, Bierman CW. Radiographic abnormalities in acute asthma in children. *Pediatrics* 54:442, 1974.
34. Towbin R, Dunbar JS. The paranasal sinuses in childhood. *Radiographics* 2:253, 1982.
35. Swischuk LE, Harden CK, Dillard RA. Sinusitis in children. *Radiographics* 2:241, 1982.
36. Tinkelman DG, Silk H. Clinical and bacteriologic features of chronic sinusitis in children. *Am J Dis Child* 143:938, 1989.
37. Goldenhersh MJ, Rachelefsky GS, Dudley J, et al. The microbiology of chronic sinus disease in children with respiratory allergy. *J Allergy Clin Immunol* 85:1030, 1990.
38. Richter JE, Castell DO. Gastroesophageal reflux: pathogenesis, diagnosis and therapy. *Ann Intern Med* 97:93, 1982.
39. McFadden ER Jr, Kiser R, de Groot WJ. Acute bronchial asthma: relations between clinical and physiologic manifestations. *N Engl J Med* 288:221, 1973.
40. Shim CS, Williams H Jr. Relationship of wheezing to severity of obstruction in asthma. *Arch Intern Med* 143:890, 1983.
41. Pratter MR, Hingston DM, Irwin RS. Diagnosis of bronchial asthma by clinical evaluation. *Chest* 84:42, 1983.
42. Polgar G, Promadhat V (eds.). *Pulmonary Function Testing in Children: Techniques and Standards.* W.B. Saunders, Philadelphia, 1971.
43. Kawabori I, Pierson WE, Conquest LL, et al. Incidence of exercise-induced bronchospasm in children. *J Allergy Clin Immunol* 58:447, 1976.
44. McFadden ER Jr, Lenner, KAM, Strohl KP. Postexertional airway rewarming and thermally induced asthma. *J Clin Invest* 78:18, 1986.
45. Smith CM, Anderson SD, Walsh S, McElrea MS. An investigation of the effects of heat and water exchange in the recovery period after exercise in children with asthma. *Am Rev Respir Dis* 140:598, 1989.
46. Eggleston PA, Guerrant JL. A standardized method of evaluating exercise-induced asthma. *J Allergy Clin Immunol* 58:414, 1976.
47. Kattan M, Keens TG, Mellis CM, Levison H. The response to exercise in normal and asthmatic children. *J Pediatr* 92:718, 1978.

48. Iikura Y, Inui H, Nagakura T, Lee TH. Factors predisposing to exercise-induced late asthmatic responses. *J Allergy Clin Immunol* 75:285, 1985.
49. Rubinstein I, Levison H, Slutsky AS, et al. Immediate and delayed bronchoconstriction after exercise in patients with asthma. *N Engl J Med* 317:482, 1987.
50. Hargreave FE, Dolovich J, Boulet LP. Inhalation provocation tests. *Semin Respir Med* IV:224, 1983.
51. Clifford RD, Pugsley A, Radford M, Holgate ST. Symptoms, atopy, and bronchial response to methacholine in parents with asthma and their children. *Arch Dis Child* 62:66, 1987.
52. Murray AB, Ferguson AC, Morrison B. Airways responsiveness to histamine as a test for overall severity of asthma in children. *J Allergy Clin Immunol* 68:119, 1981.
53. Hopp J, Bewtra AK, Nair NM, et al. Specificity and sensitivity of methacholine inhalation challenge in normal and asthmatic children. *J Allergy Clin Immunol* 74:154, 1984.
54. Galdes-Sebaldt M, McLaughlin FJ, Levison H. Comparison of cold air, ultrasonic mist and methacholine inhalations as tests of bronchial reactivity in normal and asthmatic children. *J Pediatr* 107:526, 1985.
55. Shapiro GG, Furukawa CT, Pierson WE, et al. Methacholine bronchial challenge in children. *J Allergy Clin Immunol* 69:365, 1982.
56. McLaughlin FJ, Dozor AJ. Cold air inhalation challenge in the diagnosis of asthma in children. *Pediatrics* 72:503, 1983.
57. Tal A, Pasterkamp H, Serrette C, et al. Response to cold air hyperventilation in normal and asthmatic children. *J Pediatr* 104:516, 1984.
58. Virant FS, Williams PV, Bierman CW, et al. Hyperosmolar saline challenge in children: Relationship to methacholine, exercise challenge and therapy. *J Allergy Clin Immunol* 85:259, 1990.
59. Spector S, Farr R. Bronchial inhalation challenge with antigens. *J Allergy Clin Immunol* 64:580, 1979.
60. Bronsky EA, Ellis EF. Inhalation bronchial challenge testing in asthmatic children. *Pediatr Clin North Am* 16:85, 1969.
61. Chai H, Farr RS, Froehlich LA, et al. Standardization of bronchial inhalation challenge procedures. *J Allergy Clin Immunol* 56:323, 1975.
62. Tsanckas JN, Wilson AJ, Boon AW. Evaluation of nebulizers for bronchial challenge tests. *Arch Dis Child* 62:506, 1987.
63. Cockcroft DW, Killian DN, Mellon JJA, Hargreave FE. Bronchial reactivity to inhaled histamine: a method and clinical survey. *Clin Allergy* 7:235, 1977.
64. Ryan G, Dolovich MB, Robert RS, et al. Standardization of inhalation provocation tests: Two techniques of aerosol generation and inhalation compared. *Am Rev Respir Dis* 123:195, 1981.
65. Tinkelman DG, Lutz C, Conner B. Methacholine challenges in the management of young children. *Ann Allergy* 66:225, 1991.
66. Henderson LL, Swedlund HA, Van Dellen R, et al. Evaluation of IgE tests in an allergy practice. *J Allergy Clin Immunol* 48:361, 1971.

67. Spitz E, Gelfand EW, Sheffer AL, Austen KF. Serum IgE in clinical immunology and allergy. *J Allergy Clin Immunol* 49:337, 1972.
68. Gleich GJ, Averbeck AK, Swedlund HA. Measurement of IgE in normal and allergic serum by radioimmunoassay. *J Lab Clin Med* 77:690, 1971.
69. Dorsch W, Ring J. Induction of late cutaneous reaction by skin-blister fluid from allergen-tested and normal skin. *J Allergy Clin Immunol* 67:117, 1981.
70. Talbot SF, Atkins PC, Valenzano M, et al. Correlations of in vivo mediator release with late cutaneous allergic responses in humans. *J Allergy Clin Immunol* 74:819, 1984.
71. Nelson HS. Effect of preservatives and conditions of storage on potency of allergy extracts. *J Allergy Clin Immunol* 67:641, 1981.
72. Ting S, Rauls DO, Reiman BE. Inhibitory effect of hydroxyzine on antigen-induced histamine release in vivo. *J Allergy Clin Immunol* 75:63, 1985.
73. Gendreau L, Simons KJ, Simons FER. Comparison of the suppressive effect of astemizole, terfenadine, and hydroxyzine on histamine-induced wheals and flares in humans. *J Allergy Clin Immunol* 77:335, 1986.
74. VanAsperen PP, Kemp AS, Mellis CM. Skin test reactivity and clinical allergen sensitivity in infancy. *J Allergy Clin Immunol* 73:381, 1984.
75. Menardo JL, Bousquet J, Rodiere M, et al. Skin test reactivity in infancy. *J Allergy Clin Immunol* 75:646, 1985.
76. Gleich GJ, Jones RT. Measurement of IgE antibodies by the radioallergosorbent test. II. Analyses of quantitative relationships in the tests. *J Allergy Clin Immunol* 55:346, 1975.
77. Schellenberg RR, Adkinson NF Jr. Measurement of absolute amounts of antigen-specific human IgE by radioallergosorbent rest (RAST) elution technique. *J Immunol* 115:1577, 1975.
78. Berg TLO, Johansson SGO. Allergy diagnosis with the radioallergosorbent test: a comparison with the results of skin and provocation tests in an unselected group of children with asthma and hay fever. *J Allergy Clin Immunol* 54:209, 1974.

# 12

# APPROACHES TO THE TREATMENT OF CHRONIC ASTHMA

**CHARLES K. NASPITZ**

*Escola Paulista de Medicina*
*São Paulo, Brazil*

**ALEXANDER C. FERGUSON**

*University of British Columbia*
*Vancouver, British Columbia, Canada*

**DAVID G. TINKELMAN**

*Medical College of Georgia, Augusta, Georgia,*
*and Atlanta Allergy Clinic, Atlanta, Georgia*

In this chapter we will discuss the outpatient pharmacologic approach to children with bronchial asthma whose symptoms require chronic medication to allow normal daily activity. Pharmacologic manipulation is used concomitantly with other modes of therapy, which may include environmental control, diet, physiotherapy, and immunotherapy. These nonpharmacologic approaches in the management of asthma are presented in other chapters. Our approach to treatment of the asthmatic child focuses on the physiological and psychosocial aspects, which are discussed by Fischer and Creer in their respective chapters. When a child continues to be symptomatic on a regular basis after one has attempted to effect control with these approaches, consideration should be given to the use of intermittent or continuous daily drug therapy. The goals of all therapy in bronchial asthma are the prevention of physical and psychological disability, relief of symptoms, resolution of underlying bronchial airway obstruction, maintenance of full functional ability, progress to long-term remission with the eventual withdrawal of antiasthma drugs; in other words, to ensure the child as normal a life as possible compatible with his or her age.

## DECIDING TO PLACE A CHILD ON DAILY MEDICATION

The decision to place a child on daily medication for asthma should not be taken lightly. (Fig. 1) (1). In addition to potential side effects of the medications, other factors must be considered, such as cost, the psychological impact of labeling a child as having a chronic disease that requires daily medication, and the changes in the life of the child and family that will take place by the administration of daily medication. All physicians should have some guidelines to follow to establish whether a child's asthma will require chronic daily therapy. Our own criteria for putting a child on continuous therapy include the following:

1. An average of one or more asthma attacks per month requiring the use of several medications for several days.
2. Asthma episodes less frequent but severe enough to require emergency room therapy and/or hospital admission.
3. A pattern of asthma that leads to school absences, waking up at night, or limitation of normal activities, such as running and playing.

A summary statement of these criteria might be: Daily medication should begin if the extent of asthma is associated with significant change from normal daily life. It should be noted that in the future our criteria may change as we learn more about the long-term effects of asymptomatic airway dysfunction. As more specific antiasthma medications with limited or no side effects become available in the future, we may consider daily therapy at an earlier time.

There is on the part of the physician and parents a certain reluctance to use continuous drug therapy. This probably exists because of a lack of ability to predict the negative effects of asthma on the child's physical, psychological, and social life. Unfortunately, in many instances bronchial asthma in childhood is underdiagnosed and undertreated, which may result in unnecessary emergency room visits and hospitalizations directly related to loss of time at work and school. The increase in morbidity and mortality in the last 25 years from asthma, which is discussed in the chapter by Sly, has led to the identification of a number of risk factors that include the following: underrecognition of the severity of asthma, excessive reliance on bronchodilator therapy, undertreatment with "anti-inflammatory" drugs, and delayed introduction of corticosteroid therapy in acute situations.

Education of parents and children is of crucial importance in providing optimal therapy. They require insight into the need for prophylactic medications, efficient use of drug delivery techniques, and compliance. The rationale for specific aspects of the management plan must be re-emphasized at each return visit. If parents and patients do not agree with the recommendations by their physician, all attempts at therapy will fail. Monitoring of the outcome of treatment is also critically important and should include objective assessment of airway obstruction with home peak-flow readings and office spirometry, together with a high level of sensitivity to possible adverse effects. Each child with asthma is different, and the general approach must be focused on the particular needs of the individual child.

We need to recognize that the child with asthma requires chronic therapy before there is a significant alteration in the life of the child and the family. The goals established by all concerned—parents, patients, and physicians—should be a happy child who can experience normal growth and development.

## CURRENTLY AVAILABLE DRUGS

### Beta-Adrenergic Agents

Adrenergic drugs have been known for over 5000 years since the Chinese first used the herb Ma-Huang (*Ephedra vulgaris*), a substance obtained from several plants by the Emperor Chen Nung. The active ingredient was obtained for the first time in its pure form in 1887, in the compound ephedrine, which was used by oral ingestion. The second in a long line of similarly acting preparations was epinephrine, which was initially synthesized in 1904, and shown to have bronchodilator activity. This drug, however, is not active by the oral route. It was not until 1924 that the Western world first was introduced to these agents by the work of Chen

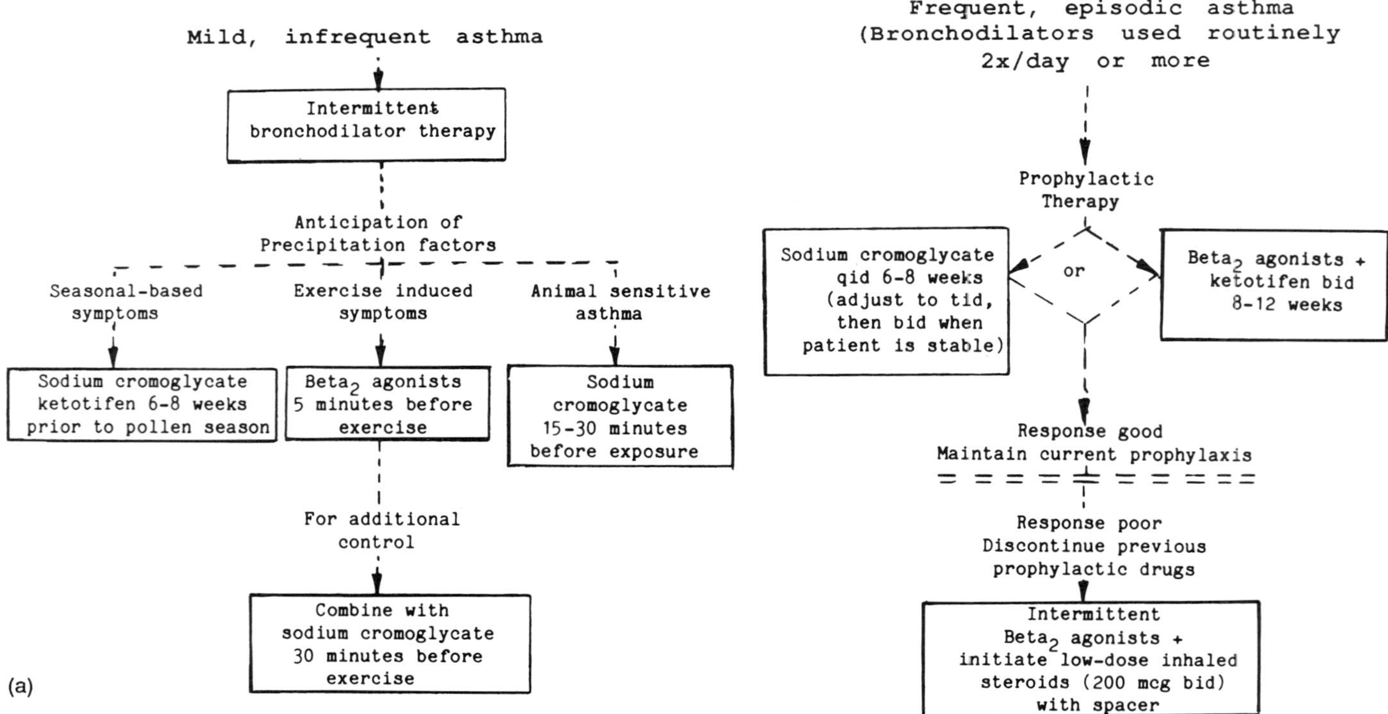
Mild, infrequent asthma
Intermittent bronchodilator therapy
Anticipation of Precipitation factors
Seasonal-based symptoms
Exercise induced symptoms
Animal sensitive asthma
Sodium cromoglycate ketotifen 6-8 weeks prior to pollen season
Beta$_2$ agonists 5 minutes before exercise
Sodium cromoglycate 15-30 minutes before exposure
For additional control
Combine with sodium cromoglycate 30 minutes before exercise
Frequent, episodic asthma (Bronchodilators used routinely 2x/day or more
Prophylactic Therapy
or
Sodium cromoglycate qid 6-8 weeks (adjust to tid, then bid when patient is stable)
Beta$_2$ agonists + ketotifen bid 8-12 weeks
Response good
Maintain current prophylaxis
Response poor
Discontinue previous prophylactic drugs
Intermittent
Beta$_2$ agonists + initiate low-dose inhaled steroids (200 mcg bid) with spacer

(a)

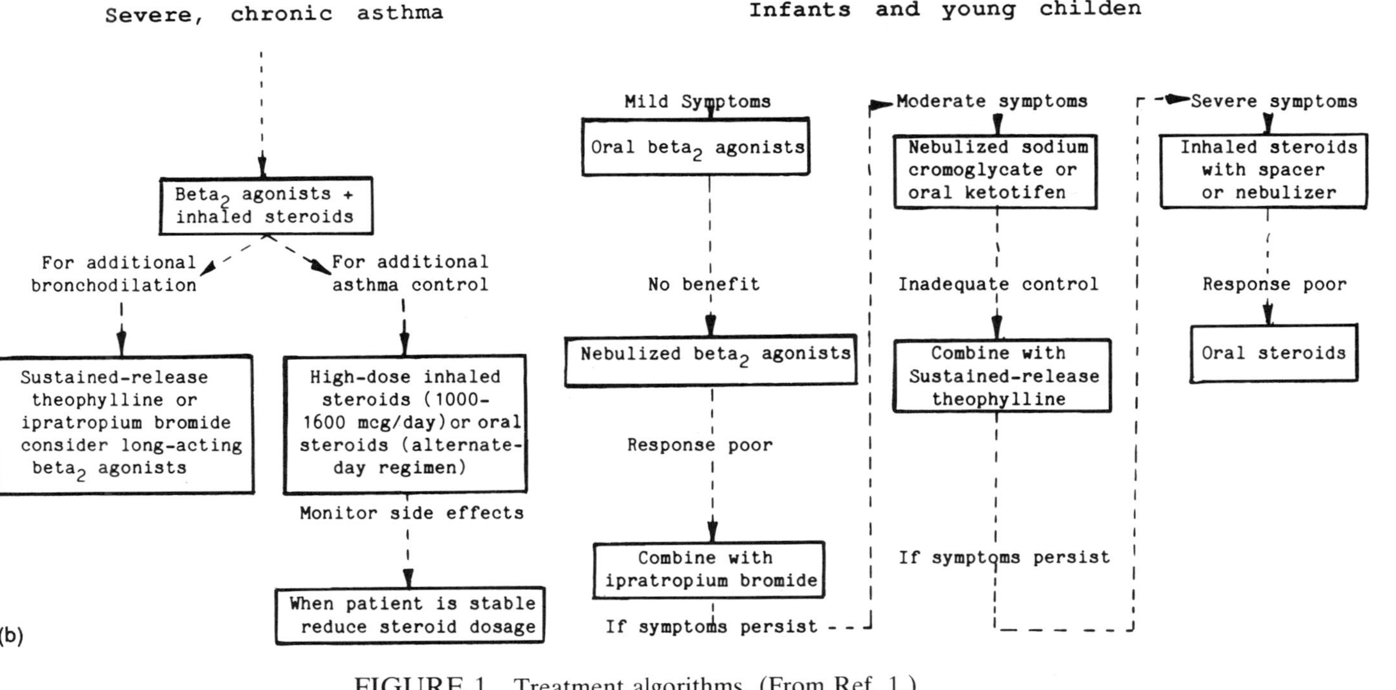


FIGURE 1 Treatment algorithms. (From Ref. 1.)

and Schmidt (2). These agents, despite their relative lack of potency, short duration of action, and toxicity from actions on both the cardiovascular and central nervous systems, remained the mainstay of therapy for asthma. A major advancement in the development of future adrenergic agents came with the description in 1948 by Ahlquist of alpha- and beta-adrenergic receptor sites responsible for the excitatory and inhibitory actions of these agents on the cardiovascular and respiratory systems (3). Another major advancement came in 1967, when Lands et al. differentiated the beta receptors into beta-1, which had their primary effect in the heart and smooth muscle of the gastrointestinal tract, and beta-2, which primarily were found in and affected the smooth muscles of the bronchi, uterus, and arteries of skeletal muscles (4). The long history of research and development of the adrenergic agents reflects the specification of the receptor activity of these agents. Isoproterenol, first developed in 1940, was the first agent not to have primary activity on the alpha-receptor sites but was noted to effect stimulation of both the beta-1 and beta-2 receptors. Metaproterenol, introduced in 1961, represented the first of the beta agonists with increased selectivity for the beta-2 receptor sites. This agent became the first agent to avoid the undesired side effects of stimulation of the beta-1 receptors of the cardiovascular system (5).

### *Relationship Between Structure and Function of the Adrenergic Bronchodilators*

Many modifications of the basic nucleus of the adrenergic agent have been introduced to allow not only a greater selectivity for the beta-2 receptor but also oral use of these medications with prolonged duration of action. Being able to understand the molecular structure of these bronchodilators will help the physician to choose the beta-adrenergic bronchodilator most suitable for a patient. The basic structure of the catecholamine compound has a benzene ring and an ethylamine side chain (Fig. 2) (6). The first agents, including epinephrine and norepinephrine, have two hydroxyl (OH) groups at the 3, 4 positions of the benzene ring. To increase sympathomimetic activity, it is necessary to have a two-carbon-atom side chain. The addition of another hydroxyl group on the beta carbon will also significantly increase the beta-agonist activity. The hydroxyl groups in the 3, 4 position are rapidly inactivated by enzymes in the intestinal wall and in the liver, thus preventing the oral use of these agents. Also, the catecholamine structure found in isoproterenol is metabolized by catechol-O-methyltransferase (COMT), which limits its duration of action. Monoamine oxidase induces degradation of the terminal amino group, decreasing the duration of bronchodilatation (Fig. 2).

To give a more prolonged duration of action and allow oral administration, the hydroxyl group in position four has been moved to position

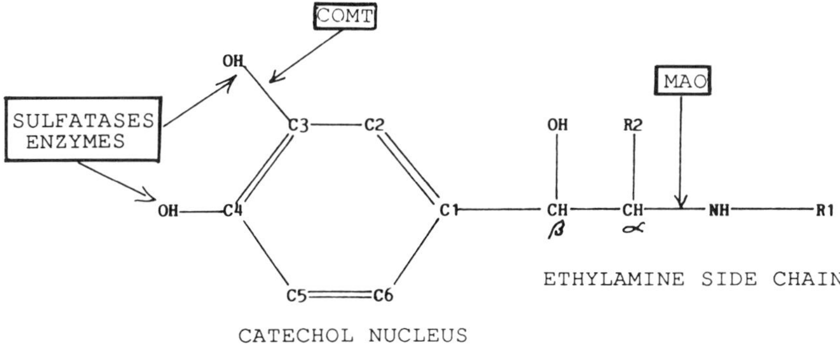


FIGURE 2 Basic structure of a catecholamine. Sites of metabolism.

five (resorcinols such as metaproterenol, fenoterol, and terbutaline) or the 3-hydroxyl is replaced by a hydroxymethyl group in the saligenins (albuterol) (Fig. 3) It has been noted that the size of the N-alkyl substitution on the ethylamine side chain determines the alpha- and beta-adrenergic activity. The larger the side chain, the less the alpha activity.

More selective beta-2 activity is enhanced or can be obtained by substituting an ethyl group on the alpha carbon (7).

Scalabrin et al. (8) studied asthmatic children during acute attacks of asthma. They found that the inhaled route is the best choice for treatment. There were no significant differences between fenoterol, salbutamol, and terbutaline, administered by nebulization, regarding onset, peak, and duration of activity as well as side effects, including tremor.

The action of these beta-2 agonists (fenoterol, salbutamol, and terbutaline) is well established. Terbutaline is safe, even in high dosages (9). Nebulized salbutamol is also safe and effective, and can be used for wheezing infants as well as for children of all ages (10). Studies in children were not able to demonstrate any effect on fine motor performance in children with chronic asthma (11). In another study in which salbutamol was administered orally in a controlled-release tablet, it was found to be a safe and effective alternative to sustained-release theophylline for management of patients with asthma (12).

In a study of young asthmatic children (mean age, 11.8 years) who demonstrated a positive bronchial challenge to *Dermatophagoides pteronyssinus*, the administration of an inhaled fenoterol was able to reverse the fall in functional expiratory volume in 1 sec ($FEV_1$) significantly during the late allergic asthmatic reaction. The authors concluded that beta-agonists probably contribute only a masking effect without truly inhibiting the late asthmatic reaction (13). Recently, Yani et al. (14) showed that the

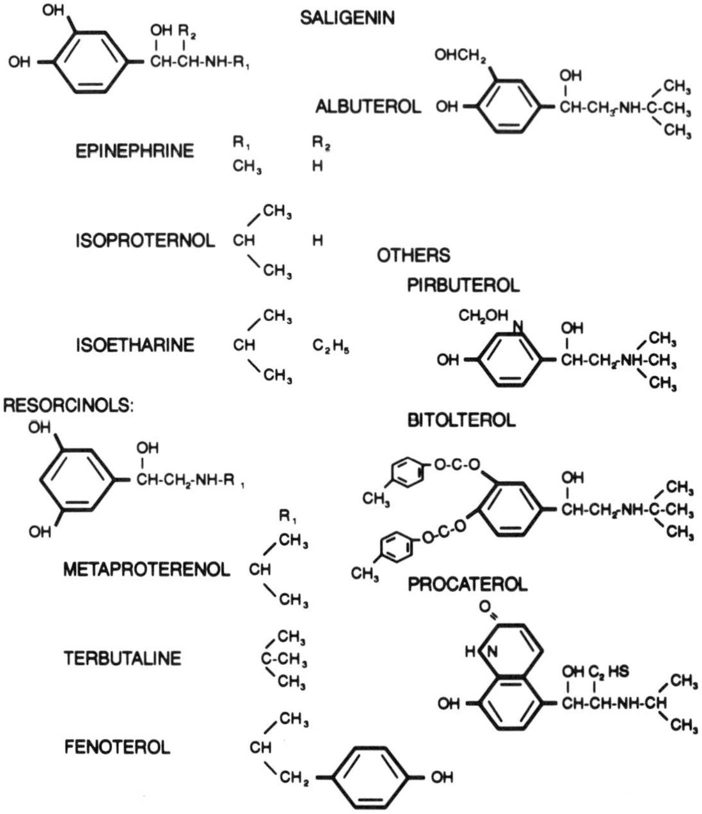

FIGURE 3 Chemical structures of catecholamines.

predominant sites of bronchodilatation from inhaled fenoterol are both the central and peripheral airways. This may or may not be the case with other beta-2 agonists. Several other beta-2 agonists have been developed in recent years. Procaterol, administered predominantly by the oral route, has been shown to have a bronchodilating effect in children with moderate to severe asthma (15). Pirbuterol, a new inhaled beta-agonist, has also been studied and found to be effective in children (16). Another mechanism to extend the half-life of the inhaled beta-agonist has been to establish a prodrug that is hydrolyzed by the lung. This is the case with bitolterol mesylate, which is hydrolyzed by lung esterases to the active preparation (16).

While increasing the beta-2 selectivity of the adrenergic agonists, there has been an enhancement of the appearance of tremor by stimulation of the beta-2 receptors in the skeletal muscle. Although it is believed that these beta-2 receptors are the same as in the bronchi, dissociation of the two effects has been achieved. After prolonged therapy the tremor appears to diminish while the bronchodilator effects continues, and this may indicate a difference in the type of receptors in these two organ systems. These differences may be either in the quality or quantity of receptors present in the these tissue sites. Despite these potential differences, it has been demonstrated that while the continuous use of beta-2 agonists increases the basal tremor it is accompanied by a decrease in the subjective perception by patients of this tremor. It was concluded in one study that one part of the tolerance appreciated by the patients may in fact be due to the increase in basal values (17). It appears that the best way to minimize the problem of tremor is to begin with a lower dosage of beta-agonists and to increase it gradually over a period of weeks (18).

Other beta-adrenergic stimulants are constantly being developed. Work on these agents has predominantly been in adults thus far. Two of these agents are broxaterol and tulobuterol (19,20).

Another issue in the development of beta-adrenergic agents is to establish a longer duration of action. Two new compounds have been developed with this in mind: formoterol and salmeterol (Fig. 4) (21), both already in clinical use. VonBerg and Berdel (22), in a group of 15 young asthmatic subjects, compared metered-dose inhaled (MDI) salbutamol with formoterol. Formoterol-induced bronchodilatation was significantly greater at 4 and 10 hr after medication administration; at 12 hr only formoterol con-

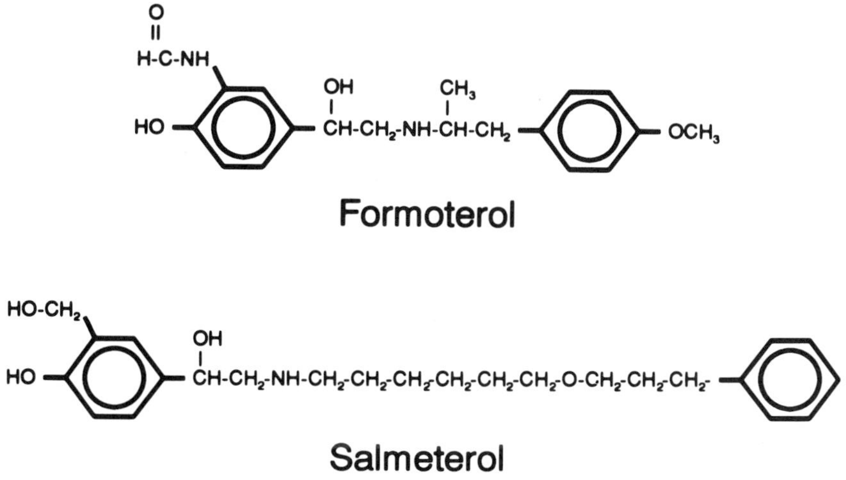

FIGURE 4 Chemical structures of formoterol and salmeterol.

tinued to give bronchodilatation. In another work with 66 children the same authors found that the best protection against exercise-induced asthma was obtained with formoterol. They also found that bronchial hyperreactivity decreased after withdrawal of formoterol, as confirmed by histamine and cold air challenges (22). Becker et al. (24) showed in 16 children that inhaled formoterol resulted in bronchodilatation and protection against methacholine challenge equivalent to that of inhaled salbutamol. However, the duration of action of formoterol was greater (12 hr vs. 3–6 hr). In another study looking at the dose relationships of formoterol, Becker and Simons (25) showed that protection from methacholine challenge by 12 or 24 μg of formoterol at 12 hr was equivalent to that of salbutamol 200 μg at 3 hr after medication. The patients receiving salbutamol achieved an $FEV_1$ of 120% of baseline at 30 min but returned to the baseline value by 3 hr. After both test dosages of formoterol the peak $FEV_1$ was 118% at 3 hr and remained significantly above baseline for the 12 hr of study. Recently, the same authors performed a double-blind study with 25 asthmatic children receiving formoterol (24 μg twice daily) or salbutamol (200 μg twice daily) for 4 weeks and then crossed the patients over to the other drug for a second 4 week study period. Peak expiratory flow rate (PEFR) and $PC_{20}$ did not change when salbutamol was administered first. PEFR and $PC_{20}$ increased significantly when formoterol was given first and this improvement was sustained for the additional 4 weeks (26). Similar protective effects of formoterol against hyperventilation with cold air have been demonstrated by Malo et al. (27). Kemp et al. (28) showed that in young asthmatic adults (mean age, 26 years) salmeterol administered every 12 hr by MDI produced bronchodilatation for 12 hr with no evidence of subsensitivity. There is some suggestion that both salmeterol and formoterol have anti-inflammatory activity, which would enhance their therapeutic advantage (29). However, more research is necessary in children before widespread use of these agents in this age group. Bambuterol can be included in the class of long-acting beta agonists. It is a prodrug of terbutaline, and when given by oral route 24 hr bronchodilatation has been observed (30).

### *Mechanism of Action*

Beta agonists induce airway relaxation by a direct effect on beta receptors located in the smooth muscle. It appears that stimulation of the beta-2 adrenergic receptor sites activates the enzyme adenyl cyclase. Activation of this enzyme will convert intracellular ATP to cyclic AMP (cAMP). The precise mechanism of action of this biochemical event may remain unknown, but it is suggested that the increase in cyclic AMP enhances the binding of intracellular calcium to the cell membrane and endoplasmic reticulum. With a reduction of available cytoplasmic calcium ion, relaxation of the smooth muscle will follow. Other effects of beta-adrenergic agents that have been described are reduction of mucous gland secretion, diminished release of mediators from mast cells in the airway, diminished release of acetylcholine from postganglionic cholinergic nerves in the airway, increase in the frequency of cilial motion, enhancement of mucociliary clearance from the lungs, suppression of cellular permeability, and increase in the flux of water and chloride ions into the bronchial lumen (31,32). There are several reports in the literature of the development of subsensitivity following the long-term administration of beta-adrenergic bronchodilators. This subsensitivity is thought to be a receptor phenomenon and is not specific for any particular beta-adrenergic agent. Tolerance in nonbronchial beta-adrenergic receptor responses in humans, including tremor, heart rate, lymphocyte and leukocyte cyclic AMP levels, and downregulation of the beta-receptor number, have been described (33,34). The development of clinically relevant tolerance after long-term treatment with a beta-2 agonist has not, however, been clearly established. Some investigators suggest that the loss of bronchodilator responsiveness affects the duration of action rather than the peak effect that has been obtained. There is ample evidence to indicate that beta-adrenergic agents continue to be effective bronchodilators with (35) or without (36) the development of subsensitivity during prolonged administration. It has also been demonstrated that the administration of corticosteroids will markedly enhance the responsiveness of beta receptors to beta-adrenergic agonists (37). This is a very important clinical finding and emphasizes the need for prompt corticosteroid therapy in patients in status asthmaticus who have been previously receiving beta-adrenergic therapy. Sears et al. (38) recently studied the effects of regular compared with on demand inhaled beta-agonist therapy in 88 adult patients. The regular use of a beta agonist (fenoterol) was associated with an increased bronchial hyperreactivity as measured by methacholine challenge, and with a more difficult control of asthma. Their recommendation was to use beta-2 agonists only for relief of acute symptoms. They also stated that high-dosage inhaled corticosteroid therapy did not prevent the development of adverse effects of beta-2 agonists.

A similar increase in bronchial hyperreactivity to histamine was observed by Schayck et al. (36) during a 1 year study of salbutamol in patients with asthma or chronic obstructive pulmonary disease (COPD). The bronchial hyperreactivity returned to baseline when the beta agonist therapy was discontinued and ipratropium bromide by inhalation was substituted for 6 months. This increase in bronchial hyperreactivity was not thought to be due to subsensitization of beta-2 adrenoreceptors.

Weinberger (39) has also expressed concern over the repeated use of sympathomimetic bronchodilators. This, however, is not universally accepted. Raes et al. (40) studied inhaled fenoterol administered for 4 months and did not find any effect on bronchial hyperreactiveness in response to histamine challenge. At present, the prudent recommendation for the treatment of children with mild to moderate asthma is that beta-2 agonists should be used on an intermittent and not continuous basis (i.e., only as rescue therapy).

### *Adverse Reactions*

Relatively nonselective beta-adrenergic agents have been associated with production of tachycardia and other disturbances of cardiac rhythm. However, it must be noted that all beta-adrenergic agents may have some side effects with systemic administration, including nervousness, irritability, insomnia, and tremor. These side effects can be markedly reduced by aerosol administration of the more selective beta-2 agonists.

Beta-2 receptor stimulation can induce metabolic responses to which tolerance has been shown to develop with chronic administration (41). Hyperglycemia can occur from glucagon release and glycogenolysis. Entrance of potassium into muscle cells can include hypokalemia, which has not been shown to be a major problem with chronic therapy. However, this has not been sufficiently studied when beta-agonists are used excessively during the acute attack. It has been shows that the $PaO_2$ can fall with ventilation–perfusion alterations during acute exacerbations of asthma. This has not been shown to be profound and is of brief duration (42). Other adverse experiences noted with beta-agonists include paradoxical bronchospasm (43), and relaxation of the gastroesophageal sphincter with oral administration (44), but there has been no evidence of a change in esophageal function with oral administration of salbutamol (44).

### *Drug Interactions*

Numerous medications commonly used by asthmatic patients can react with beta-adrenergic agents. Those discussed in this section represent the most common interactions, but it must be noted that many medications can interact with the beta-adrenergic agents or their receptors and produce untoward side effects or potentiation of action. Individuals with hypertension often have difficulty with these agents. The concomitant use of beta-agonist agents with a monoamine oxidase (MAO) inhibitor can induce severe hypertension and, rarely, death. On the other hand, adrenergic bronchodilators may be effective in patients receiving beta-receptor blockers. As mentioned above, the use of beta agonists with corticosteroids will enhance the effectiveness of the beta agonists in both their peak and duration of effects.

Some concern has been raised about the potential synergistic cardiotoxicity with the combination of beta-adrenergic agents and theophylline. This association has most recently been raised by the increase rate of deaths from asthma in New Zealand (45). However, it should be pointed out that numerous studies in the literature on the use of these agents in patients with acute and chronic asthma have indicated that with the combination of these agents there is an improved response without any evidence of significant increase in cardiovascular side effects (46), if the recommended dosages for both drugs are used. It also has been reported that no therapeutic advantage was seen with routine use of this combination (47). Nevertheless, it is common practice to combine inhaled beta-2 agonists with intravenous aminophylline for the acute management of an exacerbation of asthma. Also, combinations of inhaled beta-2 agonists with oral slow-release xanthine products have been used for patients with more severe chronic asthma (48,49).

### *Administration*

The beta-2 agonists currently available for the treatment of chronic asthma can be delivered by oral, parenteral, or inhalational routes (Table 1). The best method to administer beta-2 agonists is by inhalation (50). Proper use of MDIs or aerosol generated by nebulizers will produce a rapid onset of action with a reduction in the degree of systemic absorption and subsequent adverse effects. The duration of bronchodilatation seems to be related to the type of beta-adrenergic agent used, the dosage of medication administered, and the patient's initial physiological state. Numerous studies comparing the use of inhaled to parenteral adrenergic agents have failed to show any advantage of parenteral therapy (51,52).

Available methods of inhalation of beta-adrenergic agents are either by nebulization of an aqueous solution with an air compressor (53), or with the use of a MDI, Rotahaler, Diskhaler, or Turbuhaler. The most common problem with the MDI is incorrect technique, thus reducing the available medication for delivery to the conducting airways. With more attention being paid to education of the patient as well as the availability of spacers attached to the MDI, there is less likelihood of mistake and an increased amount of potential medication delivered (54,55). The maximum amount of medication reaching the lungs appears to be approximately 10–14%, even with most effective methods. There are at present insufficient data to determine whether a role exists for the combined use of both oral and inhaled beta agonists on a regular schedule in the treatment of asthma (56). In some children who are unable to inhale the drugs by device, the oral route can be used. The lack of suitable assays for serum concentration for these drugs means that the dosage remains somewhat empirical (57).

TABLE 1 Recommended Dosages for Beta-2 Adrenergic Agents

| Drug | Oral Route | Inhaled |
|---|---|---|
| Metaproterenol | Less than 6 years: 1.3–2.6 mg/kg/day 6–9 years: 10 mg 3 or 4 times daily More than 9 years: 20 mg 3 or 4 times daily | MDI: 650 μg/puff, 2 puffs every 3–4 hr as needed 5% nebulized solution, 0.2 ml every 4–6 hr as needed |
| Terbutaline | 0.075 mg/kg 3 times daily | MDI: 200 μg/puff, 2 puffs every 4–6 hr as needed |
| Fenoterol | 0.2 mg/kg 3 times daily | MDI: 200 μg/puff, 1–2 puffs every 4–6 hr as needed 0.5% nebulized solution, 0.01 ml/kg every 4–6 hr as needed |
| Salbutamol | 0.15 mg/kg 3 times daily | MDI: 100 μg/puff, 2 puffs every 4–6 hr as needed 0.5% nebulized solution, 0.02 ml every 4–6 hr as needed |
| Procaterol | 0.5 mg/kg tid | MDI: 10 μg/puff, 1–2 puffs every 6 hr as needed |
| Pirbuterol | 1–5 years: 3.75 mg qid more than 5 years: 7.5 mg qid | MDI: 200 μg/puff, 2 puffs every 6 hr as needed |
| Bitolterol | — | MDI: 370 μg/puff, 2 puffs every 4–6 hr as needed |

## Cromolyn Sodium

Disodium cromoglycate (cromolyn) was developed in the early 1960s from analogs of the naturally occurring *Cromone khellin* found in a Middle Eastern plant, *Ammi visnaga*. Cromolyn, which is a bis-cromone drug, is unique in having been introduced for clinical use following a very small number of clinical trials of its efficacy and safety. Initially this nonbronchodilator drug was shown to be effective in inhibiting early- and late-phase asthmatic reactions and exercise-induced asthma, and subsequently became established as an effective, safe agent for treating chronic asthma. Despite the fact that it has been available for over 20 years, its mechanisms of action remain unknown. Its ability to stabilize and prevent degranulation of mast cells, at first thought to be important, has been discounted since the later development of analogs that are potent inhibitors of mast cells proved to have little clinical effect. In recent years other mechanisms of biological activity have been suggested. Allergen–IgE-mediated activation of inflammatory cells including neutrophils, macrophages, and platelets can be inhibited by cromolyn as can nonspecific activation of neutrophils, monocytes, and eosinophils by the peptide FMLP and the polysaccharide zymosan. Nonallergenic stimulation of the bronchi with sulfur dioxide, nebulized water, cold air, and bradykinin can be inhibited by cromolyn, probably unrelated to mast cell degranulation. Inhalation of cromolyn prior to a single allergen challenge will inhibit both the early- and late-phase asthmatic responses and the development of bronchial hyperresponsiveness. The inhibitory effect of cromolyn on the late-phase asthmatic response, which is inflammatory in nature, may perhaps reflect its therapeutic effect in chronic asthma, including nonallergic asthma, since similar inhibition is evident after exposure to ozone, viral infection, and cigarette smoke.

Cromolyn is poorly absorbed orally (1%) and by inhalation, and when given parenterally under experimental conditions is excreted unchanged in the urine and bile. After inhalation its clinical half-life is 3–5 hr, peak plasma levels are present at 15 min, and 45% of total urinary excretion occurs within 1 hr.

### *Efficacy*

Cromolyn is a prophylactic agent, has no bronchodilator action, and plays no role in the management of episodes of acute severe asthma. It must be used continuously over long periods of time to have an impact on chronic asthma. Long-term studies (58) in which the criterion of efficacy was the avoidance of the need for corticosteroid therapy showed a success rate in children treated with cromolyn of 71% compared to placebo of 24% over 1 year. The success rate by the fourth and fifth years had leveled off at 65%, (Fig. 5). The majority of failures occurred within the first weeks or months, but about 33% occurred after 1 year during which good control of the asthma had been maintained. No clinical features could be clearly identified to indicate those children who would do well on cromolyn; those with more severe symptoms at a young age were less likely to respond. The presence or degree of allergy as indicated by the number of positive skin tests, IgE level, or presence of eosinophils was unrelated to the success or failure of cromolyn therapy. There is no evidence of a steroid-sparing effect in children, and follow-up of treatment failures with cromolyn indicate that few if any can effectively return to cromolyn therapy in the future.

Cromolyn inhaled before exercise can inhibit exercise-induced asthma in about 60% of affected children. Because it is so poorly absorbed there is no effect on heart rate nor any central nervous system stimulatory effect,

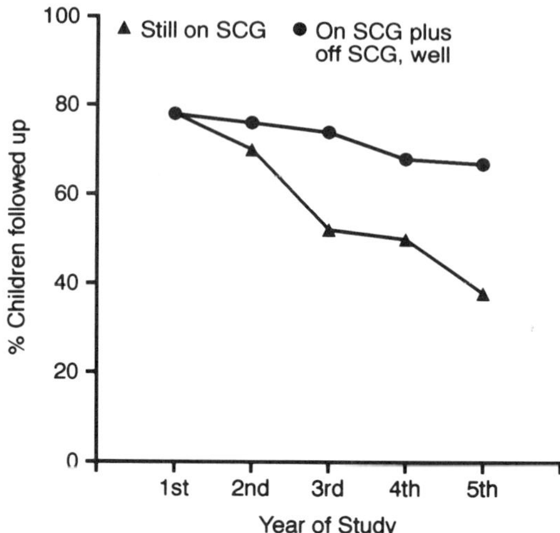


FIGURE 5 Results of the long-term follow-up of a group of asthmatic children treated with sodium cromogylcate (SCG). Two-thirds of the group remained well controlled for up to 5 years and never needed steroids. Of these SCG treatment successes, the triangle symbols (▲) show the total proportion of the whole group and the circle symbols (●) show those still needed to take SCG (From Ref. 58).

and it is widely accepted by athletic authorities. Owing to its short clinical half-life, cromolyn should be inhaled 20–30 min before exercise is commenced. Compared to inhaled beta-2-adrenergic drugs, cromolyn is much less effective in preventing exercise-induced asthma; the former drugs are usually preferred. In children who develop late-phase as well as early-phase asthmatic responses to exercise, probably an uncommon occurrence, combined therapy with albuterol and cromolyn before exercise should be considered. Tachyphylaxis with cromolyn, which occurs in rats, is not found in human tissues and is not a clinical problem.

### *Adverse Effects*

Cromolyn is one of the safest antiasthma drugs available. Short- and long-term studies with up to 10 years of treatment have shown no serious adverse effects. Transient skin rashes (2%), irritation of the throat and cough (25%), and bronchospasm, rarely, have been reported in response to the dry powdered form administered by spinhaler and, to a lesser extent, with the nebulizer solution, which is hypotonic. The bronchoconstrictive effect can be prevented by prior or concomitant inhalation of a beta-adrenergic drug. The MDI delivery system is much better tolerated, especially if the drug is inhaled via a spacer device. However, several inhalations at one time may be required to obtain the same therapeutic effect as the higher-dosage spinhaler capsule. Other very rare adverse effects include urticaria and dermatitis, myositis, gastroenteritis, upper airway obstruction, pulmonary infiltrates with cardiac failure and eosinophilia, and anaphylaxis.

*Indications*

When initially introduced cromolyn was positioned as a second-line add-on drug for use in asthma. It proved to be of little value in improving control of chronic asthma in those who were receiving corticosteroid therapy and had an overall efficacy comparable to oral sustained-action theophylline, but with minimal adverse effects (59). Theophylline, on the other hand, does modestly improve control of symptoms in some steroid-dependent asthmatic subjects. Double-blind placebo-controlled trials have subsequently substantiated the role of cromolyn in mild to moderately severe asthma as a first-line therapy used over prolonged periods to prevent asthmatic episodes. Despite several attempts to delineate clinical features that would predict a good outcome, responders cannot be clearly identified. Those with mild rather then severe asthma are much more likely to respond, but even within this large subgroup "without a trial of the drug no one can say with certainty whether or not a given patient will improve with treatment" (60). Cromolyn may be especially effective given via nebulizer as preventive therapy in younger children with frequent asthmatic episodes, which are often induced by viral infection. The effect of anticipated allergen exposure, such as upcoming pollen seasons or visits to homes with family pets, can be ameliorated and often prevented by prior treatment with cromolyn. Doses should commence four times daily 3 or 4 weeks before the pollen season or a few days before other types of allergen exposure, and continue for 1–2 weeks afterwards.

*Administration*

Cromolyn is currently available in a pure pelletized powder form (sodium $< 1.8$ mg) with a 20 mg dose inhaled via a Spinhaler or Halermatic; as a micronized powder with sorbitan trioleate as an excipient and fluorocarbons as propellants in a MDI inhaler, 1 mg/activation; and as a nebulizer solution containing 1% (20 mg) in a 2 ml ampoule of distilled water. The drug must be administered initially four times daily and an effect may be evident in some children with 2–4 weeks. Often a longer trial of 6–8 weeks is necessary before a therapeutic effect is evident. During the initial phase of preventive therapy it is important to provide symptomatic control, preferably by regular use of inhaled beta-adrenergic bronchodilator drugs, which can then be withdrawn. When a therapeutic effect is established cromolyn therapy should be continued 3–4 times daily for 6 months. Twice-daily dosing is less effective. When the drug is withdrawn, this should be done gradually over 2–4 weeks. If there has been treatment failure and the child has advanced to inhaled steroid therapy, the cromolyn can be immediately discontinued. The MDI should be used with a spacer device to minimize irritation of the airway, difficulty in co-ordinating activation and inspiration, and to enhance penetration of the drug to the lungs. The 4–5 mg dose required for a similar therapeutic effect as a single spincap or nebule may make this method of delivery more expensive and less convenient. Problems may arise with incomplete emptying of spincaps in the Spinhaler or Halermatic, loss of powder from the unit by mishandling after the capsule is punctured, and from too rapid or too slow nebulization of the nebulizer solution. Nebulizers should run for 10–15 min (2 ml volume to dryness) to ensure adequate exposure of the airway to the drug.

It is unclear whether therapy with cromolyn has a lasting effect, so careful monitoring of the patient is required to ascertain both if an initial response if forthcoming and if the improvement is maintained when the drug is withdrawn. Because of the excellent safety record, long-term therapy can be entertained.

## Nedocromil

The search for a more potent analog of cromolyn produced in the early 1980s a novel topically active derivative of pyranoquinolone dicarboxylic acid, nedocromil sodium. The drug has similar properties to cromolyn in some animal models and is more potent in others. It has been found to inhibit release of the inflammatory mediators histamine, leukotriene $C_4$, and prostaglandin $D_2$ from lung mast cells in primates, and histamine from human mast cells. Like cromolyn, nedocromil blocks the bronchoconstrictor effects of exercise, cold air, and sulfur dioxide but not the neuropeptide-releasing factor capsaicin. Nedocromil is available for inhalation via MDI and a nebulizer solution is under development.

### *Efficacy*

There are not direct comparison studies of the efficacy of cromolyn and nedocromil in patients with chronic asthma. A large multicenter, double-blind comparative group study (61) in adults with symptomatically stable asthma who were receiving combinations of oral inhaled corticosteroids, theophylline, and beta-adrenergic drugs showed a modest improvement in symptom scores, bronchodilator use, and peak flow readings. However, by the end of the 12 week treatment period only symptom scores and frequency of asthmatic episodes were significantly different, similar to a previous shorter-term study (62). A double-blind controlled study (63) of 34 subjects documented improvement in lung function (PEFR) but the use of maintenance corticosteroids was unclear. There is evidence of efficacy in adult asthmatic subjects who are not steroid dependent (64) and of inhibition of bronchial hyperresponsiveness provoked by pollen exposure in subjects allergic to grass pollen (65). There is no evidence of a steroid-sparing effect (66). In a comparative study of 202 adults with asthma, nedocromil 16 mg/day was less effective than beclomethasone 400 μg/day (67). The preventive effect and duration of action of nedocromil (4 mg) and cromolyn (20 mg) have been studied in exercise-induced asthma in adults (68). Both drugs were comparable and significantly better than placebo at 20 min after inhalation, but after 2 hr only cromolyn was effective. The efficacy of nedocromil in children with asthma remains to be defined. It will probably find a place in the management of mild to moderately severe disease.

### *Adverse Effects*

Nedocromil appears to be safe in short-term studies in adults. In one study (69), 127 subjects received nedocromil, of whom 7 withdrew mainly because of the taste of the drug, and adverse effects included nausea (13), vomiting (3), bad taste (3), throat irritation (10), and headache (9). There were no effects on hepatic, renal, hematologic functions. In a longer-term open study (64) of 12 months' duration side effects were minor and included cough, wheeze, sore throat, nausea, and bad taste. Longer-term studies of safety, and studies in children are not available.

### *Indications*

Nedocromil is a prophylactic antiasthma drug. It has been introduced as a first-line drug for use in adults with symptomatically mild to moderately severe asthma, possibly as an alternative to low-dosage inhaled steroid therapy. It may offer an alternative to cromolyn or ketotifen but there are no direct comparative studies of efficacy and it is available only as an aerosol from a metered-dose inhaler. The taste of the drug may limit its use in children. As with other drugs used in mild to moderately severe asthma there is as yet no means of identifying those who will respond without a trial of therapy.

### *Administration*

Nedocromil is available via a metered-dose inhaler, 2 mg per dose. Therapy is initiated with 4 mg four times daily routinely, with a clinical effect being evident in 2–8 weeks. It may then be possible to continue therapy with a frequency of three times or even twice daily, but long-term studies using these dosages and studies in children are not available.

## Ketotifen

Ketotifen is a benzocycloheptathiophene drug first introduced for clinical use in 1979. It was initially identified by its ability to noncompetitively block histamine ($H_1$) receptors, but evidence from studies in animals and with human tissues points to other effects that are potentially antiasthmatic. In animals the drug protects against anaphylactic shock and inhibits antigen-induced bronchoconstriction and bronchial hyperreactivity, attenuates bronchoconstriction provoked by inflammatory mediators, and prevents the influx of eosinophils to the lung. It inhibits activation of human mast cells, degranulation of eosinophils, activation of alveolar macrophages, enhances beta receptor expression on cell membranes, and modifies the priming effect of allergen on target cells. The precise mode of action in asthma remains unclear.

Taken orally, the drug is eliminated with a half-life of 21 hr, being excreted in the urine as an inactive glucuronide metabolite. The pharmacokinetics in children have not been studied, but in a group of 6 infants receiving a 1 mg dose, serum levels double those in adults receiving a 2 mg dose were observed (70). Ketotifen has no inhibitory effect on methacholine-induced bronchial responsiveness (71), but in a study of adolescents and adults it did attenuate bronchial hyperresponsiveness induced by grass pollen in allergic subjects studied during the grass pollen season (72).

### *Efficacy*

Ketotifen was first introduced for clinical use as a second-line drug to be added to regimens of preventive therapy that included cromolyn and inhaled corticosteroids. As with cromolyn, results of early studies were equivocal and confusing, with the results in retrospect often being uninterpretable. Several double-blind placebo-controlled trials in children from 1988 on have shown ketotifen to be effective in reducing the frequency of asthmatic episodes, the severity of asthmatic symptoms, and the need for theophylline and beta-adrenergic bronchodilator therapy in children with mild to moderately severe asthma. In a large study (73) of 189 children aged 2–6 years, 93 receiving active treatment, a significant improvement was found in more than half, evident within 4–8 weeks and reaching a maximum at 12 weeks. The children selected had symptoms present for 4 or more weeks prior to study, or had 3 or more episodes of cough and wheeze of greater than 2 days' duration over a 2 month period, or 5 or more episodes over a 3 month period, representing a moderately severe asthmatic population. Follow-up of younger children, aged 1–4 years, for periods of 4–12 weeks after completing a 12 week course of ketotifen to which they had responded has demonstrated persistent improvement in their asthmatic symptoms (74,75), suggesting a more fundamental change in the pathophysiology of the asthma than simply suppression of symptoms. Ketotifen appears to be more effective in reducing asthmatic symptoms in children than adults.

There are no data demonstrating a steroid-sparing effect in children, but in a study in adults (76) 24% of those taking ketotifen could be weaned from oral maintenance prednisone, compared to 7% of those receiving placebo and the mean reduction in prednisone dosage was significantly greater. Other studies in which ketotifen was added to regimens of multiple therapy including beclomethasone failed to show improvement in symptom scores or reduction in steroid use (77). Further properly designed trials are required to clarify this situation.

A number of studies have shown the antiasthmatic effect of ketotifen to be similar to cromolyn (78), and experience suggests that the same population that responds to one will respond to the other. Ways of identifying this population require further study, but the current role of ketotifen is clearly in the treatment of mild to moderate asthma, making up 75% of the asthmatic population. A recent double-blind placebo-controlled study (79) of 121 infants with atopic dermatitis without a history of cough or wheezing who received ketotifen (0.8–1.2 mg per day) for 1 year found that the incidence of asthma (defined as two separate episodes of wheezing requiring bronchodilator drugs) was significantly less in the active treatment group (13.1%) compared to the placebo group (41.6%) ($p < 0.001$). This interesting observation of successful early intervention with ketotifen suggests a truly prophylactic effect in young children and requires further study.

### *Adverse Effects*

Ketotifen has been evaluated over a prolonged period in postmarketing surveillance programs. Eight thousand asthmatic patients (adult and children) observed for up to 12 months have shown a very low incidence of adverse effects (80). Drowsiness and lethargy experienced by 14% of subjects at 3 months of treatment dropped to 4.7% at 6 months and 2.2% at 12 months. Studies in Canadian children (81) found sedation in 8% (9% on placebo), and weight gain in 5.3% (1.3%). Sedation tends to be transient in children and can often be avoided by using half doses given in the evening for the first 3 or 4 days. Excessive weight gain tends to decrease over 2–3 months of treatment and is modest; in one study (82) an average 2.1 kg for children on active treatment, 1.6 kg for placebo. Thrombocytopenia can occur with ketotifen administered in combination with oral hypoglycaemic agents, which should be avoided. Ketotifen syrup contains benzoate, which should be avoided in those with a history of adverse reactions to benzoate-containing compounds. Because of the initial sedative effect of ketotifen, concomitant administration of antihistamines, sedatives, or alcohol should be undertaken with caution.

### Indications

Ketotifen should be considered as first-line preventive therapy in children with mild to moderately severe asthma, and those with milder asthma are more likely to respond. As with cromolyn no clinical features predict a good therapeutic outcome. Because of the ease of oral administration, ketotifen is of particular value in younger children, increasing compliance and diminishing concern about the quantity of drug reaching the airway, which is a problem with inhaled drugs in patients at this age. Ketotifen is only useful when taken for periods of at least 2–3 months, and has no effect when taken just before exercise in exercise-induced asthma, or in short-term prophylaxis before allergen exposure, for which cromolyn is preferred. Preseasonal therapy continued through the pollen season will effectively prevent the seasonal increase in bronchial hyperreactivity that occurs in grass pollen sensitive asthmatic patients (63). Because of its additional antihistamine effect, ketotifen may be helpful in children who have allergic rhinitis as well as asthma. In Canada ketotifen is currently licensed for use in children aged 3 years and older, whereas in most other countries it can be used in infants as young as the first year of life.

### Administration

Ketotifen is available as a strawberry-flavored syrup, 1 mg/5ml (containing benzoate), and as a small white tablet, 1 mg (benzoate-free). The drug is taken by mouth twice daily, morning and evening, with or without food at a dose of 1 mg (2 mg/per day). Studies in infants have used 1 mg from age 1 year and older and 0.5 mg for children younger than this. Higher dosages (2 mg twice daily) in adolescents and adults have produced a more rapid onset of effect (4–6 weeks) (193), but by 12 weeks the clinical effect may be similar to the 1 mg dosage. The drug should be given as the evening dose only for the first 3–4 days to minimize daytime sedation. Excessive caloric intake should be avoided if appetite stimulation and potentially excessive weight gain occurs. If, after an initial trial of 12 weeks, no benefit is forthcoming the drug should be withdrawn. This can be done without the need for stepwise reduction. If the drug is effective a further 3 months (total 6 months) of treatment should be maintained. If treatment goals have then been reached, the drug can then be discontinued. Subsequent deterioration of disease would suggest that ketotifen therapy should be restarted. Treatment failure usually means that the child should advance to low-dosage inhaled corticosteroid therapy. Switching to cromolyn is unlikely to be effective. Other drugs (e.g., antibiotics, antipyretics) can be given with ketotifen but care should be used with the administration of alcohol-containing formulations or antihistamines, which should be given in half doses initially to prevent possible sedation.

## Inhaled Corticosteroids

The introduction of inhaled corticosteroid therapy to the treatment of asthma in 1972 marked a substantial step forward. Previous trials of inhaled hydrocortisone had shown no therapeutic advantage over oral therapy, but the development of compounds that were more specific and potent in their effect on the lung and had fewer mineralocorticoid and metabolic effects led to their firm establishment in the spectrum of treatments available. Beclomethasone and budesonide are now widely used in the treatment of children. The rationale for preferring inhaled to systemic steroids is exemplified by a study comparing the systemic and antiasthmatic effect of budesonide and prednisone (83). This showed budesonide to be almost 9 times more potent in reducing morning cortisol levels and inducing eosinopenia, whereas its antiasthma effect in reducing the frequency and severity of asthma symptoms and improving lung function was about 60 times greater. This means that a dose of inhaled budesonide one-ninth that of oral prednisone will still be six times more potent in its antiasthma effect. Very low and relatively safe dosages of inhaled steroids, therefore, have great therapeutic potential.

Pharmacokinetic studies show that inhaled steroids have low oral bioavailability and high plasma clearance compared to oral steroids. The amount of drug reaching the systemic circulation depends on the amount removed by first pass through the liver from the portion swallowed and on the amount absorbed through the lung. Newer drugs, such as budesonide, may have greater first-pass effect than beclomethasone but this may only be of marginal clinical significance.

Corticosteroids have a multiplicity of actions, many of which could be important for their beneficial effect in asthma. These include decreased IgE binding to target tissues, reduced mediator release from lung fragments, reduced eosinophil chemotaxis and adherence, transient lymphopenia, reduced T-lymphocyte responses, attenuation of IgE and IgG synthesis, reduced activation of macrophages, enhanced beta-adrenergic receptor expression, potent inhibition of inflammatory edema caused by microvascular hyperpermeability, inhibition of mucus secretion, and complex effects on the function of inflammatory cells. The precise mode(s) of action at a molecular level that are relevant to asthma in humans remain to be defined, but may be related in part to the intracellular induction of the protein lipocortin (84). This inhibits phospholipase $A_2$, an important enzyme in the metabolism of cell-membrane-derived phospholipid mediators such as leukotrienes, prostaglandins, and platelet-activating factor. There may be substantially different effects from inhaled corticosteroids depending on the type of inflammatory cell or tissue involved and on the dosage used.

This can vary widely clinically, from 200 μg to 1600 μg per day or greater, in asthmatic children.

### *Efficacy*

Inhaled corticosteroids are overall much more effective than other forms of prophylactic drug therapy in childhood asthma, but some general principles apply to their use (83). First, the efficacy and side effects are dose dependent, and there is often great variation among patients as to the dosage required. Second, aerosol treatment is not as effective as systemic therapy in patients with acute severe asthma or when substantial airway obstruction is present in patients with chronic asthma. Third, a systemic effect does occur with inhaled steroids as noted above, related to both the swallowed portion that is not removed by first pass through the liver and the portion absorbed through the lung. Fourth, inhaled steroids may be more effective in patients with chronic asthma if taken several times per day rather than once or twice.

In adults (83), a daily dosage of 400 μg of beclomethasone is equivalent in its antiasthmatic effect to 7.5 mg of prednisone. Early studies in children reported improvement in symptoms when they received dosages of 100–800 μg per day. In most children adequate control of asthma can be gained at dosages of 200–600 μg/day with those whose symptoms fall in the moderate to severe range usually needing higher dosages. Studies in adults (86) indicate that dosing frequency is important for clinical effectiveness, four times daily being more effective than twice daily. In children with mild asthma, however, 200 μg twice daily was as effective as 100 μg four times daily (87). Inhaled steroids in dosages of 100–400 μg/day may allow weaning from systemic steroid therapy (88) but treatment periods of up to 5 years may be necessary, and higher dosages of 400–800 μg/day are more effective (89).

Corticosteroids do not have any immediate effect on bronchial hyperresponsiveness, but when given in high dosage for prolonged periods, (9 months in adults), a clinically significant reduction may occur (90). In children, dosages of 600 μg/day for up to 6 months resulted in a statistically significant reduction in bronchial responsiveness to methacholine challenge (91), but the clinical relevance of this observation is unclear since the improvement was less than fourfold from baseline. A ± 2-fold change in $PC_{20}$ was found in children with stable asthma evaluated without steroid therapy over periods of months. Exercise-induced asthma can be diminished by inhaled steroids, but this requires at least 1 month of previous treatment at dosages of 200–800 μg/day, with higher dosages and more prolonged therapy being the most effective (92). Nonresponsiveness in exercise-induced symptoms is not related to the severity of asthma, and it is unclear if more prolonged treatment with increasingly high dosages would be effective.

Oral corticosteroid treatment required over long periods of time for more severe chronic asthma has usually used alternate-day prednisone therapy, with a single morning dose on the treatment day, which helped to minimize adverse effects. It is now evident that the vast majority of such children will respond to sufficiently high dosages of inhaled steroid, but a few will require the additional use of alternate-day prednisone for optimal control of their asthma with the added risk of adverse effects. The macrolide antibiotic troleandomycin, which decreases steroid metabolism, when used specifically with methylprednisolone, enhances steroid effectiveness and toxicity. There is little role for troleandomycin in children, and it is seldom used outside the United States.

It has been suggested, based on adult treatment plans, that inhaled steroids should be first-line therapy in children with asthma, especially since bronchial inflammation may be fundamental to the pathogenesis, and that their use may lead to long-term remission or even cure. This approach must be evaluated in the context of potential toxicity.

### *Adverse Effects*

The adverse effects of systemic steroid therapy have been well known for many years and should be of great concern to physicians who treat children. The risks of inhaled steroid therapy are less clear. Many studies have reported that secretion of cortisol is not suppressed by dosages of up to 800 μg/day, following stimulation with ACTH or analogues. This methodology is somewhat insensitive compared to the measurement of variation in physiological secretion of cortisol and does not test the hypothalamic–pituitary (HP) arm of the HP–adrenal (HPA) axis. Studies (93) of 24 hr urinary free cortisol, in contrast, have shown a dose-dependent decrease in 24 hr urinary free cortisol per gram of creatinine in patients receiving dosages of beclomethasone and budesonide of 200–800 μg/day for 4 weeks. The rise in serum cortisol levels following insulin-induced hypoglycemia is significantly suppressed by similar dosages. There is a dose-dependent suppression of physiological cortisol release between midnight and 6 a.m. by dosages of beclomethasone greater than 400 μg/day, suggesting that dosages up to this level are safe in most children (94). Experience suggests (95,96) that physical stress does not result in adrenal insufficiency in children receiving dosages up to 800 μg/day. This has not been described and the adrenal response to ACTH remains normal, but those studies underline the fact that inhaled steroids in dosages greater than 400μg/day do have a systemic effect, which may be more evident in other tissues. The clinical significance of a quantitative reduction in physiological secretion of cortisol is unknown and long-term evaluation of HPA function or other aspects of cortisol metabolism have not been carried out.

Many studies suggest that treatment with inhaled steroids in dosages of 400–800 μg/day is not associated with impaired growth, and indeed improved control of severe asthma may in itself allow catch-up growth to occur (97). Interpretation of such data is complicated by the observation that a substantial proportion of asthmatic children grow at a slower rate than their nonasthmatic peers but continue to grow for a longer period during adolescence. This may also be true for children with other allergic disease, not simply asthma (98). A study of asthmatic adolescents (99) treated for a mean of 2.7 years showed less rapid growth in the group receiving inhaled beclomethasone (400–800 μg/day) than in the control asthmatic group, and this has been reported in younger children. In a study (100) of inhaled budesonide in preadolescent children aged 6–13 years there was a dose-dependent suppression of growth velocity of the lower leg, measured very accurately by knemometry, with dosages of 200 μg or greater per day for 18 days. Long-term studies that evaluate children through late adolescence are required before it can be assumed that inhaled steroids in dosages commonly employed have no effect on growth.

For many years adults receiving systemic steroids have been known to be at risk for osteoporosis from even low dosages of prednisone. Inhaled beclomethasone in a dosage of 400 μg/per day in adults has been shown (101) to reduce total body calcium by 8.8%, assessed by in vivo neutron activation analysis, comparable to the 9% loss caused by prednisone at a dosage of 8.9 mg/day with calcium supplementation. The effect is not caused by excessive excretion of calcium but by reduced formation of osteocalcin bone matrix protein (102), with a comparable reduction in serum osteocalcin levels being evident for inhaled budesonide 25 μg/kg/day and oral prednisone 15 mg/day. Some adults inhaling less than 800 μg/day of budesonide had reduced osteocalcin levels comparable to those receiving 40 mg oral prednisone. Since, on a per kilogram basis, children are receiving much larger dosages of inhaled steroids, possibly modified by the use of spacers, an even greater adverse effect might be expected. There are no studies of these effects in children.

Some 20–30% of patients receiving daily oral steroid therapy will develop posterior subcapsular cataracts (103,104) and 20% of those receiving low-dose alternate day therapy will do so if treated for more than 2 years (105). Cataract formation has also be reported in some patients receiving inhaled beclomethasone (99,106). The suggested dosage of prednisone required for cataract formation is 10 mg/day for 1 year (107). This corresponds, in terms of systemic effect, to 1200 μg/day of budesonide in a 70 kg adult or 340 μg/day in a 20 kg 6-year-old child, which is well within the dosage range used in children and less than the dosage often required to control asthma. There are no systematic studies of cataract formation in children receiving inhaled steroids therapy of many months' duration.

Cough, bronchoconstriction, and hoarseness caused by an irritant effect, dysphonia from bilateral vocal cord paresis related to local steroid myopathy, and oropharyngeal candidiasis are rare in children. The latter can be avoided by rinsing the mouth and throat after inhalation, and effectively treated with oral nystatin, which permits continued steroid therapy.

Other adverse effects seem less likely, but their incidence is unclear. Bronchial mucosal atrophy has not been found with short-term inhaled steroid use (12–18 months) in adults, but there are no studies in children. Beclomethasone is absorbed more rapidly from the bronchi than skin, suggesting that mucosal effects may be less. Problems such as weight gain, hypertension, hyperglycemia, behavioral change, and immunosuppression that occur with systemic steroids have not been described.

### *Indications*

Inhaled corticosteroids are the prophylactic drugs of choice for use in children with moderate to severe asthma. From a clinical perspective this group of children, making up about 20% of the asthmatic population, is characterized by recurring episodes lasting for several days at a time with frequent loss of school time, emergency physician visits, nocturnal symptoms, and easily provoked asthmatic symptoms on exercise with a greatly restricted degree of physical activity. Dosages of beclomethasone or budesonide should begin in the intermediate range, 600–800 μg/day, inhaled two to four times daily. Four times per day dosing is more effective but may be associated with poor compliance, so that twice daily inhalations are often more practical. If the asthma is not controlled after a trial period of 4–6 weeks, the daily dosage should be increased in 200 μg steps to 1600 μg/per day at a similar intervals. If initial peak flow readings or spirometry indicate a degree of bronchial obstruction that is irreversible with inhaled bronchodilator where the PEFR or $FEV_1$ does not increase above 50% of predicted value, a 10–14 day course of oral prednisone 1–2 mg/kg/day (up to 30 mg twice daily) would be indicated. This should be followed by a reduction in dosage of 5 mg every second day, starting with the evening dose, until the prednisone is withdrawn. Inhaled steroid should be started in full dosage when the reduction in prednisone dosage commences. It is important that the PEFR or $FEV_1$ be monitored to ensure that airway obstruction has been relieved. Children with chronic asthma often have a poor perception of airway obstruction and may be apparently free of symptoms despite marked bronchial obstruction, sometimes called "silent asthma" (108).

Treatment periods with inhaled steroids may extend over months or years. Once symptomatic control and other goals of therapy have been reached, the dosage of steroid should be reduced in steps of 200 μg/day over a month at a time, with continuing monitoring for return of symptoms and evidence of falling PEFR or $FEV_1$, so that thc lowcst dosage of therapy required can be maintained. It is important that bronchodilator therapy with inhaled beta-agonists, or, less frequently, sustained-release theophylline, be used as necessary to relieve symptoms during the initial phase of inhaled steroid therapy, since the patient must be kept as functional as possible while the steroid therapy is becoming fully effective. Slit lamp examinations for cataract development every 6–12 months and height and weight measurements should be arranged for those receiving higher dosages (above 600–800 μg/day) for prolonged periods until the true incidence of adverse effects is more clearly defined.

The role of inhaled steroid therapy in those with mild to moderate asthma (about 75% of the childhood asthma population) is more controversial. In adults inhaled steroids are recommended for all except those with the very mildest symptoms because of their potential effectiveness in reversing the underlying pathogenetic mechanisms and the possibility of inducing remission. In adults there is much less concern about adverse effects in the dosages commonly used (up to 1600 μg/day). In children, for whom the dose/kg is generally much higher, the potential for beneficial versus adverse effects must be carefully weighed before a decision is made. As noted above, it is unlikely that dosages up to 400 μg/day will be associated with systemic effects, although there may be some degree of individual susceptibility. It is unclear if dosages below 400 μg/per day are any more effective in prophylactic therapy then adequate dosages of cromolyn or ketotifen, but experience suggests that dosages above this are. It is generally prudent, therefore, to initiate therapy with nonsteroidal agents in this group of children to ascertain the effect, and to move to inhaled steroids only if necessary.

About 5% of children with asthma have severe symptoms that result in frequent visits to emergency rooms, hospital admissions, grossly disturbed school, home, and social life, and the need for intermittent systemic steroid therapy. The advent of inhaled steroids has greatly enhanced the management of these children by allowing better control of asthmatic symptoms and airway obstruction, and a sparing of the requirements for oral prednisone. It is preferable to move to high dosages by the inhaled route if the oral route can be eliminated, but this may not always be possible. Careful and frequent monitoring for relief of symptoms, and development of adverse effects (slit lamp examinations for cataracts and blood pressure evaluation every 6 months) should be maintained and the patient should carry notification of their asthma and steroid use in case of emergency (e.g., Medi-alert bracelet). Reduction in systemic steroid dosage must be done slowly over periods of weeks or months, depending on the dosage and duration of therapy, to avoid adrenal insufficiency.

### *Administration*

Currently available inhaled steroid preparations are shown in Table 2. Flunisolide and triamcinolone have a more prolonged systemic effect and add little to the advantages of the original inhaled corticosteroid, beclomethasone. Budesonide is comparable in its dosing and effect to beclomethasone but may be removed slightly more rapidly from the systemic circulation, while studies of the HPA axis show a similar dose-dependent suppression of cortisol secretion.

A variety of devices are available for delivery of inhaled steroids, some being restricted to a specific drug manufacturer, and selection of an appropriate delivery method for a given patient is at least as important as the drug selected. Children from about 4 years of age and older can use a metered-dose inhaler with a spacer. The spacer should be of relatively large volume, such as a nebuhaler, but a much less expensive device that is just as efficient is a Zip-lock plastic freezer bag (109). The inhaler is placed inside a 1 L bag with a 1 inch diameter mouth piece placed in one corner. After being shaken, the inhaler is held upright inside the bag, which is inflated by a single deep breath from the child. On full expiration (bag inflated), the inhaler is activated and the aerosol released is inhaled by having the child slowly rebreathe the air in the bag three or four times. The small-volume Aerochamber is available with an infant-sized face mask, but there are few data to support its effectiveness in young children. Experience suggests the plastic bag spacer is better.

When a metered-dose inhaler is used by adolescents, it is much more effective with the open-mouth rather than closed-mouth technique (110). For this, the inhaler is held 3–4 cm from the lips. The aerosol is released just after the beginning of normal inspiration from functional residual capacity (end of tidal breathing), not full expiration. Inspiration should last at least 5 sec and the breath should be held for 10 sec at full inspiration to allow the particles to settle onto the bronchial mucosa. For those in middle childhood and those who prefer an alternative to metered-dose inhalers that contain fluorocarbons, dry powder inhalers (Beclovent Rotacaps, Beclodisk) and multidose pure drug turbuhalers (Pulmicort) are available. These are usually very well tolerated, avoid the need for good coordination of activation/inhalation, and are convenient. The turbuhaler

TABLE 2 Currently Available Inhaled Steroid Preparations

| Drug | Trade Name | Delivery System | Dosage Delivered (μg) | Formulation | Age (yrs) | Other Ingredients |
|---|---|---|---|---|---|---|
| Beclomethasone dipropionate | Beclovent/Vanceril | MDI + spacer | 50/puff | Aerosol | >4 | Fluorocarbons, oleic acid |
| | Becloforte | MDI + spacer | 250/puff | | | |
| | Beclovent | Rotahaler and capsules | 100; 200 | | | |
| | Beclodisk | Diskhaler and disk | 100; 200 Multidose disk | Dry powder | >6 | Lactose |
| Budesonide | Pulmicort | MDI | 50; 200 | Aerosol | >4 | Fluorocarbons |
| | | Turbuhaler | 100; 200 400 | Micronized powder | >6 | None |
| Triamcinolone acetonide | Azmacort | MDI (intrinsic spacer) | 200 | Aerosol | >6 | Fluorocarbons, alcohol |
| Flunisolide | Bronalide Aerobid | MDI + spacer | 250 | Aerosol | >4 | Fluorocarbons |

particularly is often preferred because of the lack of taste and the avoidance of power impacting the oropharynx. Indeed, these features may be misinterpreted by the child as indicating lack of delivery of the drug dose.

After inhalation, the mouth should be rinsed with water to avoid the possibility of oral candidiasis, but this is often unnecessary in dosages up to 400 μ/day. With all delivery systems, thorough initial training and encouragement of the child (and parents) is required, as well as re-emphasis of good technique at follow-up visits, to enhance the effectiveness of the treatment program and compliance. Very young children with severe asthma present a special challenge for delivery of inhaled steroids. For them a suspension of budesonide is available to be given via a nebulizer. Dosages of 250–500 μg two or three times per day can be given using 2 ml ampules of nebulizer solution (containing 500 μg per ml of budesonide) run to dryness over 10–15 min. This suspension can be mixed with albuterol nebulizer solution, 0.02 ml/kg/dose (max 0.5 ml) as required for bronchodilation. Budesonide suspension is available on a compassionate-release basis by application to the Health Protection Branch, Health and Welfare Canada.

### Systemic Steroids

A small proportion of asthmatic children with severe intractable symptoms that are not controlled with high-dosage inhaled steroid therapy may require continuous oral prednisone. Before initiating this therapy it is important to ensure that the potential of inhalation therapy has been fully met with four times daily dosing, optimal delivery to the airway, and short bursts of oral prednisone to ensure adequate airway patency for penetration of the drug. When the asthma has been stabilized on daily therapy (1–2 mg/kg/day, to 60 mg maximum) the dosage should be slowly reduced. This may take many months, but usually fairly rapid reduction over 4–6 weeks can be achieved to single morning doses of 30–40 mg. Thereafter it may be necessary to slow the rate of reduction to 5 mg every other day over 2 week periods, with the goal of reaching alternate-day therapy. If successful, the dose can then be reduced by 2.5 mg amounts over similar time periods. If symptoms recur, a dose three or four steps higher should be reinstituted until control is again obtained, and the reduction plan then resumed. Sometimes it proves impossible to reduce below a particular level of therapy and this dosage may have to be maintained for long periods. It is important to monitor airway obstruction objectively with daily or weekly peak flow readings by the parents and child depending on progress, and intermittent spirometry in the office to assess small airway obstruction. Concomitant inhaled steroids may allow a lower oral dosage to be reached. Any signs of recurrence of symptoms, for example, with viral upper respiratory infection in a otherwise stable steroid-dependent child, or falling PEFRs, should indicate a need for immediate escalation in dosage, often daily dosing, for 7–10 days before reducing over 4–6 weeks to the baseline level. Any continuous oral steroid therapy requires the child to have periodic checks for adverse effects, including slit lamp examinations for cataracts every 6–12 months, monitoring height, weight, and blood pressure, urinalysis for glycosuria, and assessment of pain especially in the back and hip areas.

A special group requiring short bursts of oral steroid are young infants with asthmatic symptoms of explosive onset in response to viral respiratory infection, many of whom have a prior history of acute bronchiolitis. Treatment with prednisone 2 mg/kg/day in divided doses twice daily for 48–96 hr is often enough to prevent the progress of the attack to severe respiratory distress. Response to intense bronchodilator therapy with a nebulized beta-2 agonist and ipratropium will then be adequate to permit rapid resolution of the episode. If the oral steroid therapy is initiated as early as possible, emergency treatment can often be avoided. Regular prophylactic therapy should, of course, also be emphasized.

## Theophylline

The decision to place a child on chronic bronchodilator therapy becomes more complicated with each passing year. Ten years ago theophylline was the undisputed treatment of choice in the United States for the management of chronic asthma in both adults and children. In the last 5 years, while theophylline remains one of the most commonly prescribed medications for the treatment of both infants and children with asthma, its use has been questioned both in the lay press and in the medical literature (111,112). Questions regarding the effect of theophylline on cognitive and behavioral performance (113), severe neurotoxicity and death following elevations of theophylline in the presence of acute febrile illnesses or in combination with other medications (114) leave the physician with profound reservations about its use. In addition to these questions regarding potential theophylline toxicity, recent literature has also raised certain questions concerning the mechanism of action and therapeutic potential of chronic administration of theophylline in patients with reactive airways disease (115,116).

Despite the long history of theophylline use and the multitude of studies of this particular product, its mechanism of action remains undetermined. Inhibition of the enzyme phosphodiesterase, thus preventing the degradation of cyclic AMP, once thought to be the most likely mechanism of action, does not appear to be the means by which theophylline exerts its bronchodilator activity although enzyme subgroups are presently being investigated. Other potent phosphodiesterase inhibitors have failed to produce any bronchodilatation (117). A long list of other potential mechanisms of action for theophylline, either for its bronchodilator or perhaps anti-inflammatory activity, includes such actions as blockade of adenosine receptors (118), alteration of calcium ion flow into the cytoplasmic matrix (119), alterations of eosinophil function (120), inhibition of the inflammatory reaction produced by platelet-activating factor (PAF) (121), and also suppression of leukocyte activation (122). Despite this lack of identification of the therapeutic mechanism of theophylline, major advances over the last years have occurred in determining its clinical activity, pharmacokinetics, and relationships between serum theophylline levels and its toxicity and efficacy.

In a recently completed study conducted by the American Academy of Allergy and Immunology comparing the clinical effectiveness of theophylline with inhaled beclomethasone as a first-line agent for the treatment of mild to moderate disease, there was good evidence that theophylline remains a potent bronchodilator that can indeed control the symptoms of most children with mild to moderate disease (123). This study did not seek any predetermined "therapeutic level" of theophylline, but used the patient's clinical state as a guide to dosage. The vast majority of children were adequately controlled, with limited toxicity, with peak theophylline levels less than 15 μg/ml and trough levels well below 10 μg/ml. While we now face questions regarding chronic administration of beta-agonists by inhalation or oral routes (124), the potential for growth suppression with chronic administration of inhaled corticosteroids (125,126), and limited effectiveness of cromolyn in many children with moderate to severe asthma, the use of theophylline must be considered in children who have chronic asthma requiring daily medication.

One of the issues concerning its use is the monitoring of serum theophylline levels. Methods have been developed to measure even minute quantities in the serum, and thus physicians are able to evaluate closely their management programs. Serum theophylline concentrations between 5 and 20 μg/ml have generally been accepted as consistent with effective control of wheezing with few side effects. There are children who require more or less theophylline depending on the degree of respiratory difficulty they may be experiencing. Children can vary dramatically on a daily basis in their metabolism of this agent (127) and, therefore, dosage requirements needed to maintain theophylline levels in a range therapeutic for the individual child may vary significantly from one child to another. While numerous products have been developed in the last 20 years to allow administration of medication every 6, 8, 12, and 24 hr, this must be individualized for each child because of the wide variation in metabolic rates. This variability in metabolism clearly presents the physician with problems in trying to interpret a single theophylline level even when it is obtained at the presumed peak or trough time.

Theophylline is a xanthine derivative (1,3 dimethylxanthine), related in structure to caffeine and theobromine, which are commonly found in coffee, tea, cola beverages, and chocolate. It has been combined with a variety of different bases in an effort to change its solubility, absorption rates, and possible side effects. These bases include ethylene diamine, calcium salicylate, sodium glycinate, and choline. A further attempt to alter the side effect potential for theophylline is the N-7-substituted methylxanthine, which includes the dyphylline products. These are not actually derivatives of theophylline and have a very limited potency, only approximately 10% of theophylline. As indicated above, the bronchodilator capability of theophylline has a linear relationship with serum concentration levels over a range of approximately 5–20 μg/ml. Many laboratories will label theophylline levels less than 10 as being out of the "therapeutic range." However, many of the initial studies establishing this therapeutic range were performed on individuals experiencing acute exacerbations of their asthma (128), and ample evidence exists that individuals may be clinically stable with serum theophylline levels at less than 10 μg/ml. It was suggested in the previous edition of this book that levels of theophylline between 5 and 10 μg/ml would be satisfactory for those individuals whose disease is "clinically stable," whereas those who are at higher risk of developing exacerbations of their asthma may require higher theophylline levels. This would follow the suggestion that the "therapeutic range" is actually different for different individuals, or even for the same individual at different states of asthma lability (129).

The pharmacokenetic activity of theophylline is related to three significant factors: the absorption, the metabolism, and the elimination of the product. Theophylline itself is rapidly and completely absorbed from liquid and plain uncoated tablets. The speed of absorption is effected by the coating of the tablets as well as the presence of different foods. It has been shown that a high-fat diet will increase the absorption rate of some products and decrease the absorption rate of others (130). The major factor in the rate and completeness of absorption is the rate of disintegration and dissolution of the product in the stomach. Because of wide fluctuations in serum concentrations between doses of rapid release theophylline products, the development of reliably absorbed slow-release formulations has been pursued. Differences exist in the rate and extent of absorption between various products, and it has become apparent that the rate and extent of absorption may actually vary from day to day within the same child taking the same product (127). Not only is the rate variable from day to day, but the rate of absorption also appears to be slower during the night than during the day. This should allow for a variation in dosages of theophylline being administered between the morning and evening hours. In addition, it has been suggested that administration of once daily products be done at night (131). This would have the beneficial effect of having theophylline peak levels in the early morning, to prevent the early morning fall in pulmonary function. The lower theophylline levels in the later afternoon hours would coincide with the natural increase in pulmonary function at that time (131).

The second factor affecting the serum level of theophylline is the breakdown of theophylline in the liver to inactive metabolites. This metabolism is principally performed by the microsomal enzyme system (the hepatic cytochrome P-450, which is responsible for more than 80% of theophylline clearance). Those individuals with, for any reason, decreased liver function will experience a decreased conversion of theophylline to its major metabolite, 3-methylxanthine, and are at a particular risk for theophylline toxicity (132). An acute febrile illness as well as the administration of certain other medications have been demonstrated to inhibit theophylline metabolism. This inhibition of metabolism has been associated with as much as a doubling in theophylline concentrations without a change in dosage. Infections with the influenza virus (133), respiratory syncytial virus (134), and parainfluenza virus (135) have all been associated with alterations in theophylline metabolism and elevation in serum theophylline levels. It is unclear whether the specific viral infection or the associated acute febrile reaction is the actual agent that alters the P-450 pathway of theophylline metabolism. Administration of interferon (136), which has previously been demonstrated to inhibit hepatic cytochrome P-450 enzymes, has also been associated with a reduction in theophylline metabolism.

In recognition of the effect of fever on theophylline metabolism, it is reasonable that the dosage of theophylline be reduced in half in children receiving chronic theophylline therapy who are febrile for more than 24 hr (137). This has presented a significant problem for the practicing pediatrician who often will not see the patient in the first 24 hr following a febrile illness. It is recommended to parents that they discontinue theophylline therapy completely if their child is experiencing a prolonged febrile illness and they are unable to contact their physician. Since many attacks of asthma are precipitated by viral illness, this alteration of theophylline metabolism and the potential increased wheezing with discontinuing this chronic therapy or the illness may present both the physician and parent with problems in controlling acute exacerbations of asthma. Alternative therapies must be available to the family at home should these events occur, such as beta-agonists.

### *Drug Interactions*

Numerous medications interact with theophylline and must be recognized by the physician (Table 3). Macrolide antibiotics, such as troleandomycin (TAO) and erythromycin (138), one of the most common medications administered for infections in children, will significantly decrease the clearance rate of theophylline. Cimetidine (139) will likewise decrease theophylline clearance rates while phenobarbital (140) will increase its rate of metabolism.

As indicated earlier, theophylline is used with beta-adrenergic agents and corticosteroids frequently in the treatment of asthmatic patients, both acutely and chronically. It has been demonstrated that the combination of a reduced dosage of theophylline and beta-adrenergic agent is better than a full dose of either alone with respect to its efficacy and toxicity (141). However, some children may require the full recommended dosage of both medications by oral route to achieve maximum benefit. When this is the case, attention must be paid to the potential for toxicity. However, it seems more prudent to use inhaled beta-agonists in this instance.

There is not evidence at this time of tachyphylaxis with prolonged use of theophylline. As children grow and their metabolic rates change, they will often require a higher dosage. This, however, does not reflect the development of tachyphylaxis.

### *Available Preparations*

Theophylline is currently available in a variety of forms throughout the world. There are intravenous formulations, oral preparations, including

TABLE 3 Theophylline Drug Interactions

| Agent | Effect on Levels | Reference |
|---|---|---|
| Cimetidine | Increase | CLIN PHARM 2:439, 1983 |
| Erythromycin | Increase | JACI 68:427, 1981 |
| Troleandomycin | Increase | JACI 59:228, 1977 |
| Phenobarbital | Decrease | JACI 62:27, 1978 |

liquid, tablet, and beaded capsule. Rectal solutions of theophylline are also available with absorption rates similar to oral formulations. Rectal suppositories, however, have slow and erratic absorption patterns and, thus, are potentially ineffective and very dangerous. Theophylline has not been demonstrated to work when administered by the inhaled route.

The choice of an oral preparation of theophylline should depend on the situation and patient. For patients who use theophylline intermittently for the treatment of exacerbations of wheezing, rapidly absorbed products are most appropriate, including plain uncoated tablets, liquids, and liquid-filled beads. These are all rapidly absorbed, with peak theophylline availability between 90 and 120 min, and the trough level at approximately 6 hr. For the very young child, a rectal solution can be an alternative. It should be kept in mind that inhalational therapy with beta-adrenergic agents remains the treatment of choice for acute exacerbations of wheezing. There is less risk for toxic side effects, interaction with other medications, and potential confusion when these acute exacerbations are associated with a febrile or viral illness.

For children with chronic asthma who require daily administration of medication, slow-release formulations are more suitable. Evidence exists that reducing the frequency of administration of medication from every 6 hr to every 12 hr will significantly increase the compliance rate (142). Studies using medications other than asthma products have further indicated that reduction of administration to once a day further increases compliance with medication regimens. For children who are rapid metabolizers, the best one could hope for is administration of theophylline every 8–12 hr. It must be kept in mind that there is wide variability between products and intrapatient variability on a day-to-day basis. Attention to breakthrough wheezing, signs of toxicity, and obtaining appropriate theophylline levels can help manage even the most difficult asthmatic patient who is a rapid metabolizer.

A sampling of the child's serum theophylline level should be periodically obtained, at least once a year. Before obtaining a blood specimen, the physician should know several factors: the preparation administered; its most likely time to peak and trough; the time of administration of the medication; whether any doses have been missed in the previous 2 days; time and nature of the last meal; other concomitant medications; and a history of intercurrent illness. With all that has been learned about theophylline, significant gaps still exist as to its precise mechanism of action as well as the optimal dosage, frequency, and even side effects of this product. Its use is fundamentally safe, but must be individualized and monitored closely for each child to obtain the best results with respect to efficacy and possible toxicity.

## Anticholinergic Agents

There is significant experimental evidence of increased vagal activity contributing to bronchospasm, and treatment against the parasympathetic pathways may have a role in the treatment of bronchial asthma. For years it has been recognized that the active ingredients of some herbal preparations have been employed in the treatment of asthma as cigarettes or smoking powders. These are members of the tropane family of alkaloids and have anticholinergic properties (143).

The systemic application of atropine is limited by its toxicity, and in an aerosol form there is a drying effect of the respiratory tract and retardation of mucociliary clearance. Nevertheless, in two reported studies in children, there were limited side effects, including the drying effect reported and some potential benefit. One study (144) demonstrated that atropine sulfate administered by inhalation inhibited exercised-induced bronchospasm in asthmatic children without any significant side effects other than mild xerostomia. In the other study, Hemstreet observed a bronchodilator effect of nebulized atropine in children with chronic asthma, and no adverse effects were noted (145).

The observation that quaternary derivatives of atropine retained anticholinergic activity with a decrease in central nervous system stimulatory properties was an advance in the synthesis of new compounds, such as ipratropium bromide. This compound can be administered by inhalation and is well tolerated, with limited side effects (146). It does not significantly affect production, viscosity, or clearance of mucus, problems for which atropine is suspect (147).

Atropine and ipratropium bromide are antimuscarinic agents competing with acetylcholine for receptor sites. Most investigators have considered the site of anticholinergically mediated bronchodilatation to be the large, central airways in both normal and asthmatic subjects (147,148). Since beta-adrenergic agents exert their bronchodilator effect, mainly on small airways, the inhalation of adrenergic and cholinergic agents together could be more effective than either alone. The combined use of ipratropium bromide with beta-agonist drugs, theophylline or cromolyn, could be expected to improve the results seen with individual drugs.

There have been many studies evaluating ipratropium bromide in the treatment of asthmatic children over the past 10 years. These have included evaluations of ipratropium bromide alone and with other bronchodilators in combination and in different dosages. These reports, summarized below, give a better perspective on the role of ipratropium bromide in the treatment of asthmatic children.

In 1983, Stokes et al. (149) studied ipratropium bromide treatment in infants and children with asthma. A group of 25 babies aged 5–48 weeks with acute severe bronchiolitis were evaluated after 1 nebulization with 250 μg of ipratropium bromide. Six showed improvement, suggesting that the drug may have a clinical role for some children with bronchiolitis. In another report, Milner studied airway obstruction before and 20 min after nebulized ipratropium bromide (250 μg) in 32 wheezing children between the ages of 3 months and 3 years. The treatment was effective clinically in 40% of the children. This is unlike albuterol, which rarely is an effective bronchodilator in children under the age of 18 months (150).

Although in the first year of life beta-2 stimulants are less likely to produce immediate benefit, they are recommended in the management of asthma in this age group (151). We recently showed that the combination of a beta-agonist and ipratropium bromide, administered by inhalation to 61 wheezing infants, was more effective than a beta-agonist alone in reducing wheezing and dyspnea during an acute attack (152). In wheezy infants, ipratropium bromide is the only bronchodilator that can provide benefit without the risk of hypoxemia (153). Prendiville et al. (154) evaluated pulmonary function in children between 4 and 15 months of age, before and after 250 μg of ipratropium bromide administered by inhalation. They observed improvement only in the specific airway resistance, thus confirming the action of ipratropium bromide in the large airways (147, 154). However, Davies et al. (155) evaluated asthmatic children after inhalation of various dosages of ipratropium bromide and observed an increase in the $FEV_1$ after the first dose. There was also a dose-dependent increase in the FEF25–75%, leading to the conclusion that ipratropium bromide exerted an effect on both large and small airways. This subject remains controversial; Freeman and Landau (156) considered that the addition of ipratropium bromide in addition to a sympathomimetic drug may be useful in a subgroup of asthmatic patients, particularly if there is a considerable large-airway contribution to bronchial narrowing.

The response to ipratropium bromide was not related to age in children 3–30 months. In 14 asthmatic children aged 3–6 years, the nebulization of 250 μg of ipratropium bromide produced bronchodilatation similar to that obtained with 5 mg of nebulized albuterol. The response was slower (10–30 min), however.

It must be noted that the dosage of ipratropium bromide used by Stokes et al. (157) was much higher than those usually recommended when the drug is used in a metered-dose inhaler: 40 μg, three times a day. Lin et al. (158) showed in 23 asthmatic children that ipratropium bromide was an effective bronchodilator, with an onset of effect at 15 min and a duration of action of 4 hr.

Agostini et al. (159) compared the protective effect of fenoterol spray (400 μg) to fenoterol plus ipratropium bromide spray (200 μg + 80 μg) on exercise-induced bronchospasm in children. No advantage was noted from the combination. Similar results were recently found in another study (160). Spada et al. (161) compared the action of albuterol (200 μg as a metered-dose inhaler), cromolyn (20 μg by ultrasonic nebulization), and ipratropium bromide (40 μg in a metered-dose inhaler) in preventing exercise-induced asthma in 100 children. Protection against exercise-induced bronchospasm was observed with all three agents: albuterol, 89%; cromolyn, 81%; and ipratropium bromide, 62%. They concluded that ipratropium bromide at the dose of 40 μg does not give a satisfactory level of protection against exercise-induced asthma.

Boner et al. (162) treated 12 patients with chronic asthma, aged 7–13 years, with inhalation of various dosages of ipratropium bromide on different days. All dosages gave an all-or-none protection from exercise-induced asthma. The degree of protection from exercise-induced asthma was not correlated with the bronchodilatation caused by the ipratropium bromide. They suggested that muscarinic mechanisms are only partly responsible for the pathogenesis of exercised-induced asthma in children. Wilson et al. (163) studied isocapnic hyperventilation dose–response curves in 11 asthmatic children before and after treatment with ipratropium bromide by a metered-dose inhalar. Complete protection was achieved in 6 children with 40 μg. Another 4 achieved protection with 200 μg; 1 child failed to demonstrate any protection at any dosage. No side effects were observed in the study.

Raes et al. (164) showed that long-term treatment with ipratropium bromide had no effect on bronchial hyperresponsiveness to histamine in children with asthma. On the other hand, Boner et al. (162) demonstrated that ipratropium bromide prevented the bronchoconstriction caused by methacholine.

In a study by Friberg and Graff-Lonnevig (165) looking at higher dosages of ipratropium bromide by nebulization, an increase in $FEV_1$ was observed in children with perennial asthma with dosages of 200 and 500 μg. No significant changes were demonstrated with lower dosages. This report emphasizes that ipratropium bromide has bronchodilator properties in children with asthma if given in sufficiently high dosages, without significant levels of toxicity.

Despite all these studies, the optimal dosage and frequency of administration of ipratropium bromide in children have not been well established. Further studies are necessary to establish these. The drug is available as a metered-dose inhaler (20 μg per puff) and an inhalant solution (0.025%). The dosage by solution inhalation recommended by the manufacturer is 0.05–0.1 mg (4–8 drops in 2 ml of saline). This can be administered three to five times a day, but is almost certainly too low.

Ipratropium bromide is the only anticholinergic agent now available that has potential for widespread chronic use in asthmatic children. It could be used acutely as a bronchodilator, although it is not as potent as the newer beta-adrenergic agents. It also has the potential for chronic administration as a prophylactic agent and may have added benefit for the child whose asthma is triggered by coughing spells during the night. As with other prophylactic agents, it is difficult to predict on clinical grounds who would be the best candidates for this therapy. It appears to be of benefit for the infant whose wheezing episodes are the result of viral infections, weather changes, or emotional stimuli, which do not respond well to beta-adrenergic agents. The combination of these agents may also prove to be of benefit. In older children, ipratropium bromide should be considered in those asthmatic subjects whose disease is poorly controlled by their usual medication (beta-2 agonists, theophylline, cromolyn, or ketotifen) or in those experiencing troublesome side effects from these medications.

### Troleandomycin

In patients with severe intractable asthma who have difficulty maintaining satisfactory asthma control, despite optimal conventional therapy (beta-2 agonists, theophylline, cormolyn, ketotifen, ipratropium bromide, and inhaled steroids) and high-dosage oral corticosteroids, the use of troleandomycin (TAO) has been recommended (166).

This macrolide antibiotic permits a considerable reduction in steroid dose requirements and thus produces a "steroid-sparing" effect. A double-blind study showed that TAO was "effective" in reducing steroid requirements when used concomitantly with methylprednisoline (166). The beneficial effect of TAO is observed only when associated with methylprednisolone; the combination of TAO and prednisone is less effective (166). The effect of TAO on the inhibition of corticosteriod is thus steroid specific; the inhibition of hepatic corticosteroid metabolism results in a significant decreased clearance of methylprednisolone (167). The response to the treatment with TAO and methylprednisolone is not due to the antimicrobial properties of TAO or to the concomitant inhibition of theophylline metabolism (168). The impairment of methylprednisolone "elimination" in the presence of TAO therapy is not yet established as the only mechanism of action for TAO. This effect is probably due to a change in liver metabolic function; transient elevations in liver enzymes have been described (169). TAO drug-induced hepatotoxicity seems to be related to dosage; daily TAO at a dosage of 250 mg or less in adults appears to be safe and not associated with alterations in liver function test results. The possibility of hepatotoxicity could be reduced by the alternate-day usage of TAO, which has also been found effective (169).

Zeiger et al. (169) observed that after 4–8 months' follow-up, asthma in 15 of 16 steroid-dependent patients was well controlled on TAO and methylprednisolone. The steroid requirements were reduced at least four to fivefold in most patients during TAO therapy.

The most common side effects (increased cushingoid features, weight gain, and/or fluid retention) may result from inhibition of methylprednisolone elimination or inactivation, but further reduction of steroid requirement permits partial recovery in many patients (170).

Eitches et al. (171) showed that the combination of TAO and methylprednisolone was effective in the treatment of asthmatic steroid-dependent children. After 12–28 months of treatment, using the protocol of Zeiger et al. (169), patients required fewer emergency visits and hospitalizations and missed fewer days of school. However, all patients remained on TAO and continued to be steroid dependent, although at substantially reduced dosages. The average prednisone dosage before treatment was 21.5 mg/day, and methylprednisolone dosages 1 year later averaged 3.4 mg/day.

Side effects of treatment were noted: transient elevations of serum glutamic oxaloacetic transaminase (SGOT) or serum glutamic pyruvic transaminase (SGPT), cushingoid features, and abdominal pain, which was resolved when the TAO dose was reduced.

The combined therapy of TAO and methylprednisolone should be approached cautiously in children and reserved for children with severe steroid-dependent asthma. Careful attention should be paid to all potential side effects of corticosteroid therapy as well as to liver function. The addition of any medication metabolized by the liver, such as theophylline, should be carefully monitored.

Recently, Flotte and Loughlin (172), based upon the observed increase side effects after treating 9 children (3 to 14 years) with steroid-dependent asthma using TAO and methylprednisolone, stated that further studies are necessary before this therapy can be widely used in children. Until that time, TAO must still be considered experimental therapy in children.

## Other Drugs

Methotrexate, oral gold, cyclosporine, high-dosage intravenous immunoglobulin, calcium channel blockers, potassium channel activators, nonsteroidal anti-inflammatory drugs and inhibitors or antagonists of inflammatory mediators such as PAF, 5-lipoxygenase, thromboxane A2, and leukotriene D4 are examples of the array of drugs that have been in clinical trials in adults. Even so, their roles are not yet clarified. At present, there is no evidence supporting the use of these agents in the treatment of asthma in children.

## Inhalational Devices

It is the consensus of these authors that the most expeditious way to administer medication for the treatment of asthma either acutely or chronically is by inhalation. This means of administration has become the most commonly used in patients of all ages. Despite this, difficulties in administering medication by inhalation must be considered by the physician and parent alike. This problem is especially magnified in the small child. Inappropriate delivery of medication will significantly affect its effectiveness. While the metered-dose inhaler continues to be the most frequently prescribed manner in which to deliver aerosol medication for the treatment of asthma, almost 50% of the patients have some difficulty in using it properly (173). It should be noted that even with proper patient technique, a maximum of 12% of the agent can be found in the lungs (174).

There is considerable patient variability in technique with respect to administering the metered-dose inhaler (MDI). It is generally agreed that to obtain the maximum delivery of the medication within the aerosol, the inhalation should begin from functional residual capacity within an inhalational time over several seconds and a breath holding time of 10 sec to be optimum (175). There are two general approaches to inhaler technique with the MDI. Each of these techniques has advantages and disadvantages. Some physicians prefer the open-mouth technique, with the inhaler approximately 4 cm in front of the open mouth, while others prefer placing the inhaler into a closed mouth before it is actuated (Fig. 6). The ideal technique has not been universally accepted. The theoretical advantage of the open-mouth technique is that the particles become significantly smaller as they travel from the actuator orifice to the mouth. The smaller the particle, the greater the likelihood of it reaching the smaller airways of the

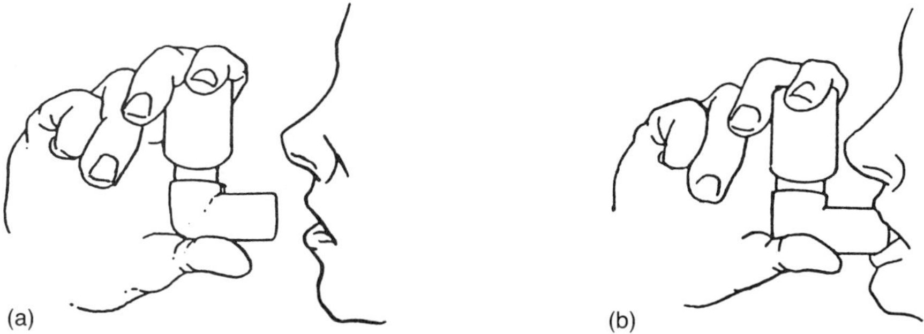


FIGURE 6 Two different methods of inhaler placement. (a) Inhaler 1–2 in. from the open mouth; (b) inhaler in the mouth.

lung. However, often with the open-mouth technique the inhaler is actuated at an angle, which prevents all of the medication from entering the mouth.

In an attempt to overcome the disadvantages of the MDI, several devices have been developed. One of these is the Gentle-haler (176), which delivers particles 1–3 μm at a lower velocity. The Rotahaler (177) delivers particles also in the same range in the form of a dry powder. The powder system requires a high flow rate for efficient delivery. Two other breath-activated inhalers are the Autohaler (178) and the Turbuhaler. These have demonstrated improvement in delivery of medication over the standard MDI. The Turbuhaler has the advantage of delivering pure drug in a very fine particle size, with no carrier powder being required. It is therefore very well tolerated.

Another means of delivering aerosol medication is through a nebulizer. This is especially common in the young child. In previous years intermittent positive pressure breathing (IPPB) was used to deliver such medications. Studies have shown IPPB has no advantage over the standard power-driven nebulizer and may even be less effective in asthmatic patients (179). Nebulizers have been used with both open and mouth closed administration (Fig. 7). Properly used metered-dose inhalers give equivalent results to nebulizers. For children who have difficulty with this technique, the nebulizer presents a significant advantage. Nebulizers also have the limitation of only having beta-agonist bronchodilators or cromolyn sodium available

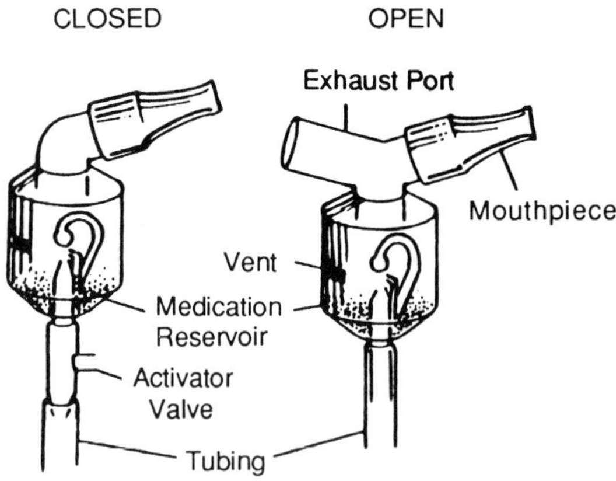


FIGURE 7 The "open" and "closed" nebulizers. The open system uses more medication and is usually used with continuous flow.

for approved administration in the United States. Other medications, including ipratropium bromide and corticosteroids, are available in other parts of the world. Nebulizers allow higher doses of medication to be administered gradually to the airways. Numerous patients use nebulizers along with their metered-dose inhalers as part of their treatment regimen for both acute and chronic asthma. Some studies with nebulizers indicate an increased intrapulmonary deposition over metered-dose inhalers, which may result from the subject's laryngeal geometry (180).

Nebulized medication can be administered either with a mouthpiece or with a mask. The mask allows inhalation through the nose as well as the mouth but also decreases the amount of medication reaching the lower airways. The inhalation should be performed through the mouth for best results, but this technique cannot be relied upon in younger children, for whom a mask is preferable.

Another effort to increase the effectiveness of inhaled medication has been the development of different types of spacing devices. These have been of different shapes, sizes, colors, and costs (Fig. 8). Definite evidence does exist that the use of a spacing device reduces the impaction of aerosol particles on the mouth and pharynx, allowing greater availability for inhalation into the lungs (181). In addition to a reduction in the impaction velocity, there is increased evaporation of propellant, which will allow smaller particle sizes to be available for inhalation into the lungs. It seems especially advantageous to use spacing devices with individuals who have difficulty timing the use of their MDI. Devices can be made using various objects found in the home. This can include a paper cup or a small food storage bag.

No matter what inhalation device is used, a slow rate of inspiration is favored over a more rapid rate. The efficacy can be shown to be increased by administering the medication in doses separated by at least 1-2 min. Proper instruction, especially to the small child, is critical and all patients should be observed administering their medication by the physician or nurse before one can assume that the patient can use the inhaled medication correctly.

## Mucolytic and Expectorant Therapy

Autopsy examination of the lungs of patients who die of asthma after several days of treatment in the hospital often shows airways blocked by sticky inspissated mucus that sometimes reaches even the most peripheral airways, despite the relative absence of goblet cells and mucous glands (182). This classic description accounts for only a proportion of autopsies, however, and deaths unrelated to endobronchial mucus suffocation also

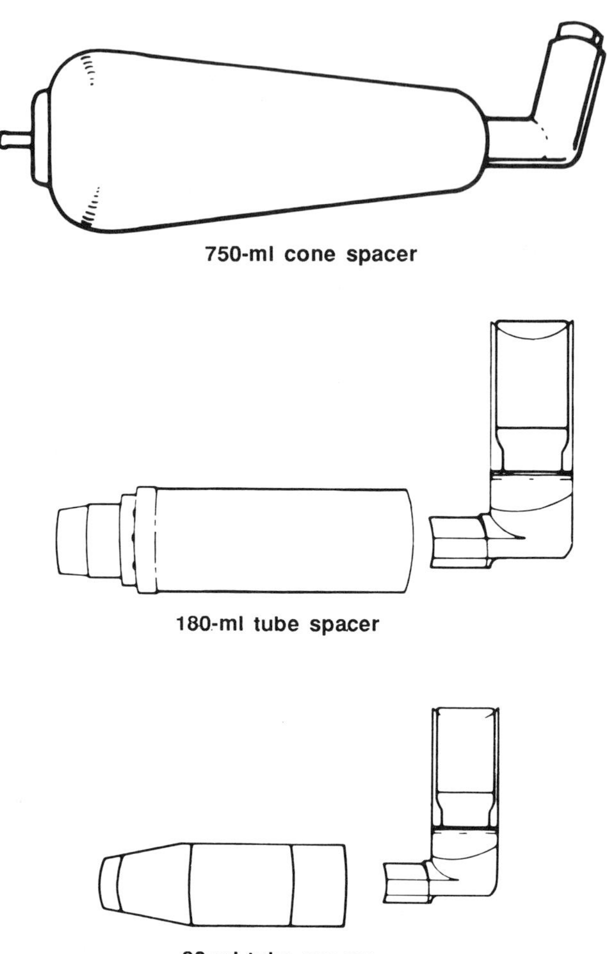


FIGURE 8 Three types of currently available spacing devices.

occur. In these patients there may be only a mild degree of mucus accumulation or the airways may be empty, suggesting that death occurred because of acute bronchoconstriction superimposed on edema and inflammation of the bronchial wall, or, possibly, cardiac arrhthmia related to hypoxia and drug therapy. Therefore, mucolytic and expectorant therapy would be expected to be of limited value in treating asthmatic subjects in whom the disease process is so diverse.

Maintaining normal hydration in patients with acute severe asthma is important to minimize adverse metabolic changes and must take into account the diuretic effects of aminophylline, if used. There is no value in overhydration and this, together with mist therapy, may be deleterious by increasing the water content of the lung interstitium and volume of the mucus in the airway. Specific drugs such as potassium iodide and glyceryl guiacolate, which are not devoid of adverse effects, have never been shown to be efficacious is asthmatic children. N-acetyl cysteine, which is highly irritating on inhalation, may provoke further broncoconstriction. Until appropriately controlled clinical trials have been conducted in carefully selected and homogeneous populations of asthmatic children, the benefits of mucolytic and expectorant therapy remain unknown. These drugs have been superseded by other antiasthma drugs of proven efficacy.

### Antihistamines

It has been well established over the last few years that mast cell mediators, including the preformed mediator histamine, play a signficant role in the production of airway inflammation and bronchial hyperreactivity. It has been over 70 years since the first association between histamine and bronchoconstriction after allergen inhalation was documented (183,184). Studies with the classic antihistamines showed equivocal results with respect to control of antigen-induced bronchoconstriction (185-187). Because higher dosages of these medications were limited by their sedative and anticholinergic effect, a question always remained as to whether anti-$H^1$-receptor agents could be used as effective medications for the treatment of acute or chronic asthma.

In the last decade attempts have been made to develop a newer generation of antihistamines that lack the sedative effect to some degree and may have activities other than pure $H^1$ blocking. These agents have been studied in a variety of models of asthma including exercise challenges, histamine challenges, methacholine challenges, and in actual clinical studies. The agents that have been studied include terfenadine, (188), astemizole (189), azelastine (190), cetirizine (191), and ketotifen (192). Although effective in some challenge systems, a lack of consistent activity in chronic asthma has been the case with many of these. Ketotifen, one of the few antihistamines with demonstrated effect in some clinical studies of chronic asthma, has been available and studied in children. Azelastine has been studied predominantly in adults, with varying degrees of success.

It is safe to say at this time that the clinical experience available is still limited, especially in children. Studies with positive results have, in many cases, been of patients with relatively mild disease. Further studies are required in patients with more severe asthma to determine whether any of these agents will be a significant addition to the currently available treatment modalities.

## REFERENCES


1. Treatment of pediatric asthma: a Canadian consensus remains. *Can Med Assoc J* In press.
2. Chen KK, Schmidt CF. The action of ephedrine, the active principle of the Chinese drug Ma Huang. *J Pharmacol Exp Ther* 24:192, 1924.
3. Ahlquist RP. A study of adrenotropic receptors. *Am J Physiol* 153:586, 1948.
4. Lands AM, Arnold A, McAuliff JP, et al. Differentiation of receptor systems activated by sympathomimetic amines. *Nature* (*Lond*) 214:597, 1967.
5. Holmes TH. A comparative clinical trial of metaproterenol as bronchodilator aerosols. *Clin Pharmacol Ther* 9:615, 1968.
6. Reed CE. Adrenergic bronchodilators. Pharmacology and toxicology. *J Allergy Clin Immunol* 78:335, 1985.
7. Devlin JP, Hargrave KD. Pulmonary and antiallergic drugs: design and synthesis. In: Devlin JP (ed.), *Pulmonary and Antiallergic Drugs*, John Wiley & Sons, New York, 1985, pp. 191–316.
8. Scalabrin DMF, Toledo EC, Oliveira CA, Solé D, Naspitz CK. Beta 2 agonists in the treatment of acute attack of asthma: Routes of administration and side effects. *J Allergy Clin Immunol* 87:255, 1991.
9. Kelly HW, McWilliams BC, Katz R, Murphy S. Safety of frequent high dose nebulized terbutaline in children with acute severe asthma. *Ann Allergy* 64:229–233, 1990.
10. Schuh, S. Cammy G, Russman JJ, Kerem E, Petric M, Levinson H. Nebulized albuterol in acute bronchiolitis. *J Pediatr* 117:633–637, 1990.
11. Mazer B, Figueroa-Rosario N, Bender B. The effect of albuterol aerosol on fine-motor performance in children with chronic asthma. *J Allergy Clin Immunol* 86:243–248, 1990.
12. Pierson WE, LaForce CG, Bell TD, MacCosbe PE, Sykes RS, Tinkelman DG. Controlled-release albuterol by oral route is a safe and effective alternative to sustained-release theophylline for management of patients with asthma. *J Allergy Clin Immunol* 85:618–626, 1990.
13. Van Bever HP, Desager KN, Stevens NJ. The effect of inhaled fenoterol, administered during the late asthmatic reaction to house dust mite (*Dermatophagoides pteronyssinus*). *J Allergy Clin Immunol* 85:700–703, 1990.
14. Yanai M, Ohrui T, Sekizawa K, Shimizu Y, Sasaki H, Takishima T. Effective site of bronchodilation by antiasthma drugs in subjects with asthma. *J Allergy Clin Immunol* 87:1080–1087, 1991.
15. Boner A, Zanotto CE, Piacentini G, Miglioranzi P, Richelli C, Sette L. Efficacy and duration of action of oral procaterol after single administration of different dosages. *J Asthma* 27:21–30, 1990.
16. *Med Lett* 33:12, 1991.

17. Ahrens RC. Skeletal muscle tremor and the influence of adrenergic drugs. *J Asthma* 27:11–20, 1990.
18. Tinkelman DG, Dejong R, Lutz C, Spangler DL. Evaluation of tremor and efficacy of oral procaterol in adult patients with asthma. *J Allergy Clin Immunol* 85:719–728, 1990.
19. Ziment I. Risk/benefit of long-term treatment with beta 2 adrenoceptor agonists. *Lung* 168(Suppl):168–176, 1990.
20. Charpin D. Long-term effectiveness of tulobuterol inhaler, a new beta 2 agonist in the treatment of asthma. *Lung* 168(Suppl):194–201, 1990.
21. Lofdahl CG. Basic pharmacology of new long acting sympathomimetics. *Lung* 168 (Suppl):18–21, 1990.
22. Von Berg A, Berdel B. Formoterol and salbutamol metered aerosols: comparison of a new and established beta 2 agonist for their bronchodilating efficacy in the treatment of childhood bronchial asthma. *Pediatr Pulmonol* 7:89–93, 1989.
23. Von Berg A, Berdel B. Efficacy of formoterol metered aerosol in children. *Lung* 168(Suppl):90–98, 1990.
24. Becker AB, Simons FER, McMillan JL Fandy T. Formoterol, a new long acting selective beta 2 adrenergic receptor agonist: double-blind comparison with salbutamol and placebo in children with asthma. *J Allergy Clin Immunol* 84:891–899, 1989.
25. Becker AB, Simons FER. Formoterol, a new long acting selective beta 2 agonist, decreases airway responsiveness in children with asthma. *Lung* 168(Suppl):99–102, 1990.
26. Becker AB, Lukowski JL, Simons FER. Formoterol modifies chronic airway hyperresponsiveness in children with asthma. *J Allergy Clin Immunol* 87:308, 1991.
27. Malo JL, Cartier, A, Trudeau RT, Ghezze H, Gontovnik L. Formoterol, a new inhaled beta 2 adrenergic agonist, has a longer blocking effect that albuterol on hyperventilation-induced bronchoconstriction. *Am Rev Respir Dis* 142:1147–1152, 1990.
28. Kemp JP, Bierman CW, Bronsky EA, Coccheto DM, DeMars DD, Justus SE, Liddle R, Orgel HA, Tinkelman DG. A one-week evaluation of salmeterol, a new long-acting beta 2 adrenergic aerosol for asthma therapy. *J Allergy Clin Immunol* 87:258, 1991.
29. Lemanske RF, Joad J. Beta 2 receptor agonists in asthma: a comparison. *J Asthma* 27:101–109, 1990.
30. Waldeck B, Olson OAT, Svensson LA. New possibilities for the beta adrenoceptor agonist bronchodilator drugs. In: O'Donell SR, Persson GA (eds.), *Directions for New Antiasthma Drugs*. Birkhauser Verlag, Basel, 1988, pp. 55–68.
31. Svedmyr N. Is beta-adrenoceptor sensitivity a limiting factor in asthma therapy? In: Morley J (ed.), *Beta-adrenoceptors in Asthma*, Academic Press, London, 1984, pp. 181–199.
32. Barnes PJ. A new approach to the treatment of asthma. *N Engl J Med* 321:1517–1527, 1989.

33. Simmonson BG. Beta 2 receptor agonists tachyphylaxis and combinations with other drugs. *Prog Respir Res* 19:315, 1986.
34. Angelici E, Delfino M, Carlone S, Serra P, Finebert NS, Farber MO. Tolerance to inhaled fenoterol. *Am Rev Respir Dis* 129:1014, 1984.
35. Kraan J, Loeter GH, Van der Mark TW, Sluiter HJ, de Vries K. Changes in bronchial hyperreactivity induced by 4 weeks of treatment with antiasthmatic drugs in patients with allergic asthma: a comparison between budesonide and terbutaline. *J Allergy Clin Immunol* 76:628–636, 1985.
36. Schayck CP, Graafsma SJ, Visch MB, Dompeling E, Well C, Hervaarden CLS. Increased bronchial hyperresponsiveness after inhaling salbutamol during 1 year is not caused by subsensitization to salbutamol. *J Allergy Clin Immunol* 86:793–800, 1990.
37. Ellis EF. Asthma in childhood. *J Allergy Clin Immunol* 72:526, 1983.
38. Sears M, Taylor DR, Print CG, Lake DC, Flannery EM, Yates DM, Lucas MK, Herbison GP. Regular inhaled beta-agonist treatment in bronchial asthma. *Lancet* 336:1391–1396, 1990.
39. Weinberger M. Antiasthmatic therapy in children. *Pediatr Clin North Am* 36:1251–1284, 1989.
40. Raes M, Milder P, Kerrejbin KF. Long term effects of ipratropium bromide and fenoterol to the bronchial hyperresponsiveness to histamine in children with asthma. *J Allergy Clin Immunol* 84:874–879, 1989.
41. Lipworth BJ, Sturthers AD, McDevitt DG. Tachyphylaxis to systemic but not to airways responses during prolonged therapy with high dose inhaled salbutamol in asthmatics. *Am Rev Respir Dis* 140:586–592, 1989.
42. Nelson HS. II. Beta-adrenergic therapy. In: Middleton E, Reed CE, Ellis EF, Adkinson NF, Yunginger JW (eds.), *Allergy—Principles and Practice*, CV Mosby, St. Louis, 1988, pp. 647–672.
43. Nicklas RA. Bronchial bronchospasm associated with the use of inhaled beta agonists. *J Allergy Clin Immunol* 85:959–964, 1990.
44. Michoud MC, Leduc T, Proulx F, Perreault S, DuSouich P, Duranceau A, Amyot R. Effect of salbutamol on gastroesophageal reflux in healthy volunteers and patients with asthma. *J Allergy Clin Immunol* 87:762–767, 1991.
45. Wilson JD, Sutherland DC, Thomas AC. Has the change to beta agonist combined with oral theophylline increased cases of fatal asthma. *Lancet* 2:1235, 1981.
46. Pierson WE, Shapiro GS, Furukawa CT, Bierman CW. Albuterol syrup in the treatment of asthma. *J Allergy Clin Immunol* 76:228, 1985.
47. Joad J, Ahrens R, Lingren S, Weinberger M. Physiological and psychological variables during therapy with inhaled albuterol and theophylline used separately and in combination. *J Allergy Clin Immunol* 73:113, 1985.
48. Warner JO, Gotz M, Landau I, Levinson H, Milner AD, Pedersen S, Silverman M. Management of asthma: a consensus statement. *Arch Dis Child* 64:1065–1079, 1989.
49. Rylance G (ed). *Drugs for Children—drugs for the Treatment of Asthma.* WHO, 1987, pp 63–67.

50. Kemp JP, Meltzer EO. Beta 2 adrenergic agonists—oral or aerosol for the treatment of asthma? *J Asthma* 27:149–157, 1990.
51. Rossing TH, Fanta CH, Goldstein DH, et al. Emergency therapy of asthma: comparison of the acute effects of parenteral and inhaled sympathomimetics and infused aminophylline. *Am Rev Respir Dis* 122:365, 1980.
52. Schwartz AL, Lipton JM, Warbutron D, et al. Management of acute asthma in childhood: a randomized evaluation of beta adrenergic agents. *Am J Dis Child* 134:474, 1980.
53. Editorial. The nebulizer epidemic. *Lancet* 2:789, 1984.
54. Adlerson SH, Warren RH. Pediatric aerosol therapy guidelines. *Clin Pediatr* 23:553–557, 1984.
55. Rachelefsky GS, Siegel SC. Asthma in infants and children—treatment of childhood asthma. *J Allergy Clin Immunol* 76:409, 1985.
56. Nelson HS. Stepwise therapy of bronchial asthma: the role of beta adrenergic agonists. *Ann Allergy* 54:289, 1985.
57. Levison H, Isler A. Response: asthma in childhood. *J Allergy Clin Immunol* 72:539, 1983.
58. Godfrey S, Balfour-Lynn L, Konig P. The place of cromolyn sodium in the long term management of childhood asthma based on a 3 to 5 year follow-up. *J Pediatr* 87:465–473, 1975.
59. Shapiro GG, Konig P. Cromolyn sodium: a review. *Pharmacotherapy* 5:156–170, 1985.
60. Toogood JH, Lefcoe NM, Wonnacott TM, et al. Cromolyn sodium therapy: predictors of response. *Adv Asthma Allergy Pulmon Dis* 5:2–15, 1978.
61. Rebuck AS, Kesten S, Boulet LP, et al. A three month evaluation of the efficacy of nedocromil sodium in asthma: a randomized double blind placebo controlled trial of nedocromil sodium conducted by a Canadian multicenter study group. *J Allergy Clin Immunol* 85:612–617, 1990.
62. Bone MF, Kubik MM, Keaney NP, et al. Nedocromil in adults with asthma dependent on inhaled steroids: a double blind placebo controlled study. *Thorax* 44:654–659, 1989.
63. Williams, AJ, Stableford D. The addition of nedocromil sodium to maintenance therapy in the management of patients with bronchial asthma. *Eur J. Respir Dis* 69(Supp 147):340–343, 1986.
64. Lal S, Malhotra S, Gribben D, et al. Nedocromil sodium: a new drug for the management of bronchial asthma. *Thorax* 39:809–812, 1984.
65. Dorward AJ, Roberts JA, Thomson NC. Effect of nedocromil sodium on histamine airway responsiveness in grass-pollen sensitive asthmatics during the pollen season. *Clin Allergy* 16:309–315, 1986.
66. Golden JG, Bateman ED. Does nedocromil sodium have a steroid sparing effect in adult asthmatic patients requiring maintenance oral corticosteroids? *Thorax* 43:982–986, 1988.
67. Bergmann K-C, Bauer C-P, Overlack A. A placebo controlled blind comparison of nedocromil sodium and beclomethasone diproprionate in bronchial asthma. *Curr Med Res Opin* 11:533–542, 1989.

68. Konig P, Hardwick NL, Kreutz C. The preventive effect and duration of action of nedocromil sodium and cromolyn sodium on exercise-induced asthma (EAI) in adults. *J Allergy Clin Immunol* 79:64–68, 1987.
69. North American Tilade Study Group. A double blind multicentre group comparative study of the efficacy and safety of nedocromil sodium in the management of asthma. *Chest* 97:1299–1306, 1990.
70. Schmidt-Redemann B, Bremeisen P, Schmidt-Redemann W, et al. The determination of pharmacokinetic parametics of ketotifen in steady state in young children. *Int J Clin Pharmacol Ther Toxicol* 24:496–498, 1986.
71. Graff-Lonnevig V, Helin G. The effect of ketotifen on bronchial hyperreactivity in childhood asthma. *J Allergy Clin Immunol* 76:59–63, 1985.
72. Dal Negro RW, Turco P, Zoccatelli O, et al. Prevention of bronchial hyperreactivity in atopic asthmatics during the period of maximal allergenic risk: a six month study. *Int J Clin Pharmacol Ther Toxicol* 24:100–103, 1986.
73. Reid JJ. Double blind trial of ketotifen in childhood chronic cough and wheeze. *Immunol Allergy Prac* 11(4):13–20, 1989.
74. Neijens HJ, Knol K. Oral prophylactic treatment in wheezy infants. *Immunol Allergy Prac* 10:17–23, 1988.
75. Volvovitz B, Versano I, Cumella JC, et al. Efficacy and safety of ketotifen in young children. *J Allergy Clin Immunol* 81:526–530, 1988.
76. Lane DJ. A steroid sparing effect of ketotifen in steroid dependent asthmatics. *Clin Allergy* 10:519–525, 1980.
77. Loftus BG, Price JF. Long term placebo-controlled trial of ketotifen in the management of preschool children with asthma. *J Allergy Clin Immunol* 79:350–355, 1987.
78. Grant SM, Goa KL, Fitton A, et al. Ketotifen. A review of its pharmacokinetic properties, and therapeutic use in asthma and allergic disorders. *Drugs* 40(3):412–448, 1990.
79. Iikura Y, Naspitz CK, Mikawa H, et al. Prevention of asthma by ketotifen in infants with atopic dermatitis. Ann Allergy 68:233–236, 1992.
80. Maclay WP, Crowder D, Spiro S. et al. Postmarketing surveillance: practical experience with ketotifen. *Br Med J* 288:911–914, 1984.
81. Rackham A, Brown CA, Chandra RK, et al. A Canadian multicentre study with Zaditen (ketotifen) in the treatment of bronchial asthma in children aged 5 to 17 years. *J Allergy Clin Immunol* 84:286–96, 1989.
82. Simons FER, Luciuk GH, Becker AB, et al. Ketotifen: a new drug for prophylaxis of asthma in children. *Ann Allergy* 48:145–150, 1982.
83. Toogood JH, Baskerville J, Jennings B, et al. Bioequivalent doses of budesonide and prednisone in moderate and severe asthma. *J Allergy Clin Immunol* 84:668–700, 1989.
84. Lundgren JD, Kaliner MA, Shelhamer JH. Mechanisms by which glucocorticoids inhibit secretion of mucus in asthmatic airways. *Am Rev Respir Dis* 141:S52–S58, 1990.
85. Reed CE. Aerosol glucocorticoid treatment of asthma. *Am Rev Respir Dis* 141:S82–S88, 1990.
86. Toogood JH, Baskerville JC, Jennings B, et al. Influence of dosing frequency

and schedule on the response of chronic asthmatics to the aerosol steroid, budesonide. *J Allergy Clin Immunol* 70:288–298, 1982.
87. Williams H, Verrier Jones ET, Silbert JR. Twice daily versus four times daily treatment with beclomethasone diproprionate in the control of mild childhood asthma. *Arch Dis Child* 41:602–605, 1986.
88. Gwynn CM, Morrison Smith J. A 1 year follow-up of children and adolescents receiving regular beclomethasone diproprionate. *Clin Allergy* 4:325–330, 1974.
89. Godfrey S, Balfour-Lynn L, Tooley M. A three to five year follow up of the use of aerosol steroid, beclomethasone diproprionate in childhood asthma. *J Allergy Clin Immunol* 62:335–339, 1978.
90. Woolcock AJ, Yan K, Salome CM. Effect of therapy on bronchial hyperresponsiveness in the long term management of asthma. *Clin Allergy* 18:165–176, 1988.
91. Kerrebijn KF, van Essen-Zandvliet EEM, Neijens HJ. Effect of long term treatment with inhaled corticosteroids and beta agonists on bronchial responsiveness in children with asthma. *J Allergy Clin Immunol* 79:653–659, 1987.
92. Hodgson SV, McPherson A, Friedman M. The effect of betamethasone valerate aerosol on exercise induced asthma in children. *Postgrad Med J* 4(Suppl):69–72, 1974.
93. Bisgaard H, Nielson MD, Anderson B, et al. Adrenal function in children with bronchial asthma treated with beclomethasone diproprionate or budesonide. *J Allergy Clin Immunol* 81:1088–1095, 1988.
94. Law CM, Marchant JL, Honour JW, et al. Nocturnal adrenal suppression in asthmatic children taking inhaled beclomethasone diproprionate. *Lancet* 2:942–944, 1986.
95. Konig P. Inhaled corticosteroids—their present and future role in the management of asthma. *J Allergy Clin Immunol* 82:297–306, 1988.
96. Kerrebijn KF. Use of topical corticosteroids in the treatment of childhood asthma. *Am Rev Respir Dis* 141:S77–S81, 1990.
97. Balfour-Lynn L. Growth and childhood asthma. *Arch Dis Child* 61:1049–055, 1986.
98. Ferguson AC, Murray AB, Tze W-J. Short stature and delayed skeletal maturation in children with allergic disease. *J Allergy Clin Immunol* 69:461–66, 1982.
99. Nassif E, Weinberger M, Sherman B, et al. Extra pulmonary effects of maintenance corticosteroid therapy with alternate day prednisone and inhaled beclomethasone in children with chronic asthma. *J Allergy Clin Immunol* 80:518–529, 1987.
100. Wolthers OD, Pedersen S. Growth of asthmatic children during treatment with budesonide: a double blind trial. *Br Med J* 303:163–165, 1991.
101. Reid DM, Nicoll JJ, Smith MA, et al. Corticosteroids and bone mass in asthma: comparisons with rheumatoid arthritis and polymyalgia rheumatica. *Br Med J* 293:1463–1466, 1986.

102. Toogood JH, Jennings B, Hodsman A, et al. Effect of inhaled budesonide on osteoblast function. *J Allergy Clin Immunol* 85:144(abstr), 1990.
103. Shapiro GG, Tattoni DS, Kelley VC, et al. Growth, pulmonary and endocrine function in chronic asthma patients on daily and alternate day adrenocorticosteroid therapy. *J Allergy Clin Immunol* 57:430–439, 1976.
104. Rooklin AR, Lampert SI, Jaegar EA, et al. Posterior subcapsular cataracts in steroid-requiring asthmatic children. *J Allergy Clin Immunol* 63:383–386, 1979.
105. Bhagat RG, Chai H. Development of posterior subcapsular cataracts in asthmatic children. *Pediatrics* 73:626–630, 1984.
106. Kewley GD. Possible association between beclomethasone diproprionate aerosol and cataracts. *Aust Paediatr J* 16:117–118, 1980.
107. David DS, Berkowitz JS. Occular effects of topical and systemic corticosteroids. *Lancet* 2:149, 1969.
108. Ferguson AC. Silent asthma. *Am J. Asthma Allergy Pediatr* 3:1–6, 1990.
109. Lee H, Evans HE. Aerosol bag for administration of bronchodilators to young asthmatic children. *Pediatrics* 74:230–232, 1984.
110. Newhouse MT, Dolovich MB. Control of asthma by aerosols. *N Engl J Med* 315:870–874, 1986.
111. Trial Lawyers of America; ATLA Alert Program. Press Conference, National Press Club, Oct. 30, 1990, Washington, DC.
112. Marks MB. Theophylline: primary or tertiary drug? A brief review. *Ann Allergy* 59:85–87, 1987.
113. Furukawa CT, DuHamel TR, Weimer L, Shapiro GG, Pierson WE, Bierman CW. Cognitive and behavioral findings in children taking theophylline. *J Allergy Clin Immunol* 81:83–88, 1988.
114. Emerman CL, Devin C, Connors AF. Risk of toxicity in patients with elevated theophylline levels. *Ann Emergency Med* 19(6):643–649, 1990.
115. Pauwels RA. New aspects of the therapeutic potential of theophylline in asthma. *J Allergy Clin Immunol* 83:548–553, 1989.
116. Pauwels R, Van Renterghem D, Van Der Straeten M, Johannessen N, Persson CGA. The effect of theophylline and enprofylline on allergen-induced bronchoconstriction. *J Allergy Clin Immunol* 76:583–590, 1985.
117. Kolbeck RC, Speir WA, Carrier GO, et al. Apparent irrelevance of cyclic nucleotides in the relaxation of trachael smooth muscle induced by theophylline. *Lung* 156:172, 1979.
118. Fredholm BB, Brodin K, Strandberg K. On the mechanism of relaxation of trachael muscle by theophylline and other cyclic nucleotide phosphodiesterase inhibitors. *Acta Pharmacol Toxicol* 43:336, 1976.
119. Ishizaka T. IgE and mechanisms of IgE mediated hypersensitivity. *Ann Allergy* 48:313, 1982.
120. Yukawa T, Kroegel C, Chanez P, Dent G, Ukena D, Chung KF, Barnes PJ. Effect of theophylline and adenosine on eosinophil function. *Am Rev Respir Dis* 140:327–333, 1989.
121. Page CP, Sanjar S, Alvemini D, Morley J. Inflammatory mediators of asthma. *Eur J Respir Dis* 68(suppl):163–189, 1986.

122. Nelson S, Summer WR, Jakab GL. Aminophylline-induced suppression of pulmonary antibacterial defense. *Am Rev Respir Dis* 131:923–927, 1985.
123. American Academy of Allergy and Immunology Beclomethasone Study Group. Aerosol beclomethasone dipropionate compared to theophylline as primary treatment for chronic mild to moderately severe asthma. In preparation.
124. Sears M, Taylor DR, et al. Regular inhaled beta-agonist treatment in bronchial asthma. *Lancet* 336:1391–1396, 1990.
125. Soderberg-Warner M, Siegel S, Katz R, Rachelefsky G. Treatment of chronic childhood asthma with beclomethasone dipropionate aerosol (BDP) IV Long term effects on growth. *J Allergy Clin Immunol* 63:(abstr 99)164, 1979.
126. Nassif E, Weinberger M, Sherman B, Brown K. Extrapulmonary effects of maintenance corticosteroid therapy with alternate-day prednisone and inhaled beclomethasone in children with chronic asthma. *J Allergy Clin Immunol* 80:518–529, 1987.
127. Rogers RJ, Szefler SJ, Wiener MB. Intraindividual variation in absorption from a sustained released theophylline formulation during continuous therapy in asthmatic children. *J Allergy Clin Immunol* 73:133, 1984.
128. Mitenko PA, Ogilvie R. Rational intravenous doses of theophylline. *N Engl J Med* 289:60, 1973.
129. Menendez R, Kelly HW. Theophylline therapy. *J Asthma* 20:455, 1983.
130. Tinkelman DG, Edelman L. DeCouto J, et al. The effect of diet on the metabolism of long acting theophylline. *Ann Allergy* 54:280, 1985.
131. D'Alonzo GE, Smolensky MH, Feldman S, et al. Twenty-four hour lung function in adult patients with asthma. *Am Rev Respir Dis* 142:84–90, 1990.
132. Jonkman JHG, Upton RA. Pharmacokinetic drug interactions with theophylline. *Clin Pharmacokinetics* 9:309–334, 1984.
133. Kraemer MJ, Furukawa CT, Koup JR, Shapiro GG, Pierson WE, Bierman CW. Altered theophylline clearance during an influenza B outbreak. *Pediatrics* 69:475–480, 1982.
134. Rao M, Ames M, Mitchell M, Bromberg K, Steiner P. Alteration of theophylline pharmacokinetics by respiratory syncytial virus infection in children. *Pediatr Res* 18:401A, 1984.
135. Koren G, Greenwald M. Decreased theophylline clearance causing toxicity in children during viral epidemics. *J Asthma* 22:75–79, 1985.
136. Renton KW. Relationship between the enzymes of detoxication and host defense mechanisms. In Caldwell J, Jakoby WB (eds.) *Biological Basis of Detoxication*, New York, Academic Press, 1983, pp. 307–324.
137. Weinberger M, Hendeles L. Theophylline use: an overview. *J Allergy Clin Immunol* 76:277–284, 1985.
138. Renton KW, Gray JD, Hung DR. Depression of theophylline elimination by erythromycin. *Clin Pharmacol Ther* 30:422–426, 1981.
139. Campbell KC, Plachetka JR, Jackson JE, Moon JF, Finley PR. Cimetidine decreases theophylline clearance. *Ann Intern Med* 95:68–69, 1981.
140. Landay RA, Gonzales MA, Taylor JC. Effect of phenobarbital on theophylline disposition. *J Allergy Clin Immunol* 62:27, 1987.
141. Wolfe JD, Tashkin DP, Calvarese B, Simmons M. Bronchodilator effects

of terbutaline and aminophylline alone and in combination in asthmatic patients. *N Engl J Med* 298:363, 1978.

142. Tinkelman DG, Vanderpool GE, Carroll MS, et al. Compliance differences following administration of theophylline at six and twelve hour intervals. *Ann Allergy* 44:283, 1980.
143. Devlin JP, Hargrave KD. Pulmonary and antiallergic drugs: design and synthesis. In: Devlin JP (ed.), *Pulmonary and Antiallergic Drugs*, John Wiley & Sons, New York, 1985, pp. 191–316.
144. Tinkelman DG, Cavanaugh MJ, Cooper DM. Inhibition of exercise induced bronchospasm by atropine. *Am Rev Respir Dis* 114:87–94, 1976.
145. Hemstreetm PB. Atropine nebulization—simple and safe. *Ann Allergy* 44:138–141, 1980.
146. Pakes GE, Brogden RN, Heel RC, Speight TM, Avery GS. Ipratropium bromide: a review of its pharmacologic properties and therapeutic efficacy in asthma and chronic bronchitis. *Drugs* 20:237–266, 1980.
147. Gross NJ, Skorodin MS. Anticholinergic, antimuscarinic bronchodilators. State of the art. *Am Res Respir Dis* 129:856–870, 1984.
148. Yanai M, Ohrui T, Sekizawa K, Shimizu Y, Sasaki H, Takishima T. Effective site of bronchodilation by antiasthma drugs in subjects with asthma. *J Allergy Clin Immunol* 87:1080–1087, 1991.
149. Stokes GM, Milner AD, Hodges IGC, Henry RL. Nebulized ipratropium bromide in wheezy infants and young children. *Euro J Respir Dis* 64(Suppl.128):494–498, 1983.
150. Milner AD. Response to bronchodilator drugs in the first five years of life. *Eur J Clin Pharmacol* 18:117, 1980.
151. Warner JO, Gotz M, Landau I, Levinson H, Milner AD, Pedersen S, Silverman M. Management of asthma: a consensus statement. *Arch Dis Child* 64:1065–1079, 1989.
152. Naspitz CK, Sole D. Treatment of acute wheezing and dyspnea attacks in children under 2 years old: inhalation of fenoterol plus ipratropium bromide vs fenoterol. *J Asthma* in press.
153. Silverman M. The role of anticholinergic antimuscarinic bronchodilator therapy in children. *Lung* 168(Suppl):304–309, 1990.
154. Prendiville A, Green S, Silverman M. Ipratropium bromide and airways function in wheezy infants. *Arch Dis Child* 62:397–400, 1987.
155. Davies A, Vickerson F, Worsley G, Mindorff C, Kazim F, Levinson H. Determination of dose–response relationship for nebulized ipratropium bromide in asthmatic children. *J Pediatr* 105:1001–1005, 1983.
156. Freeman J, Landau LI. The effects of ipratropium bromide and fenoterol nebulizer solutions in children with asthma. *Clin Pediatr* 28:556–560, 1989.
157. Stokes GM, Milner AD, Hodges IGC, Henry RL. Nebulized ipratropium bromide in wheezy infants and young children. *Eur J Respir Dis* 64(Suppl.128):494–498, 1983.
158. Lin MT, Lee-Hong E, Collins-Williams C. A clinical trial of the bronchodilator effect of SCH 1000 aerosol in asthmatic children. *Ann Allergy* 40:326–332, 1978.

159. Agostini M, Barlocco G, Mastella G. Protective effect of fenoterol spray, ipratropium bromide plus fenoterol spray, and oral clembuterol, on exercise induced asthma in children. Double blind controlled and randomized clinical trial. *Eur J Respir Dis* 64(Suppl.128)529–532, 1983.
160. Lonnerholm G, Bratteby LE, Foucard T. Ipratropium bromide and beta-2 stimulants in chronic childhood asthma. *Ann Allergy* 55:306, 1985.
161. Spada EL, Conner CF, Fracchia C, Ioli F, Patessco A, Vecchio C. A comparative evaluation of salbutamol, disodium cromoglycate and ipratropium bromide in preventing exercise induced asthma. *Respiration* 46(Suppl.1):56, 1984.
162. Boner AL, Vallone G, DeStefano G. Effect of inhaled ipratripium bromide on methacholine and exercise provocation in asthmatic children. *Pediatr Pulmonol* 6:81–85, 1989.
163. Wilson N, Dixon C, Silverman M. Bronchial responsiveness to hyperventilation in children with asthma: inhibition by ipratropium bromide. *Thorax* 39:588–593, 1984.
164. Raes M, Milder P, Kerrejbin KF. Long term effects of ipratropium bromide and fenoterol to the bronchial hyperresponsiveness to histamine in children with asthma. *J Allergy Clin Immunol* 84:874–879, 1989.
165. Friberg S, Graff-Lennevig V. Ipratropium bromide in childhood asthma—a cumulative dose response study. *Ann Allergy* 55:306, 1985.
166. Spector SL, Katz FH, Farr RS. Troleandomycin: Effectiveness in steroid dependent asthma and bronchitis. *J Allergy Clin Immunol* 54:367–379, 1975.
167. Szefler SJ, Rose JQ, Ellis EF, Spector SL, Green AW, Jusko WJ. The effect of troleandomycin on methylprednisolone elimination. *J Allergy Clin Immunol* 66:447–451, 1980.
168. Selenke WM, Leung GW, Townley RG. Nonantibiotic effects of macrolide antibiotics of the oleandomycin-erythromycin group with special reference to their "steroid sparing" effects. *J Allergy Clin Immunol* 65:454–464, 1980.
169. Zieger RS, Schatz M, Sperling W, Simon R, Stevenson DD. Efficacy of troleandomycin in outpatients with severe corticosteroid dependent asthma. *J Allergy Clin Immunol* 66:438–446, 1980.
170. Szefler SJ, Ellis EF, Brenner M, Rose JQ, Spector SL, Yurchak AM, Andrews F, Jusko WJ. Steroid specific and anticonvulsant interaction aspects of troleandomycin steroid therapy. *J Allergy Clin Immunol* 69:455–460, 1980.
171. Eitches RW, Rachelefsky GS, Katz RM, Mendoza GR, Siegal SC. Methylprednisolone and troleandomycin in treatment of steroid dependent asthmatic children. Am J Dis Child 139:264–268, 1985.
172. Flotte TR, Loughlin GM. Benefits and complications of troleandomycin in young children with steroid-dependent asthma. *Pediatr Pulmonol* 10:178–182, 1991.
173. Shim C, Williams MH. The adequacy of inhalation of aerosol from canister nubulizers. *Am J Med* 69:891, 1980.
174. Clark TJH. Factors influencing route of administration of airway therapy.

In: Sadoul P. Milic-Emili J, Simonsson BG, Clark TJH (eds), *Small Airways in Health and Disease*, Excerpta Medica, Amsterdam, 1979, p.170.
175. Newman SP, Pavia D, Clark SW. How should a pressurized beta adrenergic bronchodilator be inhaled. *Eur J Respir Dis* 62:3, 1981.
176. Symposium: Recent advances in aerosol therapy—clinical update for the 1990's. 49th Annual Meeting American College of Allergy and Immunology, November, 1989.
177. Hartley JPR, Nogrady SG, Gibby OM, Seaton A. Bronchodilator effects of drug salbutamol powder administered by Rotahaler. *Br J Clin Pharmacol* 4:673, 1977.
178. Kemp JP, Meltzer EO. Beta-2 adrenergic agonists—oral or aerosol for the treatment of asthma. *J Asthma* 27(3):149, 1990.
179. Cayton RM, Webber B, Paterson JW, et al. A comparison of salbutamol given by pressure packed aerosol or nebulization via IPPB in acute asthma. *Br J Dis Chest* 72:222, 1978.
180. Johnson JR, Schroeder RC. Deposition of particles in model airway. *J Appl Physiol* 47:947, 1979.
181. Godden DJ, Crompton GK. An objective assessment of the tube spacer in patients unable to use conventional pressurized aerosol efficiently. *Br J Dis Chest* 75:165, 1981.
182. Reid LM. The presence or absence of bronchial mucus in fatal asthma. *J Allergy Clin Immunol* 80:415–416, 1987.
183. Dale HH, Laidlaw PP. Histamine shock. *J Physiol* 52:355–390, 1919.
184. Weiss S, Robb G, Blumgart HL. The velocity of blood flow in health and disease as measured by the effect of histamine on the minute vessels. *Am Heart J* 4:664–691, 1929.
185. Casterline CL, Evans R. Further studies on the mechanism of human histamine induced asthma. *J Allergy Clin Immunol* 59:420–424, 1977.
186. Norgrady SG, Bevan C. Inhaled antihistamines—bronchodilation and effects on histamine and methacholine induced bronchoconstriction. *Thorax* 33:700–704, 1978.
187. Popa VT. Effect of an H1 blocker, chlorpheniramine, on inhalation tests with histamine and allergen in allergic asthma. *Chest* 78:442–451, 1980.
188. Rafferty P, Holgate ST. Terfenadine is a potent and selective H1 histamine receptor antagonist in asthmatic airways. *Am Rev Respir Dis* 135:181, 1987.
189. Howarth PH, Holgate ST. Astemizole, an H1 antagonist in allergic asthma. *J Allergy Clin Immunol* 75(1):166A, 1985.
190. Tinkelman DG, Bucholtz GA, Kemp J, et al. Evaluation of the safety and efficacy of multiple doses of azelastine in adult patients with bronchial asthma over time. *Am Rev Respir Dis* 141:569–574, 1990.
191. Brik A, Tashkin DP, Gong H, et al. Effect of citerizine, an new histamine H1 antagonist, on airway dynamics and responsiveness to inhaled histamine in mild asthma. *J Allergy Clin Immunol* 80:51–56, 1987.
192. Simons FER, Luciuk GH, Becker AB, et al. Ketotifen: a new drug for prophylaxis of asthma in children. *Ann Allergy* 48:145–150, 1982.
193. Weinberg E, Fourie PB, Van Niekerk CH, et al. Improved control of childhood asthma using ketotifen at higher dose. *Eur Resp J* 2(Suppl):868S, 1989 (Abstr. No. 1033).

# 13

# Assessment and Treatment of Acute Asthma

**KEVIN R. MURPHY**

*Omaha Children's Hospital*
*Omaha, Nebraska*

**THOMAS C. NILSSON**

*Midwest Allergy and Asthma Clinic*
*Omaha, Nebraska*

Despite a better understanding of the mechanisms of asthma and improved treatment regimens, acute exacerbations of asthma continue to cause frequent emergency room visits and hospitalizations. The National Center for Health Statistics has shown that from 1979 to 1987 the hospital discharge rate with asthma increased 43% among children less than 15 years of age. Asthma mortality in North America and Europe appears to be increasing, with a particular impact on the younger age group. As a potentially fatal disease asthma has been reviewed, particularly in regard to the pediatric population (1). In dealing with a common and at times life-threatening disease, it is important to determine the level of care required for each individual patient and intervene quickly in those patients who are at particular risk. The initial goals of this chapter will be the diagnosis and objective assessment of the patient, allowing one to determine the appropriate level of care required. Current concepts of treatment of the outpatient are then discussed, as well as the decision as to which patients require inhospital treatment and which can be discharged. Finally, we present assessment and medical treatment of the hospitalized patient, including issues regarding mechanical ventilation in acute respiratory failure. A recent report, Guidelines for the Diagnosis and Management of Asthma issued through the National Heart, Lung and Blood Institute, gives a current consensus outline of treatment for chronic and acute asthma (2). Physicians caring for the asthmatic patient should be familiar with that Expert Panel Report. Our review will generally reflect recommendations made by the Expert Panel.

## PATHOPHYSIOLOGICAL MECHANISMS

The mediators of asthma and pathophysiology are discussed at length in the initial chapters of this text. Airways obstruction occurs from large to small airways and involves irregular narrowing of airways due to smooth muscle spasm, mucosal edema, sloughing of epithelial cells into the airway, and diminished mucociliary transport function. One result of widespread but uneven obstruction is mismatching of alveolar ventilation relative to perfusion (decreased V/Q); this factor largely explains the frequent hypoxemia seen in patients with acute asthma. It is generally recognized that the degree of hypoxemia does not correlate well with measurements of airways obstruction. As obstruction develops, hyperventilation occurs both on a reflex basis and to meet oxygen needs. As a result of worsening obstruction and increased work of breathing, hyperventilation worsens and thus increased pressures are required to maintain adequate ventilation. The cardiovascular consequences of these large pressure changes within the thorax, as well as hyperinflation, include compromised cardiac filling and emptying. This results in an accentuated fall in systolic blood pressure with inspiration and is the basis for the clinical sign of pulsus paradoxus. With very severe airway obstruction, the work of breathing may be sufficient to fatigue the respiratory muscles and result in ventilatory failure.

The young child and infant are at particular risk for rapid progression of obstruction to respiratory failure. Differences in lung physiology that may contribute to this include (3):

1. Increased peripheral airway resistance
2. Deficient collateral channels of ventilation
3. Airway smooth muscle that extends in a spiral manner further into peripheral airways
4. Decreased elastic recoil pressure
5. Mechanically disadvantaged diaphragm

Acid base abnormalities observed are largely explained by changes in $PCO_2$. The hyperventilation of mild to moderate asthma results in respiratory alkalosis. With worsening of obstruction and decreased alveolar ventilation, respiratory acidosis may be observed as $PCO_2$ increases above 40 mmHg. Younger children will frequently have a metabolic acidosis component from lactic acidosis, as the work of breathing increases. Ketone and organic acid production may also contribute to metabolic acidosis, particularly in the child with respiratory infection, fever, and dehydration.

## OUTPATIENT ASSESSMENT

The initial assessment of the asthmatic should try rapidly to determine the severity and begin treatment immediately, if the patient is in crisis. Once the appropriate level of care is initiated, certain points of history are useful, such as the duration of worsening and whether any trigger factors can be identified, including specific allergens or respiratory infections. The more prolonged the attack, the more likely it is that recovery will be slow and more intense therapy necessary (4). It is necessary to know all medicines being used, particularly the requirement for corticosteroids. The patient may be at risk for severe asthma and prolonged intensive treatment if there is history of previous hospitalizations, frequent emergency room visits, chronic corticosteroid use or recent withdrawal from systemic steroids, and history of intensive care unit management or mechanical ventilation. Psychosocial problems, particularly in inner city teenagers, have been shown to pose an increased risk for sudden death and severe hospital courses (5,6).

## PHYSICAL EXAMINATION

The initial physical examination seeks to determine rapidly the severity of airflow obstruction, identify complications, and should be repeated periodically after each treatment intervention is instituted. An initial impression of the patient's status would include alertness, a general impression of the level of respiratory distress, and color. Cyanosis or confusion suggests respiratory failure. In infants, observe overall alertness, responsiveness to the environment, ability to feed or suckle, and the quality of cry. The cry will become softer and shorter as airway obstruction increases.

The level of dyspnea should be noted, as well as use of accessory muscles of respiration. Heart rate and respiratory rate should be documented in the medical record. Diaphoresis and inability to lie supine as well as fragmented speech in the older child correlate with marked airflow obstruction (7). Attempts should be made to measure paradoxical pulse, since this correlates in children with significant obstruction (8). This value reflects the difference in fluctuation of systolic blood pressure between inspiration and expiration. It is measured as the difference in systolic blood pressure, between the pressure at which an observer first hears sporadic faint pulse sounds and the pressure at which all sounds are heard. If the pulse difference is greater than 20 mmHg, moderate to severe obstruction is present. Infants and children may have intercostal retractions, because of chest wall compliance, reflecting moderate airway obstruction.

Auscultation of the chest will generally reveal prolongation of the expiratory phase, as well as variable degrees of wheeze and decreased air exchange. It is well known that if the chest is relatively quiet, marked airways obstruction may be present. The "silent chest" will still demonstrate marked prolongation of the expiratory phase. Chest auscultation and examination should evaluate the possibility of complications such as atelectasis, pneumothorax, and pneumomediastinum. Palpation of supraclavicular and suprasternal areas may suggest pneumomediastinum, if present.

Studies in adults have shown that patients may have a better sense of the level of asthma present than the physician with physical examination, using pulmonary function testing as the standard (9). Even when symptoms and physical findings are minimal, considerable air flow limitation may be present, leaving those patients at risk for worsening after discharge. In addition, patients may have different levels of perception of asthma, and this may be modified by psychological factors such as denial. In infants and young children, whose condition may deteriorate most quickly, observation and physical examination may not give an adequate assessment of gas exchange. These points make it mandatory that some objective measurements be made to assess adequately the acute asthmatic patient.

## LUNG FUNCTION INVESTIGATIONS

Measurement of air flow obstruction should be made by peak expiratory flow rate (PEFR), measured with a peak flowmeter, or forced expiratory volume in 1 sec (FEV1). These measures correlate fairly well and peak flowmeters may be simply and economically used in office or emergency room settings. Adequate peak flow measurement can be made by most patients 5 years or older, but requires some patient cooperation in making a maximal expiratory effort. PEFR measures primarily large airway function and it should be recognized that diffuse airways disease may be present even with near-normal PEFR values. By the time wheezing can be detected with a stethoscope, PEFR is already decreased by 25% or more (10). Objective measurement of lung function should be used as part of the assessment of asthma severity and to measure response to initial medical therapy. It is also used as part of the overall appraisal of need for hospitalization or discharge and the need for stepped-up medical treatment as an outpatient, such as with corticosteroids.

Measurement of PEFR has eliminated the need for arterial blood gas studies in many asthmatic subjects, since only those with flow rates less than 25% of predicted had hypercarbia or acidosis (11). In addition to those with flow rates less than 25% of predicted, arterial blood gases (ABG) should be measured in the patient in extremis, if intubation and mechanical ventilation are being considered, or if pulmonary function testing cannot be performed and respiratory failure is suspected. In general, ABG measurements can be deferred until the patient's response to initial treatment is appraised. The use of this study in patients in status asthmaticus is discussed below.

Another useful study in the objective assessment is pulse oximetry measurement of arterial oxygen saturation. This can be done in patients who are too ill or too young to cooperate with pulmonary function tests. It has been shown that peak flow values improve before oxygen saturation values, probably because the flow rates reflect large airway obstruction, and oximetry may reflect a more diffuse airway narrowing and ventilation–perfusion inequality. The use of peak flow and oximetry will be discussed below with regard to decision making regarding admission or discharge.

## OTHER LABORATORY STUDIES

Other laboratory studies are generally not indicated on a routine basis. A white blood cell (WBC) assessment might be obtained if there are questions about infection, such as fever or purulent sputum in the unusually ill child. Measurement of electrolytes is not justified in the outpatient setting; however, the hospitalized child may be hypokalemic as a result of beta-agonist and corticosteroid therapy, which may predispose to cardiac rhythm disturbances.

If there has been any history of theophylline use, a blood level of theophylline should be determined to rule out theophylline toxicity in case the patient has taken extra medicine when their symptoms worsened. This would also serve as a baseline value if oral or intravenous theophylline is to be continued during inpatient management. The acute care physician should not assume noncompliance because of low theophylline blood levels in the acute situation, since metabolism and absorption may change with acute illness (12). Changes in maintenance theophylline dosages should be deferred to the primary care physician to avoid increases in dosage that may cause toxicity.

## CHEST RADIOGRAPHS

It has been determined that a chest x-ray should not be done on a routine basis in children with acute asthma in the emergency room (13). In that study of 371 children presenting during first attacks of asthma, 94% of radiographs were compatible with uncomplicated asthma. Patients with positive findings were more likely to have a respiratory rate above 60/min or a pulse rate above 160/min, localized rales or decreased breath sounds, and/or temperature greater than 38.3° C. No patient had an unsuspected pulmonary disease (e.g. cystic fibrosis or foreign body) and a posteroanterior and lateral chest x-ray does not reliably exclude the presence of inhaled foreign bodies (other radiographic studies are required to investigate this). A chest x-ray may be indicated as a baseline for intensive care if the diagnosis of asthma is unclear, particularly in a young child, and to evaluate for the presence of atelectasis, pulmonary infiltrates, pneumomediastinum, or pneumothorax. These conditions may be present if the patient has physical findings suggestive of these complications, deteriorates rapidly, or if problems in gas exchange are greater than expected. Pneumothorax can be a disastrous complication in the patient with acute asthma, but is fortunately much less common than the other conditions.

## INITIAL TREATMENT IN THE OFFICE OR EMERGENCY ROOM

A treatment protocol is presented that is appropriate for the majority of patients seen. We cannot overemphasize the need to evaluate expeditiously the level of care that will be required and to make sure that those with severe or life-threatening asthma are quickly identified and treatment initiated. An algorithm has been developed by the National Asthma Education Program Expert Panel Report. These recommendations are a guide to therapy, modified by specific circumstances and the physician's judgment (see Figs. 1, 2).

## Oxygen

The majority of patients seen for acute asthma care will have some level of hypoxemia. Oxygen at a rate of 3–6 liters/min should be started, so that arterial oxygen saturation is maintained at greater than 92%. Beta-agonist therapy may lead to intermittent dips in saturation, based on changes in V/Q matching, but it is not clear that this is clinically very important. Oxygen therapy should be initiated promptly and gas exchange then assessed by oximetry or measurement of blood gases as indicated clinically. Arterial oxygen saturation is monitored by pulse oximetry if the child requires admission to the hospital.

## Beta-2 Agonist Bronchodilators

The current standard for initial treatment of acute asthma is aerosolized selective beta-2 agonists. It is generally believed that the long-acting selective beta-2 agonists, such as albuterol and terbutaline, may have fewer side effects and better duration of action than the older agents. Administration by the aerosol route is favored, since this delivers the drug to the site of action in the lung with lower dosages and fewer side effects than parenteral therapy. Of available agents we recommend albuterol because there is no evidence that terbutaline provides any greater bronchodilatation or longer duration of action. Conventional initial dosages would be 0.5 ml of a 0.5% solution diluted with 3 ml normal saline. This dose is administered every 20 min for three doses by compressor nebulizer, depending on the patient's initial status and response to treatment. Higher-dosage beta-agonist therapy and continuous nebulization are discussed below under treatment of inpatient status asthmaticus. If the patient responds well to initial treatment, the frequency of aerosols may be decreased as plans for discharge are made. If there continues to be wheeze, dyspnea, and peak flow measurement is 40–70% of predicted, aerosols may be continued every 20–30 min, for 3 or 4 doses, as the patient's status is continually monitored. In this group hospitalization will often be required and corticosteroids should be considered when response is not prompt. Prolonged emergency room treatment of ill patients should be avoided.

There have been several reports of emergency room beta-agonist therapy using metered-dose inhalers (MDI) alone, showing that this is successful (14–19). The advantages of doing this include quicker initiation of treatment, since respiratory care services need often to be mobilized for

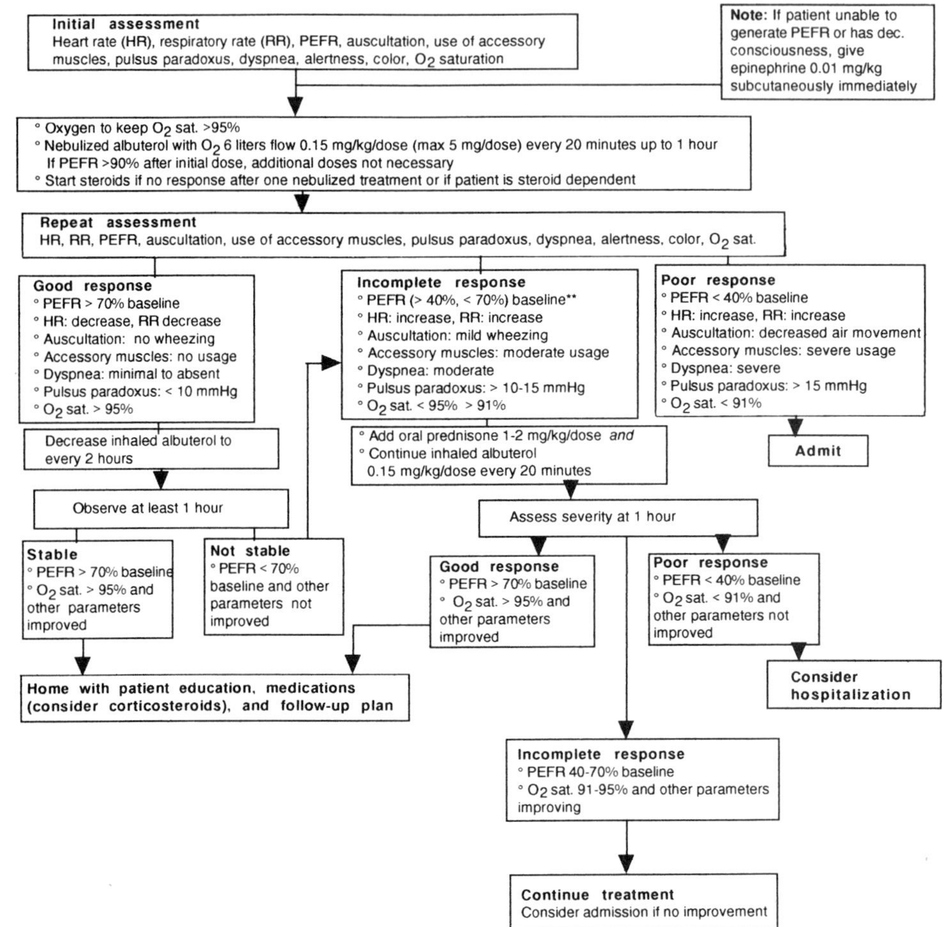


FIGURE 1 Acute exacerbations of asthma in children: emergency department management. Therapies are often available in a physician's office. However, most acutely severe exacerbations of asthma require a complete course of therapy in an emergency department. PEFR % baseline refers to the norm for the individual, established by the clinician. This may be percentage predicted based on standardized norms or patient's personal best (From Ref. 2.)

nebulizer treatment. Costs involved are also lower and equal amounts of drug may be administered. Despite these advantages of MDI therapy, the majority of studies done to date have been in adults. It has not yet been clearly shown that young children can cooperate or develop the flow rates necessary for this treatment to be effective. As of now the standard of care continues to be compressor–nebulizer delivery.

### Epinephrine

Aqueous epinephrine has both alpha- and beta-adrenergic agonist effects and the alpha-adrenergic effect may have some beneficial effects on mucosal edema as well as the beta-bronchodilator mechanism. However, as initial treatment for asthma, epinephrine has been displaced by the beta-agonist bronchodilators. Current preference for the inhaled route is based on slightly lower effectiveness of sequential epinephrine, greater side effects (20), and because injections are painful for children. Epinephrine may have a role as immediate therapy in a patient who presents in crisis and may not be able to inhale a beta-agonist. There may also be patients who respond to epinephrine when initial beta-agonist therapy does not seem to be helping (21). In the obstructed patient with asthma, epinephrine doses do not significantly affect pulse and blood pressure; the benefit of improved air flow tends to balance out any stimulant cardiovascular effects.

### Aminophylline

Although for many years intravenous aminophylline was a cornerstone of the initial emergency room care of acute asthma, the rational basis for its use has not been substantiated (22–23). In studies comparing injected epinephrine, repetitive beta-agonist aerosols, and intravenous aminophylline in accepted blood levels, aminophylline was a significantly less effective bronchodilator that the other treatments. When used in combination with sequential beta-agonist aerosols, no improvement was seen in bronchodilatation with combination therapy compared to beta-agonist therapy alone. Side effects were significantly higher in the aminophylline-treated group (24). At this time there is no evidence that aminophylline should be used in the first 4 hours of acute care for asthma.

In light of the strong support in the literature for avoiding aminophylline in emergency room treatment, a recent article is of interest. In a series of adults treated with metaproterenol and intravenous prednisolone, with or without aminophylline, the aminophylline-treated group had a significantly lower hospital admission rate than those who received placebo (25). An editorial accompanying this paper reflects on the role of aminophylline in asthma therapy (26). This study is of interest, but should not at present change the role of aminophylline in the emergency room care of acute asthma.

### Corticosteroids

It is well established that corticosteroid therapy is of benefit in hospitalized patients whose obstruction does not resolve with emergency room bronchodilator therapy (27,28). It is somewhat more difficult to decide precisely when steroids should be administered to the emergency room patient. In general, there is a correlation between the extent of obstruction found in initial assessment and the time course of improvement. It has likewise been shown in children that slow recovery is expected when peak expiratory flow responds slowly to injected and inhaled sympathomimetics (29). It is likely that the more obstructed patients who respond slowly to initial treatment have diffuse inflammatory changes that will require anti-inflammatory therapy with steroids. The current recommendation is to administer oral prednisone 1–2 mg/kg if the patient is not responding to the initial treatment with sequential aerosols. Either oral prednisone or intravenous methylprednisolone may be administered, with no evidence that the parenteral route is more effective if comparable steroid dosages are used (30,31). Intramuscular administration of steroid in infants and toddlers has also been shown to be effective (75).

Studies in adults have been somewhat conflicting as to whether early corticosteroids reduce the need for hospital admissions in patients with acute asthma: one study showed a benefit (32) and a subsequent study failed to show a decrease in admission rates (33). Considering the slow onset of corticosteroid action (1–8 hr) and the slow time course for resolution of obstruction in more severely affected patients, it is not unexpected that steroids may not have a significant short-term impact. The value of steroid therapy in the emergency room setting is to initiate that treatment in the patient likely to need admission and to prevent relapse in the patient with milder disease after he or she leaves the hospital.

The majority of children with acute asthma will be discharged to home care. Which of these discharged children should receive short-course corticosteroids remains poorly defined. In 28 children who were discharged after outpatient therapy and received treatment with methylprednisolone or placebo, short-term corticosteroid therapy accelerated resolution of asthma compared to the placebo-treated group, without significant suppression of adrenal function (34). Studies in adults have shown that short-course oral prednisone in patients discharged from emergency room reduced early relapse rates, measured as return to the emergency room or persisting symptoms (35). It remains to be determined whether the less ill patient whose course reverses completely based on examination and PFTs needs corticosteroid therapy. We would be inclined to use corticosteroids in children who have required regular medical therapy for asthma, if there were a viral infection trigger, or other past history suggests risk for relapse. The steroid-treated outpatient is generally given 1–2 mg/kg/day of prednisone as initial dosage, with tapering of the dosage over 5–10 days.

## INDICATIONS FOR HOSPITAL ADMISSION

A recent study from Toronto analyzing emergency room visits over a 16 month period showed that 74% of patients were discharged, with 26% admitted to the hospital; 83% of these children admitted were less than 10 years of age (36). Attempts have been made to predict which patients will require hospital care and who can be discharged. No predictive index has been reliable in predicting patient outcome. Levison and colleagues recently presented information that was helpful in deciding who required admission, based on a clinical score derived from standard physical examination (37). Factors measured included heart rate, respiratory rate, pulses paradoxus, subjective impression of dyspnea, accessory muscle use, and wheezing (see Table 1). Patients with a clinical score over .45 on disposition were likely to be hospitalized. It has been suggested in another study that patients with $SAO_2$ equal to or less than 91% should be hos-

TABLE 1 Clinical Scoring System

| | Score = 0 | Score = 1 |
|---|---|---|
| Heart rate (/min) | $<120$ | $\geq 120$ |
| Respiratory rate (/min) | $<30$ | $\geq 30$ |
| Pulsus paradoxus (mm Hg) | $<15$ | $\geq 15$ |
| Dyspnea[a] | Absent or mild | Moderate or severe |
| Accessory muscle use | Absent or minimal | Moderate or severe |
| Wheezing | Absent[b] or end-expiratory only | Throughout expiration[b] or expiratory + inspiratory |

[a]Dyspnea was defined as the investigator's impression of the degree of the child's breathlessness.

[b]A patient with absent wheezing but who was in respiratory distress was assigned a score of 1.

*Source*: Kerem E, Canny G, Tibshirani R, Reisman J, Bentur L, Schuh S, Levison H. Clinical–Physiologic correlations in acute asthma of childhood. *Pediatrics*. 87:4, 481, 1991.

pitalized (38). Only 38% of the Toronto children who were hospitalized had $SAO_2$ values less than 91%. The authors state that no protocol can be relied on absolutely and clinical judgment remains as important as any predictive index. They also make the important point that the decision for hospitalization or discharge may be determined by nonmedical factors such as patient and parental compliance, parents' understanding of the disease, and adequate monitoring, should worsening occur at home.

Patients requiring admission will generally continue to have peak flows less than 50% of predicted despite initial therapy, decreased air exchange and expiratory wheezes on physical examination, continued signs of increased work of breathing, and $SAO_2$ less than 91% following treatment. The emergency department management algorithm in Figure 1 outlines a reasonable approach to disposition. If in doubt, it is prudent to admit the patient, particularly toddlers or infants who may require more careful monitoring and specialized treatment.

## TREATMENT AFTER EMERGENCY ROOM DISCHARGE

A child should not be sent home on the same treatment program that failed to control symptom worsening; some intensification of treatment is necessary. There should be a discussion about careful compliance with medicines, not overusing beta-agonist therapy, and consideration given to a course of corticosteroids as discussed above. A peak flowmeter should preferably be used on a regular basis to ensure improvement in lung function. No patient should leave the emergency room (ER) without outpatient follow-up within 3–10 days. At follow-up, the exacerbation should be reviewed and the treatment program refined to try to intervene before symptoms worsen so that ER care is required. In patients who have had emergency room visits and been hospitalized, referral to an asthma specialist appears to reduce the rate of relapse very significantly, as measured by fewer returns to the hospital and better asthma control. This was due in part to greater use of inhaled steroids and cromolyn in the referred group (39). Management and monitoring of the outpatient asthmatic patient are discussed in another chapter of this text.

## INPATIENT MANAGEMENT OF STATUS ASTHMATICUS

Status asthmaticus, or acute severe asthma that is resistant to appropriate outpatient therapy, can be life-threatening and requires prompt, systematic, and aggressive management in the hospital. The younger child is at increased risk for both status asthmaticus and rapid deterioration leading to acute respiratory failure (40). The assessment of asthma severity, especially in younger children, thus becomes paramount, followed by initiation of early and appropriate bronchodilator therapy.

## Assessment of Severity

The child with status asthmaticus should be managed either in the intensive care unit or pediatric unit so that the patient's overall clinical course, vital signs, physical findings, and symptoms can be monitored closely. The management of each child with status asthmaticus should be individualized; however, certain general principles apply to all patients (see Fig. 2).

An appropriate history should be obtained and physical examination performed. Information on previous acute exacerbations of asthma can be quite helpful in deciding an approach to therapy, as well as predicting a response to treatment. In assessing the severity of the asthma attack, specific historical points are of importance and include the duration of the episode, therapy prior to admission to the hospital, and other associated medical disorders. Pertinent physical findings include overall level of consciousness, respiratory rate, use of accessory muscles of respiration, and air exchange. Lung function assessment should include peak flow measurements and in most cases is reliably measured in children over 5 years of age. Noninvasive measurement of oxygen saturation with pulse oximetry is safe, reliable, and should be performed on all patients admitted to the hospital. In the past clinical pulmonary indexes or severity scoring systems have been recommended (41). Most recent data suggest that the use of peak flow measurements in combination with oxygen saturation can be highly predictive of outcome and in determining the degree of severity of the attack (11). These noninvasive assessments of asthma severity usually are sufficient to obviate the need for more invasive evaluation including blood gas measurements (see Table 2). Peak flow measurements in patients with acute asthma showed that no patient with a peak flow of greater than 25% predicted had a $PCO_2$ greater than 45 mm Hg, or a pH less than 7.35. The converse was true: patients with a peak flow less than 25% predicted were at risk for significant acid-base imbalance and would require measurement of blood gas levels (11).

Hypoxemia is almost always present during acute exacerbations of asthma. With the availability of pulse oximeters, oxygen saturation should be measured in all children with an acute asthma attack. If the oxygen saturation is less than 90%, an arterial blood gas or capillary blood gas evaluation should then be obtained to measure $PACO_2$, as well as to evaluate acid–base status more closely (42). Chest radiographs should be considered on an individual basis. If both tachypnea and fever are present, a chest x-ray can be helpful (13,43).

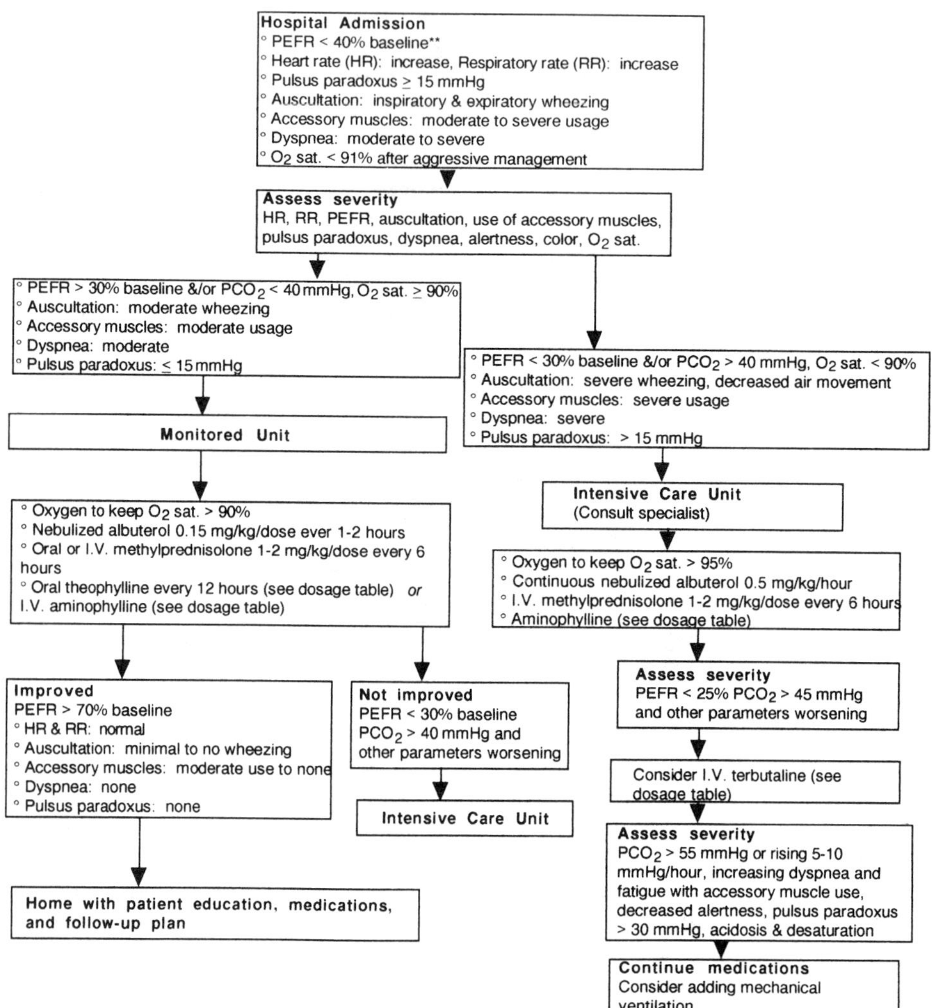


FIGURE 2 Acute exacerbations of asthma in children: hospital management. PEFR % baseline refers to the norm for the individual, established by the clinician. This may be percentage predicted based on standardized norms or % patient's personal best. (From Ref. 2.)

TABLE 2 Estimation of Severity of Acute Exacerbations of Asthma in Children

| Sign/Symptom | Mild | Moderate | Severe |
|---|---|---|---|
| Respiratory rate (see Table 3) | Normal to < 1 standard deviation from the norm (S.D.) for age | Normal to < 2 S.D. for age | Normal to > 2 S.D. for age |
| Alertness | Normal | Normal | May be decreased |
| Dyspnea | Absent or mild; speaks in complete sentences | Moderate; speaks in phrases or partial sentences | Severe; speaks only in single-word or short phrases |
| Pulsus paradoxus (mm Hg) | <10 | 10–20 | 20–40 |
| Accessory muscle use | No intercostal to mild retractions | Moderate intercostal retraction with tracheosternal retractions; use of sternocleidomastoid muscles | Severe intercostal retractions, tracheosternal retractions with nasal flaring |
| Color | Good | Pale | Possibly cyanotic |
| Ascultation | End-expiratory wheeze only | Wheeze during entire expiration and inspiration | Breath sounds becoming inaudible |
| Oxygen saturation (%) | >95 | 90–95 | <90 |
| $PCO_2$ | <35 | <40 | >40 |
| PEFR | 70–90% predicted or personal best | 50–70% predicted or personal best | <50% predicted or personal best |

Source: Ref. 2.

Most children admitted to the hospital with status asthmaticus can be monitored and treated on the pediatric floor. Those patients with more severe symptoms should be managed in the intensive care unit. The use of peak flow measurements and blood gas determination, in combination with the examination, can be helpful in determining the need for more intensive care monitoring and management (see Table 2).

## Oxygen Therapy

Oxygen administration is required for almost all children admitted to the hospital with status asthmaticus, with the goal of keeping $O_2$ saturation greater than 95%. Humidified oxygen can be delivered by nasal cannula, face mask, or through a mechanical ventilator. Flow rates of oxygen during acute asthma are critical. Low flow rates, including use of nasal prongs, are inadequate when a patient is hyperventilating. Due to the increased work of breathing with acute asthma, flow rates, as well as oxygen concentration, need to be high (44).

TABLE 3 Normal Resting Respiratory Rate (Breaths/min)

| Age (Years) | Boys (Mean ± SD) | Girls (Mean ± SD) |
|---|---|---|
| 0–1 | 31 ± 8 | 30 ± 6 |
| 1–2 | 26 ± 4 | 27 ± 4 |
| 2–3 | 25 ± 4 | 25 ± 3 |
| 3–4 | 24 ± 3 | 24 ± 3 |
| 4–5 | 23 ± 2 | 22 ± 2 |
| 5–6 | 22 ± 2 | 21 ± 2 |
| 6–7 | 21 ± 3 | 21 ± 3 |
| 7–8 | 20 ± 3 | 20 ± 2 |
| 8–9 | 20 ± 2 | 20 ± 2 |
| 9–10 | 19 ± 2 | 19 ± 2 |
| 10–11 | 19 ± 2 | 19 ± 2 |
| 11–12 | 19 ± 3 | 19 ± 3 |
| 12–13 | 19 ± 3 | 19 ± 2 |
| 13–14 | 19 ± 2 | 18 ± 2 |
| 14–15 | 18 ± 2 | 18 ± 3 |
| 15–16 | 17 ± 3 | 18 ± 3 |
| 16–17 | 17 ± 2 | 17 ± 3 |
| 17–18 | 16 ± 3 | 17 ± 3 |

Source: Waring WW. The history and physical examination. In Kendig, Cherniak (eds.), *Disorders of the Respiratory Tract in Children*, WB Saunders, Philadelphia, 1983, p. 63.

TABLE 4 Guidelines for Intravenous Fluid Therapy in Status Asthmaticus

Hydration (initial)
5% glucose in normal saline, 12 ml/kg or 360 ml/$m^2$ for first hour
Depletion Repair
Normal saline, 10–15 ml/kg or 300–500 ml/$m^2$ in 24 hr
Water (5% glucose in water), 10–15 ml/kg or 300–500 ml/$m^2$ in 24 hr
Maintenance
Fluids: 5% glucose in water, 50 ml/kg or 1500 ml/$m^2$ in 24 hr, depending on age
Electrolytes: Potassium, 2 mEq/100 ml of maintenance IV fluid
Sodium, 3 mEq/100 ml of maintenance IV fluids
Buffers
If pH is below 7.30 and base deficit is greater than 5 mEq/L, correct to normal range with IV sodium bicarbonate according to the following calculation: bicarbonate (mEq) = negative base excess (mEq) × 0.3 × body weight (kg)
Administer half the calculated dose initially and the other half after repeating blood gas determinations.

Source: Ref. 46.

## Intravenous Fluids

Children admitted to the hospital with worsening chest symptoms often have inadequate fluid intake and increased insensible water loss. Administration of intravenous fluids thus often becomes essential for appropriate hydration. In cases of dehydration, rehydration at a rate of 1-1/2 times the usual maintenance level can be safely initiated with the use of 5% glucose, sodium 3 mEq/100 ml, and potassium 2 mEq/100 ml. Electrolytes need to be monitored, especially sodium and potassium. Hypokalemia can occur and is thought to be secondary to frequent beta-adrenergic therapy (45). Inappropriate antidiuretic hormone secretion has been reported during acute asthma with the findings of hyponatremia with continued renal excretion of sodium. A guide for intravenous fluid therapy in status asthmaticus (see Table 4) is designed to replace fluid deficits as well as to provide appropriate normal maintenance requirements (46).

## Medications

### *Beta-Agonists*

Adrenergic agonists, with their refinement and more specific beta-2 effect, have become the mainstay in treatment of acute asthma. The various medications available for clinical use have been classified into nonspecific catacholamine derivatives, which include ephedrine, epinephrine, and isoproterenol, and specific beta-2 agonists, which include metaproterenol, terbutaline, fenoterol, and albuterol.

Beta-agonists can be administered orally, parentally, or by aerosol. Multiple studies have compared these methods of administration and find that inhaled nebulized beta-agonists are more effective, and in certain instances have fewer side effects. Albuterol has been shown to be effective in a group of children 5–17 years of age with moderate to severe asthma treated with standard (0.15 mg/kg) and high-dosage (0.3 mg/kg) hourly aerosols. The higher dosage is usually not required, however it produced better improvement in FEV 1.0, without greater side effects, than the standard dosage (47). Administration of nebulized albuterol every 20 min produces a significantly greater improvement in lung function than a higher dosage given every hour (48). When clinically indicated, the more frequent administration of albuterol is appropriate, safe, and without associated increased side effects. Beta-adrenergic therapy can be accomplished with the use of a metered-dose inhaler (MDI), ultrasonic or jet nebulizer. Aerosol therapy, delivered either by MDI or nebulizer, is effective in treatment of acute asthma. When using an MDI during acute exacerbations of asthma, the dosage should be increased (six times the maintenance dose) and delivery enhanced with the use of a spacer device attached to the inhaler (49–51).

### *Methylxanthines*

For years aminophylline has been the bronchodilator choice for treating patients with status asthmaticus. In many centers, methylxanthines are still commonly used. It is clear that methylxanthines have (some) bronchodilator effect in acute exacerbations of asthma; however, in adult studies it has been difficult to show added benefit when aminophylline is used in conjunction with maximal dosage of inhaled beta-agonists and steroid (52,53). In addition, the side effects of methylxanthines are numerous and include tachycardia, nausea, vomiting, as well as irritability, restlessness, and headache. Aerosolized beta-agonist therapy in children is the standard for emergency room care. In hospitalized children only one double-blind placebo-controlled trial of intravenous aminophylline has been carried out, which demonstrated a clear benefit for aminophylline (54). Until further studies have been performed in children, aminophylline continues to be an appropriate adjunct to first-line beta-agonist therapy. When aminophylline is administered intravenously, an initial bolus is frequently used to obtain therapeutic blood levels; however, initial bolus therapy may be unnecessary in those patients already receiving daily oral theophylline. Bolus and maintenance therapy should only be started after theophylline blood level is known. Due to the variable half-life of this agent from patient to patient, the infusion dosage must be individually adjusted to maintain blood levels in the suggested therapeutic range of 10–20 μg/ml (55). It is mandatory to monitor signs of toxicity including tachycardia, headache, nausea, vomiting, seizures, and cardiac arrhythmias (see Fig. 3).

**Guideline For Intravenous Aminophylline Therapy in Status Asthmaticus**

Give aminophylline bolus (over 30 min),
Every 1 mg/kg aminophylline increases serum
theophylline level 2 μg/ml; then follow
with constant intravenous aminophylline

| *Age* | *Infusion Rate* |
|---|---|
| 1-6 months | 0.5 mg/kg/hr aminophylline |
| 6 mo-1 year | 1.0 mg/kg/hr aminophylline |
| 1-9 years | 1.5 mg/kg/hr aminophylline |
| 10-16 years | 1.2 mg/kg/hr aminophylline |

obtain serum **theophylline level** 1 hour post bolus

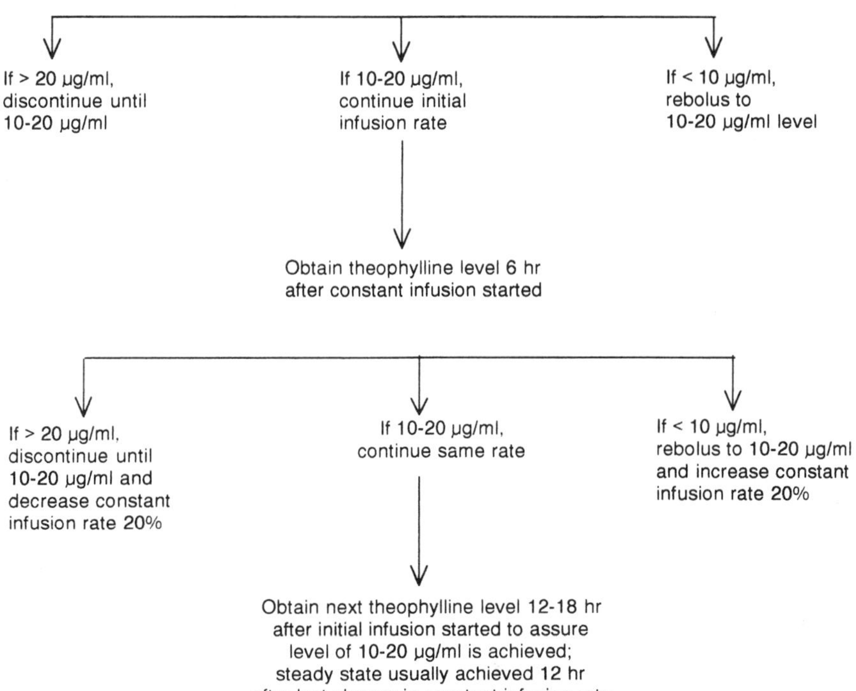


FIGURE 3 Algorithm for therapy with intravenous aminophylline. (Adapted from Ref 55.)

### *Anticholinergics*

Anticholinergic drugs produce bronchodilatation by inhibiting cholinergic-mediated bronchospasm. They primarily affect the central airways and have a slower onset of action than beta-agonist drugs. Ipratropium bromide (Atrovent) is available as an MDI and is less lipid-soluble than atropine, thus avoiding atropine's side effects, such as dryness, flushing, and tachycardia. Studies have shown added bronchodilatation when anticholinergics are combined with beta-agonist during acute exacerbations of asthma (56). However, that initial improvement averages upward to 15% and it is not yet clear that this leads to improved clinical outcome. Benefits of ipratropium have not yet been evaluated against high-dosage frequent beta-agonist aerosols (57).

### *Corticosteroids*

It is well accepted that corticosteroids are effective and necessary in the treatment of acute asthma. Corticosteroids, when started early in treatment, have been shown to reduce both morbidity and mortality (58,23). The mechanisms of steroid activity are thought to be primarily a reduction in the inflammatory process. This occurs through various pathways, including inhibition of phospholipase $A_2$ activity, thus inhibiting release of inflammatory mediators. Corticosteroids also increase the number and affinity of beta-receptors, and inhibit both the early and late asthmatic response. Some studies have shown benefits of higher dosages of steroids, however in the only pediatric trial there was no advantage to a high dosage over a moderate dosage of intravenous steroids (59). Methylprednisolone can be administered safely in a dosage of 1–2 mg/kg every 6 hr, and some patients may require higher dosages. Methylprednisolone has less mineralocorticoid effect and thus is recommended over other steroid preparations.

### *Other Medications*

Various other medications and modes of therapy have been suggested for the treatment of acute exacerbations of asthma. Antibiotics are rarely indicated, since most infectious exacerbations of asthma are secondary to viral disease. Certainly the exception is *Mycoplasma pneumoniae* and this should be considered, particularly during times of community outbreaks (60). Erythromycin is used with caution if simultaneous methylxanthines are being administered, since this antibiotic affects the pharmacokinetics and half-life of methylxanthines. The use of alkalizing agents, specifically sodium bicarbonate, is indicated for the more critically ill child with mixed respiratory metabolic acidosis (61). Sodium bicarbonate administration is indicated when the pH is less than 7.30. Administration should be in a dosage equal to the base deficit $\times$ 0.3 $\times$ body weight in kilograms (see

Table 4). In children with pH above 7.30, acidosis is usually corrected with appropriate use of beta-agonists and corticosteroids.

## Intensive Care Management

In children with poor response to initial therapy, or those who present or develop persistent hypoxemia, exhaustion, or change in state of consciousness, admission to the intensive care unit is required. A number of asthma scores include blood gas findings, chest examination, and state of consciousness to define impending or acute respiratory failure. It is generally agreed upon that a $PCO_2$ greater than or equal to 55 mmHg defines impending respiratory failure and a $PCO_2$ greater than 65 mmHg signifies respiratory failure. Depending on the degree of hypoxia, a patient may well be in impending respiratory failure with a rising $PACO_2$ less than 55 mmHg. It is difficult to obtain information about the mortality of severe life-threatening asthma that requires intensive care treatment. It has been estimated that as many as two-thirds of asthma deaths could possibly be avoided if the patient was given early and appropriate therapy (62). Thus the importance of aggressive management of acute exacerbations of asthma cannot be overemphasized, particularly a severe asthma attack with associated hypoxemia and respiratory distress.

### *Continuous Beta-Agonist Nebulization*

A number of investigators have shown that individuals with severe airways obstruction will improve significantly with continuous nebulized beta-agonist, after standard therapy has failed (63–65). The safety and efficacy of continuous nebulized terbutaline has gained acceptance over the last few years. Terbutaline can be continuously nebulized at a dosage between 1 and 12 mg/hr. A simple and effective approach consists of administering 0.25–3.0 mg of terbutaline (1 mg/ml) in saline to give a total volume of 3 ml every 15 min, to a maximal dose of 12 mg/hr, or until clinical improvement occurs (64). It has been suggested that terbutaline offers no advantage over albuterol and is more dilute (1 mg/1 ml) than albuterol (5 mg/ml). Albuterol is available as a nebulizer solution administered at a dosage of 0.5 mg/kg/hr, with a maximal dosage of 15 mg/hr (2).

### *Intravenous Beta-Agonist Infusion*

In children with severe airways obstruction and low inspiratory flow rates, continuously inhaled bronchodilators may be ineffective. In this case, an arterial line should be placed and intravenous terbutaline initiated. This is recommended over administration of intravenous isoproterenol, because cardiac complications have been reported to occur with isoproterenol. Intravenous terbutaline is initiated with an infusion rate of 0.4 μg/kg/min, with an increase in the infusion rate of 0.2 μg/kg/min every 15 min, to a maximum of 3–6 μg/kg/min, or until there is a fall in PACO2 with improved findings on a chest examination (67,68).

### *Controlled Ventilation*

Only when asthma cannot be controlled with conventional therapy, including aggressive ICU management, should mechanical ventilation be employed. A volume-cycled ventilator is recommended, with a low rate and long expiratory time. End-expiratory pressure should be minimal, and tidal volume estimated to keep peak airway pressure less than 40–50 cm $H_2O$. This can be accomplished usually only with heavy sedation or muscle paralysis. All medications used before controlled ventilation should be continued. In those individuals who do not improve with mechanical ventilation, general anesthesia with halothane or ketamine has been shown in some individuals successfully to relieve severe airway obstruction unresponsive to all other measures (69–71).

## AFTERCARE AND PREVENTION OF STATUS ASTHMATICUS

Deaths from asthma as well as life-threatening exacerbations appear to be related to overreliance on bronchodilators, delay in seeking treatment, and underutilization of oral corticosteroids as symptoms worsen (72). Some deaths have been attributed to undertreatment following recent symptom flares (73,74). At the time of follow-up after severe asthma, a medical plan needs to be developed that better recognizes the warning signs of asthma. There should be regular monitoring of peak flows in any high-risk patient and medical contact should be made if predetermined peak flow declines to a certain level, even if the patient does not seem particularly symptomatic. At follow-up, psychosocial issues need to be identified and appropriate intervention instituted. The family should have available a physician they can contact and emergency room observation and care should be sought before crises occur. Dr. Richard Farr has said that status asthmaticus should be treated 3 days before it happens; this should be the continuing goal of the physician who helps patients and families to manage asthma.

## REFERENCES

1. Strunk RC. Identification of the fatality-prone subject with asthma. *J Allergy Clin Immunol* 83:477–485, 1989.
2. Sheffer A. *Guidelines for the Diagnosis and Management of Asthma*. National Institutes of Health, National Asthma Education Program, Bethesda, Maryland, Publication No. 91-3042.

3. Isles AF, Levison H. Pediatric asthma in: *Bronchial Asthma: Mechanisms and Therapeutics*, 2nd ed. (Little, Brown: Boston) 1985, pp. 838–859.
4. Fanta CH, Rossing TH, McFadden ER Jr. Emergency room treatment of asthma. *Am J Med* 72:416–412, 1982.
5. Fritz GK, Rubinstein S, Lewiston NJ. Psychological factors in fatal childhood asthma. *Am J Orthopsychiatry* 57(2):253–257, 1987.
6. Rea HH, Scragg R, Jackson R, Beaglehole E, Fenwick J, Southerland D. A case-controlled study of deaths from asthma. *Thorax* 41:833–839, 1986.
7. Brenner BE, Abraham E, Simm R. Position and diaphoresis in acute asthma. *Am J Med* 74:1005–1009, 1983.
8. Galant SP, Grancy CE, Shaw KC. The value of pulsus paradoxus in assessing the child with status asthmaticus. *Pediatrics* 61:46–51, 1978.
9. Shim CS, Williams MH Jr. Evaluation of the severity of asthma: patients versus physicians. *Am J Med* 68:11–13, 1980.
10. Shirri CS, Williams H. Relationship of wheezing to the severity of obstruction in asthma. *Arch Intern Med* 143:890–892, 1983.
11. Martin TG, Elenbaas RM, Pingleton SH. Use of peak expiratory flow rates to eliminate unnecessary arterial blood gases in acute asthma. *Ann Emerg Med* 11:70–73, 1982.
12. Weinberger M. The pharmacology and therapeutic use of theophylline. *J Allergy Clin Immunol* 73:525–540, 1984.
13. Gershel JC, Goldman HS, Stein R, Shelov SP, Ziprkowski M. The usefulness of chest radiographs in first asthma attacks. *N Eng J Med* 1983; 309:336–339.
14. Shim CS, Williams HM. Effect of bronchodilator therapy administered by cannister versus jet nebulizer. *J Allergy Clin Immunol* 387–390, 1984.
15. Turner JR, Corkery KJ, Eckman D, Gelb A, et al. Equivalence of continuous flow nebulizer and metered dose inhaler with reservoir bag for treatment of acute airflow obstruction. *Chest* 93:476–481, 1988.
16. Morgan MDL, Singh BV, Frame MH, Williams SJ. Terbutaline aerosol given through pear spacer in acute severe asthma. *Br Med J* 285:849–850, 1982.
17 Madsen EB, Bundgard A, Hidinger KG. Cumulative dose-response study comparing terbutaline pressurized aerosol administered via a pear-shaped spacer and terbutaline in a nebulized solution. *Eur J Clin Pharmacol* 23:27–30, 1982.
18. Morley TF, Marozsan E, Zappason SJ, Griesback R, Guidice JC. Comparison of beta-adrenergic agents delivered by nebulizer versus metered dose inhaler in hospitalized asthmatic patients. *Chest* 94:1:51S, 1988.
19. Hodder RV, Calcutt LE, Leech JA. Metered dose inhaler with spacer is superior to wet nebulization for emergency room treatment of acute, severe asthma. *Chest* 94:1:52S, 1988.
20. Becker AB, Nelson NA, Simons FER. Inhaled albuterol versus injected epinephrine in the treatment of acute asthma in children. *J Pediatr* 102:465–469, 1983.
21. Appel D, Karpel JP, Sherman M. Epinephrine improved expiratory flow rates in patients with asthma who do not respond to inhaled metaproterenol sulfate. *J Allergy Clin Immunol* 84:90–98, 1989.

22. Rossing TH, Fanta CH, Goldstein DH, Snapper JR, McFadden ER Jr. Emergency therapy of asthma: comparison of the acute effects of parenteral and inhaled sympathomimetics and infused aminophylline. *Am Rev Respir Dis* 122:365–371, 1980.
23. Fanta CH, Rossing TH, McFadden ER Jr. Emergency room treatment of asthma: relationships among therapeutic combinations, severity of obstruction, and time course of response. *Am J Med* 72:416–422, 1982.
24. Siegel D, Sheppard D, Gelb A, Weinberg PF. Aminophylline increases the toxicity but not the efficacy of an inhaled beta-adrenergic agonist in the treatment of acute exacerbations of asthma. *Am Rev Respir Dis* 132:283–286, 1985.
25. Wrenn K, Slovis CM, Murphy F, Greenberg RS. Aminophylline therapy for acute bronchospastic disease in the emergency room. *Ann Intern Med* 115:241–247, 1991.
26. McFadden ER Jr. Methylxanthines in the treatment of asthma: the rise, the fall, and the possible rise again. *Ann Intern Med* 115:323–324, 1991.
27. Ratto D, Alfaro C, Sipsey J, Glovsky MM, Sharma OP. Are intravenous corticosteroids required in status asthmaticus? *JAMA* 260:527–529, 1988.
28. Fanta CH, Rossing TH, McFadden ER. Glucocorticoids in acute asthma: a critical controlled trial. *Am J Med* 74:845–851, 1983.
29. Lewis JE, Richards W, Church JA, Haftel A, Keens TG. Therapy of acute asthma I. Evaluation of successive bronchodilator treatments. *Ann Allergy* 55:472–475, 1985.
30. Ratto D, Alfaro C, Sipsey J, Glovsky MM, Sharma OP. Are intravenous corticosteroids required in status asthmaticus? *JAMA* 260:527–529, 1988.
31. Jonsson S, Kjartansson G, Gislason D, et al. Comparison of the oral and intravenous routes for treating asthma with methylprednisolone and theophylline. *Chest* 94:723, 1988.
32. Littenberg B, Gluck EH. A controlled trial of methylprednisolone in the emergency treatment of asthma. *N Eng J Med* 314:150–152, 1986.
33. Stein LM, Randolph PC. Early administration of corticosteroids in emergency room treatment of acute asthma. *Ann Intern Med* 112:822–827, 1990.
34. Shapiro GG, et al. Double blind evaluation of methylprednisolone versus placebo for acute asthma episodes. *Pediatrics* 71:510–514, 1983.
35. Chapman KR, Vercheek PR, White JG, Rebuck AS. Effect of a short course of prednisone in the prevention of early relapse after the emergency room treatment of acute asthma. *N Eng J Med* 324:788–794, 1991.
36. Canny GJ, Rebuck AS, Levison H. Acute asthma: observations regarding the management of a pediatric emergency room. *Pediatrics* 83:507–512, 1989.
37. Kereni E, Levison H, et al. Predicting the need for hospitalization in children with acute asthma. *Chest* 98:1355–1361, 1990.
38. Geelhoed GC, Landau LI, LeSouef PN. Predictive value of oxygen saturation in emergency evaluation of asthmatic children. *Br Med J* 297:395–396, 1988.
39. Zeiger RS, Schatz M, et al. Facilitated referral to asthma specialist reduced relapses in asthma emergency room visits. *J Allergy Clin Immunol* 87:1160–1168, 1991.

40. Arnold AG, Lane DJ, Zapata E. The speed of onset and severity of acute severe asthma. *Br Dis Chest* 76:257, 1982.
41. Galant SP. *Childhood Asthma: Pathophysiology and Treatment*, Marcel Dekker, Inc., New York, 1987.
42. Geelhoed GC, Landau LI, LeSouef PN. Predictive value of oxygen saturation in emergency evaluation of asthmatic children. *Br Med J* 297:395–396, 1988.
43. Rushton AR. Role of chest radiograph in the management of childhood asthma. *Clin Pediatr* 21:325–328, 1982.
44. Goldstein RS, Young J, Rebuck AS. Effect of breathing pattern on oxygen concentration received from standard face masks. *Lancet* 2:1188–1190, 1982.
45. Haalboon JRE, Deenstra M, Struyvenberg A. Hypokalaemia induced by inhalation of fenoterol. *Lancet* 1:1125, 1985.
46. Bierman CW, Pearlman DS. *Allergic Disease from Infancy to Adulthood*, 2nd ed., WB Saunders, Philadelphia, 1988.
47. Schuh S, Reider MJ, Canny G et al. Nebulized albuterol in acute childhood asthma: comparison of two doses. *Pediatrics*. 86:509–513, 1990.
48. Robertson CF, Smith F, Beck R, et al. Response to frequent low doses of nebulized salbutamol in acute asthma. *J Pediatr* 106:672–674, 1985.
49. Freelander M, Van Asperen PP. Nebuhaler versus nebulizer in children with acute asthma. *Br Med J* 288:1873–1874, 1984.
50. Dolovich MB, Ruffin RE, Roberts R, et al. Optimal delivery of aerosols from metered dose inhalers. *Chest* 80:911S–915S, 1981.
51. Konig P. Spacer devices used with metered dose inhalers: breakthrough or gimmick? *Chest* 88:276–284, 1985.
52. Littenberg B. Aminophylline treatment in severe acute asthma—a meta-analysis. *JAMA* 259:1678–1684, 1988.
53. Self T, Abou-Shala N, Burns R, et al. Inhaled albuterol and oral prednisone in hospitalized adult asthma: does the theophylline add any benefit? *Am Rev Respir Dis* 141(2):A21, 1990.
54. Pierson WG, Bierman CW, Stamm SJ, et al. Double-blind trial of aminophylline in status asthmaticus. *Pediatrics* 48:642–646, 1971.
55. Weinberger M, Hendeles L. In: Weiss EB, Segal MS, Stein M (eds.), *Bronchial Asthma, Mechanisms and Therapeutics*, Little, Brown, Boston, 1985.
56. Reisman J, Galdes-Sebalt M, Fazim F, et al. Frequent administration by inhalation of salbutamol and ipratropium bromide in the initial management of severe acute asthma in children. *J Allergy Clin Immunol* 81:16–20, 1988.
57. Kelly HW, Murphy S. Should anticholinergics be used in acute severe asthma? *Ann Pharmacother* 24:409–411, 1990.
58. Johnson AJ, Nunn AJ, Somner AR, et al. Circumstances of death from asthma. *Br Med J* 288:1870–1872, 1984.
59. Harfi H, Hanissian AS, Crawford LV. Treatment of status asthmaticus in children with high doses and conventional doses of methylprednisolone. *Pediatrics*. 61:829–831, 1978.
60. Seggev JS, Lis I, Siman-Tov R, et al. *Mycoplasma pneumoniae* is a frequent cause of exacerbation of bronchial asthma in adults. *Ann Allergy* 57:263–265, 1986.

61. Menitove SM, Goldring RA. Combined ventilator and bicarbonate strategy in the management of status asthmaticus. *Am J Med* 74:898–901, 1983.
62. Edelson JD, Rebuck AS. The clinical assessment of severe asthma. *Arch Intern Med* 145:321–323, 1985.
63. Moler FW, Hurwitz ME, Custer JR. Improvement in clinical asthma score and PaCO2 in children with severe asthma treated with continuously nebulized terbutaline. *J Allergy Clin Immunol* 81:1101–1109, 1988.
64. Portnoy J, Aggarwal J. Continuous terbutaline nebulization for the treatment of severe exacerbations of asthma in children. *Ann Allergy* 60:368–371, 1989.
65. Kelly HW, McWilliams BC, Katz R, Murphy S. Safety of frequent high dose nebulized terbutaline in children with acute, severe asthma. *Ann Allergy* 64:229, 1990.
66. Rubin BK, Marcushamer MD, Priel I, App E. Emergency management of the child with asthma. *Pediatr Pulmonol* 8:45–57, 1990.
67. Williams SJ, Winner SJ, Clark TJH. Comparison of inhaled and intravenous terbutaline in acute severe asthma. *Thorax* 36:629–631, 1981.
68. Hill JH. Acute severe asthma. In: Blumer JL (ed.), *A Practical Guide to Pediatric Intensive Care*, 3rd ed., Mosby–Year Book, St. Louis, 1990.
69. O'Rourke PP, Crone RK. Halothane in status asthmaticus. *Crit Care Med* 10:341–343, 1982.
70. Rosseel P, Lawers LF, Baute L. Halothane treatment in life-threatening asthma. *Intens Care Med* 11:241–246, 1985.
71. Schwarz SH. Treatment of status asthmaticus with halothane. *JAMA* 2688–2689, 1984.
72. Benatar SR. Fatal asthma. *N Eng J Med* 314:423–429, 1986.
73. Stableforth D. Death from asthma, *Thorax* 38:801–805, 1983.
74. Kravis LP, Kolski GB. Unexpected Death in childhood asthma. *J Allergy Clin Immunol* 80:467–473, 1987.
75. Tal A, Levy N, Bearman JE. Methylprednisolone therapy for acute asthma in infants and toddlers: a controlled clinical trial. *Pediatrics* 86:350–356, 1990.

# 14

# Problems in the Diagnosis and Management of the Asthmatic Adolescent

**THOMAS J. FISCHER**

*Cincinnati Children's Hospital Medical Center and University of Cincinnati College of Medicine Cincinnati, Ohio*



Adolescence is a special but confusing time in the life of every developing child. When the adolescent is confronted with a chronic illness like asthma, the burden placed upon him or her and the parents can appear overwhelming. Likewise, the health care professional caring for this patient must develop an intelligent and compassionate strategy to help the adolescent effectively and to avoid being "part of the problem" rather than part of the solution.

Although adolescence typically occurs between 10 and 18 years of age, recent insights in the field of child development recognize that adolescence is not a homogeneous state defined only by age in years. Tanner (1) described five physical stages of puberty that occur at different stages or rates in boys and girls, and differ from individual to individual. Coupled with varying degrees of cognitive awareness and psychological insights, the physically changing adolescent patient with asthma does not always fit a general concept of "the model asthmatic patient."

This chapter explores the problems of asthma in the adolescent patient, both in terms of diagnosis and management.

## NATURAL HISTORY OF ASTHMA IN ADOLESCENCE

The common adage that the "asthmatic child outgrows asthma" might better read that "the asthmatic child outgrows his or her pediatrician." The frequency with which asthma progresses into adult life has been reviewed in a number of prospective studies (see Chap. 4). In brief, approximately only 25–30% of childhood asthmatic subjects are completely wheeze-free as adults (2,3). In addition, Kelly et al. showed that 44% of patients with infrequent wheezing at age 21 years had a worsening of their symptoms by age 28 years (4). Even in adults free of clinically apparent asthma, persistent pulmonary function abnormalities can be noted (2,5).

Appropriate counseling of the adolescent with asthma would include the need for him or her to have a continued awareness into adulthood of factors that can trigger or reactivate hyperreactive airways, such as cigarette smoking (active or passive), allergen exposure in the workplace (occupational exposures) or home (e.g., new pets), exercise/cold air, viral infections or emotional stress.

Another common concern of asthmatic adolescents, worried about their body image, and their parents is the effect of asthma on growth and development. Balfour-Lynn (6) reviewed 13 reports that studied growth retardation in children with asthma. Although nine of these studies concluded that asthma caused growth retardation, a careful and more detailed analysis indicates that carefully done longitudinal studies (in contrast to cross-sectional studies) were more reliable methods of observing growth. These carefully done longitudinal studies indicate that once puberty (which can be significantly delayed in asthma) has finally begun, complete "catch-up" growth results in the attainment of predicted adult height. However, during this period of pubertal delay, emotional stress about this issue can occur in an already emotionally fragile adolescent. This added stress can decrease asthma control and compliance with the treatment regimen. In addition, significant growth retardation does occur if daily administered oral corticosteroids are taken on a regular basis (7–10). The introduction of single-dose, oral, alternate-day therapy and, in recent years, inhaled corticosteroids, has usually permitted better control of the asthma "without growth impairment" (6).

In practice, the physician caring for the patient with severe asthma should be aware that frequent steroid "bursts" may mitigate the effects of alternate-day regimens or inhaled corticosteroids. The frequency of these "bursts" should be carefully monitored (11). Likewise, a rare patient (12) may have an unusual degree of systemic sensitivity even to an inhaled corticosteroid. Finally, in Shohat's study of the military records of 2,252 boys and 1,158 girls who were inducted into the Israeli army at age 17, they noted that mildly affected asthmatic children are actually taller and heavier than adolescents without asthma. They speculate that because normal children who mature late are likely to present a slightly taller structure (compared to those who mature early), these children with asthma, with their delay in bone age, will mature later with a slightly taller stature (13).

## DIAGNOSIS

The physician makes the diagnosis of asthma based upon a detailed medical history, careful physical examination, and supporting laboratory tests. The need to take a careful history cannot be overemphasized. Topics to cover during history taking include (14): symptoms and conditions known to be associated with asthma (e.g., rhinitis); pattern of symptoms; precipitating or aggravating factors; long-term development and progress of the asthma; a profile of a typical exacerbation including prodromal signs, temporal progress, usual management, and usual outcome; environmental conditions; family history; general medical history; the impact of the asthma on patient and family; and an assessment of the family's and the patient's perception of this illness.

Effective communication between physicians and adolescents and their families can be a challenge, which, if unmet, can pose a significant obstacle to precise history taking, accurate diagnosis, and, ultimately, effective treatment. Physicians caring for the adolescent with asthma must be aware of their own biases, develop the techniques of active listening and mutual participation, and understand the impact of cognitive and developmental issues during adolescence (15,16).

Health care providers must be aware of their own values but attempt, as much as possible, to avoid making value or moral judgments during the interview. In fact, a sensitive adolescent can often sense the reactions of the caregiver and, adversely affected, can respond by refusing to communicate effectively. On the other hand, a sensitive health care provider does not need to be the adolescent's friend ("cool"), but rather be friendly and genuinely interested in the adolescent world. This "being friendly but not a friend" approach also allows the physician to develop a mutual advocacy relationship with both the adolescent and the adolescent's parents (15).

An awareness of adolescent development and behavior can also improve the chances for effective communication. The younger adolescent usually uses concrete operational thinking: the ability to reason about the world and life is tied to observable properties. The transition to formal operational thinking or abstract thinking usually occurs at 14–15 years of age but can be initially limited to certain areas. For example, the adolescent can exhibit abstract thinking in math class but not when dealing with the complexity of asthma.

Effective interview techniques with adolescents must be based upon the principle of "actively listening" by the health care professional. These techniques, summarized in Table 1, are essential for the accurate collection of data during the initial history but are also required on a continuing basis during later treatment phases. When treatment is offered, a mutual participation model is most appropriate: both patient and physician actively participate in therapy (avoiding the "guidance–cooperation mode," in which the physician is the authority figure and the patient "cooperates").

TABLE 1 Guidelines for Effective Interviews with Adolescent Patients

1. During the initial interview, make introduction both to adolescent and parent.
2. Begin appointments on time; avoid interruptions.
3. Allow patient to begin conversation and avoid "bombarding" with questions or allowing insufficient time to answer.
4. Ask open-ended questions: "Tell me how you use your inhaler" rather than "Do you know how to use your inhaler?"
5. Use indirect questions to elicit information ("I wonder how you're feeling about that problem").
6. Avoid assuming to know what the adolescent is thinking: check assumptions by restating what was heard.
7. Respond to inflammatory remarks by responding to the emotional content rather than the remark itself (acknowledge that the patient is upset and angry).
8. Avoid false reassurances, unrealistic promises, or the implication of constant availability to the patient.
9. Request specific information in response to vague reports (respond to "I used a lot of puffs on my inhaler" by asking the patient to specify how many is "a lot").
10. Clarify the meaning of the phrase "I don't know." Does it mean lack of understanding of the question or a desire not to answer? Be patient.

Source: Adapted from Ref. 15.

## Physical Examination

Although the physical examination of a patient with chronic asthma focuses on the upper respiratory tract, chest, and skin, other aspects should not be overlooked. Nutritional status, weight, height, and phase of maturation (using Tanner scale [1]) should be noted. The adolescent, often easily embarrassed by a request to disrobe and use a gown, should be gently encouraged to undress in order to allow a complete examination, especially during the initial consultation.

## Laboratory Diagnosis

Individual selection of diagnostic procedures is mandatory (see Chap. 11) to confirm the diagnosis of asthma as well as further classify the severity of the disease (14,17). The differential diagnosis of asthma in the adolescent include entities seen more commonly in adults including hyperventilation syndrome, mitral valve prolapse, chest pain with exercise, and laryngeal stridor (physical or psychological) (18).

Hyperventilation syndrome can be mistaken for asthma or coexist with it (18,19). In this situation, careful evaluation of the teenage patient is mandatory to avoid overlooking an organic cause of dyspnea or overtreating a psychologically based hyperventilation syndrome. In hyperventilation syndrome, the patient is usually anxious, complains of marked shortness of breath and air hunger despite excellent air exchange on auscultation, has no wheezing on auscultation, demonstrates normal pulmonary function tests, and normal oxygen saturation. Acute treatment consists primarily of reassurance and having the patient rebreathe into a paper bag to elevate $pCO_2$.

"Laryngeal wheezing" is another condition that can mimic asthma, often of a refractory nature. These patients typically have dyspnea, inconsistent with the clinical picture of asthma, and wheezing heard loudest over the larynx. They often possess a strong psychological overlay. Laboratory testing demonstrates no bronchial hyperreactivity when challenged with methacholine, no flattening of the inspiratory flow volume loop suggesting extrathoracic obstruction, normal arterial–alveolar oxygen gradients during an attack, and a lack of response to usual treatment modalities (20,21). Other laryngeal syndromes must be excluded including epiglottitis, anaphylaxis, tumors of the larynx or vocal cords, abscesses of the hypopharynx or larynx, laryngeal trauma, vocal cord paralysis, and foreign body aspiration. Accurate diagnosis of vocal cord dysfunction requires careful otolaryngologic exam with laryngoscope or laryngeal mirror to document paradoxical vocal cord motion during the acute "attack." Treatment of paradoxical vocal cord movement is multidisciplinary, with best results obtained with speech therapy and psychological counseling (21).

Adolescents will commonly complain of shortness of breath on exertion and/or chest pain and discomfort. On the one hand, these complaints of pain may be severe enough to prompt referral to a cardiologist to exclude cardiovascular abnormalities. Conversely, wheezing may be so subtle and not immediately prompt concerns about exercise-induced asthma. Nudel et al. (22) studied 180 patients with chest pain ranging in age from 5 to 22 years (mean, 13.2 years). All patients had normal cardiovascular exams, electrocardiograms, chest x-rays, and two-dimensional echocardiograms. Maximal exercise tests were performed on a treadmill or bicycle ergometer, measuring pulmonary functions (forced expiratory volume in 1 sec [FEV1], FEF25-75%, peak expiratory flow rate, and flow volume loops), and pulmonary gas exchange including minute ventilation, $CO_2$ production, and respiratory ratio. These exercise tests revealed no cardiovascular abnormalities. However, 14 patients with chest pain and 7 patients with dyspnea on exertion developed exercise-induced asthma, with postexercise decreases in peak flow of 26.2 ± 3.7% for patients with chest pain and 34.4 ± 8.9% for those with dyspnea on exertion.

Despite the lack of cardiovascular abnormalities noted in Nudel's study, cardiovascular abnormalities are occasionally found. For example, patients with mitral valve prolapse can have symptoms of chest pain during or following strenuous exercise. These complaints might prompt a diagnosis of exercise-induced asthma. These patients with mitral valve prolapse typically are slender, asthenic adolescents, often female, and on auscultation have systolic "clicks" heard in the mitral area. Echocardiography is used to confirm the mitral valve prolapse (23).

## THERAPEUTIC PROBLEMS

The management of asthma in the teenager, as in the child and adult, is directed toward several goals, which include prevention of symptoms, the maintenance of normal activity levels (including exercise), the maintenance of normal or near-normal pulmonary function measures, the prevention of recurrent flares of asthma, and the avoidance of the adverse effects of asthma medications. Treatment regimens should be designed to avoid asthmatic triggers (environmental controls), provide step-care pharmacologic therapy, and provide psychological support and resources for the patient, family, and school.

If the diagnosis of teenage asthma can be hampered by the special problems of adolescence, successful treatment can be jeopardized even more by the turmoils and pressures of being adolescent. Problems can arise in one or multiple areas of asthma treatment. Because of lack of information or noncompliance, or a combination of both, the teenager with asthma may fail to monitor carefully or recognize highly unstable labile airflow obstruction pattern. These patients can fail to recognize or purposely expose themselves to provoking environmental health hazards such as cigarette smoke, animal danders, occupational exposures in low-paying manual jobs, or excessive exercise. With medication, their lack of understanding and noncompliance is almost "proverbial." Psychologically immature and stressed, they often suffer psychological problems such as depression, denial, or low self-esteem. The combination of these factors can merge, producing the high morbidity of adolescent asthma and, at times, tragic consequences such as asthma deaths.

Asthma, as with any chronic illness with a protracted course, poses obstacles to the accomplishment of several psychological and physical tasks, including the development of independence in health care behavior. When the assessment of self-care agency (the power to care for one's self in relation to health) was studied in chronically ill adolescents with asthma, diabetes, or convulsive disorders (24), there actually appeared to be very few disease-specific differences. Likewise, Seigel et al. demonstrated that adolescents with chronic disease (sickle cell, asthma, or diabetes) have statistically higher depression scores and lower self-esteem than healthy age-matched controls. Of note, there is no statistical difference between depression, self-esteem, and life events among the three diverse groups (25). These findings suggest commonalities among diseases that may provide useful information for the development of clinical practices and health policy decisions that can help to support successful health behaviors in teenagers.

The ability to develop and practice successful health behaviors requires three components: knowledge (information, skills, and beliefs), resources (equipment, supplies, and access to health care), and motivation (positive incentives, peer approval, social sanctions) (26). In caring for adolescents, the health care provider often traditionally supplies knowledge but falls short in providing resources and motivation. Successful care of the asthmatic teenager must aim to provide in all these areas.

## ASTHMA TRIGGERS: AVOIDANCE, ELIMINATION, CONTROLS

Avoidance measures are reviewed in detail in Chapter 17. However, two areas of elimination or control especially relevant to teenagers require special mention.

Cigarette smoking has been identified as the single most preventable cause of excessive morbidity and mortality in the United States. Since 90%

of all smokers begin smoking as teenagers, the asthmatic adolescent must be targeted early (100,000 preteens are reported to smoke) to avoid cigarette smoking. Peak initiation of smoking occurs between the ages of 14 and 16 years. By the senior year of high school, 29% of teenagers smoke, 18% of them on a daily basis. Teenagers smoke for many reasons including the influence of parents who smoke, peer pressure (the first cigarette is almost always smoked with a friend), and the need for social status and to appear "more adult." Cigarettes have also been labeled a "gateway" drug because their use can predate other risk-taking behaviors, including alcohol and other drug use and sexual experimentation. For the asthmatic teenager, such behaviors obviously pose added obstacles to successful asthma control. Interventions in the office or clinic are summarized in Table 2 (26).

Strategies to deal with exercise as a trigger factor must also be developed to allow adolescents with asthma the opportunity to participate in any activity they choose without experiencing asthma symptoms. Athletic conditioning can improve muscle and exercise efficiency and thereby decrease the level of ventilation (although it does not modify exercise-induced asthma for a given level of ventilation) (27). Added benefits for exercise and

TABLE 2 Intervention Checklist to Prevent Smoking

1. Ask about the use of cigarettes and smokeless tobaccos (including use by close friends). The message should be "don't start" or "quit now."
2. If the patient is not smoking, provide pamphlets or other educational materials to reinforce that choice.
3. If the patient is smoking, set target date to quit.
4. If parents smoke, motive them to quit or at least commit to a smoke-free home.
5. Provide both self-help materials and referral to smoking-cessation groups for all smokers in the family.
6. Discard magazines containing tobacco advertising in your office or put labels such as "don't fall for this" on ads for tobacco products.
7. Emphasize the immediate negative consequences: stained teeth, bad breath odor, reduced sports performance, and peer disapproval.
8. Emphasize the benefits of quitting smoking (better sports performance, food tastes better, and dates prefer nonsmokers).
9. Initiate role playing, saying "no" to peer pressure if friends smoke.
10. Reinforce nonsmoking behaviors (e.g., personal letter of commendation).
11. Encourage alternatives, especially exercise and sports.
12. Advocate local laws to eliminate teenagers' access to cigarette machines.
13. Support smoke-free schools and no-smoking policies everywhere.

Source: Adapted from Ref. 26.

participation in sports include improvement in self-image and enhanced psychological outlook for the adolescent patient. Because of the obvious benefit of exercise, participation by teenagers is encouraged but only with appropriate education of the patient, family, school personnel, and coaches. Among these groups, especially parents, considerable anxiety exists about the potential dangers of exercise to the adolescent athlete with asthma. However, reports of exercise as the precipitating event of a fatal episode of asthma are not noted in several reviews (28–36) of adolescent asthma deaths. Ausdenmoore reported a fatality in a teenager secondary to exercise-induced anaphylaxis (37). His report and McFadden's (38) editorial review of asthma fatalities, however, also indicate that there have been no published reports of fatal outcomes from exercise-induced asthma. Nonetheless, possible coexisting factors such as allergens (39) or air pollutants (40) may lower the threshold to exercise-induced wheezing and potentiate a severe attack of asthma. Of note, 8 of the 11 patients (one of the 2 who died) reported by O'Holloren (39) were teenagers. All of these patients demonstrated evidence of IgE-mediated sensitivity to *Alternaria alternata*, a mold with high exposures in the midwestern part of the United States from June through November.

Physicians caring for teenagers with asthma should approach the topic of exercise using the following guidelines (41):

1. Equip and instruct patients and parents on appropriate medications (usually inhaled beta-agonists and/or inhaled cromolyn), correct delivery, and timing (see Chap. 12).
2. Warn the adolescent with asthma about complicating factors that may accentuate exercise-induced asthma, for example, respiratory tract infections, including sinusitis; pollen, mold, and air pollution exposure; and the use of beta blockers.
3. Advise appropriate physical training to increase resting airway function in order to allow a larger margin of vital capacity before the patient participates in the athletic event.
4. When appropriate (and under supervision), plan a vigorous warm-up strategy to induce a refractory state to exercise-induced asthma.
5. Observe diet, especially 2 hr before exercise. Specific foods that have been shown to be related to exercise-induced asthma or anaphylaxis include shellfish, celery, and melon.
6. Advise the adolescent to choose a sport where warm, humid air is inhaled (e.g., swimming, water polo). Warm air induces less bronchoconstriction with the same amount of exercise. Likewise, encourage the use of a face mask for rebreathing warmed air.
7. Notify teachers, coaches, and other school officials that the teenager has exercise-induced asthma. Provide appropriate counseling and ed-

ucational materials to these educators. When appropriate, support the practice of allowing the teenager to carry his or her inhaled medications for more immediate and optimal management. Position papers supporting this concept have been published (42,43).

8. For the highly competitive athlete, check all medications with the appropriate regulatory bodies, for example the U.S. Olympic Committee (44).

## COMPLIANCE WITH MEDICATION

The development and improved understanding of several classes of antiasthma medication over the last decade have allowed new opportunities for the pharmacologic control of this chronic disease. However, if the patient with asthma does not comply or adhere to the planned treatment protocol, success will not occur. Overall estimates of noncompliance in childhood asthma range from 12 to 66% (45–48). Rates of noncompliance of adolescents may be even higher. Miller reported that only 10% of teenage patients, 12–17 years of age, had serum theophylline levels in the therapeutic range (49), while Christiaanse et al. noted in their study of 38 children (ages 7–17 years) that increasing age correlated with percentage of noncompliant theophylline levels (50). This pattern is found in adolescents taking chronic medication for other chronic illnesses (51).

Many additional factors can influence compliance, including the complexity of the treatment regimen, the physician–patient relationship, the patient's belief in the effectiveness of the treatment, and the presence of a social support system for the patient (52). Even in apparently highly motivated patients enrolled in clinical research studies, compliance was poor (37–39%) as measured by highly sophisticated microprocessor monitoring devices capable of recording each actuation of the inhaler (52) or opening and closing of the pill bottle (53). Attempts to modify noncompliant behavior in adolescents with asthma can be of several types (54). Asthma self-management programs can stress improved cognitive knowledge (patient education) of the disease and at the same time attempt to instill behavior modification strategies to aid decision-making, especially concerning the response during an acute asthma attack. For example, Tehan et al., in a pilot project of self-management education at Dartmouth College Student Health Service, showed improved compliance with the asthma treatment recommendations (55).

Another intervention strategy to improve compliance in the adolescent patient is to simplify the medication regimen. For example, Bierman et al., studying 21 patients aged 12–18 years, showed that once a day dosing with Uniphyl tablets compared with twice daily Theodur tablets led to higher mean morning theophylline levels (13.1 vs. 9.6 μg/ml, $p=0.02$), and similar symptom scores, morning and evening pulmonary function test values, and the need for supplemental use of aerosol bronchodilators (56). For patients with mild to moderate asthma who are not tolerant of theophyllines, controlled-release albuterol tables (taken twice a day) may provide ease of administration over conventional, immediate-release tablets administered every 6–8 hr (57). Likewise, less frequent dosing can be considered, if tolerated and appropriate, for other treatment modalities such as inhaled corticosteroids or sodium cromolyn.

Improving patient compliance in the adolescent with asthma requires improved understanding for physicians about the basic relationship between physician and patient. Compliance is often assumed ultimately to be "under control" by the physician. Sbarbaro (58) notes that researchers in social sciences who study chronic diseases from the patients' perspective have found that patients visiting physicians is only one of a wide range of strategies to control or tolerate an illness. Another strategy to assert control over the disease is to attempt independent adjustment of dosage and scheduling of the medications. From the viewpoint of patients, especially teenagers, this approach is not "noncompliance" but an attempt to regulate their own lives and to reconcile their therapy with their understanding of the disease.

## SPECIAL CONCERNS OF THE ADOLESCENT GIRL WITH ASTHMA

The teenage girl with asthma can have additional problems or complications from her asthma. Eliasson et al. (59) have reported that of 57 women with asthma 19 (33%) had significant worsening ($p=0.006$) of total pulmonary symptom scores during either their premenstrual period, the menstrual period, or both. The maximal increase in dyspnea, wheezing, and chest tightness occurred during the premenstrual period ($p=0.002$). The other 38 (66%) women noted no such changes in their asthma. The investigators noted that both dysmenorrhea scores and premenstrual syndrome scores correlated significantly with baseline pulmonary function scores in the group who had symptoms of asthma during the premenstrual period. In both groups there was no history of a predictable effect on asthma symptoms with either pregnancy or use of oral contraceptives. Also, although not clearly documented in their article, there was no strong evidence of aspirin or other nonsteroidal anti-inflammatory medications being used that might exacerbate wheezing. Although the exact mechanism of this worsening is not known, it appears that a subgroup of patients with asthma may suffer from premenstrual asthma (PMA). Eliasson also noted that two of their indexed patients had recurrent respiratory failure caused by exacerbation of their asthma during menstruation. Barkman (60) also reported the sudden death from asthma of two sisters who both died at the same time of their menstrual cycle just after the onset of puberty.

Because asthma is more common in adolescents than other adults of the reproductive age, asthma may often complicate adolescent pregnancy more frequently than pregnancies in general. The combination of asthma and pregnancy in an asthmatic teenager can generate multiple problems during gestation, both for the teenager and her baby. Apter et al. (61) studied 28 pregnancies in a series of 21 pregnant adolescents with severe asthma. Fifty-six exacerbations of asthma were recorded, including 22 hospitalizations and 20 emergency room visits. Eighteen of these pregnancies required outpatient systemic corticosteroids, while 29% received inhaled corticosteroids. Known exacerbating factors include respiratory tract infections (59%) and noncompliance with medical therapies (27%). Although no maternal or fetal deaths or evidence of intrauterine growth retardation was reported, two infants were premature, one experiencing acute respiratory distress syndrome. Adequate management includes careful ambulatory care with close monitoring. They advised seeing patients frequently, at least monthly, and whenever possible by the same physician. These patients were given a telephone number to reach a physician on call 24 hr a day if any problems arose. Likewise, care was coordinated with the obstetrician to provide optimal management.

## SUBSTANCE ABUSE AND THE TEENAGE ASTHMATIC/ALLERGIC PATIENT

Drugs of abuse can induce a variety of respiratory symptoms and signs that can mimic allergic respiratory disease or complicate existing disorders such as asthma. Because almost any illicit drug can be administered via the respiratory mucosa, this technique is often the "route of choice" for adolescents and other individuals experimenting with drugs (62). Inhaled cannabinoids, stimulants (intranasal cocaine or inhaled crack cocaine), or volatile inhalants can produce respiratory tract effects that might be ignored by the user but obvious to an observer. These illegal drugs can produce symptoms by their irritant effect, vascular effects (e.g., cocaine), or as a true allergic response.

Diagnosis of substance abuse can be difficult, especially in an adolescent patient distrustful of an adult health care provider. Patients are reluctant to volunteer a history of drug use (63). As such, a high index of suspicion is required, especially in patients who fail to improve with the usual antiallergy therapy. Especially for chronic nasal symptoms, the appearance of a red raw mucous membrane, nasal crusts or scabs, recent nosebleeds, coupled with medication failure should prompt a nonthreatening inquiry (e.g., "Do you party?") (64).

Because of the epidemic proportions of substance abuse and the large number of allergic/asthmatic adolescents, the physician must be aware that drug dependency can complicate successful management of these patients' respiratory disorders and be willing to help develop appropriate health care behaviors in all aspects of the teenager's life.

## REFERENCES


1. Rauh JL, Brookman RR. Adolescent developmental stages. In: Johnson TR, Moore WM, Jeffries JE (eds.), *Children Are Different: Developmental Physiology*, Ross Laboratories, Columbus, OH, 1978, pp. 25–29.
2. Blair H. Natural history of childhood asthma. *Arch Dis Child* 52:613–619, 1977.
3. Kuzemko JA. Natural history of childhood asthma. *J Pediatr* 97:886–892, 1980.
4. Kelly WJ, Hudson I, Phelan PD, Pain MCF, Olinsky A. Childhood asthma in adult life: a further study at 28 years of age. *Br Med J* 294:1059–1062, 1987.
5. Friberg S, Bevegard S, Graff-Lonnevig V, Hallback I: Asthma from childhood to adulthood—a special follow up study of 20 subjects with special reference to work capacity and pulmonary gas exchange. *J Allergy Clin Immunol* 84:183–190, 1989.
6. Balfour-Lynn L. Effect of asthma on growth and puberty. *Pediatrician* 14:237–241, 1987.
7. Van Metre TE Jr, Pinkerton HL Jr. Growth suppression in asthmatic children receiving prolonged therapy with prednisone and methylprednisolone. *J Allergy* 30:103–113, 1959.
8. Spock A. Growth patterns in 200 children with bronchial asthma. *Ann Allergy* 23:608–615, 1965.
9. Falliers CH, Szentivanyi J, McBride M, Bukantz SC. Growth rate of children with intractable asthma. *J Allergy* 32:420–434, 1961.
10. Blodgett FM, Burgin L, Lezzoni D, Gribetz D, Talbot ND. Effect of prolonged cortisone therapy on statural growth, skeletal maturation and metabolic studies of children. *N Engl J Med* 254:636–641, 1956.
11. Dolan L, Keserwala HH, Fischer TJ. Short-term high-dose systemic steroids in children with asthma. The effect on the hypothalamic–pituitary–adrenal axis (HPAA). *J Allergy Clin Immunol* 80:81–87, 1987.
12. Hollman GA, Allen DB. Overt glucocorticoid excess due to inhaled corticosteroid therapy. *Pediatrics* 81:452–455, 1988.
13. Shohat M, Shohat T, Kedem R, Mimmouni M, Davon YL. Childhood asthma and growth outcome. *Arch Dis Child* 62:63–65, 1987.

14. Guidelines for the Diagnosis and Management of Asthma. National Heart, Lung, and Blood Institute National Asthma Education Program Expert Panel Report. *J Allergy Clin Immunol* 88 (no. 3, part 2):433, 1991.
15. Rosenthal SL, Biro FM. Communication with adolescents and their families. *Adolesc Pediatr Gynecol* 4:57–61, 1991.
16. Kreipe R, Jack M. Communicating with adolescents who have behavior problems. *Semin Adolesc Med* 5(2):127, 1987.
17. Weinberger M. Pharmacologic management of asthma. *J Adolesc Health Care* 8:74–83, 1987.
18. Bierman CW, Pearlman DS. Asthma. In Chernick V, Kendig EL Jr (eds.), *Disorders of the Respiratory Tract in Children*, W.B. Saunders, Philadelphia, 1990, pp. 557–601.
19. Sher TH. Recurrent chest tightness in a 28-year-old woman. *Ann Allergy* 67:310–314, 1991.
20. Downing ET, Braman SS, Fox MJ, et al. Factitious asthma—physiologic approach to diagnosis. *JAMA* 248(21):2878, 1982.
21. O'Hollaren MT: Masqueraders in clinical allergy: laryngeal dysfunction causing dyspnea. *Ann Allergy* 65:351–356, 1990.
22. Nudel DB, Diamant S, Brady T, et al. Chest pain, dyspnea on exertion, and exercise-induced asthma in children and adolescents. *Clin Pediatr* 26:388–392, 1987.
23. Devereaux RB, Perloff JK, Reichele N, Josephson MF. Mitral valve prolapse. *Circulation* 54:3, 1976.
24. Gaut DA, Kieckhefer GM. Assessment of self-care agency in chronically ill adolescents. *J Adolesc Health Care* 9:55–60, 1988.
25. Seigel WM, Golden NH, Gough JW, et al. Depression, self-esteem, and life events in adolescents with chronic diseases. *J Adolesc Health Care* 11:501–504, 1990.
26. Shafer MAB (ed): Priority health behaviors in adolescents. Adolescent health update. Section on Adolescent Health. *J Am Acad Pediatr* 3:1–8, 1991.
27. Nickerson BG, Bautista DB, Namey MA, Richards W, Keens TG. Distance running, improves fitness in asthmatic children without pulmonary complications or changes in EIB. *Pediatrics* 71:147–152, 1983.
28. Miller BD, Strunk RC. Circumstances surrounding the deaths of children due to asthma. *Am J. Dis Child* 143:1294–1299, 1989.
29. Kravis, LP. An analysis of fifteen childhood asthma fatalities. *J Allergy Clin Immunol* 80:467–472, 1987.
30. Strunk RC. Asthma deaths in childhood: identification of patients at risk and intervention. *J Allergy Clin Immunol* 80:472–477, 1987.
31. Sears MR, Rea HH. Patients at risk for dying of asthma: New Zealand experience. *J Allergy Clin Immunol* 80:477–481, 1987.
32. Rubinstein S, Hindi RD, Moss RB, Blessing-Moore J, Lewiston NJ. Sudden death in adolescent asthma. *Ann Allergy* 53:311–318, 1984.
33. Birkhead G, Attaway NJ, Strunk RC, Townsend MC, Teutsch S. Investigation of a cluster of deaths of adolescents from asthma: evidence of implicating

inadequate treatment and poor patient adherence with medications. *J Allergy Clin Immunol* 84:484–491, 1989.
34. Sly RM. Mortality from asthma in children 1979–1984. *Ann Allergy* 60:433–443, 1984.
35. Lewiston NJ, Rubinstein S. The young Damocles: the adolescent at risk for serious or fatal status asthmaticus. *Clin Rev Allergy* 5:273–284, 1987.
36. Friday GA, Fireman P. Morbidity and mortality of asthma. *Pediatr Clin North Am* 35:1149–1162, 1988.
37. Ausdenmoore RW. Fatality in a teenager secondary to exercise-induced anaphylaxis. *Pediatr Asthma Allergy Immunol* 5:21–24, 1991.
38. McFadden ER. Fatal and near-fatal asthma. *N Engl J Med* 324:409–411, 1991.
39. O'Hollaren MT, Yuninger JW, Offord KP, Somers MG, O'Connell EJ, Ballard DJ, Sachs MI. Exposure to aeroallergen as a possible precipitating factor in respiratory arrest in young patients with asthma. *N Engl J Med* 324:359–363, 1991.
40. Koenig JQ, Covert DS, Hanley QS, Van Belle G, Pierson WE. Prior exposure to ozone potentiates. Subsequent response to sulfur dioxide in adolescent asthmatic subjects. *Am Rev Respir Dis* 141:377–380, 1980.
41. Pierson WE. Exercise-induced bronchospasm in children and adolescents. *Pediatr Clin North Am* 35:1031–1039, 1988.
42. Kemp JP, et al. Position statement. The use of inhaled medications in school by students with asthma. *J Allergy Clin Immunol* 84:400, 1989.
43. Healy A, et al. Policy Statement. Children with health impairments in schools. *Am Acad Pediatr News*, July, 1990.
44. U.S. Olympic Committee. *Drug Free*. 1989–1992, pp. 34–35.
45. Radius SM, Becker MH, Rosenstock JM, et al. Factors influencing mother's compliance with a medication regimen for asthmatic children. *J Asthma Res* 15:133–149, 1978.
46. Kleiger JH, Dirke JF. Medication compliance in chronic asthmatic patients. *J Asthma Res* 16:93–96, 1979.
47. Sublett JL, Pollard SJ, Kadlec GJ, et al. Non-compliance in asthmatic children: a study of theophylline levels in the pediatric emergency room population. *Ann Allergy* 43:95–97, 1979.
48. Wood PR, Casey R, Kolski GB, et al. Compliance with oral theophylline therapy in asthmatic children. *Ann Allergy* 54:400–404, 1985.
49. Miller KA. Theophylline compliance in adolescent patients with chronic asthma. *J Adolesc Health Care* 3:177–179, 1982.
50. Christiaanse ME, Lavigne JV, Lerner CV. Psychosocial aspects of compliance in children and adolescents with asthma. *J Dev Behav Pediatr* 10:75–80, 1989.
51. Litt IF, Cuskey WR. Compliance with medical regimens during adolescence. *Pediatr Clin North Am* 27:3–15, 1980.
52. Mawhinney H, Spector SL, Kinsman RA, Siegel SC, Rachelefsky GS, Katz RM, Rohr AS. Compliance in clinical trials of two non-bronchodilator, anti-asthma medications. *Ann Allergy* 66:294–299, 1991.

53. Cramer JA, Mattson RH, Prevey ML, Scheyer RD, Ouellette UL. How often is medication taken as prescribed? A novel assessment technique. *JAMA* 261:3273–3277, 1989.
54. Jerome A, Wigal JK, Creer TL. A review of medication compliance in children with asthma. *Pediatr Asthma Allergy Immunol* 1:193–211, 1987.
55. Tehan N, Sloane BC, Walsh-Robart N, Chamberlain MD. Impact of asthma self-management education of the health behavior of young adults. *J Adolesc Health Care* 10:513–519, 1989.
56. Bierman CW, Pierson WE, Shapiro GG, Furukawa CT. Is a uniform round-the-clock theophylline blood level necessary for optimal asthma therapy in the adolescent patient. *Am J Med* 85(Suppl 1B):17–20, 1988.
57. Pierson WE, LaForce CF, Bell TD, MacCosbe PE, Sykes RS, Tinkelman D. Long-term, double-blind comparison of controlled-release albuterol versus sustained-release theophylline in adolescents and adults with asthma. *J Allergy Clin Immunol* 85:618–626, 1990.
58. Sbarbaro JA. Non-compliance with medications: vintage wine in new (pill) bottles. *Ann Allergy* 66:273–275, 1991.
59. Eliasson O, Scherzer HH, DeGraff AC. Morbidity in asthma in relation to the menstrual cycle. *J Allergy Clin Immunol* 77:87–94, 1986.
60. Barkman RP. Sudden death in asthma. *Med J Aust* 1:316, 1981 (letter).
61. Apter AJ, Greenberger PA, Patterson R. Outcome of pregnancy in adolescents with severe asthma. *Arch Intern Med* 149:2571–2575, 1989.
62. Dax EM. Drug dependency in the differential diagnosis of allergic respiratory disease. *Ann Allergy* 64:261–262, 1990.
63. Snyder RD, Snyder LB. Intranasal cocaine abuse in an allergists' office. *Ann Allergy* 54:489–492, 1985.
64. Schwartz RH, Estroff T, Fairbanks DNF, Hoffman NG. Nasal symptoms associated with cocaine abuse during adolescence. *Arch Otolaryngol Head Neck Surg* 115:63–64, 1989.

# 15

## Exercise-Induced Asthma

**PEYTON A. EGGLESTON**

*The Johns Hopkins Medical School*
*Baltimore, Maryland*



Most asthmatic subjects wheeze after exercise, that is, they experience exercise-induced asthma (EIA). Exercised-induced asthma is an example of the abnormal responsiveness to a nonimmunologic stimulant and in almost every case exercise is only one of a variety of triggers (allergens, respiratory infections, weather changes, emotional stress, or irritants such as dust, pollutants or chemicals,) that will induce an asthma attack. Of these EIA is the best studied and is so well characterized that it is thought, mistakenly, to be a unique asthmatic syndrome.

## ASTHMATIC RESPONSE TO EXERCISE

Most of what is known about EIA is the result of controlled exercise challenges (1–3). Volunteers are asked to avoid their usual medications that might interfere with the asthmatic response for several hours before exercise. The exercise itself is brief (5–8 min), and intense (adequate to raise heart rate and $O_2$ consumption to 70–80% of maximum). EIA following such a challenge is typical of any asthma attack, with wheezing, coughing, dyspnea, and hyperventilation. Symptoms generally worsen for 5–10 min after exercise and resolve spontaneously within 30–60 min. During and immediately after brief exercise, existing obstruction is actually relieved (1,3), and the improvement is most striking when obstruction is more severe before exercise. This effect presumably is related to the adrenergic response to exertion (4). With more prolonged exercise, the attack may begin before completion of the effort (1).

The airway response involves both large and small airways (5–8) and appears functionally similar to attacks following other stimuli (7,9). Residual volume may increase 200% in an average attack and provides the most sensitive indicator of obstruction (5,8). All measures of airflow are diminished to a similar extent, so that two relatively simple measures, the peak expiratory flow rate (PEFR) and the forced expiratory volume in 1 sec ($FEV_1$), are generally used to assess the response. Although the majority of asthmatic subjects show this picture of widespread obstruction, it has been shown that in approximately 40% maximal expiratory flow rate is significantly improved on breathing helium–oxygen mixtures, which suggests that large airway obstruction predominates (6,7). Arterial $pO_2$ is depressed during the attack (6,10), probably as a consequence of obstruction and ventilation-perfusion abnormalities. Arterial pH is also depressed at the height of the attack (10,11), at the same time serum lactic acid levels are increased. Late-phase obstruction may be seen at 4–8 hr after exercise (12), but is generally much less severe than that seen following allergen challenge (13) and is not accompanied by the expected increase in bronchial hyperresponsiveness.

The severity of obstruction depends on several factors. In part, the status of the person exercising: a person with more severe asthma as defined by medication requirements, resting airflow obstruction, frequency of attacks or symptom scores has a more severe response to exercise (15). It should be emphasized that this is a rough correlation and that asthmatic persons with apparently mild disease or persons who are unaware of their diagnosis of asthma may have quite significant EIA (16). The degree of obstruction present at the time of exercise influences the severity of symptoms seen during the attack. In general, an asthmatic subject who begins exercise with airflow obstruction will endure greater obstruction at the nadir of the attack than another asthmatic person who begins unobstructed.

The severity of the attack also depends on the exercise conditions (3,17,18). For reasons discussed below, the severity of an attack increases with increasingly strenuous exercise. The relationship to the duration of exercise is more complex. The severity of obstruction increases with longer exercise, up to 6–8 min, but usually diminishes with more prolonged exercise as subjects begin to “”run through” their attack. Exercise in cold, dry air induces more severe attacks than similar exercise in warmer air (19,20). Air pollutants, especially $SO_2$, increase airway response (21). The response is greater during a symptomatic pollen season (22), presumably because inflammation already present in the lower airway increases bronchial hyperresponsiveness.

## PATHOPHYSIOLOGICAL FINDINGS

Our current understanding of the pathophysiology of EIA may best be understood if one classifies the process into four components: 1) initiating stimulus, 2) translational event, 3) obstructive response, and 4) modulating factors.

### Initiating Stimulus

The initiating stimulus has proven to be the environmental stress imposed upon the lower airways by the need to heat and humidify large volumes of air during exercise (23). This relationship was suggested by early observations that obstruction was less severe with swimming than with other forms of exercise and that exercise during the winter led to more severe EIA (19,20). The definitive experiments identifying ventilatory adaptation as the intiating stress demonstrated that EIA could be reproduced by hyperventilation and that both hyperventilation- and exercise-induced asthma could prevented by having subjects breathe humidified air during exercise (24–27).

Alveolar air is 37°C and fully saturated with moisture (44 mg/liter). Even in summer, ambient air is cooler and rarely contains more than 25 mg/ml water; and in the winter at subfreezing temperatures, air containing 2 mg/liter is fully saturated. During respiration, ambient air is heated and humidified in the upper airway (nose, trachea, bronchi) before it reaches the alveoli (34,35). Water and heat losses are minimal during quiet respiration but still occur; this is obvious in the condensed breath seen during winter. Because of this net loss of heat and water the tracheal surface is 2–3°C cooler (29) and airway fluid osmolarity is 50–100 mOsm/kg higher (30,31) than core body conditions. In adapting to exercise, respiration increases quickly (32), and may double during quiet walking or increase 30-fold with jogging or more strenuous exercise (33). With this degree of hyperventilation, tracheal surface temperatures may decrease by several more degrees, and segmental bronchi, which are normally at core body temperature, are cooled as well (29). Surface osmolarity changes have not been measured under similar conditions but are likely to change as well.

The relative importance of heat and water loss as initiating stimuli is controversial. Airway surface temperatures clearly are depressed during hyperventilation and the intensity of this depression correlates with the severity of EIA (29). When airway heat loss is calculated, this also correlates closely with the asthmatic response. However, more than 80% of the heat loss from the airway relates to evaporation (34,35), so that water loss correlates just as closely with EIA (28). Furthermore, exercising while breathing hot (50°C) dry air still causes EIA (35); and, although this has never been confirmed with direct measurements at the airway surface, there is no heat loss by indirect measurements under these conditions. Inhaled hyperosmolar aerosols may induce obstruction that shares many characteristics with EIA (36). Thus, most of the available evidence favors exercise-induced water loss as the initiating stimulus, although it does not exclude a contribution by thermal stress.

### Translational Events

The translation of this physiological stress into airway obstruction requires an intervening step, the nature of which is not currently known. The hypotheses that best explain the experimental data include either pulmonary mast cell mediator release or direct effects of cooling on bronchial or vascular smooth muscle.

The evidence for mast cell mediator release includes the ability of cromolyn to inhibit EIA, since the drug has no known effect on bronchial smooth muscle and inhibits mast cell activation. However, cromolyn inhibits mast cell activation only at very high concentrations (37), and has been demonstrated to prevent bronchoconstrictive responses to inhaled histamine (41) and to sulfur dioxide (42) through mechanisms that are unlikely to involve mast cell activation. A second piece of evidence is that plasma histamine and neutrophil chemotactic factor (NCF) increase during EIA (40). However, the changes that have been reported are small, are seen during the asthmatic response to exercise rather than during exercise, have not found by all investigators (39), and can be explained in part by the increased numbers of basophils found in the circulation after exercise. Late-phase obstruction, thought to be characteristic of mast cell-dependent reactions, may be seen following EIA (12). However, the change is comparatively modest, is seen in a minority of subjects, and is not accompanied by the period of increased airway responsiveness characteristic of allergen-inducc late-phase reactions.

Some of the most convincing evidence to date that mast cells are activated comes from experiments that show that when dry air is insufflated through the nose for 5–10 min, histamine, prostaglandins, TAME esterase and other mast cell mediators are found in subsequent nasal lavage fluids (43). The amounts of these mediators are very similar to that found after allergen challenge, and their appearance is accompanied by functional changes (increased vascular permeabilty) similar to those seen in allergen challenge. The osmolarity of nasal mucus increases slightly in proportion to the changes in mast cell products. Additional evidence that mast cells could be activated during hyperventilation comes from in vitro studies showing that isolated mast cells can be activated by increases in osmolarity (44). Thus, both of these experiments are consistent with the hypothesis that hyperventilation increases airway water loss, which then increases local osmolarity and activates mucosal mast cells.

An alternative hypothesis is that airway cooling directly alters vascular and bronchial smooth muscle. Beta-adrenergic receptors on bronchial smooth muscle are altered by cooling and are activated by alpha-adrenergic (bronchoconstrictor) stimuli (50). There is little direct evidence that this occurs in the airway. It has also been proposed that airway obstruction in EIA occurs secondary to vasodilation of mucosal vessels (46). When the skin is cooled, local vasoconstriction occurs, and with rewarming, constricted vessels not only return to baseline tone but develop reactive hyperemia. It has been proposed that submucosal vessels in the lower airway respond in much the same way, based on the observation that obstruction occurs after exercise is completed, and experiments showing that maneuvers that delay rewarming of the airways will inhibit EIA. Thus, the reactive hyperemia would decrease the airway diameter and lead to the obstructive response interpreted as exercise-induced bronchoconstriction.

### Obstructive Response

The obstructive response requires hyperresponsive airways (48). Normal subjects do not develop airway obstruction with the same stress that causes bronchoconstriction in asthmatic subjects. EIA is more severe in the subjects with most severe asthma, and the severity of EIA correlates well with other measures of increased airway responsiveness, such as the sensitivity to inhaled histamine or methacholine (48). Hyperventilation-induced asthma also correlates with response to these stimuli (49). The increased severity in EIA that occurs during a pollen season (22) or following a cold (86) may be explained by the increased airway responsiveness that accompanies these conditions.

### Modulating Factors

Many exercise-related changes could modulate these responses. Although hyperventilation maintains arterial $PO_2$, tissue oxygen utilization is less efficient, resulting in a metabolic acidosis (largely lactic acid) that is apparent when oxygen consumption is 50% of maximum or greater (33). Arterial pH may fall to 7.10–7.20 and acidosis may continue for 15–30 min after exercise. This time course coincides with the abnormal pulmonary response to exercise and could contribute to airway obstruction. Plasma catecholamine concentrations increase 5–10 fold during exercise and generally return to baseline by 10 min after exercise (10), suggesting that they may contribute to the transient bronchodilation seen during exercise. Airway smooth muscle preparations become less responsive to beta-adrenergic (bronchodilatory) stimuli when cooled and more responsive to alpha-adrenergic (bronchoconstrictive) stimuli, so the airway cooling noted during exercise may enhance the response to translational events or to circulating catecholamines (50). Core body temperature is elevated 1°C or more during strenuous exercise (27), and may affect pulmonary water loss or vascular response. Muscle metabolites such as adenosine increase in venous blood during vigorous exercise; since adenosine may cause bronchoconstriction when inhaled (23), it is possible that increased concentrations in venous plasma presented to the lungs may augment obstruction following exercise.

## REFRACTORY PERIOD

In about 50% of persons with asthma, EIA is followed by a period of 30–90 min during which further exercise is followed by a shorter, less severe asthmatic response; by 2 hr this refractoriness has waned (51). The degree of refractoriness is related to the intensity of initial EIA; when the initial exercise is strenuous and induces more severe EIA, a second exercise period induces milder EIA even if the exercise is equally strenuous. A similar refractory period does not follow hyperventilation-induced asthma. Exercise while breathing air with a high moisture content is not followed by EIA, but does induce a refractory period in most subjects. Response to histamine or methacholine do not change during the refractory period (51).

The mechanism of the refractory period is not known, and most hypotheses such as smooth muscle desensitization, mast cell mediator depletion, and circulating catecholamines have not been supported experimentally. Studies with the airway response to inhaled hyperosmolar aerosols (36) and adenosine (23) have recently provided unexpected clues. These aerosols cause bronchoconstriction with several characteristics that are similar to EIA: inhibition by cromolyn and nedocromil and the induction of a refractory period. During the adenosine-induced refractory period, subjects are also refractory to EIA (23). Furthermore, pretreatment with indomethacin interferes with adenosine-induced bronchoconstriction (53) and with the refractory period following EIA (54). While there is no evidence directly linking adcenosine with EIA, these experiments suggest that the two stimuli may induce bronchoconstriction through mechanisms that share one or more steps.

## EPIDEMIOLOGICAL CHARACTERISTICS AND DIAGNOSIS

Exercise challenges have been suggested as a useful method of diagnosing asthma in questionable clinical settings and as a method of perfoming epidemiological surveys of asthma. Techniques for studying EIA have been well described and can be safely utilized in children or young adults, especially if the exercise stress is increased gradually over the first 2 min. Exercise is performed on a treadmill or cycloergometer, or with stereotyped running in a hallway or on a stairwell. Exercise continues for 6–8 min and is strenuous enough to raise the heart rate to 70–90% of the maximum predicted for age and minute ventilation above 60 liters/min. Peak expiratory flow rate (PEFR) or forced expiratory volume in 1 sec ($FEV_1$) is measured before and frequently after exercise, and a 15% fall in PEFR or a 10% fall in $FEV_1$ is considered abnormal.

These challenge procedures have allowed us to demonstrate that a history of EIA correlates poorly with the response to challenge (16). Abnormal exercise responses are seen not only with asthma but also in children with chronic cough (55), in patients with cystic fibrosis (56), allergic rhinitis (16), a past history of asthma (58), a past history of bronchiolitis (59), and in relatives of persons with asthma (61,62).

In comparison with other bronchial challenge procedures such as inhalation of methacholine and histamine, exercise challenge can be said to be more specific (less likely to be positive in persons without asthma) but less sensitive. Only 70–80% of current asthmatics have abnormal responses, whereas virtually all asthmatic subjects respond abnormally to inhalation of histamine or methacholine (48,49). Both exercise and inhalation challenges procedures are reasonably reproducible, with a coefficient of variation of about 30% with repeat testing (17,18).

## DRUG EFFECTS

Many drugs have been shown to affect EIA when given immediately before exercise. Table 1 lists those drugs whose effects have been documented with placebo-controlled challenges. Placebo treatment itself may reduce EIA by 20–30% (62) and hypnotic suggestion that exercise is effortless can be even more effective (63). Not only does this demonstrate the interrelationship between emotional and physical precipitants of asthma but

TABLE 1 Drugs Shown to Affect EIA

| Agent | Bronchodilation | EIA | Comments |
|---|---|---|---|
| *Beta-adrenergic agonists* | | | |
| Oral (64–66) | + | 0 to ± | 1–2 hr duration |
| Inhaled (65,66,72) | + | + | 1–2 hr duration |
| *Methylxanthines* (64,68,69) | + | + | 2–4 hr duration Serum level > 10 μg/ml |
| *Anticholinergic agents* (6,47,72) | + | 0 to ± | Effective in 25% |
| *Mast cell stabilizers* (67,70,71) | 0 | + | Ineffective in 30% 1 hr duration |
| *Antihistamines* (73,75) | ± | ± | |
| *Alpha-adrenergic antagonists* (79) | ± | ± | Effective by inhalation |
| *Calcium antagonists* (80) | 0 | ± to + | |
| *Nonsteroidal anti-inflammatory agents* (54) | – | 0 | |
| *Corticosteroids* | | | |
| Oral (76) | 0 | ± | Therapy slowly improves baseline functions |
| Inhaled (77,78) | 0 | + | |
| *Others* | | | |
| Propranolol (79) | – | 0 | |
| Vasoactive intestinal peptide (82) | – | 0 | |
| MK 571 (83) | 0 | + | $LTD_4$ inhibitor |
| Furosemide (81) | 0 | + | |

it also emphasizes that at least a 30% inhibition must be achieved by a drug to be considered truly capable of inhibition EIA.

Orally administrered adrenergic agonists are effective bronchodilators, but the reported studies on the effects of oral treatment with metaproterenol, terbutaline, and albuterol on EIA are conflicting, with some showing clear inhibition and others showing only bronchodilation at similar doses (64–66). Inhibition, when seen, generally lasts for 2 hr. Inhaled doses of the same agents not only are just as effective as bronchodilators but they also will effectively inhibit EIA in more than 90% of persons and reduce the mean response to exercise by over 80% (65,66,72). In addition, they have a more rapid onset of action (minutes) and a comparable duration of action at one-twentieth of the dosage. The lower effective dosage is obviously associated with less severe toxicity, which may be an especially important advantage when cardiovascular risks must be minimized, such as in competitive athletes and adults with coronary vascular disease, or when toxic effects such as skeletal muscle tremor prevent the use of oral doses.

Methylxanthines, both theophylline and dyphylline, effectively inhibit EIA and also act as bronchodilators (64,68,69). Although some effects of theophylline may be seen with serum levels less than 10 μg/ml, protection is significantly greater at higher levels.

Cromolyn has no bronchodilating properties, but pretreatment with a single 2 mg dose can prevent EIA for up to an hour (67,70,71). The effect is not increased with chronic therapy, and the drug is not effective if given during or immediately after exercise. It is not uniformly effective and most studies show that EIA is not significantly inhibited in 25–30% of asthmatic subjects. Its effects are additive with beta-adrenergic agonists, so that it is the second drug of choice in EIA, especially in the small proportion of patients whose EIA is not treated effectively by inhaled beta-adrenergic drugs. Nedocromil has similar properties.

Cholinergic antagonists (atropine, ipratropium) are potent bronchodilators but are generally less effective inhibitors of EIA (6,47,72,73). In 25–30% of asthmatic subjects, EIA is significantly reduced. Subjects in whom atropine inhibits EIA exhibit predominantly large airway obstruction after exercise (6).

Although antihistamine and corticosteroids are generally said to have little effect on EIA, only recently have blinded, controlled studies on either class of drug been published (73–78). Moderate dosages of terfenadine partially inhibit EIA (75); similar effects by inhaled clemastine and chlorpheniramine (73,74) are of less practical significance. In a controlled study of steroids, prednisone 12.5–40 mg daily for 1 week was associated with small but statistically significant inhibition in a group of nine subjects with asthma; the change in baseline spirometry was much more striking and of more practical importance since maximal obstruction following exercise was proportionally reduced as well (76). Recent studies with inhaled steroids have shown similar improvement of resting obstruction, with modest reduction of the percentage change in spirometry (77). In one study, the effectiveness of beta-adrenergic pretreatment was enhanced (77). An interesting finding was that treatment with intranasal steroids has effects comparable to pulmonary treatment; they presumably act by maintaining nasal patency and allowing patients to avoid mouth breathing during exercise (78).

Beta blockers generally increase obstruction in asthmatic persons but have no significant effect on the response to exercise (79). Calcium channel blockers have a weak inhibitor effect (80). Nonsteroidal anti-inflammatory agents may precipitate obstruction in asthmatic persons, but they have no effect on EIA (54). Remember, however, that indomethacin has been shown to interfere with the refractory period to exercise. This effect may have practical implications for athletes who may be receiving these drugs fo pain relief, and who may at the same time have developed a warm-up routine designed to induce a refractory state for an athletic event. Recent studies demonstrating inhibition by furosemide (811) and by prostanoid inhibitors (83) contribute to our understanding of the pathophysiology of EIA, and may someday be important therapeutic options.

## CLINICAL MANAGEMENT

The most important step in the management of EIA is recognition. Pediatricians and family practitioners need to be aware that the prevalence of asthma is between 5 and 10% of the pediatric population, so any child with a cough or unusual dyspnea related to exercise should be suspected of having EIA, and be given an appropriate therapeutic trial to confirm the suspicion. Any patient with lung disease should be questioned about cough, wheezing, and dyspnea after exercise, and appropriate treatment begun. These sound like simple steps, but studies of competitive athletes at the college and Olympic level have documented that as many as one-third of atheletes with EIA are not diagnosed and appropriately treated.

The differential diagnosis of EIA is limited and listed in Table 2. A careful history is the most important step. Normal dyspnea or the exercise limitation imposed by other lung disease creates dyspnea during, not after, exercise, and resolves with a few minutes of rest. A history of stridor suggests exercise-induced laryngospasm. This uncommon disorder occurs most commonly in the early teens and is more common in girls. Stridor, dysphonia, and respiratory distress begin abruptly during exercise and stops

TABLE 2 Differential Diagnosis of Exercise-Induced Asthma

| |
|---|
| Normal exercise-related hyperpnea |
| Chronic heart or lung disease |
| Exercise-induced laryngospasm |
| Exercise-induced anaphylaxis |

within minutes when the patient rests. Pretreatment with inhaled adrenergic agonists is not helpful. Exercise-induced anaphylaxis may present with wheezing and respiratory distress, but this is not typical of the syndrome. However, EIA with urticaria should bring this diagnosis to mind. There is no safe method of confirming the diagnosis, since life-threatening anaphylaxis occurs erratically, and may be induced by the exercise challenge.

Even though an exercise challenge is a more reliable way to detect EIA, it is indicated in clinical situation because it is less sensitive than inhalation challenge tests, there is a certain degree of unavoidable risk, and the comparable confirmation of a clinical history may be obtained more easily with a therapeutic trial. The primary indications for the test are to determine disability, evaluate for participation by asthmatic patient in some high-risk activity such as athletics or military service, and in confusing clinical situations such as a poor drug response in a known asthmatic subject or an unusual clinical history.

In most cases, the presence of EIA indicates that a patient's asthma is poorly controlled. It is important to remember that exercise is part of normal functioning, especially in the child, and one of the major goals of asthmatic therapy is to restore the patient to normal function. It is therefore incumbent upon the pracititoner to ask about exercise functioning and to encourage children to participate in the extent of their interest and ability, whether this includes only physical education class and play activities or competitive athletics. It may be helpful to give examples of successful athletes with asthma, to provide the child with a role model. Premedication, even if required on a regular basis, is preferable to avoiding exercise, with the risk of exclusion from a peer group or establishing sedentary habits that may increase the health risk later in life.

The medication of choice currently is an adrenergic agonist by inhalation taken 4–5 min before exercise. Exercise induced asthma will be inhibited immediately, while the bronchodilating effect of the agonist generally takes several minutes to maximize and to contribute to the effect of the treatment. To avoid complicating the drug regimen of an asthmatic subject already taking a bronchodilator, however, it is appropriate first to adjust the dosage and/or timing of the current medication to inhibit the response whenever possible rather than adding another drug. Cromolyn is usually substituted in a drug regimen only when there is some concern about the cardiovascular side effects of other drugs during exercise. On the other hand, when treatment with a beta-adrenergic agonist is partially effective, the addition of cromolyn as a second drug just before exercise is appropriate. Follow-up, if only by telephone, is essential to evaluate the benefits and side effects of therapy.

For recreation, patients should be advised to pursue activities that are less likely to induce asthma, such as swimming. A porous mask (3 M Cold Weather Mask) increases the humidity of inspired air and reduces EIA (84); a muffler probably has the same effect. Consciously breathing through the nose reduces EIA (85) and most patients can be trained to use this technique when engaging in mild to moderate exercise. The asthmatic response is more severe in patients with more severe asthma (15), especially with resting airway obstruction (1). Patients should be aware that during a pollen season (22), following a cold (86) or asthma attack, or during exposure to pollution (21), they may exprience more EIA and may need to increase medication, modify exercise, or both. Thus, some patients must avoid exercise without extra medication and all patients must take extra medication or limit exercise on some days.

In asthmatic athletes, special problems are encountered. Coaches as well as team physicians at any level of competition must be made aware of the diagnosis; the athlete will usually turn to them for advice before asking his or her own physician. They and their coaches should be aware of the potential danger of abusing adrenergic aerosol (especially epinephrine sold over the counter as Primatine Mist or Bronchaid Mist) in a youngster rendered acidotic by exercise (arterial pH at the end of a marathon is in the range of 7.00!) and hypoxic by asthma. The coach should also be aware that performance will be suboptimal on cold days or when concomitant chest symptoms occur; the athlete should certainly not be penalized or derided as a malingerer.

In addition, the competitive drive of athletes must be acknowledged. Whether driven by team spirit or by their own desire to be the best, most athletes have a strong desire to excel, and view EIA as an obstacle to be ignored or overcome. If these drives can be enlisted by providing the athlete with an understanding that performance can be enhanced with proper treatment, treatment will be more successful.

The usual drug of first choice for asthmatic athletes is a selective beta-adrenergic agonist, but here cromolyn has clear indications and is an equally good choice in many patients. Whenever recommending inhaled drugs, observe the patient administer them and be quick to recommend a spacer device for any patient with suboptimal technique. In those patients whose asthma requires regular medication, these drugs should be used optimally. Inhaled steroids may be added to improve control during an athletic season. Drugs are officially restricted only at the Olympic level of competition (87). Here, inhaled beta-agonists (albuterol, bitolterol, and terbutaline), cromolyn, and theophylline are allowed. Inhaled corticosteroids are allowed but written notification must be given the International Olympic Committee Medical Commission or the U.S. Olympic Committee Drug Control Program, since these drugs may be confused with banned steroids in urine samples. At the National Collegiate Athletic Assocation and high school level, drugs recommended by a physician are allowed.

Several general measures can be recommended. Early in an athletic child's career, it may be possible to select sports in which EIA will create less disadvantage, such as swimming, or those that emphasize skill, hand-eye coordination or strength (i.e., baseball, golf, field events) rather than endurance (track, soccer, football, basketball, hockey). Later, it may be possible to select positions that require less endurance (i.e., goalie). In addition to being aware of the benefit of nasal breathing, athletes should be aware of the refractory period after EIA. Repeated short sprints (7 successive 30 sec sprints) are an effective way of inducing this refractory period without first inducing asthma (88). A portable peak flowmeter is half as expensive as a pair of athletic shoes, and can provide invaluable feedback to the athelete in designing a warm-up program or adjusting medications.

In summary, a knowledge of the relationship of asthma to exercise, the pathophysiology and control of the attack, and its clinical implications is important to the physician caring for any asthmatic person, but especially in the care of youngsters during the most physically active phases of their lives.

## REFERENCES

1. Anderson SD, Silverman M, Konig P, Godfrey S. Exercise-induced asthma. *Br J Dis Chest* 69:1–39, 1975.
2. Eggleston PA, Rosenthal RR, Anderson SA, Anderton R, Bierman ER, Chai H, Cropp GJ, Johnson JD, Konig P, Morse J, Smith LJ, Summers RJ, Trautlein JJ. Guidelines for the methodology of exercise challenge testing of asthmatics. Study Group on Exercise Challenge, Bronchoprovocation Committee, American Academy of Allergy. *J Allergy Clin Immunol* 46:42–45, 1979.
3. Silverman M, Anderson SD. Standardization of exercise tests in asthmatic children. *Arch Dis Child* 47:882–889, 1972.

4. Zielinski J, Chodosowska E, Radumyski A, Araszkiewicz Z, Kozolowski S. Plasma catecholamines during exercise-induced bronchoconstriction in bronchial asthma. *Thorax* 35:823–827, 1980
5. Anderson SD, McEvoy JDS, Bianco S. Changes in lung volumes and airway resistance after exercise in asthmatics subjects. *Am Rev Respir Dis* 106:30–36, 1972.
6. McFadden ER Jr, Ingram RH Jr, Haynes RL, Wellman JJ. Predominant site of flow limitation and mechanism of post exertional asthma. *J Appl Physiol* 42:746–752, 1977.
7. Chan-Yeung M, Abboud R, Tsao MS, McClean L. Effect of helium on maximum expiratory flow in patients with asthma before and during induced bronchoconstriction. *Am Rev Respir Dis* 113:433–443, 1976.
8. Haynes RL, Ingram RH Jr, McFadden ER Jr. An assessment of the pulmonary response to exercise in asthma and an analysis of the factors influencing it. *Am Rev Respir Dis* 114:739–752, 1976
9. McFadden ER Jr, Kiser R, deGroot WJ. Acute bronchial asthma: relations between clinical and physiologic manifestations. *N Engl J Med* 288:221–226, 1973.
10. Anderson SD, Silverman M, Walker SR. Metabolic and ventilatory changes in asthmatic patients during and after exercise. *Thorax* 27:718–725, 1972.
11. Chan Yeung MMW, Vyas MN, Grzybowski. Exercise induced asthma. *Am Rev Respir Dis* 104:915–924, 1971.
12. Bierman CW, Spiro SG. Characteristics of the late response in exercise-induced asthma. *J Allergy Clin Immunol* 74:701–709, 1984.
13. Stearns Dr, McFadden ER Jr, Breslin FJ, Ingram RH Jr. Reanalysis of the refractory period in exertional asthma. *J Appl Physiol* 50:503–508, 1981.
14. Martin A, Landau LI, Phelan PD. Lung function in young adults who had asthma in childhood. *Am Rev Respir Dis* 122:609–616, 1980.
15. Sly RM. Exercise related changes in airway obstruction: frequency and clinical correlates in asthmatic children. *Ann Allergy* 28:1–15, 1970.
16. Kawabori I, Pierson WE, Conquest LL, Bierman CW. Incidence of exercise-induced asthma in children. *J Allergy Clin Immunol* 58:447–455, 1976.
17. Eggleston PA, Guerrant JL. A standardized method of evaluating exercise induced asthma. *J Allergy Clin Immunol* 58:414–425, 1966.
18. Godfrey S, Silverman M, Anderson SD. Problems of interpreting exercise-induced asthma. *Allergy Clin Immunol* 59:199–209, 1972.
19. Strauss RH, McFadden ER Jr, Ingram RH. Enhancement of exercise induced asthma by cold air. *N Engl J Med* 297:743–747, 1977.
20. Bar-Or O, Neuman I, Dolan R. Effects of dry humid climates on exercise-induced asthma in children and preadolescents. *J Allergy Clin Immunol* 60:163–168, 1977.
21. Sheppard D, Saisho A, Nadel JA, Boushey HA. Exercise increases sulfur-dioxide-induced bronchoconstriction in asthmatic subjects. *Am Rev Respir Dis* 123:286–291, 1981.
22. Eggleston PA. Exercise-induced asthma in children with intrinsic and extrinsic asthma. *Pediatrics* 56(suppl):856–859, 1975.

23. Fitch KD, Morton AR. Specificity of exercise in exercise-induced asthma. *Br Med J* 4:577–581, 1971.
24. Chen WY, Horton DJ. Heat and water loss from the airways and exercise-induced asthma. *Respiration* 34:305–313, 1977.
25. Deal EC Jr, McFadden ER Jr, Ingram RH Jr, Stauss RH, Jaeger JJ. Role of respiratory heart exchange in the production of exercise-induced asthma. *J Appl Physiol* 46:467–475, 1979.
26. Deal EC Jr, McFadden ER Jr, Ingram RH Jr, Jaeger JJ. Hyperpnea and heat flux: initial reaction sequence in exercise-induced asthma. *J Appl Physiol* 46:476–483,
27. Deal EC Jr, McFadden ER Jr, Ingram RH Jr, Jaeger JJ. Esophageal temperature during exercise in asthmatic and non-asthmatic subjects. *J Appl Physiol* 46:484–490, 1979.
28. Hahn A, Anderson SD, Morton AR, Black JL, Fitch KD. A reinterpretation of the effect of temperature and water content of the inspired air in exercise-induced asthma. *Am Rev Respir Dis* 130:575–579, 1984.
29. McFadden ER Jr, Denison DM, Waller JF, Assoufi B, Rescock A, Sopwith T. Direct recording of the temperature in the tracheobronchial tree in normal man. *J Clin Invest* 69:700–705, 1982.
30. Man SFP, Adams GK III, Proctor DF. Effects of temperature, relative humidity and mode of breathing on canine airway secretions. *J Appl Physiol* 46:205–209, 1979.
31. Boucher RC, Stutts MJ, Bromberg PA, Gatzy JT. Regional differences in airway surface liquid composition. *J Appl Physiol* 50:513–520, 1981.
32. Asmussen E, Nielsen M. Studies on the regulation of respiration during muscular work. *Acta Physiol Scand* 6:353–358, 1943.
33. Shephard RJ, Allen C. Renade AJS, Davies CTM, di Pompero PE, Hedman R, Merriman JE, Myhre K, Simmons R. Standardization of submaximal exercise tests. *Bull WHO* 38:765–766, 1968.
34. McFadden ER Jr, Ingram RH Jr. Exercise-induced asthma: observations on the initiating stimulus. *N Engl J Med* 301:763–769, 1979.
35. Anderson SD. Issues in exercise-induced asthma. *J Allergy Clin Immunol* 76:763–771, 1985.
36. Shoeffel RE, Anderson SD, Altounyan REC. Bronchial hypereactivity in response to inhalation of ultrasonically nebulized solutions of distilled water and saline. *Br Med J* 283:1285–1287, 1981.
37. Sheard P, Blair AMJN. Disodium cromoglycate. Activity in 3 in vitro modes of the immediate hypersensitivity reaction in lung. *Int Arch Allergy Appl Immunol* 38:217–225, 1970.
38. Finnerty JP, Polosa R, Holgate ST. Repeated exposure of asthmatic airways to inhaled adenosine 5′monophosphate attenuates bronchoconstriction provoked by exercise. *J Allergy Clin Immunol* 86:353–359, 1990.
39. Deal EC Jr, Wasserman SI, Soter NA, Ingram RH Jr, McFadden ER Jr. Evaluation of the role played by the mediators of immediate hypersensitivity in exercise-induced asthma. *J Clin Invest* 65:659–665, 1980.

40. Lee TH, Nagy L, Nagakura T, Walport MJ, Kay AB. Identification and partial characterization of an exercise-induced neutrophil chemotactic factor in bronchial asthma. *J Clin Invest* 69:889–899, 1982.
41. Woenne R, Kattan M, Levison H. Sodium cromoglycate-induced changes in the dose–response curve of inhaled methacholine and histamine in asthmatic children. *Am Rev Respir Dis* 119:927–931, 1979.
42. Sheppard D, Nadel JA, Boushey HA. Inhibition of sulfur dioxide induced bronchoconstriction by disodium cromoglycate in asthmatic subjects. *Am Rev Respir Dis* 124:257–259, 1981.
43. Togias AG, Naclerio RM, Proud D, Adkinson NF Jr, Kagey-Sobotka A, Lichtenstein LM. Nasal challenge with cold dry air results in the release of inflammatory mediators. *J Clin Invest* 76:1373–1381, 1983.
44. Eggleston PA, Kagey-Sobotka A, Lichtenstein LM. A comparison of the osmotic activation of basophils and human lung mast cells. *Am Rev Respir Dis* 135:1043–1048, 1987.
45. Godfrey S, Konig P. Inhibition of exercise-induced asthma by different pharmacologic pathways. *Thorax* 31:137–143, 1976.
46. McFadden ER Jr, Jenner CW, Strohl KP. Postexertional airway rewarming and thermally induced asthma. *J Clin Invest* 78:18–25, 1988.
47. Breslin FJ, McFadden ER Jr, Ingram RH Jr, Deal EC Jr. Effects of atropine on respiratory heat loss in asthma. *J Appl Physiol* 48:619–623, 1980.
48. Eggleston PA. A comparison of the asthmatic response to methacholine and exercise. *J Allergy Clin Immunol* 63:104–110, 1979.
49. Bleecker ER, Chatham M, Smith PL, Mason PL, Norman PS. Airways responses to conditioned air, methacholine, histamine and exercise in asthmatics and normals. *Am Rev Respir Dis* 125:72, 1982.
50. Souhrada M, Souhrada JF. The direct effect of temperature on airway smooth muscle. *Respir Physiol* 44:311–323, 1981.
51. Edmunds AT, Tooley M, Godfrey S. The refractory period after exercise-induced asthma: its duration and relation to the severity of exercise. *Am Rev Respir Dis* 117:247–254, 1978.
52. Hahn AG, Nogrady SG, Tumulty DM. Histamine reactivity during the refractory period after exercise induced asthma. *Thorax* 39:919, 1984.
53. Crimin N, Palermo F, Polsa R. The role of cyclooxygenase derived mediators on adenosine-induced bronchoconstriction. *J Allergy Clin Immunol* 83:921–925, 1989.
54. O'Byrne PM, Jones GL. The effect of indomethacin on exercise-induced bronchoconstriction and refractoriness after exercise. *Am Rev Respir Dis* 134:69–72, 1988.
55. Cloutier MM, Loughlin GM. Chronic cough in children: a manifestation of airway hyperreactivity. *J Pediatr* 67:6–12, 1981.
56. Day G, Mearns MB. Bronchial lability in cystic fibrosis. *Arch Dis Child* 48:355–359, 1973.
57. Konig P, Godfrey S, Abrahamov A. Exercise induced bronchial lability in children with a history of wheezy bronchitis. *Arch Dis Child* 48:513–517, 1973.

58. Martin AJ, Landau LI, Phelan PD. Lung function in adults who had asthma in childhood. *Am Rev Respir Dis* 122:609–616, 1980.
59. Kattan M, Keens, TG, Lapierre J-G, Levison H, Bryan AC, Reilly BJ. Pulmonary function abnormalities in symptom-free children after bronchiolitis. *Pediatrics* 59:683–688, 1977.
60. Konig P, Godfrey S. Prevalence of exercise-induced bronchial lability in families of children with asthma. *Arch Dis Child* 48:942–951, 1973.
61. Konig P, Godfrey S. Exercise-induced bronchial lability in monozygotic (identical) and dizygotic (non-identical) twins. *J Allergy Clin Immunol* 45:280–287, 1974.
62. Godfrey S, Silverman M. Demonstration of placebo response in asthma by means of exercise testing. *J Psychom Res* 17:293, 1973.
63. Ben-Zvi Z, Spohn WA, Young SH, Kattan M. Hypnosis for exercise-induced asthma. *Am Rev Respir Dis* 125:392–395, 1982.
64. Eggleston PA, Beasley PP, Kindley RT. The effects of oral doses of theophylline and fenoterol on exercise-induced asthma. *Chest* 79:399–405, 1981.
65. Anderson SD, Seale JP, Rozea R, Bandler L, Theobald G, Lindsay DA. Inhaled and oral salbutamol in exercise induced asthma. *Am Rev Respir Dis* 114:493–500, 1976.
66. Konig P, Eggleston PA, Serby CW. Comparison of oral and inhaled metaproterenol for prevention of exercise-induced asthma. *Clin Allergy* 11:597–604, 1981.
67. Silverman M, Andrea T. The time-course of disodium cromoglycate in asthmatic children. *Arch Dis Child* 47:419–427, 1972.
68. Simons FER, Bierman CW, Sprenkle AC, Simons KJ. Efficacy of diphylline (dihydroxy propyltheophylline) in exercise-induced bronchospasm. *Pediatrics* 56(supplement) 916–918, 1975.
69. Bierman CW, Shapiro GG, Pierson WE, Dorsett CS. Acute and chronic theophylline therapy in exercise-induced bronchospasm. *Pediatrics* 60:845–849, 1977.
70. Eggleston PA, Bierman CW, Pierson WE, Stamm SJ, Van Arsdel PP. A double blind trial of the effect of cromolyn sodium on exercise induced bronchospasm. *J Allergy Clin Immunol* 50:57–61, 1972.
71. Latimer KM, Roberts R, Morris MM, Hargreave FE. Inhibition by sodium cromoglycate on bronchoconstriction stimulated by respiratory heat loss: comparison of pressurized aerosols and powder. *Thorax* 39:277–281, 1982.
72. Yeung R, Nolan GM, Levison H. Comparison of the effects of inhaled SCH 1000 and fenoterol on exercise-induced bronchospasm in children. *Pediatrics* 66:109–114, 1980.
73. O'Byrne PM, Thomson NC, Morris M, Roberts R, Daniel EE, Hargreave FE. The protective effect of inhaled chlorpheniramine and atropine on bronchoconstriction stimulated by airway cooling. *Am Rev Respir Dis* 128:611–617, 1983.
74. Zielinski J, Chodosowaka E. Exercise-induced bronchoconstriction in patients with bronchial asthma: its prevention with an antihistaminic agent. *Respiration* 34:31–35, 1977.

75. Patel JR. Terfenadine in exercise-induced asthma. *Br Med J* 288:1496–1497, 1984.
76. Konig P, Jaffe P, Godfrey S. Effect of corticosteroids on exercise-induced asthma. *J Allergy Clin Immunol* 45:14–19, 1974.
77. Henrickson JM, Dahl R. Effects of inhaled budesonide alone and in combination with low-dose terbutaline in children with exercise-induced asthma. *Am Rev Respir Dis* 1128:993–997, 1983.
78. Henricksen JM, Wenzel A. Effects of an intranasally administered corticosteroid (budesonide) on nasal obstruction, mouth breathing and asthma. *Am Rev Respir Dis* 130:1014–1019, 1984.
79. Sly RM, Heimlich EM, Busser RJ, Strick L. Exercise-induced bronchospasm: effect of adrenergic and cholinergic blockade. *J Allergy* 40:93–99, 1967.
80. Corris PA, Nariman S, Gibson GJ. Nifedipine in prevention of asthma induced by exercise and histamine. *Am Rev Respir Dis* 128:991–997, 1983.
81. Bianco S, Vagh A, Robuschi M, Pasargiklian M. Prevention of exercise-induced bronchoconstriction by inhaled furosemide. *Lancet* 2:252–255, 1988.
85. Bundgaard A, Enehjelm SD, Aggestrup S. Pretreatment of exercise-induced asthma with inhaled vasoactive intestinal peptide (VIP) *Eur J Respir Dis* 64:427, 1983.
83. Manning PJ, Watson PM, Mangoskee DJ, Williams VC, Schwartz JJ, O'Byrne PM. Inhibition of exercise-induced bronchoconstriction by MK-571, a potent leukotriene $D_4$ receptor antagonist. *N Engl J Med* 323:1736–1739, 1990.
84. Schachter EN, Lach E, Lee M. The protective effect of a cold weather mask on exercise-induced asthma. *Ann Allergy* 46:12–16, 1981.
85. Shturman-Ellstein R, Zeballos RJ, Buckley JM, Souhrada JF. The beneficial effect of nasal breathing on exercise-induced bronchoconstriction. *Am Rev Respir Dis* 118:65-73, 1978.
86. Aquilina AT, Hall WJ, Douglas GR Jr, Utell MJ. Airway reactivity in subjects with viral upper respirattory tract infections: the effects of exercise and cold air. *Am Rev Respir Dis* 122:3–10, 1980.
87. U.S. Olympic Committee. *Drug Free.* 1989–1992, pp. 34–35.
88. Schnall RP, Landau LI. Protective effects of repeated short sprints in exercise-induced asthma. *Thorax* 35:828–832, 1980.

# 16

## Sinusitis and Reactive Airway Disease

**ROGER M. KATZ, GARY S. RACHELEFSKY, and SHELDON C. SIEGEL**

*Allergy Research Foundation, Inc., and*
*UCLA School of Medicine*
*Los Angeles, California*



Sinusitis is common in children and is often overlooked as a possible diagnosis in children who have acute and chronic respiratory symptoms. It is estimated that up to 5% of upper respiratory tract infections and 50% of children with allergic rhinitis have their sinuses involved with inflammation. The natural history of chronic sinusitis is not clearly defined. However, complications of the sinuses can involve the lower respiratory tract with resultant reactive airway disease (RAD). Establishing a diagnosis of sinusitis and the appropriate management of this disease are important to control both the lower and upper respiratory tract complications. The linkage between sinusitis and reactive airway disease has been suggested by various authors (1–4). Recovery of the lower respiratory tract problems occurs when the upper respiratory tract problems are well managed.

## ANATOMICAL RELATIONSHIPS

Sinuses develop anatomically as outpouchings from the nasal mucosa. Thus, their mucosal linings are similar to that of the nose. At birth, the ethmoid and maxillary sinuses are developed whereas the frontal and sphenoid sinuses remain rudimentary until at least 3 years of age and the frontal sinuses seem to pneumatize at about 8 years of age (5). All the sinuses communicate to the nose through ostial openings from the sinuses to the nasal antrum.

The nose consists of three turbinates in each nostril that protrude from the lateral wall. The prominent inferior turbinate is separate, but the middle and superior turbinates are actually portions of the ethmoid bone, and the ostia from the perinasal sinuses are hidden in the meatus between the middle and superior turbinates, (i.e., the middle meatus beneath the middle turbinate contains the ostia of the maxillary sinuses, whereas the superior meatus beneath the superior turbinate contains the ethmoid ostia). On the other hand, the sphenoid sinus ostium is located in the sphenoethmoid recess, superiorly and posteriorly within the nose.

Cilia of the maxillary sinuses beat upward, carrying the mucus up and out of the sinus cavity, whereas the frontal sinus drainage flows through the ethmoid sinuses causing the mucus blanket to drain directly by gravity.

Like the cilia of the nose, those of the sinus function automatically as long as cytoplasm remains attached to them. The cilia movement is synchronous, in unison, and one-directional, causing the secreted mucus to move through the ostia and into the nose. Drying (local evaporation) and increased mucus viscosity lead to stasis of the mucus blanket whereas low temperature (35°C) and low pH (6.4) can decrease cilia activity immensely. Patent ostia are extremely important, along with normal cilia function, to remove mucus and allow proper function of the sinuses.

The membranes in the nose are richly vascularized and are continuous with the linings of the perinasal sinuses. The inflammation of this tissue will block the drainage through the ostia from the sinuses. Edema of the ostia or edema of the tissue surrounding the ostia can occur as well, from upper respiratory tract infections, allergic reactions, air pollution, trauma, foreign bodies, polyps, tumors, or adenoid hypertrophy. Abuse of topical decongestants can cause rebound vasodilation and resultant edema. In addition, this can cause narrowing of the nasal passages and consequently affect the mucociliary floor.

The vessels of the nasal and sinus respiratory mucosa are greatly influenced more readily than other blood vessels of the body by amino amines such as histamine. These vessels have very porous fenestrations and continuous singular endothelial basilar elastic membrane that responds readily to the amino amines (histamine, other mediators) released from the nasal mast cells. The single cell membrane acts as a minimal barrier between the circulatory system and that of the mucosal membrane, thus making it much easier for edema to occur. The venous system of the nose is valveless and, consequently, nasal congestion stasis develops.

The anterior and posterior ethmoid nerve supply to the sinuses and nose are similar. The sensory receptor cells (sense of smell) form small nerve fibers that pass through the cryptiform plate into the brain, whereas pain, temperature, and touch are supplied by branches of the ophthalmic division of the trigeminal nerve. The facial nerve, on the other hand, supplies the parasympathetic impulse and also passes through to the sphenopalatine ganglion and the fine fibers distributed to the glandular epithelium within the nose, which, in turn, results in the secretions from the mucosal glands. The sympathetic spinal nerve fibers, T1–T3, of the sphenopalatine gland stimulate vasal constriction. Both autonomic and parasympathetic impulses help to regulate the mucus secretion of vascular responses.

There are many symptoms of sinus disease (Table 1), but cough seems to be the most relevent. Cough may also be related to reactive airway disease (RAD).

## COUGH

Although the physiology of cough reflex is not defined, it does involve intricate responses of the receptor sites, both the afferent and efferent

TABLE 1 Clinically Suspected Sinusitis

| Symptoms | Signs |
|---|---|
| Headache | Erythema/edema of the nasal turbinates |
| Postnasal drip | Discharge seen on PE (rhinoscopy) |
| Jaw ache | Tenderness over sinuses |
| Toothache | Polyps (nasal) |
| Facial pain | |
| Facial swelling | |
| Rhinorrhea (other than clear) | |
| Cough | |
| Fever | |
| Ear pain or fullness | |
| Eye pain | |
| Nasal obstruction | |
| Taste change | |
| Smell change | |
| Hearing change | |

nerve pathways. The upper airway cough receptors are located in the paranasal sinuses, ear canals, tympanic membranes, nasal passageways, and pharynx. Stimulation of these receptors creates a nerve impulse that travels through the afferent pathway to the medullary cough center, which, in turn, stimulates the efferent nerve pathways such as the vagus, phrenic, and possibly spinal motor nerves. Another concept of cough physiology involves the view that irritation of mucosal receptors initiates bronchospasm as a direct reflex.

Cough is commonly present and seems to occur both day and night as the major symptom in sinusitis (6). Sinus disease may present as a chronic cough as early as 2 months of age. The dry and irritative cough occurs during sleep and does not necessarily awaken the child, as does the cough associated with asthma. A concomitant nasal discharge (thick postnasal drip), pharyngeal irritation, and sinus congestion with pain in the teeth or jaw may be present, especially in older children. Coughing from the lower respiratory tract, however, is usually deep, paroxysmal, hacking, and often nonproductive. It may be associated with a wheeze or with chest tightness when the small airways are involved. Cough with asthma will often awaken the child.

Cough may also be induced by the release of histamine, particularly after exposure to allergens or irritants (smoke, noxious gas, dust, fumes, scents, and chemicals). Respiratory irritants or physical factors such as cold air, high humidity, and dry inhaled air induce reflex coughing due to the activation of the vagal receptors in the upper airway. This cough may be initiated from the middle ear or sinuses and is enough to interfere with sleep.

## UPPER AND LOWER RESPIRATORY TRACT LINKAGE

### Experimental Evidence

A link between the upper and lower respiratory tracts has been demonstrated in one experimental model. Cats have increased lower airway resistance after their noses are stimulated with an irritant such as sulfur dioxide (6). Other animal studies have suggested the presence of a nasal bronchial reflex. This was done by mechanical and electrical stimulation of the nasal mucous membrane and then abolishment of the response by sectioning the vagus nerve. In humans, resection of the trigeminal nerve results in a significant decrease in pulmonary resistance. This suggests the presence of a reflex arc via the vagal pathway to the bronchi (7). Other links to the lower respiratory tract involve casual relationships between the sinus, nose, and pulmonary tree. In healthy persons with normal pulmonary function, silica, a substance that irritates mucosal membranes when blown into the nasopharynx, causes increased lower airway resistance (7). Other nerve reflex phenomena can be shown by applying a cold stimuli in the nose, thus obtaining an increased airway resistance that in turn can be blocked by an anticholinergic drug (8).

Irritation of the upper respiratory tract and consequent stimulation of the nervous system can be compared to gastroesophageal nerve reflex. The gastric contents splash into the esophagus, stimulate the vagus nerve, and in turn trigger bronchospasm. It has consequently been suggested that when sinus membranes are irritated, stretched, or inflamed, a reflex pathway occurs to the brain and subsequently to the vagus nerve resulting in bronchospasm.

In opposition to the reflex mechanism, when the vagus nerve in dogs has been blocked either by atropine or vagotomy, bronchoconstriction was not inhibited by stimulation by either cold or chloroform applied to the nose. In humans, some studies have likewise shown no lower respiratory tract response to the application of known sensitizing antigens to the nasal membranes (9).

Viral infections of the upper respiratory tract may also cause sinusitis. These infections may induce epithelial damage, thus increasing hyperreactivity and sensitivity at the irritant receptors (10). Viral infections may also interfere with sensory neurons and smooth muscle beta-adrenergic responses, which, inturn, affect bronchial tone. Impaired beta-receptor responses have also been found in the lymphocytes and polymorphonuclear leukocytes during the viral infection. Along with the impaired beta-receptor response, there is an enhancement of the lower airway hyperreactivity. As examples, bronchial challenge with nonspecific agents such as methacholine and histamine during the viral upper respiratory tract involvement causes a hyperreactive smooth muscle response, but the lower airway resistance can be attenuated with the use of aerosolized atropine. These corrections suggest the nerve impulse reflex theory as being causative of RAD. To counter the reflex theory, McFadden notes no causality and no evidence of the sinobronchial reflex. Thus, how can sinusitis cause an increase in lower airway reactivity? He further notes that the incidence of sinus x-ray abnormalities does not correlate with the severity of asthma.

Another proposed mechanism for sinusitis and asthma as a correlative-associated measure is the possibility of eosinophils acting as affector cells in chronic inflammation of the whole respiratory tree. The histopathologic nature of the paranasal respiratory epithelium from patients with chronic sinusitis is similar to that of patients with bronchial asthma with the presence of eosinophils. Studies by Harlin et al. (11) substantiate the correlation. Measurements of the mediators in the maxillary sinuses with fluid obtained during surgery showed that these washings contained large amounts of leukotrienes, histamine, and sulfidopeptides that may relate to inflammation and local irritant receptor stimulation (12). Chronic bronchitis secondary to bacterial seeding (a postnasal drip from infected sinuses) has been suggested as hypersensitivity to the bacterial byproducts or bacterial endotoxins. These events would result in adrenergic blockage and refractory bronchospasm. Despite the plausible mediator theory of bronchial hyperreactivity, many patients with sinus disease also have lower respiratory tract problems such as cystic fibrosis, and patients with bronchitis usually do not have the additional asthmatic components.

## Clinical Studies

The studies in which sinusitis and asthma occurred note a range of a 40–60% incidence of associated sinusitis with asthma. Are they the same process involving a similar inflammation or does sinusitis itself trigger asthma? Evidence of a convincing nature is still required. However, refractory asthma in patients who had sinusitis definitely improved when the concurrent sinusitis was treated properly.

In adults, several studies have been published noting an association of sinus disease and reactive airways. Treatment of the sinus involvement with antibiotics for infection and lavage or surgical drainage for fluid retention or surgical extrapolation of diseased sinus tissue has generally resulted in improvement of the lower respiratory tract symptoms and reduction of medication for control of asthma. Most recently, a 5 year follow-up study was reported in patients who had concomitant asthma and sinus disease. This study in particular noted decreased airway hyperresponsiveness and requirement of medication for asthma including steroids (13). Two studies done in children reported that when sinusitis-associated asthma was treated with appropriate antibiotics, significant improvement in the asthma occurred. In one study 78% of the children were able to show resolution of the asthma concomitant with resolution of the sinus disease (Table 2) (4). Of importance is the substantially reduced dependence on bronchodilator medication. We believe that these clinical studies present convincing evidence of the causes of the sinus-bronchial relationship.

Sinuses become obstructed, followed by the signs and symptoms of nasal discharge, cough, malodorous breath, fever, headache, facial pain, peri-

TABLE 2 Pulmonary Function Tests and Need for Medication in 48 Children with Sinusitis and Reactive Airway Disease

| | Before Treatment | After Treatment |
|---|---|---|
| Pulmonary function testing abnormal (%) | 100 | 33 |
| Bronchodilator treatment needed (%) | 100 | 21 |

orbital or facial swelling, sore throat, and other symptoms such as malaise, irritability, headaches, and poor performance in school. These complaints may suggest acute or chronic sinusitis and may be associated with fluid retention and bacterial infection. Bacterial agents within the sinuses do not seem to be associated with the cause and effect of asthma. These bacterial infections often follow viral upper respiratory tract infections that result in either decreased immunity or increased inflammation of the sinuses. The proper use of antibiotics (and decongestants?) may relieve the problems of both the upper and the lower respiratory tract. When the sinusitis is properly treated, the concurrent asthma symptoms disappear and the pulmonary function tests return to normal.

Treatment of chronic sinus disease and its relationship to RAD require the same approach as chronic sinusitis without RAD. To confirm the diagnosis, imaging techniques are most appropriate. These would include plain radiographs, computed tomography, and magnetic resonance imaging (MRI). Depending upon the location of the sinus disease (maxillary versus ethmoid, frontal, sphenoid), the cost of the procedures and their proper use should be the deciding factors. Recent studies have shown a high correlation of fiberscopic rhinoscopy (with a flexible endoscope) with MRI findings consistent with sinusitis. Edema, drainage, and inflammation had a 95% correlation with positive MRI findings of fluid, opacification, and mucosal thickening. Thus, fiberscopic rhinoscopy is useful, nonradiologic technique to evaluate this often perplexing problem. Among the imaging techniques, MRI is most useful for soft tissue swelling and fluid retention but the tomogram may be more readily available and less expensive with often similar findings. Young children need to be sedated for these procedures. Radiographs for maxillary sinus disease (Water's view) can alleviate the need for other imaging techniques in a child younger than 1 year. Patients in whom you suspect sinusitis or who have concomitant asthma require an evaluation for sinusitis (Table 3).

TABLE 3 Evaluation for Sinusitis in Patients with Asthma

| |
|---|
| Patient presents with asthma |
| Check for sinusitis |
| Consider |
|   Fiberoptic rhinoscopy |
|   Nasal smear |
|   Sinus radiograph |
|   Sinus MRI |
|   Sinus CT scan |
| Treat for asthma and/or sinusitis |

TABLE 4 Antibiotic Treatment of Sinusitis

| Drug | Dosage | |
|---|---|---|
| | Children (mg/kg/day) | Adults |
| Amoxicillin | 40 | 500 mg three times daily |
| Trimethoprim–sulfamethoxazole | 8–40 | 1 Septra DS twice daily |
| Erythromycin and sulfisoxazole | 50–150 | |
| Cefaclor | 40 | 500 mg three times daily |
| Amoxicillin–clavulanate | 50 | 500 mg three times daily |

The cultures of maxillary sinuses in both adults and children from whom sinus aspirates had been obtained, revealed *Streptococcus pneumoniae*, *Branhamella catarrhalis*, *Staphylococcus aureus*, *Staphylococcus pyogenes*, and *Peptostreptococcus bacteroides* as well as *Haemophilus influenzae* as predominant organisms. Therapy with appropriate antibiotics results in the best responses (Table 4). Therapy only with decongestants or antibiotics that are not bactericidal results in equally poor responses. Because beta-lactamase-producing organisms are common, one must always consider an antibiotic that would be effective in this situation.

## REFERENCES

1. Gottlieb MJ. Relation of intranasal disease in the production of bronchial asthma. *JAMA* 85:105–107, 1925.
2. Berman JZ, Matlison DA, Stevenson DD, Asselman JA, Shore S, Tan EM. Maxillary sinusitis and bronchial asthma: correlations of recent roentgenogram, cultures, and thermograms. *J Allergy Clin Immunol* 53:311–317, 1974.
3. Phipatanakul CS, Slavin RG. Bronchial asthma produced by paranasal sinusitis. *Arztl Otolaryngol* 100:109–112, 1974.
4. Rachelefsky GS, Katz RM, Siegel SC. Chronic sinus disease with associated reactive airway disease in children. *Pediatrics* 73(4):526–529, 1984.
5. Bernstean L. Pediatric sinus problems. *Otolaryngol Clin North Am* 4:127, 1971.
6. Rachelefsky GS, Goldberg M, Katz RM, et al. Sinus disease in children with respiratory allergy. *J Allergy Clin Immunol* 61:310–314, 1978.
7. Kaufman J, Chen JC, Wright GW. The effect of trigeminal resection on reflex bronchoconstriction after nasal and nasopharyngeal irritation. *Am Rev Respir Dis* 101:768–769, 1970.
8. Berger D, Nolte D, Reichenkall B. On nasobronchial reflex in asthmatic patients. *Rhinology* 17:193–198, 1979.

9. Hoehn JH, Reed CE. Where is the allergic reactor's in rag weed asthma? *J Allergy Clin Immunol* 80:268–273, 1987.
10. Empey DW, Laitinen LA, Jacobs L, et al. Mechanisms of bronchial hyperreactivity in normal subject and upper respiratory tract infections. *Am Rev Respir Dis* 113:131–134, 1976.
11. Harlin BL, Ansel DG, Lane SR, et al. A clinical and pathologic study of chronic sinusitis: the role of eosinophil. *J Allergy Clin Immunol* 81:867–875, 1988.
12. Stone BD, Georgitis JW, Mathews B. Inflammatory mediators in sinus lavage fluid (abst). *J Allergy Clin Immunol* 85:222, 1990.
13. Slavin RG, Cannon RE, Friedman WH, et al. Sinusitis and bronchial asthma. *J Allergy Clin Immunol* 66:256–257, 1980.

# 17

# Nonpharmacologic Approaches to the Management of Asthma

**MICHAEL J. WELCH, NANCY K. OSTROM, ELI O. MELTZER, and H. ALICE ORGEL**

*Allergy and Asthma Medical Group and Research Center and Children's Hospital*
*San Diego, California*

Pharmacologic management of asthma in children has become highly effective, given the many potent and well-tolerated medications available to the physician. However, nonpharmacologic measures for asthma control must not be overlooked. In fact, the ideal management plan should combine these two complementary types of intervention. In this chapter, we will discuss some nonpharmacologic approaches to asthma including environmental control, immunotherapy, physical training, and breathing exercises.

## ENVIRONMENTAL CONTROL

Our environment can be classified into the abiotic environment, with climatic factors such as wind, temperature, humidity, radiation, and nonliving contents of the air; and the biotic environment, which includes all living or recently living plant and animal materials. Numerous environmental substances precipitate or aggravate asthma by immunologic or nonimmunologic mechanisms; minimizing contact with them is the treatment referred to as environmental control.

### Abiotic Environment

#### *Climate*

Multiple meteorologic factors create our climate. It is not always easy to assess the effect of individual factors such as wind velocity, humidity, temperature, and barometric pressure on a child's asthma because their complex interaction influences the quality of air and its allergens and irritants. Low wind velocity leads to accumulation of pollutants, whereas high velocity and turbulence disperse particulates and may decrease their concentration. High wind velocity can, however, increase outdoor allergen concentration by dispersing pollen and mold spores.

Variations in humidity can alter factors that may trigger asthma symptoms in susceptible patients. High humidity is generally detrimental to asthmatic patients (1). This may be due to the adverse effect of altering mucosal osmolality (2), the result of increased numbers of mites and pollen-producing plants, or greater mold sporulation and release under conditions of high humidity. Dry windy weather can also disperse mold spores over long distances.

Changes in temperature seem to be troublesome for asthmatic patients. In particular, a sudden decrease in temperature can precipitate attacks of asthma (3). Laboratory studies have shown that all conditions that extract heat from the airway cause a fall in specific airway conductance in normal subjects and even more profoundly in asthmatic individuals (2). The use of indoor heating systems at the onset of cold weather can also contribute to environmental irritants affecting asthma. It is likely that the reactive airway problems are due to a combination of the cold air and the allergen exposure from the circulated dust and mold spores (4).

Barometric pressure changes have long been associated with an increase in the frequency of asthma attacks. In 1933, laboratory studies documented an increase in symptoms associated with sudden barometric pressure drops (5). Other investigators have reported an increase in asthma during days of high barometric pressure (6). Major epidemics of asthma in New Orleans have occurred with the combination of rising barometric pressure, decreasing temperature and relative humidity, plus minimal wind velocity (7). It would appear, therefore, that barometric pressure changes may aggravate asthma, perhaps under different conditions in different locations.

Considerable interest in the past has been given to the possible effect of atmospheric ions on the airway. Current data suggest that negative or positive ionization does not play a significant role in the aggravation of asthma (8).

### *Outdoor Air Pollution*

Asthma exacerbated by air pollution is a problem of growing magnitude with increasing urbanization. Air pollution is defined as the atmospheric accumulation of substances to a degree that becomes injurious to humans, animals, or plants. Although the overall concentrations of outdoor pollutants have decreased since the Clean Air Act was passed in 1970, certain communities are still experiencing an increase in environmental air pollution. There are two main outdoor types of pollution: industrial smog (sulfur dioxide–particulate complex), and photochemical smog (ozone and nitrogen dioxide). The first results from the combustion of solid or liquid sulfur-containing fossil fuel (e.g., coal and oil for heat and power) and the second from the chemical reaction of sunlight with automobile exhaust emissions. Photochemical oxidants are most prevalent in cities where auto use is high, sunshine is abundant, and there is little wind. Ozone can also be the product of the action of sunlight on hydrocarbons and nitrogen oxides emitted from industrial processes, power plants, and the petroleum industry. Recent air quality data indicate that more than 50% of the United States population lives in an area where there is potential exposure to peak ozone concentrations that exceed National Ambient Air Quality Standards (NAAQS) (9).

These two types of pollution can coexist in a given area. The levels of air pollutants are affected by many weather conditions, but low wind velocity in particular hinders their horizontal dispersion and high barometric pressure and temperature inversions limit their vertical dispersion. Local geographic features that confine pollutants emitted into the air also contribute to air stagnation.

Numerous studies have implicated various pollutants as aggravating asthma. Investigators analyzing the problem of pollution have utilized either controlled chamber exposure experiments or epidemiological studies. In the laboratory, ozone has been found to induce an increase in nonspecific airway hyperreactivity, thereby placing children with asthma at increased risk for adverse effects (10). Significant decrements in respiratory function have been noted in controlled clinical studies in children and adolescents exposed to as little as 0.12 parts per million (ppm) of ozone (equal to the NAAQS safety standard) while exercising at moderate levels. Although children experience reduced respiratory mechanics after ozone exposure, in contrast to adults, they often are asymptomatic (11,12). Exercise clearly potentiates the ozone effect on lung function since it lowers the exposure concentration necessary to induce abnormalities (13).

Controlled chamber exposure experiments have shown that asthmatic children have even more exquisite sensitivity to sulfur dioxide than oxone (13). Whereas exposure to high sulfur dioxide concentrations (>5 ppm) is necessary to induce bronchoconstriction in normal children, patients with asthma or atopy alone may have marked bronchoconstriction after inhaling sulfur dioxide at concentrations as low as 1 ppm at rest, and 0.5 ppm during moderate exercise. Sulfur-dioxide-induced effects are not only increased by exercise but also may be potentiated by the prior inhalation of ozone (14) and the concomitant administration of cold air (15). The mechanism by which sulfur dioxide aggravates asthma may be more than just a direct airway irritant effect. Animal experiments showing enhancement of IgE formation with sulfur dioxide exposure lend support to the theory that pollutants may potentiate allergen sensitization, resulting in hyperreactivity of the airways (16). Finally, although nitrogen dioxide has known irritating properties on airways, it is a curious finding that asthmatic subjects respond with little, if any, clinically significant decrements in lung function following acute controlled exposure to nitrogen dioxide (17).

Numerous epidemiological studies have been performed to investigate the role of air pollution in asthma. Studies such as these are fraught with difficulties due to confounding variables including meteorologic conditions, season of the year, aeroallergens, and infection. It is therefore not surprising that the results of epidemiologic studies attempting to link the incidence of asthma with ambient pollution have been inconclusive (18). There is some information suggesting that an association exists between ambient air pollution (particularly sulfur dioxide) and emergency room visits for asthma (19,20). However, other studies have shown either no relationship (21) or an inverse relationship of sulfur dioxide and photochemical oxidant levels with asthma-related hospitalizations and emergency room visits (22, 23). Given these inconclusive findings, it is possible that chronic low level pollution exposure may predispose to lower respiratory disease in a more subtle and complicated manner.

There is currently no proven therapy for patients with asthma to block the respiratory effects of pollution. However, the Weather and Air Pollution Committee of the American Academy of Allergy and Immunology has developed the following guidelines for asthmatic patients during air pollution episodes (24):

1. Avoid unnecessary physical activity. Cold temperature and low humidity are additionally stressful to the asthmatic patient who exercises under conditions of high air pollution (25).
2. Avoid smoking and smoke-filled rooms.
3. Avoid exposure to dust and other irritants such as hair spray, paint, exhaust fumes, or smoke from any fire.
4. Avoid exposure to persons with respiratory infections.
5. Try to stay indoors in a clean environment. Air conditioning and other filters may be helpful.
6. If it appears that the air pollution episode will persist or worsen, it may be desirable to leave the polluted area temporarily.
7. The physician and patient should formulate specific plans to be followed with regard to medication use and medical evaluation at the office or emergency room.

### *Indoor Air Pollution*

Multiple factors relating to both indoor and outdoor pollutants may potentiate the development of respiratory disease, particularly in atopic families. Indoor air pollution frequently involves different contaminants, sources, and atmospheric dynamics than outdoor pollution. Even in areas where the outdoor quality is good, indoor pollution is an important health factor since the great majority of children may spend up to 20 hr of each day inside a building. The prevalence of indoor pollution may be greater than in the past because modern construction techniques have made structures more resistant to indoor–outdoor air exchange. Mobile homes, prefabricated housing units, and energy-efficient homes are especially prone to indoor air problems. Potential indoor air quality problems include: outgassing of materials, return of air through flues and sanitation vents, and moisture build-up that leads to mold and fungus growth (26). Turnover of indoor air in newer and better insulated structures is generally only 50% that of the average house. Inadequate fresh air make up, poor distribution of air, or infiltration of outdoor contaminants occasionally leads to the "sick building syndrome," in which occupants develop such symptoms as irritation of mucous membranes and chest pains.

In about 50% of homes in the United States, natural gas or liquid propane is used for cooking (27). The combustion of these fuels can be a source of carbon monoxide, carbon dioxide, sulfur dioxide, formaldehyde, hydrocarbons, and nitrogen oxides. Numerous studies have reported elevated indoor levels of carbon monoxide, carbon dioxide, nitrogen monoxide, and nitrogen dioxide in homes with unvented appliances (28). Gas cooking commonly leads to nitrogen dioxide concentrations that are higher than the outside air by two to four times in the bedroom and five to six times in the kitchen. Three percent of homes exceed the 100 $\mu g/m^3$ safety standard, which is a nitrogen dioxide level exceeded outdoors in only one or two locations in the United States. There has been a national trend away from cleaner space-heating fuels such as gas and electricity and a resurgence of wood and coal-burning stoves, along with kerosene heaters (29). The number of wood-burning stoves is in excess of 1.5 million and there are over 13 million kerosene heating units in use during the winter months. Emissions from these heating appliances contain toxic and carcinogenic particles and gases. Indoor heating with wood burning stoves has been associated with increased frequency and severity of cough and wheezing compared with children whose homes are heated by other means (30). In this study, 84% of children in the wood-burning-stove group reported the occurrence of at least one severe symptom, compared to only 3% of the control group. Major pollutant emission byproducts of wood combustion in these stoves included carbon monoxide, nitrogen dioxide, sulfur dioxide, and respirable particulates.

Formaldehyde exposure from building materials such as plywood and particle board, furnishings, and some types of foam insulation has also been problematic. Outgassing of formaldehyde from these products can occur over a considerable time, with the half-life for emissions between 2 and 5 years. Adverse effects may result from inhalation, ingestion, or contact. Formaldehyde at concentrations of 1.2–2.5 $mg/m^3$ has been demonstrated to cause asthma in 5% of occupationally exposed persons. Whether the lower ambient levels (0.4 $mg/m^3$), which are not uncommon in homes, can also cause asthma remains to be determined (31).

A large percentage of children have significant respiratory exposure to the approximately 30% of adult Americans who smoke (32). Tobacco combustion contributes to concentrations of respirable particles, polycyclic hydrocarbons, carbon monoxide, nicotine, nitrogen dioxide, and acrolein. About 75% of the smoke from a cigarette wafts into the air without being inhaled by the smoker. This sidestream smoke burns hotter and is considerably more toxic than the smoke inhaled by the cigarette user; for example, the concentration of ammonia is 50 times greater. Homes with two or more smokers often have particle concentrations that exceed the federal standards set for outdoors.

The adverse effects of passive smoking are most clear in fetuses. Maternal smoking has a definite, dose-dependent association with decreased birth weight and increased preterm births and perinatal mortality (33,34). It has also been correlated with an increased incidence of placenta previa and abruptio placentae. The mechanism of action for these effects is unknown, but it is believed that they result from a combination of placental vasoconstriction due to nicotine and fetal tissue hypoxia caused by carbon monoxide in cigarette smoke.

Sidestream smoke inhaled by nonsmokers from active smokers is particularly irritating to respiratory mucosa. Conjunctival irritation, nasal discomfort, cough, sore throat, and sneezing have all been noted in nonsmokers exposed to cigarette smoke (35). Other more severe changes in small airway function have also been reported in nonsmokers who are exposed to smoke (36).

Animal studies, using lambs, have shown measurable respiratory effects of passive smoking on the young animals (37). Numerous human studies of the effects of parental smoking on respiratory health in children show an association with increased respiratory morbidity, especially during the first 2 years of life (38–44). In a prospective study of the first year of life, it was found that tracheitis and bronchitis occurred more frequently in infants exposed to cigarette smoke in the home. Maternal smoking imposed greater risks upon the infant than paternal smoking, and a family history of respiratory illness (chronic cough or bronchitis) significantly increased the incidence of bronchitis in the child (45). For children beyond the age of infancy whose mother smoked there was a 20–35% excess of respiratory problems such as wheezing, coughing, and bronchitis compared with children living in homes without smokers. Paternal smoking was associated with smaller but still substantial increases in such respiratory problems. Illness and symptom frequencies were linearly related to the number of cigarettes smoked by the child's mother. Rates of illness were higher for children of current smokers than for children of former smokers. The forced expiratory volume in 1 sec ($FEV_1$) was significantly lower for children of current smokers than for children of nonsmokers. The decrease in the $FEV_1$ was linearly related to daily cigarette consumption. Maternal smoking of one pack per day is estimated to reduce $FEV_1$ by 0.6–0.8% (46). These results provide strong support of a causal effect of sidestream cigarette smoke on increased respiratory illness and reduced pulmonary mechanics in preadolescent children.

At present, the mechanism by which passive smoking causes decreased lung function is uncertain. Some hypothesize that the smoke damages the airway epithelium, making it more susceptible to a higher frequency and severity of respiratory infections, which in turn lead to decreased lung function. The issue of whether tobacco smoke sensitivity is at all due to an allergic mechanism or is entirely irritant is yet to be resolved. Nonetheless, it is clear that tobacco smoke exerts numerous deleterious effects on host defense mechanisms. These include denudation of ciliated epithelium with squamous metaplasia of the epithelium, toxic effects on ciliary function with decrease in mucociliary clearance of inhaled materials, depression of alveolar macrophage phagocytic and bactericidal activity, and increase in overall bronchial irritability.

Other unprocessed tobaccos including clove cigarettes and marijuana have great potential for irritation of the respiratory mucosa and triggering of asthma symptoms in susceptible individuals. A wide variety of additional irritants are known to affect certain patients with asthma. In addition to those already mentioned are insecticides, aerosols, paint, laundry detergents, cooking fumes, and cosmetics. With chronic exposure, increased susceptibility to their effect is possible, due in part to sensitization of tracheobronchial vagal receptors (47). This results in exaggerated bronchoconstrictor responses and may be a significant factor in the airway hyperreactivity of asthma.

## Biotic Environment

### *Environmental History*

The number of substances found in our environment that induce allergic reactions is legion. Environmental control depends on the identification of allergens that may play a role in triggering any particular patient's asthma symptoms. A thorough history is the first step in this determination. Considerations should include those outlined below.

- Home: Structural considerations
  - Location: city, suburb, rural
  - Outdoors: landscaping, adjacent lots and structures
  - Age of home and length of time in residence
  - Rental vs. ownership of property
  - Construction:
    - Type: house, condominium, apartment
    - Material: stone, brick, frame, stucco, other
    - Basement, crawl space, or attic
  - Heating: forced air, electric, wall/floor furnace, space heater, radiator, fireplace, stove, other
  - Cooling: central, window, swamp cooler
  - Filtration: forced air, electrostatic, high-efficiency particulate air (HEPA), frequency of filter change

Patient's bedroom
- Location: basement, main floor, upper floor
- Number of family members sharing room and number of beds
- Type of beds and bedding:
  - Pillow: feather, foam, polyester, kapok
  - Mattress: fiber, foam, water
  - Springs: open or box
  - Bedding: synthetic, wool, cotton, feather
- Furniture:
  - Easily cleaned: dresser, desk, simple chairs, night stand, lamps, electrical equipment
  - Difficult to clean: stuffed furniture, books, toys, stuffed animals, bric-a-brac
- Flooring: wood, tile or linoleum, area rug, wall-to-wall carpet (age and type), pad (type)
- Window covering: shades, curtains, blinds, drapes
- Closet: clothing, toys, storage
- Heating vent: location

Home: Special considerations
- Cleaning for dust: broom, mop, vacuum, frequency
- Moisture/mold:
  - Condensation: windows, walls, bath, basement
  - Humidifiers: furnace, room, frequency of cleaning
  - Exhaust fans: kitchen, bathrooms
  - Plants: number, location
- Pets: number, type, extent of range in home
- Pollutants: tobacco, hobbies

Away from home
- Locations: school, workplace, babysitters, day care, relative's home, vacation home
- Outside: climate, geography
- Vehicle used for traveling
- Change of symptoms in different locations or environments

### *General Measures for Controlling the Environment*

Environmental control measures must be based on the suspected or known sensitivities of the patient and developed through discussion and cooperation with the family. The first suggestions should be those that will be easiest to accomplish and least likely to necessitate a change in behavior, relationships, or priorities. Further steps may be necessary if symptoms persist in the partially modified environment. These must take into consideration expense, lifestyle changes, and the impact on the whole family, and require an understanding and a reasonable expectation that these will benefit the patient, and thus the wellbeing of the family.

Since allergic reactivity to various substances is a matter of degree, it may be sufficient to reduce exposure rather than totally eliminate the substance from the environment. Emphasis, therefore, should be placed on the known exacerbating factors and on those areas, such as the bedroom, where a patient spends the greatest amount of time.

For the patient with more severe symptoms, more extensive measures may be needed in the entire house, in the babysitter's home, in the school room, and other frequently encountered environments. With recalcitrant problems, a visit to the home may uncover unexpected environmental factors (48). The neighborhood geography, age and nature of the house, quality of housekeeping, presence of animals or irritant odors, and compliance with previous recommendations may be directly assessed. In addition to information gathering, the effect of the home visit is to underscore the importance of the instructions for controlling the environment.

House dust has been described as an allergen since 1920 and was for many years thought to be a conglomerate composed of tiny particles of wool, cotton and cottonseed, kapok, feathers, hair, dirt, plaster, paint, cosmetics, and dander from humans and animals. In 1967, the house dust mite, *Dermatophagoides*, was shown to be the major source of the house dust allergen (49). Measures to minimize the exposure of asthmatic patients allergic to house dust and dust mite have for many years been advocated as a fundamental part of therapy (50). An extensive review of the role of dust and dust mite in asthma with recommendations for therapy is found in Chapter 18.

Fungi are classified as two types, molds and yeasts, both of which can act as airborne allergens. There is no way to separate completely the indoor air of any dwelling from the outside air, whether the structure is a home, office, or farm building. The types and quantity of outdoor and indoor airborne fungi in any locality are affected by the meteorologic conditions, the flora and fauna of the area, and the type of neighborhood in which they are found (farmland, industrial area, seashore, suburb, etc.). Fungi are most prominent throughout the growing season in temperate areas, with peak spore levels occurring in late summer and autumn, particularly during hot breezy periods when dry spore forms are especially abundant. Spore levels are higher closer to the ground. Therefore, hiking, lawn mowing, raking leaves, and grain harvesting are activities of high exposure.

The influence of the outdoor fungi on the indoor environment is more prominent in conventionally ventilated homes than in homes where the windows and doors are airtight and cooling and heating are accomplished through central closed systems. Once spores enter a home, part will be circulated back to the outdoor atmosphere; part will stay in the indoor air for a long period of time; part will be circulated through the home's air systems, be filtered, or settle and germinate in the ducts or fluids of these systems to form colonies; part will settle on household products (e.g., bread, fruit) and form colonies; part will settle on surfaces, cracks, and, if adequate humidity is present, form colonies; part will combine with dust and mites, in or on objects (e.g., carpets, mattresses, books, plants, pets) and either become nonviable or form colonies; and part will be inhaled by occupants of the home (51). Dark, humid, and poorly ventilated areas are optimal for indoor fungal growth. Such sites include the basement, crawl spaces, the washer and dryer area, stored furniture, rubber carpet underpads soiled by leaks or by urine from animals, suitcases, bathroom walls, shower stalls, window sills, and sinks. The kitchen refrigerator's contents are also a source of mold and thousands of spores may be released into the air when the door is opened. Fungi can grow very well within the systems used for cooling, heating, or humidification (52). The water container of portable and central humidifiers should be changed frequently and be treated with chemicals to eliminate fungal growth. High shade level, poorly maintained landscaping, large quantities of organic debris near the home, and house plants, fish tanks, and paper products may also contribute to indoor mold growth (53).

The best remedy for reducing the number of viable or nonviable fungal spores within the indoor environment is the removal or cleaning of dusty, mold-laden objects. Keeping every place and every item in the house well ventilated is the second important factor. The third requirement is maintenance of low humidity. Air conditioning, which both reduces humidity and filters large fungal spores, lowers the mold and yeast count indoors (54). Preventing a home from becoming moldy is considerably easier than trying to eliminate the sites of fungal growth.

Major allergenic windborne pollens from trees, grasses, and weeds are so prevalent outdoors throughout the lower atmosphere that avoidance measures can only curtail excessive exposure. Common sense attention to meteorologic conditions can be helpful since low pollen counts prevail after a prolonged rain, while extended warm, dry weather promotes dispersion. Brisk winds also promote pollen transport, which can extend over 100 miles. Awareness that morning hours are the time of peak pollen emission and that there are seasonal variations for certain pollen exposures will also aid a patient in avoiding them. Greater concentrations of pollen can be found in parks, fields, vacant lots, unpaved parking areas, construction sites, wooded lots, and in rural environments. Hobbies and activities such as hiking, camping, team sports, horseback riding, dirt bike riding, and yard work need to be evaluated in relationship to an individual's sensitivities and severity of symptoms.

Indoor pollen levels may be reduced effectively by closing windows. Forcing these particles off their natural course will usually reduce their entrance into a car or a building. Air conditioning effectively removes pollen and mold spores from rooms, resulting in much lower counts than in rooms that are not air conditioned (55).

Virtually any fur-bearing species of animal can sensitize a patient, but the degree and frequency of exposure remain critical factors in determining the level of a child's symptoms. It is the dandruff or skin scale, serum, saliva, and urine from the animals, rather than the hair, that is believed to be responsible for stimulating IgE production. Although some animals, notably the cat and the horse, tend to be more allergenic, none is hypoallergenic. Sensitivity to a species of an animal appears to include sensitivity to all varieties of that species. Despite the myth that poodles and chihuahuas do not trigger asthma, when it comes to allergenicity, a dog is a dog. Animal exposure is most frequent with the child's family pet. It should, therefore, be kept outside the allergic child's home. If the child is not yet allergic to a pet, its indoor presence promotes the development of this new sensitivity.

### *Specific Measures for Controlling the Environment*

Patient's Bedroom. 1. (See Fig. 1.) Bedroom clothing should be kept in a closet, with the door shut. The closet should not be used for storage of toys, equipment, luggage, or out-of-season clothing (Fig. 1).

2. Heavy curtains and fiber blinds should be avoided. Horizontal blinds are particularly good dust collectors. Window shades or frequently laundered curtains should be used instead. If the child is allergic to pollen or molds, windows should remain closed as much as possible.

3. Upholstered furniture should be eliminated from the bedroom. Plain wood or plastic chairs should be used.

4. Pillows should be encased in zippered, airtight covers, or synthetic polyester pillows that can be washed monthly and replaced yearly should be used. A patient should pack this pillow for use when traveling.

5. Water bed mattresses support mite growth least. When mite counts were compared from three types of fiber mattresses, foam rubber appeared preferable for mite-sensitive atopic subjects. The surface of kapok mattresses averaged twice and innerspring mattresses three times the number of mites found in foam rubber (56). Brushing and suction cleaning of a mattress reduces the number of live and dead mites by over 90%. The mattress and box springs should be encased in zippered airtight covers (possible sources include Allergy Control Products, Ridgefield, CT; or

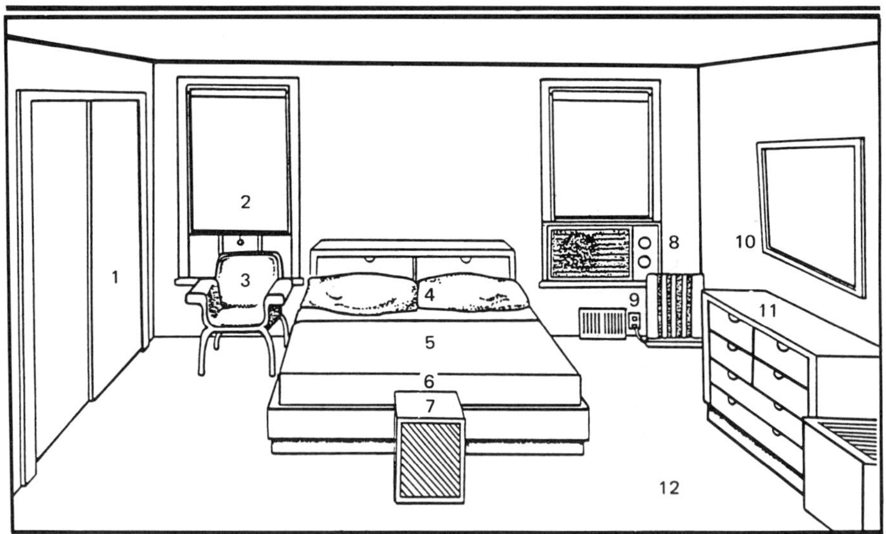


FIGURE 1 Dust control in bedroom. For numbers, see text.

Sears) and the zipper of the encasing sealed with tape to prevent leakage. If there is more than one bed in the room, all should be encased. If there are bunk beds, it is preferable to have the patient sleep on the top one or to split the bunks so that the patient does not sleep under a canopy.

6. Washing and airing of bedding normally removes a significant proportion of the mites. The water must be hot (over 70° C) to kill the mites. Warm or cold water, with or without detergents, will not kill mites and washing living mites out of fabric is not possible (57). Since we shed 0.5–1 g of skin scales a week, the sheets should be washed weekly and the mattress pads and synthetic blankets every 2 weeks. Wool blankets, chenille spreads, and down comforters should be avoided.

7, 8, 9. Both central and portable (e.g., floor model) filtering systems are available. The simplest type of filtering system is mechanical, employing closely knit fibers that sift out particles as small as 5–10 μm. These are adequate for most pollens and mold spores (see Fig. 2), and the major allergen associated with house dust mites (which is found in highest concentration in fecal particles between 10 and 25 μm). A commonly used mechanical filter is a HEPA unit. It functions by drawing air through charcoal prefilters and then distributing the air flow in a laminar fashion through the various-sized glass fibers that compose the HEPA filter. This filter can also be coated with chemicals that kill bacteria or viruses borne on dust particles. These very effective filters catch all particulates greater

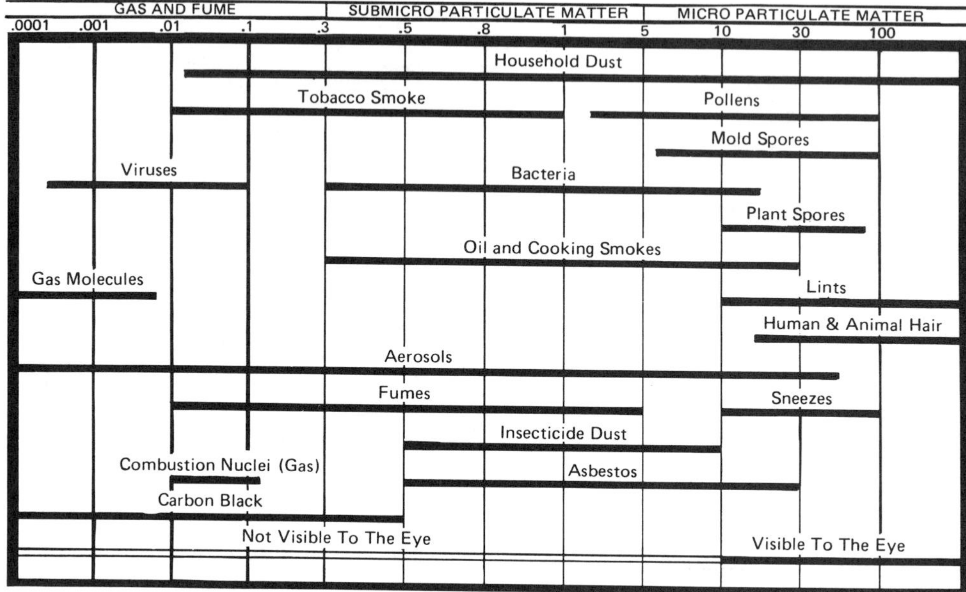


FIGURE 2 Size of more common air pollutants.

than 0.3 μm and, because the filters act like a blotter, they become more efficient with use. The HEPA filters can maintain high efficiency for 2–5 years. Using a portable HEPA filter in the bedroom can filter airborne allergens, most efficiently within 48 inches of the filtration unit (58). This may be of particular benefit in patients who have nocturnal asthma flares and morning symptoms.

The negative ion generator is a room air purifier that imparts a negative charge to particles dispersed in room air. The particles are attracted to walls and floors, which carry a positive charge. The disadvantages of this equipment are the production of ozone, which may be a respiratory irritant; removal of only particulate, not gaseous matter; soil deposition on surfaces; and the easy resuspension of particles.

Room air filtration can also be accomplished with the use of electrostatic filters, which charge particles in an electric field, trapping them on an oppositely charged filter plate. Because they may produce ozone, room electostatic filters could potentially intensify asthma in some patients. All electrostatic filters require a mechanical prefilter and a carbon filter to remove gaseous particles. They should be cleaned manually every 1 or 2 months.

At flows equal to several air changes per hour, both the electrostatic and the HEPA filters remove particles 0.5 μm in diameter and larger with an efficiency of approximately 85% (59). However, air filtration can only remove airborne allergens, and most dust allergen becomes airborne only during cleaning and then falls rapidly (60). In fact, 96% of all dust particles will precipitate from the air within 5–15 min after the area is disturbed. Thus while air filtration is theoretically helpful, it can fail at times to alter significantly the patient's symptoms. One cause for lack of improvement is the failure to keep windows and doors of the bedroom entirely closed to ensure that these units work effectively. To circumvent this problem, central filter units (i.e., part of the forced air system of the house) are available, ideally combining a mechanical and an electrostatic filter, with added carbon filters as needed. These units, however, can be a significant financial investment and require that the forced air system be operating the majority of time in the house with the windows closed.

10. Wall pennants, macrame hangings, toys, models, books, plants, and other dust collectors and fungus producers should be avoided. Small objects such as knick-knacks and trophies should be placed in drawers or closed cabinets.

11. Closets and drawers can be cleaned with a damp cloth and used for storing only laundered clothes. Any fungal growth that appears should be eliminated immediately, with caution taken not to disperse the mold spores while disposing of them. The growth should first be soaked gently and generously with an antifungal agent such as Clorox for at least 15 min prior to cleaning. Avoid using Lysol spray since it only eliminates the moldy smell, but does a poor job of actually killing fungi. Wet firewood, dried plants, and house plants should be avoided since they tend to promote mold growth.

12. All carpeting in the room should be removed, if possible. Even repeated vacuum cleaning is ineffective for removing mites from carpets, where they are present in abundance (61). Wood, linoleum, or tile floor should be cleaned with a damp or oiled mop daily. Antistatic surface sprays can be used on other areas.

Patient's Home. Home cooling systems include fans and air-conditioning systems. Exhaust fans that pull outside pollens, fungi, and dust through the house are not acceptable. Others that cool by circulating air through the attic are helpful. Evaporative coolers ("swamp coolers") can be a source of mold growth when the water cooled is not completely enclosed in the system. The ideal type of air conditioning is the refrigeration type. A central refrigerator unit is reasonably efficient in filtering larger allergens and irritants. It can also prevent the high heat and humidity that stimulate mite and fungal growth (62). Although central air conditioning is preferable, window units can be helpful. The windows and doors to the room should be shut and the air conditioner operated with its vent closed. The major mechanism in reducing spore counts in air conditioned homes is the closed windows, although the lower relative humidity and perhaps filtration are also associated with lower spore counts (54).

There are three basic types of controlled heating systems: forced air, in which air is heated and then blown throughout the house through a duct system; electric heat, with separate units in each room; and hot water, distributed via pipes to individual rooms and then heating by radiation and convection. Electric and hot water radiant systems are cleaner sources of heat for the allergic individual, since a forced air system promotes dust circulation. However, forced air is relatively inexpensive, and consequently, is utilized in many modern homes. In such homes, vents in the child's bedroom should be closed and sealed to prevent dust-laden air from filling the room during furnace operation. Adequate heat can still be maintained by use of a radiant space heater, electric blanket, or heated water bed. Dacron or electrostatic furnace filters are more efficient than the standard fiberglass filter and can be used as a substitute in the furnace. High-efficiency central filter units can be installed, but these can be a costly investment.

High concentrations of mite allergen may be present in upholstered furniture and carpets outside the bedroom. Minimizing the dust mite allergen level in the remainder of the house is also helpful. Vacuuming with an industrial vacuum cleaner will partially remove surface dust and fecal pellets, but not live mites. A typical home vacuum cleaner with inadequate suction and/or a leaking bag will cause allergens to become airborne. Allergic individuals can protect themselves from exposure by wearing a mask while cleaning, avoiding rooms where dust is being raised, and allowing it to settle for at least 1 hr before entering. While simple house cleaning does not reduce the existing level of mite antigen, the failure to clean a house results in a sizable increase in mite antigen level and, therefore, routine home cleaning measures are important.

Several chemicals have become available for use in killing mites. These acaricides have been shown to reduce levels of *D. pteronyssinus* antigen $P_1$ in carpets by up to 75% and by more than 50% in soft furniture following a single application (63). Thus, while routine cleaning is insufficient to reduce the mite allergen level and lead to consequent clinical improvement, acaricides hold this promise.

Use of humidifiers and vaporizers is generally not recommended, but if their use is absolutely necessary, overhumidification should be avoided. Humidifiers and vaporizers must be cleaned regularly to control fungal growth, which can be a major source of airborne spores. For normal function of human mucous membranes, a humidity level of 25–40% is considered optimal. Mold grows best in humidity greater than 50% and at temperatures above 37°C. Mites grow best at 75–80% relative humidity. Mite allergen levels will remain high with relative humidity above 50%. Keeping relative humidity below 50% is the single most important factor in reducing mold and mite numbers (64,65). If the relative humidity remains above 50%, air conditioning or a dehumidifier, a potent acaricide, or moving to a house that is structurally less humid should be considered. Sources of dampness such as leaking pipes, defective walls or roofs should be repaired. If the house is built on soil that becomes waterlogged, the walls may become damp by water rising from the ground through capillary action.

Respiratory irritants such as cigarette smoke, and cleaning, cooking, and cosmetic fumes should be eliminated from the home environment or confined to well-ventilated areas.

Patients with animal allergies react to epidermal scales, urine, and saliva that are readily dispersed throughout the home, when dry. Severe allergy to animals may improve dramatically within weeks or months after removing an offending pet. Specific sensitivity should be demonstrated (e.g., skin testing) before this avoidance measure is undertaken. Mild sensitivities may be resolved satisfactorily by keeping the pet outside or confined to the utility room when in the house.

Patient's Location. Some environments can be responsible for intractable symptoms in a given child. The mechanism may be severe sensitivity to pollens and mold on a ranch or farm, air pollution from a nearby factory causing bronchial irritation, or increased airway reactivity due to a cold, damp climate. In these circumstances, a change in geographic location can be considered. Although such a move may provide short-term benefit for the patient (66), little improvement will result if the family pet cat continues to sleep with the child, if new sensitivities in the new environment are acquired, or if the psychosocial and financial well-being of an entire family are compromised. Therefore, a 1 or 2 month trial period should precede any permanent decision and only in rare circumstances is the move indicated.

## IMMUNOTHERAPY

Immunotherapy, first introduced by Noon in 1911 for the treatment of hay fever, is now well accepted as effective therapy for allergic rhinitis caused by some inhaled allergens, and for hypersensitivity to venoms. It is less well established as a therapeutic modality for asthma due to the small number of acceptable, placebo-controlled trials in which benefit has been demonstrated. These are discussed below. The natural history of asthma in children, with its tendency to spontaneous improvement and multiple causative and precipitating factors, has added to the difficulties of designing, conducting, and interpreting such trials. However, the growing recognition of allergen exposure as a significant factor in the development of childhood asthma (67) reinforces the need for continued study of this treatment modality, which has the potential to reduce inflammatory mediator release and bronchial irritability (68–72).

### Studies in Childhood Asthma

To investigate whether immunotherapy has a beneficial effect on childhood asthma, a proper clinical study should have the following characteristics:

1. Adequate numbers of appropriate subjects whose asthma is thought to be directly triggered by allergens to which they are sensitive
2. Random assignment
3. Placebo control
4. Adequate dosage
5. "Blind" evaluation
6. Sensitive index of response
7. Adequate analysis of data

Studies that satisfy most of these criteria and could be considered acceptable are listed in Tables 1 and 2.

The first three studies listed (73–75) showed significant improvement in symptoms of asthma in children treated with ragweed or mixed pollen antigens. In the long-term prospective study (75), 72% of children receiving active treatment and only 22% of those receiving saline were free of asthma symptoms by the age of 16 years. This percentage of patients responding to the placebo injections is lower than in most reports. Since nearly one-third of the total 210 patients were unavailable for follow-up at the end of the study, this may represent a flaw in the analysis.

In 1971, Aas conducted a study of children who reacted on bronchial challenge to house dust extracts. He showed that bronchial reactivity was significantly decreased in the patients receiving active treatment compared with those receiving placebo; symptoms were also decreased more in the active treatment group but the difference was not statistically significant (76).

In a study by Warner et al. (77), a tyrosine-absorbed extract of *Dermatophagoides pteronyssinus* was used for immunotherapy; the effect on bronchial reactivity, symptom scores, and medication requirements in asthmatic children was evaluated. The immediate response to bronchial challenge was unaltered in most children after 1 year of treatment, but in those who had a late bronchial reaction, it was absent in 10 of 22 receiving active treatment compared with only 1 of 15 children receiving placebo. The loss

TABLE 1 Placebo-Controlled Studies of Immunotherapy for Childhood Asthma Showing Efficacy

| Authors | Year (Duration in Months) | Allergens | Evaluation Method | Significance (p) |
|---|---|---|---|---|
| Johnstone (73) | 1957 (12–36) | Ragweed | Symptoms | <0.001 |
| Johnstone and Crump (74) | 1961 (48) | Mixed | Symptoms | <0.001 |
| Johnstone and Dutton (75) | 1968 (up to 168) | Mixed | Symptoms | <0.01 |
| Aas (76) | 1971 | Dust | Bronchial challenge | <0.01 |
| Warner et al. (77) | 1978 (12) | Mite (modified) | Delayed response to bronchial challenge | <0.05 |
| | | | Medications | <0.007 |
| | | | Symptoms | <0.015 |
| Price et al. (year 2 of above) (78) | 1984 (24) | Mite (modified) | As above | |
| Valovirta et al. (79) | 1984 (10–12) | Dog | Bronchial challenge | <0.1 |
| | | | Conjunctival challenge | <0.001 |

TABLE 2 Placebo-Controlled Studies of Mold Immunotherapy for Childhood Asthma

| Author | Year (Duration in months) | Allergens | Evaluation Method | Significance (p) |
|---|---|---|---|---|
| Dreborg et al. (80) | 1986 (10) | Mold (*Cladosporium*) | Symptoms | n.s. |
| | | | Medications | <0.01 |
| | | | Bronchial challenge | <0.05 |
| Karlsson et al. (81) | 1986 (10) | Mold (*Cladosporium*) | Specific IgE | <0.05 |
| | | | IgG/IgE | <0.05 |
| Horst et al. (82) | 1990 (12) | Mold (*Alternaria*, standardized) | Self evaluation | <0.001 |
| | | | Symptoms | |
| | | | Medication | <0.005 |
| | | | Nasal challenge | <0.05 |

of the late reaction correlated with a decrease in symptom scores. Medication use was also significantly reduced in the group receiving active extract. This study was continued for a second year (78). At that time, patients who had received active treatment were randomized double-blind to receive another year of active therapy or to placebo treatment. In those 12 children in whom therapy was withdrawn in the second year, there was first a deterioration in lung function and then an increase in drug requirements. Late responses also recurred in three of the four children who had lost them after 1 year of treatment. Of the children who had received placebo for the first year, 21 completed a year of active treatment. There was also improvement but it was less impressive than in the group receiving active treatment in the previous year. It was concluded that treatment was effective in reducing symptoms of asthma, bronchial reactivity, and medication usage; asthma deteriorated when treatment was discontinued; and *D. pteronyssinus* was a major allergen causing perennial asthma in children.

A placebo-controlled study of immunotherapy with "standardized" dog antigen in 27 children in Finland showed significant improvement in conjunctival sensitivity in the active treatment group by comparison with placebo. Improvement in bronchial reactivity was also detected in 6 of 15 active and two of the 12 placebo-treated patients ($p < 0.1$). Subjectively, half of each treatment group reported decreased sensitivity, emphasizing the need for objective measurement, especially in emotionally charged situations such as exposure to pets (79).

A few recently published studies have shown the efficacy of mold immunotherapy in asthma patients as measured by various immunologic and clinical parameters (Table 2). Treatment for a 10 month period with *Cladosporium herbarum* produced improvement in medication scores as well as bronchial and nasal challenge sensitivity compared with a placebo-treated group (80). With use of the same antigen, changes measured as specific IgG, IgE, and the IgG/IgE ratio following treatment also showed a theoretically favorable response in a group of actively treated patients compared to a group treated with placebo (81). In a group of children and adults treated with standardized *Alternaria* extract for a 1 year period, both specific IgG and clinical parameters including self-evaluation, symptom and medication scores, and nasal challenges showed a significantly improved response compared with a group of placebo-control subjects (82). These initial studies showing efficacy of immunotherapy with mold antigens may add to the treatment armamentarium available for the large number of patients with asthma affected by allergy to this ubiquitous antigen (83).

Double-blind placebo-controlled studies in adults show that immunotherapy for asthma is effective for the following allergens: dust (81), mite (85,86), grass (87,88), and cat (89,90). Immunotherapy with *Alternaria* antigen has also been shown to decrease the late asthmatic response in sensitive patients (91).

There is no reason to believe that the mechanisms of action of immunotherapy differ in children and adults and it seems reasonable to assess the evidence for children and adults together. This review has concentrated on placebo-controlled studies that show the efficacy of immunotherapy. Negative studies exist but, on critical review, many of these "failures" can be explained by problems with study design, antigen selection, and dosage.

In summary, there is clearly a need for additional well-controlled trials of immunotherapy in asthma. To date, most acceptable trials have shown improvement in symptoms, bronchial reactivity on challenge, or medication requirements, for control of asthma symptoms. Immunologic changes that characterize satisfactory responses have also been documented. Despite the remaining controversy regarding the effectiveness of immunotherapy for the alleviation of asthma, it remains the only modality of treatment known to reduce the immunologic response of the individual to specific allergens that are likely significant triggers for both acute and chronic asthma symptoms.

## Mechanism of Action

The modes of action of immunotherapy are not completely understood but certain changes have been well documented:

1. An initial rise in specific IgE antibodies followed, after several years of therapy, by a gradual decrease. Treated patients had blunting or absence of the seasonal increase in IgE seen in untreated populations (92–95).
2. An increase in specific "blocking" IgG antibodies in serum (96) and secretions and an increase in specific secretory IgA (97). In serum, $IgG_4$ is an important component of the immunologic response (88,98).
3. A decrease in the reactivity of mediator cells in many patients with decrease in antigen-induced leukocyte histamine release (99).
4. A decrease in in vitro antigen-induced T lymphocyte proliferation, probably due to generation of suppressor T cells (100) and other changes (101).
5. A decrease in target organ sensitivity to the specific allergens (76,77,79,102).
6. Changes in the late-phase reaction to bronchial challenge (77,91). It is probable that additional changes are induced and that a combination of interacting mechanisms is involved (103, 104). This would explain, for example, the poor correlation between the concentration of specific

"blocking" antibodies and the clinical response following immunotherapy.

### Selection of Patients and Antigen

The allergic reactions that cause asthma in children are probably exclusively IgE mediated. Diagnosis depends on a careful history and correlation of symptoms with exposure to suspected allergens. Sensitivities should be identified by skin tests or assay of specific serum IgE antibodies. While every effort should be made to treat with only those antigens that appear relevant based on both history and testing, this may be impossible. Of particular difficulty is the child with perennial asthma who has large positive skin test reactions to many locally prevalent allergens but for whom causative correlations are difficult to identify. If known exposure is perennial or lasts many months, these antigens are customarily included in treatment sets. Triggers of bronchial hyperreactivity appear to be additive; not only exposure to allergen(s) but also nosnpecific irritants and infections all play a role to different degrees at different times in any patient's asthma.

The antigens should be obtained from reputable sources and should be standardized by modern methods. Many of the allergens available for immunotherapy at the present time are nonstandardized extracts that vary from one manufacturer to another, and even from lot to lot. On the other hand, when crude allergenic extracts are purified to contain only "major" allergens, efficacy of immunotherapy may be reduced (105,106), suggesting that optimal results are obtained when the extract contains most of the identifiable antigens. Since efficacy of immunotherapy correlates with the dosage of antigen administered, the availability of antigens of known potency is essential for safe and successful treatment. The Food and Drug Administration is encouraging the use of modern methods of immunologic standardization and, as a result, the quality of extracts should improve in the future.

There is no indication for immunotherapy with food antigens. Bacterial vaccines have been shown to be ineffective and not recommended.

At the pesent time, children who are suitable candidates for immunotherapy should have the following characteristics:

1. Documented IgE-mediated hypersensitivity to prevalent and unavoidable antigens
2. Significant illness: considerable interference with sleep, exercise, school, and play, or more
3. Increasing severity of disease, despite optimal environmental measures and pharmacotherapy

## Preparation and Administration

The formulation of individual extract mixtures for a particular patient requires special training and experience. The mixtures should contain all significant allergens. Allergens to which the patient is extremely sensitive should not be mixed with others to which he or she has lesser sensitivity, since they will limit the amount of other allergens that can be administered. The antigens are suitably diluted depending on the degree of sensitivity and given in increasing amounts (usually a 50% increase) each week. Dosages may need to be decreased during periods of increased airborne allergen exposure, for example, during the grass or ragweed seasons. Maintenance dosage is usually defined as the maximum dosage the patient can tolerate without experiencing serious adverse effects or, arbitrarily, as 0.3–0.5 ml of the most concentrated antigen(s). When a fresh supply of antigen is prepared, the maintenance dosage should be reduced by 25–50% and then gradually increased again to the maintenance level. The interval between injections may be increased at the maintenance level from weekly dosing to every 2, then 3, then 4, then every 6 weeks. A typical course of immunotherapy is continued for 2–5 years.

## Adverse Reactions

The patient should receive the injections in the physician's office and remain there for at least 20–30 min for observation and treatment of local or systemic reactions. Local reactions consist of swelling, redness, and itching and occur frequently. Reactions larger than 2 cm in diameter or persisting longer than 24 hr, and any type of systemic reaction, indicate that the dosage of the next injection should be reduced.

Systemic reactions may consist of generalized erythema, itching, tingling or urticaria, angioedema, laryngeal edema, bronchospasm, or cardiovascular collapse. They may occur unpredictably at any time, even following a long period of administration of the maintenance dosage. Any office or medical facility administering immunotherapy should be supplied and trained to deal with an anaphylactic reaction. Treatment of local and systemic reactions is reviewed below.

## Management of Reactions

Local reactions should be treated with local application of ice pack and oral antihistamine and topical steroids as needed. The dosage schedule should be reviewed.

Systemic reactions should be treated as follows:

1. 0.01 ml/kg up to 0.2 ml aqueous epinephrine 1:1000 subcutaneously *at the site of the injection of allergens*

2. 0.01 ml/kg up to 0.3 ml aqueous epinephrine at another site
3. Diphenhydramine intravenously or intramuscularly 1.25 mg/kg up to 50 mg
4. Tourniquet above the site of the injection
5. Observation in the office until it is clear that the patient is stable.

Other treatments may be required: For bronchospasm: inhaled beta-agonists, intravenous hydrocortisone, oxygen; laryngeal edema: oxygen, intubation, tracheostomy; hypotension: intravenous fluids, vasopressors; cardiac arrest: resuscitation. The dosage schedule should also be reviewed.

## Duration of Therapy

Duration of treatment depends on the response of the patient, which should be monitored with regular evaluations. Treatment is often continued, if benefit is demonstrated, until the patient is symptom-free for 1–2 years. It may then be stopped. In some patients, the relief from symptoms continues; in others, symptoms recur. Recurrent symptoms may be mild and can be managed by environmental controls and medications, but sometimes it is necessary to reinstitute immunotherapy.

## Modified Allergens

There have been various modifications to the antigens, with a view to decreasing the number of injections required to attain the immunotherapeutic dose and to minimize adverse reactions (107). They have been evaluated primarily in patients with hay fever. Alum precipitation is effective for grass pollen but not for ragweed pollen (possibly because ragweed antigen E is denatured by the process). Conjugation of antigen with polyethylene glycol (PEG) or with D-glutamic acid and D-lysine (D-GL) is only moderately successful in increasing immunologic responses while decreasing reactions (107).

Antigen extracts modified by mild formalin treatment are known as "allergoids." They are effective in decreasing symptoms, increasing IgG-blocking antibodies, and decreasing the number of injections required to reach maintenance dose from approximately 25 to less than 10. Booster injections may be given at 6–12 week intervals instead of the usual 4–6 week schedule required for standard aqueous antigens (108,109). Since each antigen must be investigated separately, additional evaluations are still required before these new preparations can be released to the practicing clinician.

The delay in availability is also true for glutaraldehyde-modified tyrosine-absorbed preparations now used in Europe and tested in the United States (110,112). All these modified antigens have been shown to retain immunogenicity and reduce allergenicity (107–112). At this time, modified allergens of this type have the most promise for improving allergen immunotherapy.

## PHYSICAL TRAINING

The development of highly effective, protective medications has made it possible for many asthmatic children to participate in a wide range of physical activities, including physical training. This is true even for those with significant disease. Although physical training has not been clearly shown to improve asthma per se, it appears to have several benefits. These include increased physical fitness, enhanced tolerance of attacks, and greater social and psychological independence. Asthmatic children are no longer required to "sit on the sidelines," but can participate fully in the exercise or sports activity of their choice. Children with asthma should be inspired by the 53 U.S. Olympic athletes with asthma who were able to win a total of 16 medals in various events during the 1988 World Olympics.

### Impact of Physical Training Programs

It is generally accepted, on an intuitive basis, that exercise is good for patients with lung disease, but the extent to which it alters the asthmatic condition is not clearly established. Measurements of exercise endurance, tolerance, and oxygen consumption have clearly indicated that children with asthma are not as fit as their peers without asthma (113,114). Therefore, it is not surprising that numerous studies conclude that asthmatic children benefit in multiple ways from participation in specially designed physical fitness programs (115–120). One important physiological gain from a sustained exercise program is improved peak work capacity and aerobic fitness, which can lead to better exercise tolerance and apparently less exercise-induced asthma (121,122). This is not, however, the result of direct improvement in lung function. Basic pulmonary function parameters such as the forced vital capacity (FVC), $FEV_1$, and $FEF_{25-75}$ have not been noted to change after exercise programs in asthmatic patients (113,119,120). It is theorized that the improved aerobic capacity in the conditioned state leads to decreased ventilatory requirements for a given work-load. This results in less airway cooling and/or evaporative losses, creating what appears to be less exercise-induced bronchoconstriction. However, when maximal oxygen uptake ($VO_2$) is controlled for, the degree of exercise-induced hyperreactivity after physical training is unchanged (123).

Improvements in posture, lean body mass, cardiac output, and muscle strength have been reported in asthmatic patients after undergoing training programs. In addition, frequency of asthma symptoms, medication requirements, and school absenteeism decrease in association with physical conditioning (116,119,124–125). In retrospect, many of these studies were not rigorously designed and they often lacked a proper control group, making it difficult to reach any firm conclusions about cause and effect. Physical training does have the theoretical benefit of increasing the endurance of the asthmatic child, giving him or her additional reserves for coping with episodes of severe respiratory airway obstruction or respiratory failure.

Psychosocial benefits of physical conditioning in the asthmatic child are at least as important as the physiological ones. Although not well documented, it is believed that physical training can improve self-esteem and confidence. By developing a positive personal image through physical activity, the child is less likely to have the self-perception of being "sick" or "weak." This leads to less social isolation and better acceptance by peers. The child's parents are also affected and often react by becoming less protective and imposing fewer restrictions.

### Selecting the Type of Exercise or Sport

With proper medical management, most children with asthma can participate fully in any type of exercise or competitive activity they desire. This includes contact sports, team sports, solo competition, or simple physical conditioning. However, certain sports offer greater chances of success than others. Swimming has been shown to be less asthmagenic than running or cycling (127). This has been attributed to the high humidity of the air near the surface of the water, which reduces evaporative cooling of the airway mucosa. However, Inbar et al. (128) demonstrated that swimming produces little asthma, even when subjects breathe relatively dry air from an external source. Swimming training in children may also lead to improved posture and fitness, reduced fat folds, and decreased need for chronic asthma medications, but the frequency and severity of exercise-induced asthma following other activities is not altered (124). Because swimming seems to provoke less exercise-induced asthma, it is not surprising that many of the Olympic medals won by asthmatic patients have been won by swimmers and divers.

Interrupted or spurt exercise, in which running or exertion is of short duration, is also better tolerated (125). Examples of sports with intermittent activity include baseball, wrestling, racquet sports, and sprinting. Although running is generally regarded as the most asthmagenic form of exercise, children with even severe chronic asthma can often successfully participate in distance running training programs when receiving adequate therapy; they can also obtain measurable physiological benefits in ventilatory muscle strength and endurance (120). Therefore, if sensibly and flexibly approached, the popular activity of jogging can usually be enjoyed by those with asthma.

In school, the problem of exercise-induced asthma occurs during physical education (PE) class or on the playground. PE teachers and coaches may not realize that a student has asthma or that excessive exercise may induce asthma symptoms in some students who are otherwise healthy. If so, the affected student may be penalized or pushed beyond his or her capacity to exercise, thus precipitating asthma. At the other extreme, the student with asthma may be inappropriately transferred to adaptive PE. With few exceptions, most children with asthma should be able to participate fully in regular PE activities provided there is adequate understanding by the instructor of the potential limitations of the patient, and that, when indicated, medication is allowed prior to and/or following exercise. As stated by the American Academy of Pediatrics Committee on Children with Disabilities regarding children with asthma: "Every effort should be made to minimize restrictions and to invoke them only when the condition of the child makes it necessary." (129). The PE coach should be made aware that long distance running (e.g., "running laps") poses the greatest problem for the child with asthma; activities with repeated short bursts of running are better tolerated. Permission should be requested for the student to premedicate before exertion with either an inhaled beta-agonist, cromolyn, or both. This usually permits full participation in most strenuous physical activity. Physicians managing children with asthma should rarely need to excuse a child permanently from PE or enroll them in adaptive PE due to asthma. It is helpful to meet with a patient and parents at the beginning of the school year to discuss asthma control in the school setting, to educate regarding premedication before exercise, and to provide the family with a form for the PE instructor that explains the child's medical problem and how it can be effectively managed in the PE class (see Fig. 3). A small number of children with asthma use their illness to avoid certain physical activities at school for reasons unrelated to the issue of exercise-induced asthma. They have learned to manipulate overprotective parents and unwary physicians. PE and exercise are beneficial to children with asthma, and any decision to modify a school PE program should only be made following a reasonable consultation with the physician, parent, child, and school. The ideal situation is a trusting relationship between the student and the PE instructor. The student should be allowed to assess his or her asthma control and either modify exercise activity accordingly or take medication before, during, or after exercise.

### Warming Up

It has been suggested that a "warm-up" may reduce exercise-induced asthma by gradually discharging the bronchial mast cells, thereby inhibiting subsequent development of exercise-induced asthma (130). There is still an absence of research evidence to substantiate this theory (131). Nevertheless, warm-up activities are currently recommended for asthmatic athletes for possible respiratory benefit, as well as any general benefits related to reducing injury and assisting flexibility. The warm-up period should include activities in which the intensity can be controlled by the patient, thereby enabling the patient to discover his or her own exercise tolerance level and limits. A 20 min warm-up incorporating short sprints, jumping, and gymnastic activities has been recommended to provide protection from exercise-induced asthma (125). A similar "warming down" has also been suggested at the end of exercise to help reduce exercise-induced bronchospasm (132).

## BREATHING EXERCISES AND CHEST PHYSIOTHERAPY

### Breathing Exercises

Breathing exercises have been advocated to help asthmatic patients increase diaphragmatic breathing, increase tidal air volume, and prevent deformities (133,134). Rehabilitation programs, which included breathing exercises, have resulted in an improvement in asthma severity in some patients (135). However, the general consensus is that breathing exercises for purposes of training the respiratory apparatus are of little use in children with asthma (136,137). The overall gain from these types of exercises is usually too minimal to warrant the time and energy necessary for such a training program. Furthermore, since asthmatic episodes provide sufficient exercise to respiratory muscles, the respiratory apparatus of asthmatic children needs very little special training or conditioning. Breathing training may have some use if viewed as as relaxation technique (138). The teaching of slow, diaphragmatic, and lower costal breathing can sometimes facilitate relaxation in a child who is having an acute asthma episode.

### Chest Physiotherapy

Although no careful studies yet demonstrate that chest physiotherapy clearly benefits the asthmatic patient, this modality is still used on occasion for the patient who has difficulty expectorating tenacious secretions (138,139). In selected patients, postural draining with chest percussion and vibration has been helpful in relieving secretional obstruction and supplementing the inhalation of $beta_2$ aerosols. Since the patient with a severe exacerbation

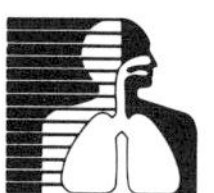

**Allergy & Asthma Medical Group**
**& Research Center**
PEDIATRIC ALLERGY MEDICAL GROUP

JAMES P. KEMP, M.D. • ELI O. MELTZER, M.D. • H. ALICE ORGEL, M.D. • MICHAEL J. WELCH, M.D. • NANCY K. OSTROM, M.D.

AMERICAN BOARD OF ALLERGY AND IMMUNOLOGY AMERICAN BOARD OF PEDIATRICS

Dear Physical Education Instructor: Date: ______________, 19 ______

______________________________ is under my care for ASTHMA.
(Name of student)

Because exercise is important for the asthmatic child, both physically and psychologically, I am providing information and instructions concerning this child's **participation in physical education.**

1 He/she should be permitted to remain in regular PE classes and should be able to engage in *regular* physical education activities most of the time. However, during asthma episodes (characterized by cough, wheeze, shortness of breath) activities may have to be *temporarily* curtailed.

2 Each asthmatic child has a different limit of exercise tolerance. In particular, asthmatics may have difficulty "running laps" and playing competitive soccer and basketball; please do not "force" the child, but let the student participate at his/her own level. Swimming is usually well-tolerated and an excellent activity for asthmatics.
*Please permit the youngster to set his/her own pace on a daily basis.* If you feel inappropriate choices are being made, please contact the parent so that we can all help the student maintain as normal an activity level as possible.

3 Warm-up exercises are often useful in warding off wheezing episodes.

4 We do not wish the student with asthma to feel "different." Please do what is necessary toward accomplishing this end.

5 If this student does have some problem with "endurance" sports, please permit him/her to take the following medication*: ______________________ ***before*** participating to ***prevent*** symptoms.

6 In case of breathing difficulty, talk to the child reassuringly and calmly; have the child take prescribed medication (______________________).*
If the treatment is ineffective or symptoms are severe, notify the school nurse or parent immediately.

We welcome your suggestions regarding these recommendations.

*The student's parent has been given a "school medication authorization" form to transmit to the school. Where indicated, permit the child to medicate herself/himself if authorized by physician and parent.

Sincerely,

______________________ ______________________
(Parent's Signature) (Physician's signature)

______________________
Address

______________________
City, State, & Zip Code

______________________
Telephone

*Modified from recommendations developed by The American College of Allergists.*

3444 KEARNY VILLA ROAD, SUITE 100
SAN DIEGO, CA 92123
(619) 292-1144

A PROFESSIONAL CORPORATION
CARING FOR CHILDREN AND YOUNG ADULTS

215 S. HICKORY STREET, SUITE 102
ESCONDIDO, CA 92025
(619) 480-0799

FIGURE 3 Sample of instructions to physical education instructor.

of asthma will usually have a major problem with mucus plugging, and since such patients will usually be hospitalized, it is in the inpatient setting where this therapeutic modality is of most value. In particular, the patient with increased asthma due to a chest infection (e.g., localized pneumonia) may benefit from chest physiotherapy. However, the vigorous maneuvers of chest percussion and vibration should be avoided when the asthmatic child is first hospitalized and in significant respiratory distress. Chest manipulation at that time may further upset the already agitated child and increase the chance of respiratory failure. Most patients can tolerate physiotherapy after 1–2 days of hospital management of status asthmaticus. At that point, mobilization of mucus may be facilitated by chest physiotherapy. However, the lack of evidence supporting its efficacy makes it difficult to advocate as a routine method in asthma management, and indeed, it is usually not necessary for most hospitalized asthmatic children.

## REFERENCES


1. Lopez M, Salvaggio JE. Climate-weather-air pollution. In: Middleton E Jr, Reed CE, Ellis EF (eds.), *Allergy: Principles and Practices*, C.V. Mosby, St. Louis, 1983, p. 1203.
2. Aitken ML, Marini JJ. Effect of heat delivery and extraction on airway conductance in normal and in asthmatic subjects. *Am Rev Respir Dis* 131:357–361, 1985.
3. Tromp S. Influence of weather and climate on asthma and bronchitis. *Rev Allergy* 22:1027, 1968.
4. Greenburg L, Field F, Reed JI, Erhardt CL. Asthma and temperature change. *Arch Environ Health* 8:642–647, 1964.
5. Nelson T, Rappaport BZ, Walker WH: Asthma and weather. *JAMA* 100:1385, 1933.
6. Girsh LS, Shubin E, Dick C, Schulaner FA. A study on the epidemiology of asthma in children in Philadelphia: the relation of weather and air pollution to peak incidence of asthmatic attacks. *J Allergy* 39:347–357, 1967.
7. Salvaggio J, Hasselblad V, Seabury J, Heiderscheit LT. New Orleans asthma II. Relationship of climatologic and seasonal factors to outbreaks. *J Allergy* 45:257–365, 1970.
8. Davis JB. Review of the scientific information on the effect of ionized air on human beings and animals. *Aerospace Med* 34:35–42, 1963.
9. Lippman M. Health effects of ozone: a critical review. *J Air Pollut Control Assoc* 39:672–695, 1989.
10. Paulo M, Gong H. Respiratory effects of ozone: whom to protect, when, and how? *J Respir Dis* 12:482–499, 1991.
11. Avol EL, Linn WS, Shamoo DA, et al. Respiratory effects of photochemical oxidant air pollution in exercising adolescents. *Am Rev Respir Dis* 132:619–622, 1985.

12. McDonnell WF, Chapman RS, Leigh MW, et al. Respiratory responses of vigorously exercising children to 0.12 ppm ozone exposure. *Am Rev Respir Dis* 132:875–879, 1985.
13. Gong H. Effects of outdoor air pollutants on exercise performance. *Clin Rev Allergy* 6:361–384, 1988.
14. Koenig JQ, Covert DS, Hanley QS, et al. Prior exposure to ozone potentiates subsequent response to sulfur dioxide in adolescent asthmatic subjects. *Am Rev Respir Dis* 141:377–380, 1990.
15. Sheppard D, Eschengacher WL, Boushey HA, Bethel RA. Magnitude of the interaction between the bronchomotor effects of sulfur dioxide and those of dry (cold) air. *Am Rev Respir Dis* 130:52–55, 1984.
16. Osebold JW, Gerschwin LJ, Zee YC. Studies on the enhancement of allergic lung sensitization by inhalation of ozone and sulfuric acid aerosol. *J Environ Pathol Toxicol* 3:221–234, 1980.
17. Avol EL, Linn WS, Peng RC, et al. Experimental exposure of young asthmatic volunteers to 0.3 ppm nitrogen dioxide and to ambient air pollution. *Toxicol Ind Health* 5:1825–1834, 1989.
18. Richards W. Effect of air pollution on asthma. *Ann Allergy* 65:345–347, 1990.
19. Bates DV, Baker-Anderson M. Sizto R. Asthma attack periodicity: a study of hospital emergency visits in Vancouver. *Environ Res* 51:51–70, 1990.
20. Imai M, Yoshida K, Kitabatake M. Mortality from asthma and chronic bronchitis associated with changes in sulfur oxides air pollution. *Arch Environ Health* 41:29–35, 1986.
21. Goldstein IF, Weinstein AU. Air pollution and asthma: effects of exposure to short-term sulfur dioxide peaks. *Environ Res* 40:332–345, 1986.
22. Tseng RYM, Li CK. Low level atmospheric sulfur dioxide pollution and childhood asthma. *Ann Allergy* 65:379–383, 1990.
23. Richards W, Azen SP, Weiss J, et al. Los Angeles air pollution and asthma in children. *Ann Allergy* 47:348–354, 1981.
24. Slavin RG, Claman LN, Kailin EW, et al. Guidelines for the asthmatic patient during air pollution episodes. *J Allergy Clin Immunol* 55:222–223, 1975.
25. Linn WS, Shamoo DA, Anderson KR, et al. Effects of heat and humidity on the response of exercising asthmatics to sulfur dioxide exposure. *Am Rev Respir Dis* 131:221–225, 1985.
26. Spengler JD. Indoor air pollution. *N Engl Reg Allergy Proc* 6:126–134, 1985.
27. Samet JM, Marbury MC, Spengler JD. The Fourth Annual Aspen Allergy Conference. Respiratory effects of indoor air pollution. *J Allergy Clin Immunol* 79:685–700, 1987.
28. *National Research Council Committee on Indoor Pollutants*. National Academy Press, Washington, D.C., 1981.
29. Pierson WE, Koenig JQ, Bardana EJ. Potential adverse health effects of woodsmoke. *West J Med* 151:339–342, 1989.
30. Honicky RE, Osborne JS III, Akpom CA. Symptoms of respiratory illness

in young children and the use of wood-burning stoves for indoor heating. *Pediatrics* 75:587–593, 1985.

31. Nordman H, Keskinen H, Tuppurainen M. Formaldehyde asthma—rare or overlooked? *J Allergy Clin Immunol* 75:91–99, 1985.
32. Office on Smoking and Health. *The Health Consequences of Involuntary Smoking: A Report of the Surgeon General.* US Public Health Service, Rockville, MD, 1986.
33. Meyer MB. Effects of maternal smoking and altitude on birth weight and gestation. In: Reed DM, Stanley FJ (eds.), *The Epidemiology of Prematurity*. Urban and Schwarzenberg, Baltimore, 1977, pp. 81–104.
34. Shiono PH, Klebanoff MA, Rhoads GG. Smoking and drinking during Pregnancy. The effects on preterm birth. *JAMA* 255:82–84, 1986.
35. US Department of Health, Education and Welfare. *Smoking and Health, A Report of the Surgeon General.* Publication (PHS) 79-50066, 1979.
36. White JR, Froeb HF. Small airways dysfunction in nonsmokers chronically exposed to tobacco smoke. *N Engl J Med* 302:720–723, 1980.
37. Stecenko A, McNicol K, Sauder R. Effect of passive smoking on the lung of young lambs. *Pediatr Res* 20:853–858, 1986.
38. Tager IB, Weiss ST, Rosner B, Speizer FE. Effect of parental cigarette smoking on the pulmonary function of children. *Am J Epidemiol* 110:15–26, 1979.
39. Weiss ST, Tager IB, Schenker M, Speizer FE. The health effects of involuntary smoking. *Am Rev Respir Dis* 128:933–942, 1983.
40. Fergusson DM, Hons BA, Horwood LJ. Parental smoking and respiratory illness during early childhood. *Pediatr Pulmonol* 1:99–106, 1985.
41. Murray AB, Morrison BJ. The effect of cigarette smoke from the mother on bronchial responsiveness and severity of symptoms in children with asthma. *J Allergy Clin Immunol* 77:575–581, 1986.
42. White JR, Froeb JF. Small-airways dysfunction in nonsmokers chronically exposed to tobacco smoke. *N Engl J Med* 302:720–723, 1980.
43. Weitzman M, Gortmaker S, Klein Walker D, Sobol A. Maternal smoking and childhood asthma. *Pediatrics* 85:505–510, 1990.
44. Tager IB, Weiss ST, Munoz A, et al. Longitudinal study of the effects of maternal smoking on pulmonary function in children. *N Engl J Med* 309:699–703, 1983.
45. Pedreira FA, Guandolo VL, Feroli EJ, et al. Involuntary smoking and incidence of respiratory illness during the first year of life. *Pediatrics* 75:594–597, 1985.
46. Ware JH, Dockery DW, Spiro A, et al. Passive smoking, gas cooking and respiratory health of children living in six cities. *Am Rev Respir Dis* 129:366–374, 1984.
47. Nadel JA, Salem H, Tamplin B, Tokiwa Y. Mechanism of bronchoconstriction during inhalation of sulfur dioxide. *J Appl Physiol* 20:164–170, 1965.
48. Wiseman RD, Wiseman JR. Value of home visits in the treatment of the allergic patient. *NY State J Med* 64:1948–1951, 1964.

49. Voorhorst S, Spieksma FThM, Varekamp H, et al. The house-dust mite (*Dermatophagoides pteronyssinus*) and the allergen it produces. Identity with the house-dust allergy. *J Allergy* 39:325–339, 1967.
50. Maunsell K, Wraith DG, Cunnington AM. Mites and house-dust allergy in bronchial asthma. *Lancet* 1:1267–1270, 1968.
51. Al-Doory Y. The indoor airborne fungi. *N Engl Reg Allergy Proc* 6:140–149, 1985.
52. Solomon WR. Fungus aerosols arising from cold-mist vaporizers. *J Allergy Clin Immunol* 54:222–228, 1974.
53. Kozak PP Jr, Gallup J, Cummins LH, Gillman SA. Factors of importance in determining the prevalence of indoor molds (abstr). *J Allergy Clin Immunol* 61:185, 1978.
54. Hirsch DJ, Hirsch SR, Kalbfleisch JH. Effect of central air conditioning and meteorologic factors on indoor spore counts. *J Allergy Clin Immunol* 62:22–26, 1978.
55. Chafee FH. Pollen studies in a hospital air conditioned room *N Engl Reg Allergy Proc* 6:150–157, 1985.
56. Abbott J, Cameron J, Taylor B. House dust mite counts in different types of mattresses, sheepskins and carpets, and a comparison of brushing and vacuuming collection methods. *Clin Allergy* 11:589–595, 1981.
57. Platts-Mills TAE. Dust mite avoidance in the treatment of asthma. *Ann Allergy* 55:419–420, 1985.
58. Zwemer RJ, Karibo J. Use of laminar control device as adjunct to standard environmental control measures in symptomatic asthmatic children. *Ann Allergy* 31:284–290, 1973.
59. Bowler SD, Mitchell CA, Miles J. House dust control and asthma: a placebo-control trial of cleaning air filtration. *Ann Allergy* 55:498–500, 1985.
60. Tovey ER, Chapman MD, Wells CW, Platts-Mills TAE. The distribution of house dust mite allergen in the houses of patients with asthma. *Am Rev Respir Dis* 124:630–635, 1981.
61. Carpenter GB, Win GH, Furumizo RG, et al. Air conditioning and house dust mite (abstr). *J Allergy Clin Immunol* 75(suppl):121, 1985.
62. Arlian LG, Appleton GL, Bernstein IL, Gallagher JS. Effect of home environmental factors on the abundance of house dust mites (abstr). *J Allergy Clin Immunol* 65:211, 1980.
63. Mitchell EB, Wilkins S, McCallum Deighton J, Platts-Mills TAE. House dust mite reduction in the home use of an acaracide (abstr). *J Allergy Clin Immunol* 75(suppl):146, 1985.
64. Korsgaard J. Preventive measures in house dust allergy. *Am Rev Respir Dis* 125:80–84, 1982.
65. Villaveces JW. The dehumidifier: its indoor use in controlling molds and mold asthma—a personal case history. *Ann Allergy* 29:93–98, 1971.
66. Skoogh BE, Simonsson BG, Berggren AG, et al. Climate and environment change in patients with chronic airway obstruction. *Arch Environ Health* 31:15–20, 1976.

67. Sporik R, Holgate S, Platts-Mills T, Cogswell J. Exposure to house-dust mite allergen and the development of asthma in childhood. *N Engl J Med* 323:502–507, 1990.
68. Creticos P. Immunotherapy in asthma. *J Allergy Clin Immunol* 83:554–562, 1989.
69. Bousquet J, Hejjaoui A, Michel F. Specific immunotherapy in asthma. *J Allergy Clin Immunol* 86:292–305, 1990.
70. Norman PS. Immunotherapy. *Prog Allergy* 32:318–346, 1982.
71. Ohman JL. Allergen immunotherapy in asthma: evidence for efficacy. *J Allergy Clin Immunol* 84:133–140, 1989.
72. Zeiger RS, Schatz M. Immunologic approach to the management of asthma. *J Asthma* 20(5):391–409, 1983.
73. Johnstone DE. Study of the role of antigen dosage in the treatment of pollenosis and pollen asthma. *Am J. Dis Child* 94:1–5, 1957.
74. Johnstone DE, Crump L. Value of hyposensitization therapy for perennial bronchial asthma in children. *Pediatrics* 27:39–44, 1961.
75. Johnstone DE, Dutton A. The value of hyposensitization therapy for bronchial asthma in children. A 14-year study. *Pediatrics* 42:793–802, 1968.
76. Aas K. Hyposensitization in house dust allergy asthma. *Acta Paediatr Scand* 60:264–268, 1971.
77. Warner JO, Soothill JF, Price JF, Hey EN. Controlled trial of hyposensitization of *Dermatophagoides pteronyssinus* in children with asthma. *Lancet* 2:912–915, 1978.
78. Price JF, Warner JO, Hey EN, et al. A controlled trial of hyposensitization with tyrosine-absorbed *Dermatophagoides pteronyssinus* antigen in childhood asthma: in vivo aspects. *Clin Allergy* 14:209–219, 1984.
79. Valovirta E, Koivikko A, Vanto T, et al. Immunotherapy in allergy to dog: a double-blind clinical study. *Ann Allergy* 53:85–88, 1984.
80. Dreborg S, Agrell B, Foucard T, et al. A double-blind, multicenter immunotherapy trial in children, using a purified and standardized Cladosporium herbarum preparation: clinical results. *Allergy* 41:131–140, 1986.
81. Karlsson R, Agrell B, Dreborg S, et al. A double-blind, multicenter immunotherapy trial in children, using a purified and standardized *Cladosporium herbarum* preparation: in vitro results. *Allergy* 41:141–150, 1986.
82. Horst M, Hejjaoui A, Horst V, et al. Double-blind, placebo-controlled rush immunotherapy with a standardized *Alternaria* extract. *J Allergy Clin Immunol* 85:460–472, 1990.
83. Licorish K, Novey HS, Kozak P, et al. Role of *Alternaria* and *Pennicillium* spores in the pathogenesis of asthma. *J Allergy Clin Immunol* 76:819–825, 1985.
84. Bruun E. Control examination of the specificity of specific desensitization in asthma. *Acta Allergol* 2:122–128, 1949.
85. Smith, AP. Hyposensitization with *Dermatophagoides pteronyssinus* antigen: trial in asthma induced by house dust. *Br Med J* 4:204–206, 1971.
86. Davies D. A trial of house dust mite extract in bronchial asthma. *Br J. Dis Chest* 73:260–270, 1979.

87. Frankland AW, Augustin R. Prophylaxis of summer hay-fever and asthma. A controlled trial comparing crude grass-pollen extracts with the isolated main protein component. *Lancet* 1055–1057, 1954.
88. Ortolani C, Pastorello E, Moss RB, et al. Grass pollen immunotherapy: a single year double-blind, placebo-controlled study in patients with grass pollen-induced asthma and rhinitis. *J Allergy Clin Immunol* 73:283–290, 1984.
89. Taylor WW, Ohman JL. Lower FC. Immunotherapy in cat-induced asthma. Double-blind trial with evaluation of bronchial responses to cat allergen and histamine. *J Allergy Clin Immunol* 61:283–287, 1978.
90. Ohman JL, Findlay SR, Leiterman SB. Immunotherapy in cat-induced asthma. Double-blind evaluation of in vivo and in vitro responses. *J Allergy Clin Immunol* 74:230–239, 1984.
91. Metzger WJ, Donnelly A, Richerson HB. Modification of late asthmatic responses (LAR) during immunotherapy for alternaria-induced asthma. *J Allergy Clin Immunol* 71:119, 1983.
92. Lichtenstein LM, Ishizaka K, Norman PS, et al. IgE antibody measurements in ragweed hay fever. Relationship to clinical severity and the results of immunotherapy. *J Clin Invest* 52:472–482, 1973.
93. Foucard T, Johansson SGO. Allergen-specific IgE and IgG antibodies in pollen-allergic children given immunotherapy for 2–6 years. *Clin Allergy* 8:249–257, 1979.
94. Berg T, Johansson SGO. In vitro diagnosis of atopic allergy IV: seasonal variations of IgE antibodies in children allergic to pollens. *Int Arch Allergy* 41:452–462, 1971.
95. Levy DA, Osler AG. Studies on the mechanism of hypersensitivity phenomena: XVI. In vitro assays of reaginic activity in human sera: effect of therapeutic immunization on seasonal titer changes. *J Immunol* 99:1068–1077, 1967.
96. Lichtenstein LM, Norman PS, Winkenwerder WL. A single year of immunotherapy for ragweed hay fever. *Ann Int Med* 75:663–671, 1971.
97. Platts-Mills TAE, von Maur RK, Ishizaka K, et al. IgA and IgG anti-ragweed antibodies in nasal secretions. Quantitative measurements of antibodies and correlation with inhibition of histamine release. *J Clin Invest* 57:1041–1050, 1976.
98. Adler TR, Beall GN, Heiner DC, et al. Immunologic and clinical correlates of bronchial challenge responses to Bermuda grass pollen extracts. *J Allergy Clin Immunol* 75:31–36, 1985.
99. Pruzansky JJ, Patterson R. Histamine release from leukocytes of hypersensitive individuals. II. Reduced sensitivity of leukocytes after injection therapy. *J Allergy* 39:44–50, 1967.
100. Rocklin RE, Sheffer AL, Greineder DK, Melmon KL. Generation of antigen-specific suppressor cells during allergy desensitization. *N Engl J Med* 302:1213–1219, 1980.
101. Hsieh KH. Altered interleukin-2 (IL-2) production and responsiveness after hyposensitization to house dust. *J Allergy Clin Immunol* 76:188–194, 1985.

102. Tuchinda M, Chai H. Effect of immunotherapy in chronic asthmatic children. *J Allergy Clin Immunol* 51:131–138, 1973.
103. Rocklin RE. Clinical and immunologic aspects of allergen-specific immunotherapy in patients with seasonal allergic rhinitis and/or allergic asthma. *J Allergy Clin Immunol* 72:323–334, 1983.
104. Lichtenstein LM, Valentine MD, Norman PS. A re-evaluation of immunotherapy for asthma. *Am Rev Respir Dis* 129:659–659, 1984.
105. Osterballe O. Immunotherapy with grass pollen major allergens. Clinical results from a prospective 3-year double-blind study. *Allergy* 37:379–388, 1982.
106. Osterballe O, Lowenstein H, Norn S, et al. Immunotherapy with grass pollen major allergens. Immunological results from a prospective 3-year double-blind study. *Allergy* 37:491–501, 1982.
107. Grammer LC, Shaughnessy MA, Patterson R. Modified forms of allergen immunotherapy. *J Allergy Clin Immunol* 76:397–401, 1985.
108. Marsh DG, Lichtenstein LM, Campbell DH. Studies of allergoids prepared from naturally occurring allergens. Assay of allergenicity and antigenicity of formalinized rye group I component. *Immunology* 18:705–722, 1970.
109. Norman PS, Lichtenstein LM, Kagey-Sobotka A, Marsh DG. Controlled evaluation of allergoid in the immunotherapy of ragweed hay fever. *J Allergy Clin Immunol* 70:248–260, 1982.
110. Metzger WJ, Dorminey HC, Richerson HB, et al. Clinical and immunologic evaluation of glutaraldehyde-modified tyrosine-absorbed short ragweed extract: a double-blind placebo-controlled trial. *J Allergy Clin Immunol* 68:442–448, 1981.
111. Hendrix SG, Patterson R, Zeiss CR, et al. A multi-institutional trial of polymerized whole ragweed for immunotherapy of ragweed allergy. *J Allergy Clin Immunol* 66:486–494, 1980.
112. Grammer LC, Shaughnessy MA, Suszko IM, Patterson R. A double-blind histamine placebo controlled trial of polymerized whole grass for immunotherapy of grass allergy. *J Allergy Clin Immunol* 72:448–452, 1983.
113. Orenstein DM, Reed, ME, Gorgan FT, Crawford LV. Exercise conditioning in children with asthma. *J Pediatr* 106:556–560, 1985.
114. Strunk RC, Rubin D, Kelly L et al. Determination of fitness in children with asthma: use of standardized tests for functional endurance, body fat composition, flexibility and abnormal strength. *Am J Dis Child* 142:940–944, 1988.
115. Millman M, Grundon WG, Kasch F, et al. Controlled exercise in asthmatic children. *Ann Allergy* 23:220–225, 1965.
116. Petersen KH, McElhenney TR. Effects of a physical fitness program upon asthmatic boys. *Pediatrics* 35:295–299, 1965.
117. Itkin IH, Nacman M. The effect of exercise on the hospitalized asthmatic patient. *J Allergy* 37:253–263, 1966.
118. Hyde JS, Swarts CL. Effect of an exercise program on the perennially asthmatic child. *Am J Dis Child* 116:383–396, 1968.

119. Sly RM, Harper RT, Rosselot I. The effect of physical conditioning upon asthmatic children. *Ann Allergy* 30:86–94, 1972.
120. Nickerson BG, Bautista DB, Namey MA, et al. Distance running improves fitness in asthmatic children without pulmonary complications or changes in exercise-induced bronchospasm. *Pediatrics* 71:147–152, 1983.
121. Oseid S, Haaland K. Exercise studies on asthmatic children before and after regular physical training. In Eriksson B, Furberg B (eds.), Baltimore, 1978, *Swimming Medicine IV*. University Park Press, pp. 32–41.
122. Bundgaard A, Ingemann-Hansen T, Schmidt A, Kristensen J. Effect of physical training on peak oxygen consumption rate and exercise-induced asthma in adult asthmatics. *Scand J Clin Lab Invest* 42:9–13, 1982.
123. Fitch KD. Sport, physical activity and the asthmatic. In: Oseid S, Edwards AM (eds.), *The Asthmatic Child in Play and Sport*. Pitman Press, London, 1983, pp. 254–255.
124. Fitch KD, Morton AR, Blanksby BA. Effects of swimming training on children with asthma. *Arch Dis Child* 51:190–194, 1976.
125. Morton AR, Fitch KD, Han AG. Physical activity and the asthmatic. *Physician Sportsmed* 9:51, 1981.
126. Strunk RC, Mascia AV, Lipkowitz MA, Wolf SI. Rehabilitation of a patient with asthma in the outpatient setting. *J Allergy Clin Immunol* 87:601–611, 1991.
127. Fitch KD. Comparative aspects of available exercise systems. *Pediatrics* 56:904–907, 1975.
128. Inbar O, Dotan R, Dlin RA, et al. Breathing dry or humid air and exercise-induced asthma during swimming. *Eur J Appl Physiol* 44:43–50, 1980.
129. American Academy of Pediatrics Committee on Children with Handicaps. The asthmatic child and his participation in sports and physical education. *Pediatrics* 45:150–151, 1970.
130. Godfrey S. Clinical variables of exercise-induced bronchospasm. In: Dempsey JA, Reed CE (eds.), *Muscular Exercise and the Lung*. University of Wisconsin Press, Madison, 1977, pp. 247–263.
131. Lindsay D. The benefits of warm-up for asthmatic children. In: Oseid S, Edwards AM (eds.), *The Asthmatic Child in Play and Sport*. Pitman Press, London, 1983, pp. 305–311.
132. McFadden ER, Lenner KAM, Strohl KP. Post exertional airway rewarming and thermally induced asthma: new insights into pathophysiology and possible pathogenesis. *J Clin Invest* 78:18–25, 1986.
132. Dorinson SM. Breathing exercises for bronchial asthma and pulmonary emphysema. *JAMA* 156:931–933, 1954.
134. Scherr MS, Frankel L. Physical conditioning program for asthmatic children. *JAMA* 168:1996–2000, 1958.
135. Hyde JS, Swarts CL. Effect of an exercise program on the perennially asthmatic child. *Am J Dis Child* 116:383, 1968.
136. McNeill RS, McKenzie JM. An assessment of the value of breathing exercises in chronic bronchitis and asthma. *Thorax* 10:250–252, 1955.

137. Herxheimer H. *A Guide to Bronchial Asthma*. Academic Press, London, 1975, p. 86.
138. Haas A, Castillo R, Lustig F. The application of rehabilitation medicine to bronchial asthma. In: Weiss EB, Segal MS (eds.), *Bronchial Asthma—Mechanisms and Therapeutics*, Little, Brown and Company, Boston, 1976, pp. 1081–1106.
139. Levy SE. Respiratory therapy modalities in asthma. In Weiss EB, Segal MS, Stein M. (eds.), *Bronchial Asthma—Mechanisms and Therapeutics*. Little, Brown and Company, Boston, 1985, pp. 910–911.

# 18

## Indoor Allergens and Asthma

**RICHARD SPORIK and PETER W. HEYMANN**

*University of Virginia Health Sciences Center*
*Charlottesville, Virginia*

**ENRIQUE FERNANDEZ-CALDAS**

*University of South Florida College of Medicine*
*Tampa, Florida*

**THOMAS A. E. PLATTS-MILLS**

*University of Virginia Health Sciences Center*
*Charlottesville, Virginia*

## INTRODUCTION

The association between hypersensitivity to inhalant allergens and asthma in children has long been recognized. Increasing evidence about the nature of allergen exposure and the immune (or inflammatory) response of the lung has recently supported the view that there is a direct causal link between exposure to these allergens and asthma. The idea that inhalants cause asthma is not new (1), however it has been increasingly appreciated that this response is limited to those children who develop an IgE antibody response; the nature of the response and the levels of exposure can now be accurately measured, and there is extensive evidence that the problem is very large. The strong association of hypersensitivity to allergens and asthma has been shown in case–control studies, cross-sectional studies of school children and prospective studies (2–13). This association does not become clear in children until after the age of 3, suggesting that other factors are of greater importance in the precipitation of wheeze in infancy and early childhood (13–15). In some areas of the world house-dust mites of the genus *Dermatophagoides* are completely dominant, with up to 85% of asthmatic children having positive skin tests to mite allergens (16). In other areas cat, dog, or cockroach allergens are also important (13,17). The importance of allergens other than the house-dust mite is underscored by the presence of asthma, albeit at a reduced prevalence, in many areas where mites will hardly grow at all, and by epidemics of asthma related to grass pollen in Northern California, to the fungus *Alternaria alternata* in the American Midwest and to cockroach in inner city patients (18–20). However, as our understanding of allergens improves and better surveys are undertaken it becomes increasingly obvious that exposure to allergens plays a very important role in childhood asthma.

Asthma among children is common and appears to be getting more common. More school children are being treated chronically for asthma in the United States than for any other chronic illness. Given the dominant association between house-dust mite sensitivity and asthma in Northern Europe, the Gulf coast and Pacific Northwest of America, New Zealand, coastal Australia, and Japan it seems difficult to believe that the reported increases in the prevalence and morbidity are unrelated to an allergic mechanism. A possible explanation is that childhood exposure to allergens has increased. It is probable that increasing warmth and humidity in our homes have significantly improved the conditions for mite growth. Children are also spending increasing amounts of time indoors, lured by the dubious attractions of television, and parental concern over their safety. Another explanation is that the increase may be related to overreliance on bronchodilators, which has lead to increasing severity of asthma (21). However the observations about bronchodilators also have several possible explanations. Bronchodilation could have harmful effects because it allows patients to inhale larger quantities of allergen and that increased bronchial reactivity is a consequence of this increased exposure. The bronchodilators themselves may also have a direct effect on the lung that increases bronchial hyperreactivity. However it is clear that this effect can only appear in children who are treated with bronchodilators, that is, those in whom some primary cause of asthma has already induced symptoms.

The importance of diagnosing allergen sensitization in children depends on the effectiveness of allergen specific therapy. Indeed many primary care physicians do not request skin testing on asthmatic children because they are not convinced of the benefits of immunotherapy. Identifying allergen sensitization has three roles, the first is education; parents and children need to understand the difference between bronchospasm and the underlying bronchial hyperreactivity. They need to understand the factors that can influence this and the purpose of different forms of treatment. The second objective of allergen-specific diagnosis is to design avoidance therapy. It is important to stress that the primary anti-inflammatory treatment for asthma is allergen avoidance. Dramatic improvements in symptoms and bronchial reactivity have been produced in almost all studies that have reduced exposure. A distant third comes allergen-specific immunotherapy. Although allergen immunotherapy can be effective in patients with asthma, it clearly is not without risk and this risk may well be greatest among the brittle asthmatics who tend to be put on treatment because other measures are not working. Finally, the ability to measure allergen exposure in houses has greatly increased our understanding of allergic asthma. Monoclonal antibody assays have been developed to measure house-dust mite allergens by four different laboratories and the results are all standardized relative to the World Health Organization (WHO) international standard (22). These assays have made it possible to propose threshold levels for exposure. The main role of defining thresholds is educational. That is, these are levels of exposure above which there is a definite increase in the risk of developing asthma and they represent target levels for reducing exposure. It is also possible to measure cat, dog, and cockroach allergens and these assays are being used, in a similar manner, to define threshold levels and to design effective techniques for reducing exposure (23–25).

## EVIDENCE FOR A CAUSAL RELATIONSHIP

Although many different allergens are associated with asthma, the major epidemiological studies have related to the house-dust mite allergens. A number of studies have shown a direct link between the quantity of house-dust mite allergen exposure and both sensitization and asthma (Fig. 1). It is very difficult to prove a causal relationship for an exposure that is as common and continuous as house-dust mite. However, the evidence from a wide range of studies can now be considered to have fulfilled all of the

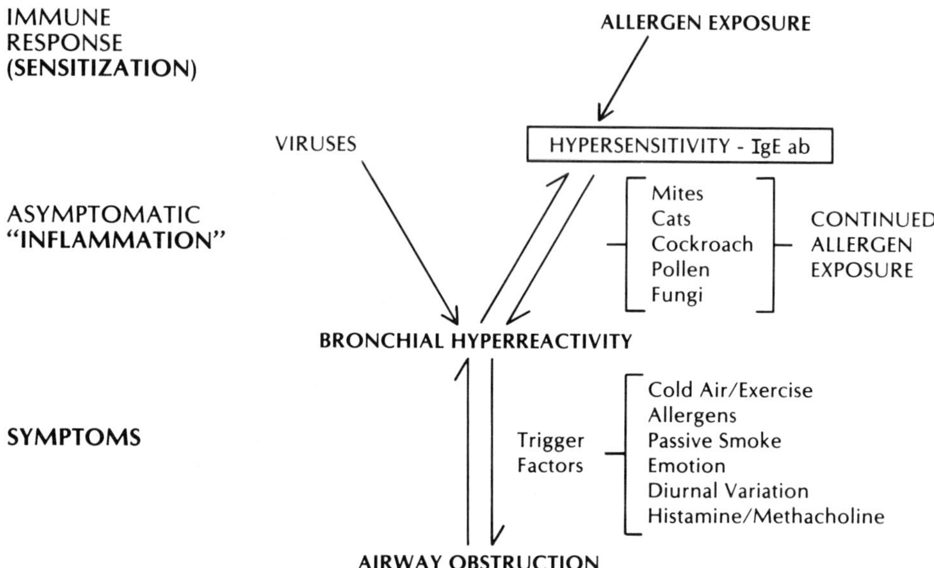


FIGURE 1 Model for the role of allergens in childhood asthma.

criteria proposed by Hill to differentiate between association and causation. These are that 1) the strength of association is large; 2) repeated observations in different populations, under different conditions have consistent findings; 3) a cause leads to a specific effect; 4) the cause precedes the effect in time; 5) there is experimental evidence; 6) there is a dose–response gradient; 7) there are analogous explanations; 8) the mechanism is biologically plausible (26).

Sensitization to an allergen is dependent on exposure to that particular allergen and an innate ability to react to allergens in general. This explains why many individuals may be exposed to high levels of allergen and do not become sensitized, in much the same way that not all children suffer from hay fever despite being exposed to approximately the same levels of allergen. Sensitization appears to be dose dependent (3,11,12,27,28) and there is a suggestion that allergen exposure in infancy enhances subsequent sensitization (29,30). Indeed, when areas within countries with different mite exposures are compared (e.g., inland to coastal Australia, high-altitude to coastal France, northern to southern Sweden, inland northern California and Virginia), the prevalence of sensitization increases with increasing exposure (11,31) (Fig. 2).

In areas of high mite exposure it has been repeatedly demonstrated that most children with asthma have positive skin tests and serum IgE antibodies to dust mites (2,4,10,31). In these areas the association of positive skin

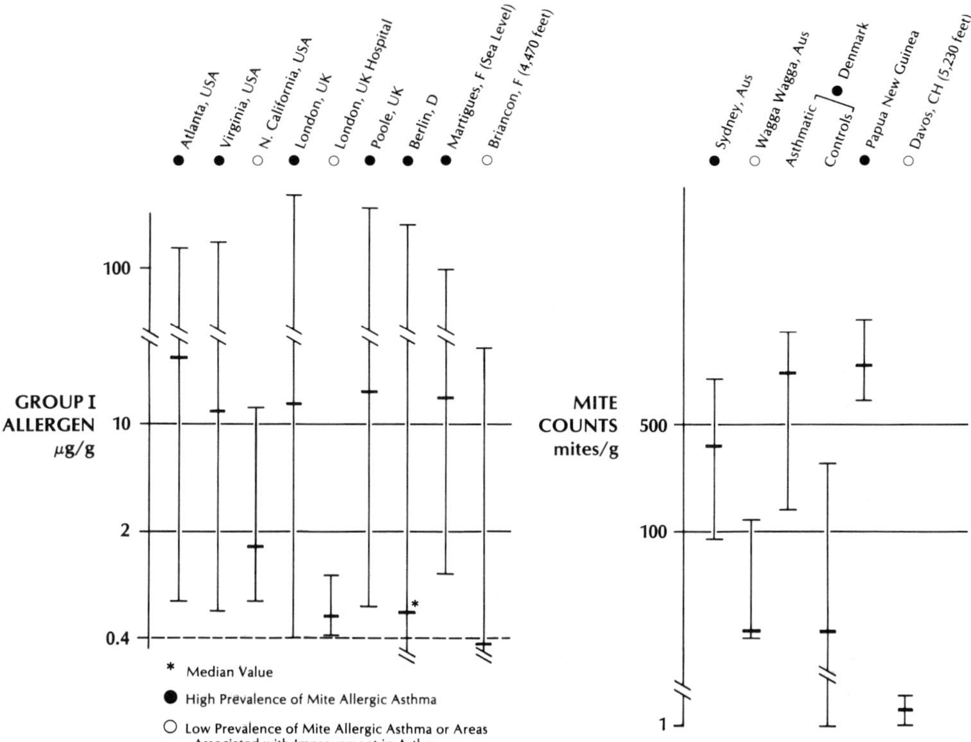


FIGURE 2 House-dust mite allergen levels and house-dust mite numbers (mean and range). Group I allergen levels above 2 μg/g dust (~100 mites/g) have been proposed as a level above which there is a risk for the development of IgE antibody and persistent bronchial reactivity; above 10 μg/g (~500) represents a risk for acute asthma and a level at which most mite allergic patients will experience symptoms. The limit of detection of the assay is ~0.4 μg/g.

tests and asthma is strongest in children, with up to 85% showing evidence of sensitization. In a prospective study of children at risk of developing immediate hypersensitivity, 94% of the asthmatic children were mite sensitized and those children who were mite sensitized had a 19-fold increased risk of developing asthma (12). In a study of children attending the Emergency Room in Florida with exacerbations of asthma, 90% were sensitized to mite compared to 36% of a control population (6). In a similar study from England more than 80% of the children were mite sensitized (this increased to 91% if children under 3 years were excluded) and 60% were both sensitized and exposed to high levels of house-dust mite (33). An additional finding was that the risk of readmission was significantly higher in those children who continued to be exposed to high levels of mite allergens. In studies of Brazilian children, 60% of asthmatic children are house-dust mite sensitized, and it has recently been demonstrated that the children with positive skin tests were exposed to high concentrations of house-dust mite allergen (9). In areas of low mite exposure, the level of sensitization is correspondingly lower and other allergens appear to be of more importance (13,18,19). Observations of low levels of mite sensitization have been reported in natives from several dry areas: northern Sweden; Saskatoon, Canada; Briançon (altitude 4470 feet), France; and Los Alamos (alt. 7200 feet), New Mexico. There is also some evidence to suggest that the prevalence of asthma in some of these areas is reduced (11).

Allergens derived from the house-dust mite have only been proposed to have one specific effect on the lung: to induce asthma. Furthermore it appears to be harmless for a nonsensitized person to inhale even large quantities of this allergen. It should also be noted that in all studies there is a minority of children who have evidence of sensitivity to mites who are nevertheless without symptoms.

Temporal evidence that acute exposure to mites results in symptoms in sensitized individuals comes from areas with seasonal fluctuations in mite populations. In a study from Virginia, an increase in symptoms was found to follow an increase in mite allergen levels in sensitized subjects (34). Studies from Papua New Guinea, where good conditions for mite growth were inadvertently introduced, reported a subsequent increase in the prevalence of asthma, a previously rare condition (35). In the majority of children measurable sensitization to aeroallergens does not occur until after 3 years of age. There is some animal evidence that localized sensitization of the lung can occur, prior to systemic evidence, and this may happen in younger children (36). Wheezing episodes that occur in children of this age are more likely to be caused by factors such as viral infections than allergic mechanisms (14,37–39). However, in long-term follow-up studies only the children who develop sensitization continue to wheeze (13,15).

Experimental evidence of the induction of symptoms by exposure to mite allergens comes from bronchial provocation studies in which both early and late reactions can be induced following inhalation of mite allergens, albeit in large quantities (40–44). On a population basis, pollen asthma, although well recognized, is not a major problem. However, it affords a useful model of asthma following the inhalation of allergen in a sensitized person. Pollen inhalation causes not only acute bronchospasm but also long-term increases of bronchial reactivity in sensitized individuals (52). This provides a direct analogy for what happens following inhalation of mite allergen in a sensitive person. It has been clearly shown that experimental allergen exposure can produce the inflammatory changes in the lung that are now considered to be the underlying cause of bronchial hyperreactivity (45,46). Evidence that mite avoidance results in an improvement in the symptoms of asthma comes from a number of studies. A traditional treatment for asthma has been the removal of individuals to high altitudes. Studies of children in these environments show that bronchial reactivity of the mite-allergic patients is, at least, a partially reversible phenomenon and that reductions in bronchial reactivity take 6 weeks or more (47). Similar findings have been duplicated in young adults in the "allergen-free" environment of a hospital (48) and it has been suggested that admission to this environment is one of the main benefits of hospital admission for patients with asthma. Reported studies on the use of avoidance measures in the home have produced conflicting results, although in some studies it was thought that the measures recommended were not "aggressive" enough and in fact did not cause a measurable fall in allergen exposure. Reductions in bronchial reactivity occur only under conditions that include very extensive avoidance regimens. However, a Canadian study provided clear evidence that mite avoidance measures in the child's bedroom were not only practical but also effective at reducing bronchial hyperreactivity and medication usage (49). It is interesting to compare the effects of pharmacologic treatment on bronchial hyperreactivity with those obtained from allergen avoidance. The effect of beta-agonists on bronchial hyperreactivity is lost within hours. The effects of inhaled steroids likewise appear to be largely reversed within 6 weeks (50,51). The implication is that all pharmacologic approaches are only suppressing the inflammation. Thus allergen avoidance could be considered the best approach to maintaining decreases in bronchial hyperreactivity for long periods of time.

It is relatively easy to propose a credible mechanism by which allergen inhalation could cause an increase in bronchial reactivity (invoking surface IgE on mast cells, mediator release, cell migration, and subsequent bronchoconstriction), with allergen stimulation being the driving force behind the "inflammatory" changes of asthma (45,46). There is also some evidence to suggest that following sufficient inflammation of this kind, structural changes occur that in some cases result in irreversible increases in airway reactivity so that asthma becomes, at least in part, independent of further allergen exposure.

## INDOOR ALLERGENS

### House-Dust Mites

These are sightless, photophobic, eight-legged arthropods roughly a third of a millimeter long and are members of the order Acaridae (53). They are close relatives of storage mites, ticks, chiggers, and distant relatives of spiders and scorpions. The principal mite species are the pyroglyphid mites *D. pteronyssinus*, *D. farinae*, *D. microceras*, and *Euroglyphus maynei*, which usually account for more than 90% of the mite species in house dust from temperate regions. The presence of house-dust mites has been confirmed on a worldwide basis, with studies from Europe, the Far East, Southeast Asia, Australia, and North and South America. Each species has found an ecologic niche. *D. pteronyssinus* is more susceptible to dessication but is usually the dominant mite in constantly damp climates, such as Northern Europe, Brazil, and the Pacific Northwest. In very humid areas *Euroglyphus maynei* is also of importance. *D. farinae* is the most prominent house-dust mite in areas of North America where there is a

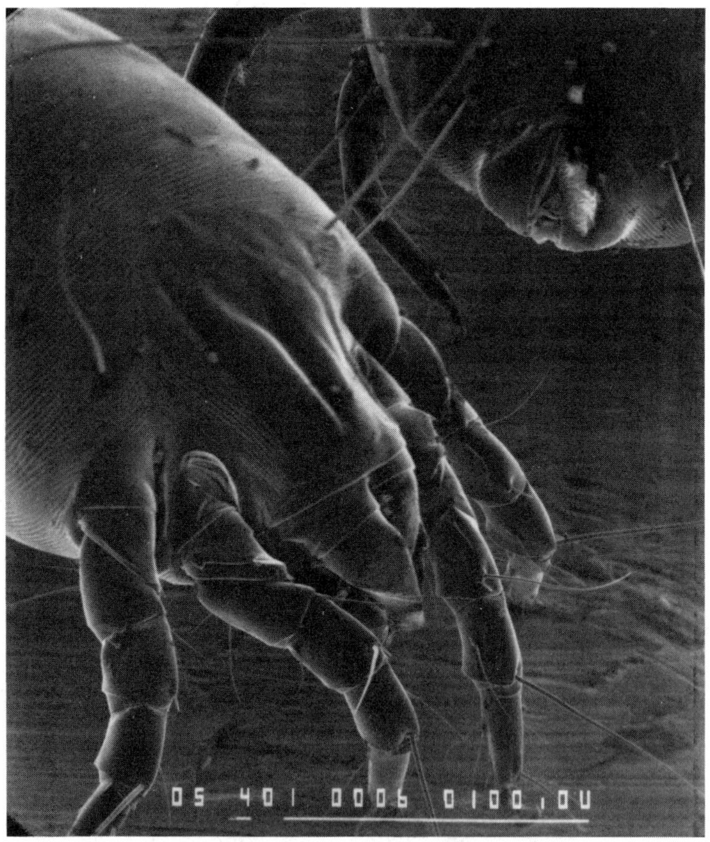


Two *Dermatophagoides pteronyssinus*, front and rear. 400×.

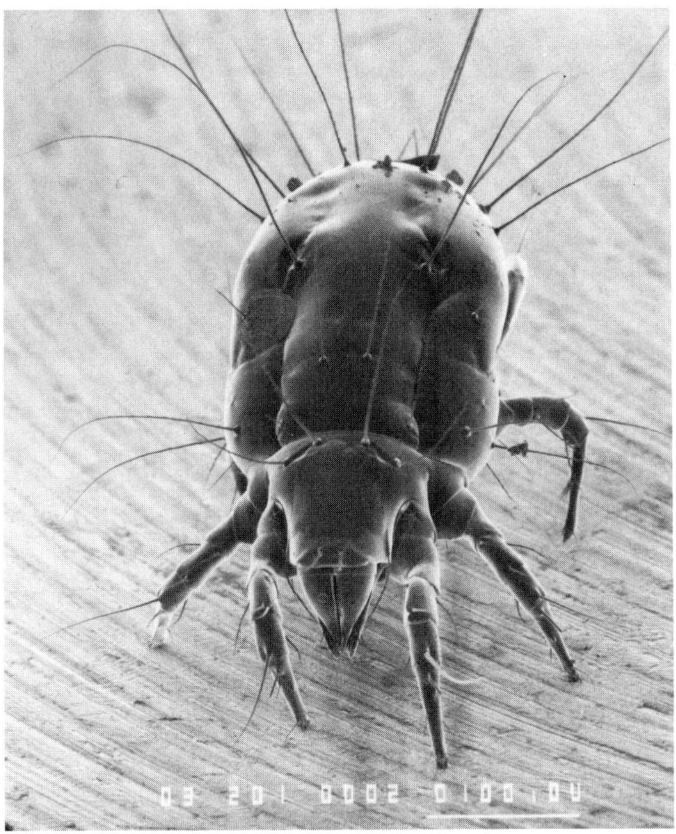

*Tyrophagus putrescientae*. 200×.

prolonged dry winter. *Blomia tropicalis* is found in houses in tropical and subtropical areas such as Brazil and Florida (9).

The main determinants of mite growth are temperature and humidity (54). Optimal conditions for mite growth are a temperature between 70 and 80°F and an absolute humidity > 8 g/kg (which corresponds to a relative humidity of approximately 70%). Humidity is probably the most important determinant of mite numbers, since they have a very limited ability to search for or consume water. In the northcentral United States the humidity is often below this level. In the south east, or Gulf coast, mean outdoor absolute humidity is often as high as 13 g/kg in the summer. Under those conditions humidity can only be controlled by air conditioning. In areas with a suboptimal climate for growth, mite numbers follow the seasonal

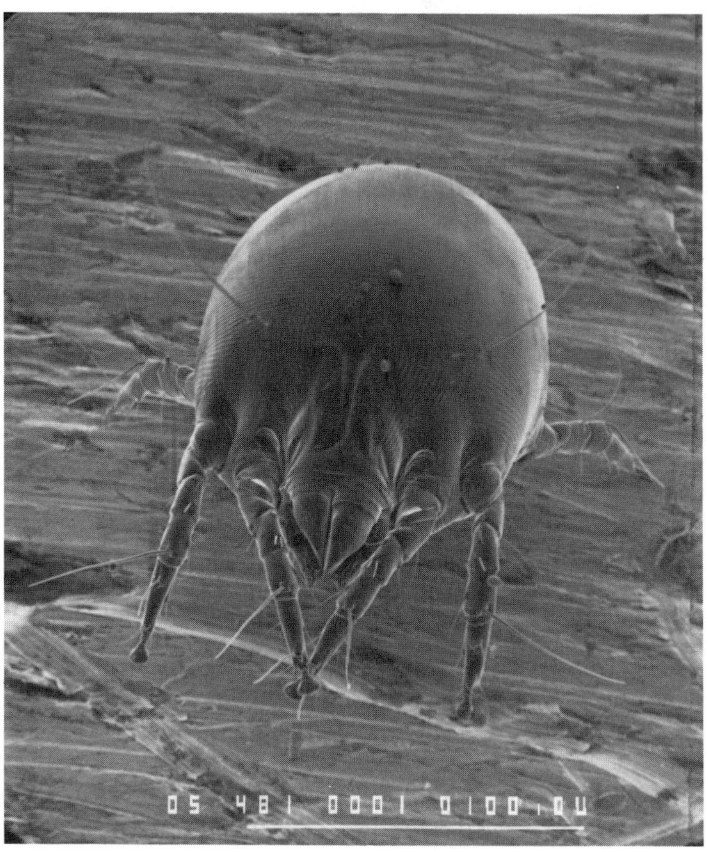

*Dermatophagoides pteronyssinus* larva. 480×.

variations in humidity and temperature, giving rise to a "mite season" in the late summer and fall. Humidity falls progressively with altitude and above 6,000 feet the air is generally too dry for mite growth. In Europe indoor humidity tends to be higher than that outdoors, especially when ventilation is poor. This is because considerable moisture is released by breathing, sweating, cooking, and washing. The humidity of the "micro" environment in which the mites live is determined not only by the ambient humidity but also by local factors. Mites tend to bury themselves deep in carpets, mattresses, and soft furnishings. Sofas and mattresses, because of their depth of padding, take much longer to dry out and remain a good environment for mite growth. In many studies, mattresses have the highest

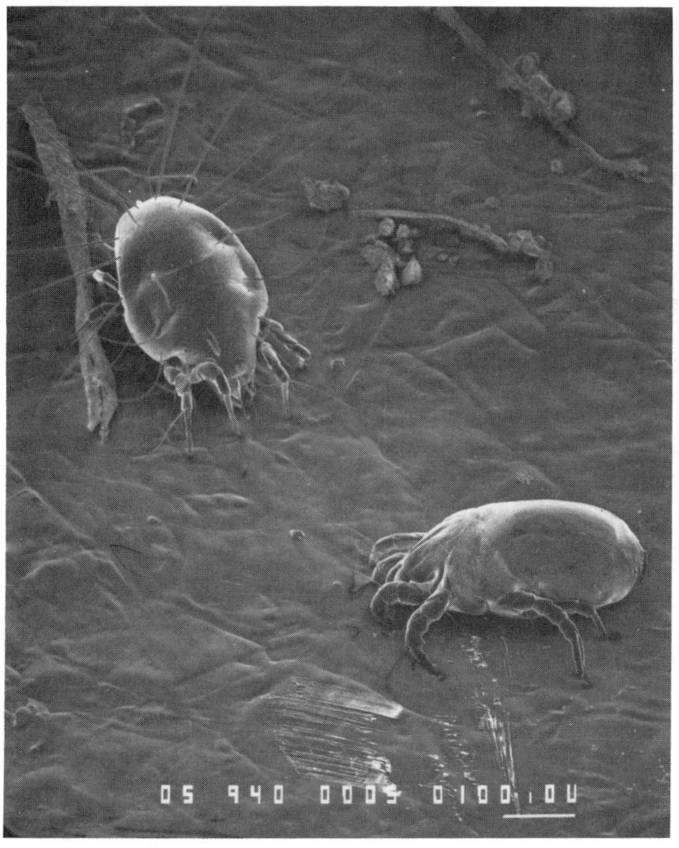

*Blomia tropicalis* (top) and *Dermatophagoides pteronyssinus* (bottom). 94×.

mite levels in the house, which probably reflects the combination of perspiration (up to 1½ pints each night) and continuous warmth in beds.

The first allergen purified from *Dermatophagoides pteronyssinus* was Der p I (previously antigen pI) (Table 1) (55). There are probably more than 20 allergens produced by mites; however, the two main groups, group I and group II, account for most of its allergenicity (56,57). There is very high cross-reactivity between allergens of the same group derived from different species. The group I (molecular weight [mw] 24,000 daltons) allergens are heat and pH sensitive proteins occurring in very high concentration in mite feces (~0.2 ng/particle; ~10 mg/ml) and they elute from feces very rapidly (i.e., 90% within 2 min) (58). Both common and species-specific epitopes have been identified on Der p I, Der f I, and Der m I.

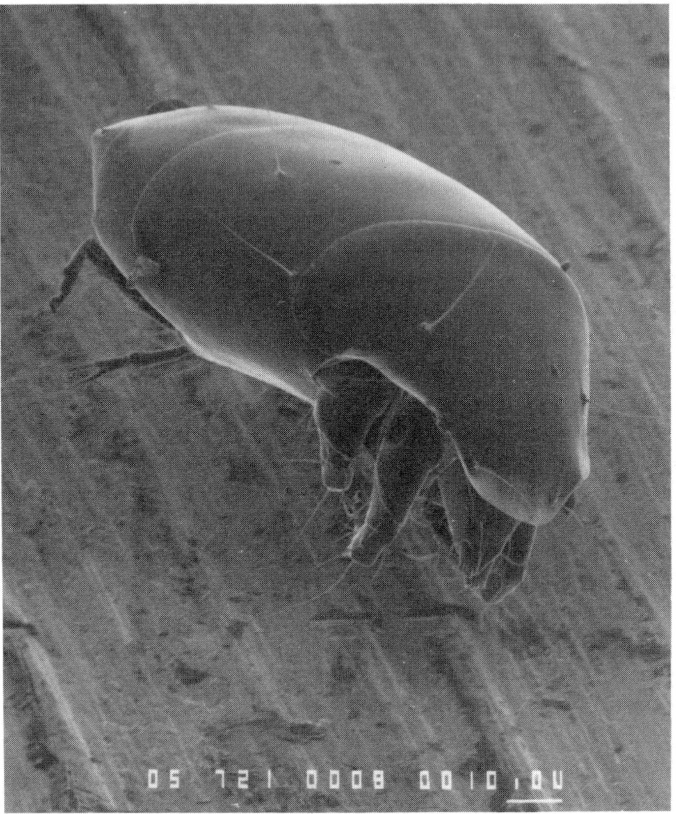

*Tarsonemus* spp. 720×.

They are proteolytic enzymes secreted in the mite digestive tract and show protein sequence homology to thiol proteases (e.g., papain). Since mites are probably coprophagic (i.e., they reingest fecal pellets), it is possible that the presence of these enzymes allows a more extensive digestion to occur ex vivo (personal communication, TG Merrett). The group II (mw 14,000) allergens are derived from both mite bodies and feces. They are heat and pH resistant and, in a surprising finding, show no sequence homology with other known proteins. Der f I and Der f II, and Der p I and Der p II have recently been sequenced and cloned (59,60). The group III allergens (mw of 29,000) have been partially sequenced and show sequence homology with serine proteases such as trypsin and chymotrypsin. The relative importance of group I and group II allergens is supported by measurements of these allergens in house dust; by contrast, very little group

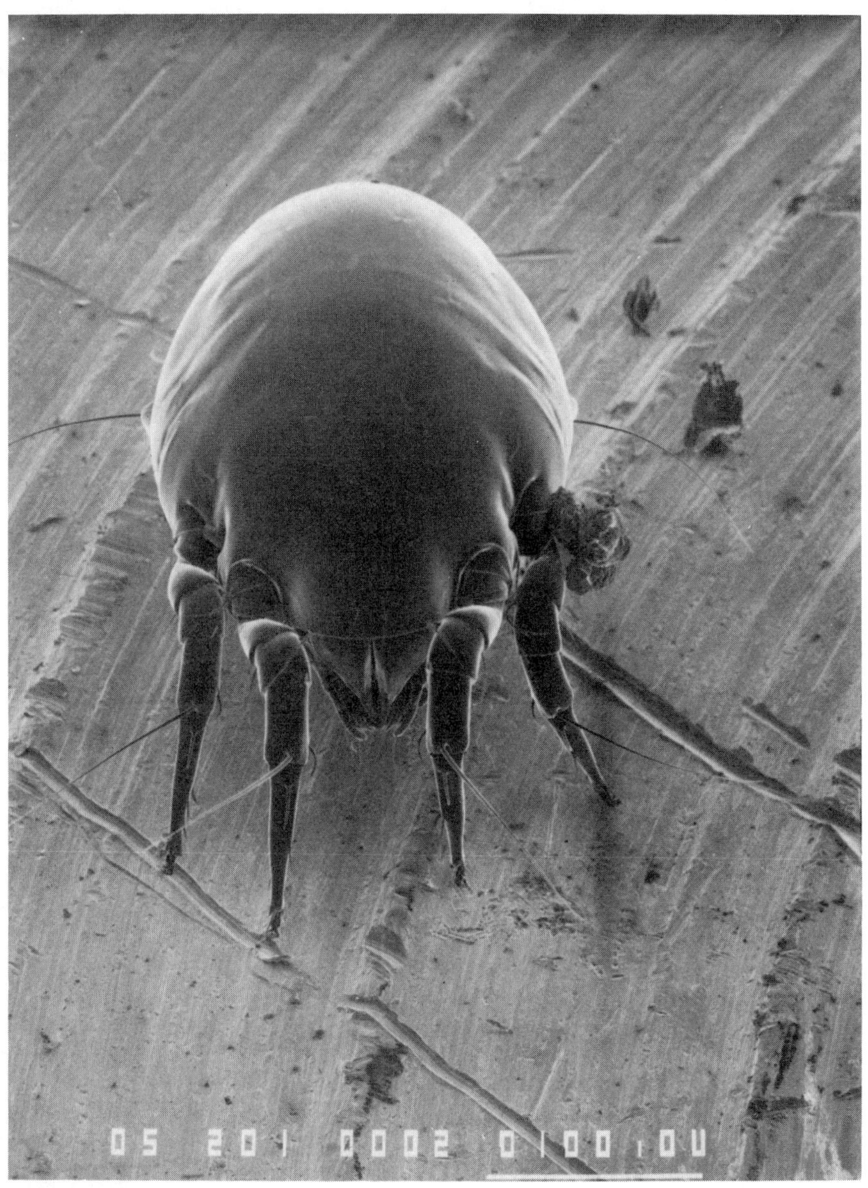


*Chortoglyphus arcuatus*. 200×.

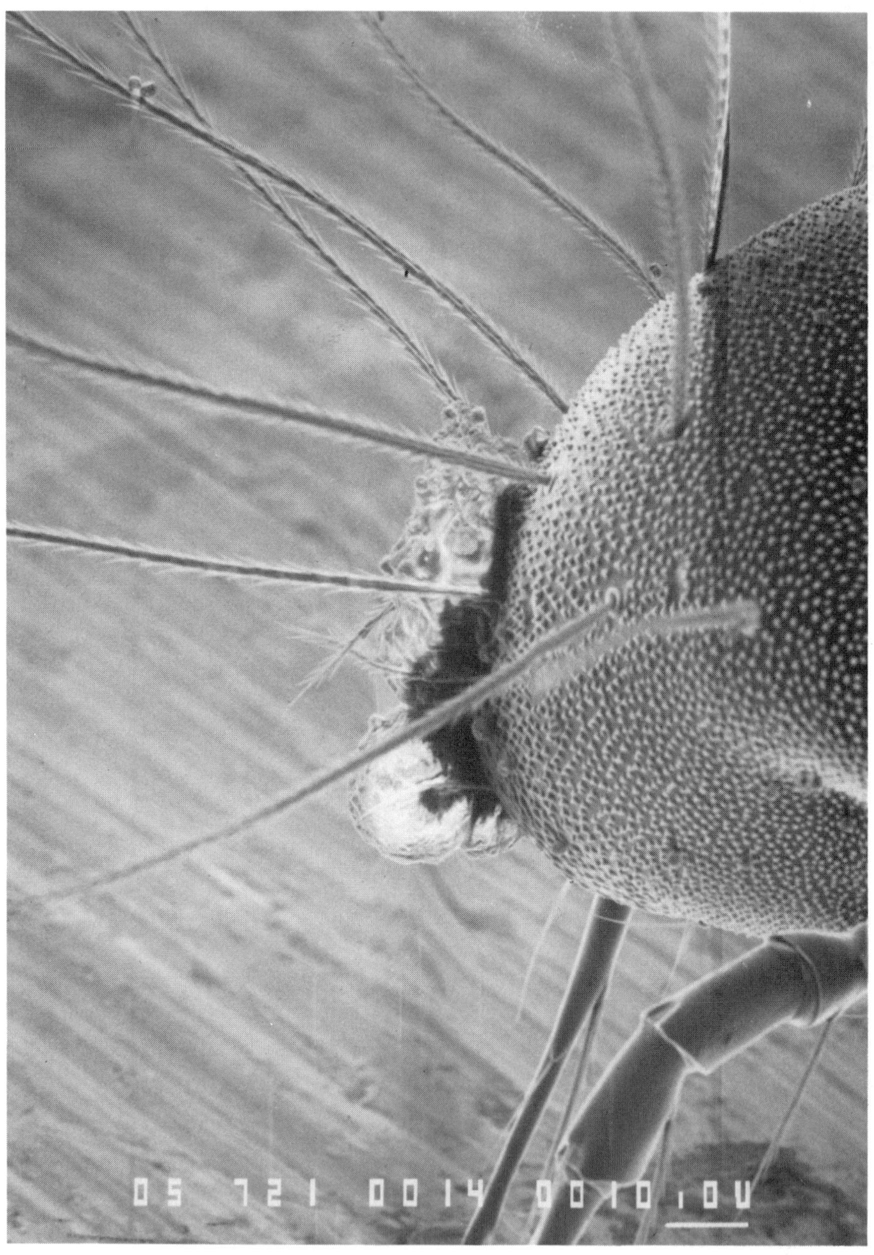


Rear end, *Blomia tropicalis* with fecal pellet. 720×

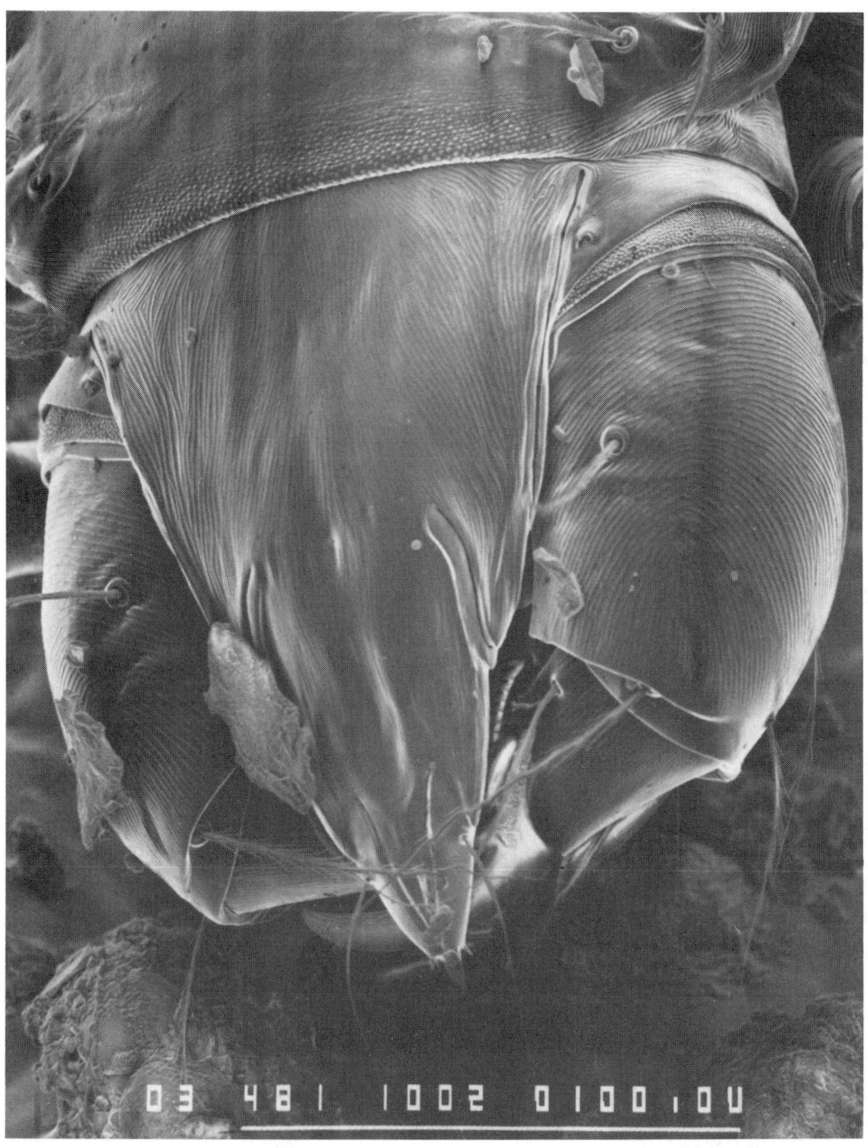


*Cheyletus malaccensis*. 480×.

TABLE 1 Defined Indoor Allergens

| Source | Allergen | Monoclonal assay available |
|---|---|---|
| House-dust mite | | |
| *Dermatophagoides pteronyssinus* | Der p I (55) | Yes |
| | Der p II (56) | [a] |
| *Dermatophagoides farinae* | Der f I (57) | Yes |
| | Der f II (56) | [a] |
| Cockroach | | |
| *Blattella germanica* | Bla g I (25) | Yes |
| | Bla g II (25) | Yes |
| *Periplaneta americana* | Per a I (75) | [a] |
| Cat | | |
| *Felis domesticus* | Fel d I (77) | Yes |
| Dog | | |
| *Canis familiaris* | Can f I (24, 97) | [a] |
| Mouse | | |
| *Mus musculus* | Mus m I (102) | [a] |
| Fungus | | |
| *Aspergillus fumigatus* | Asp f I (104) | [a] |

[a]Assay developed, but use limited to research laboratories.
WHO allergen nomenclature is used: genus, species initial, purification order.

III allergen ($\leq$0.5 μg/g) has been found in dust. It has been proposed that exposure to >2 μg Der p I/g of sieved house dust is a risk factor for the development of mite sensitization and asthma, and >10 μg Der p I/gm for the development of acute exacerbations of wheeze (16). These proposed threshold values are based on prevalence studies and the exposure and sensitization of adults and children visiting emergency rooms for exacerbations of asthma.

### Cockroach

Sensitization to allergen derived from cockroach is being described with increasing frequency in asthmatic children. In some locations and among some ethnic groups, sensitization to cockroach allergen may even be more common than for the house-dust mite. There certainly appears to be an excess of sensitization to this allergen among asthmatic patients in urban areas in the United States (e.g., New York, Washington D.C., Chicago, Detroit, Atlanta, and Boston) and African-American uninsured inhabitants, a group with a rapidly increasing prevalence and morbidity from asthma (17,20,62–66), appear to be at exceptional risk. Indeed, a recent study of patients attending the emergency room for treatment of asthma in Delaware showed that 28% of blacks studied were cockroach sensitive compared with only 4% of whites (67). In contrast to sensitization to house-dust mites, which may have increased with increasing affluence (e.g., as a result of wall-to-wall carpets, better heating, and "tighter" houses), cockroach sensitization is associated with poverty. Sensitization to cockroach has also been described in a variety of studies: among laboratory workers who handled cockroaches and also in case studies from many parts of the world, especially in the tropics (68–72). In sensitized children, nasal challenges and bronchial challenge have provoked nasal obstruction and both early and late asthmatic responses (70,73).

Most species of cockroaches live in tropical climates and do not flourish in colder climates. Central heating has, however, enabled them to thrive outside their normal habitat. The three most common species in North America and Europe are the American cockroach (*Periplaneta americana*), the German cockroach (*Blattella germanica*), and the Oriental cockroach (*Blatta orientalis*). The national designations are a misnomer since all three species originated in Africa (74). The American cockroach is the largest and is found in urban areas and in the southern United States. The German cockroach is the smallest and is found in all parts of the United States and Europe. The Oriental cockroach commonly occurs in damp, "below-ground" structures. Cockroach allergens have only recently been described and are poorly characterized, although provisional data on exposure to these allergens are emerging. The allergens derived from the German and American cockroach have been the most extensively studied. A series of cross-reacting and species-specific allergens has been identified. Two of these (a mw 35,000 heat-stable and a mw 36,000 heat-sensitive protein) have been provisionally designated Bla g I and Bla g II respectively, and another (mw 33,000–35,000) Per a I (25,75). Monoclonal antibodies have been raised against these and their presence in house dust can be measured (76).

## Cat

Sensitization to allergens derived from the domestic cat is frequently seen. The principal cat allergen is Fel d I (*Felis domesticus* allergen I), which is responsible for most of the allergenic activity of cat dander extract (77–79). It is present in sebaceous glands of the skin and also in sublingual salivary glands; however, saliva is not the major source of cat allergen. The pelt is very rich in allergen from these sources, the sebaceous secretions being probably the most important. It is not present in urine obtained by bladder puncture but is present in voided urine from male cats (79–83).

In contrast to mite allergen, a significant proportion (~25%) of airborne Fel d I is found in association with small particles (≤2.5 μm) (84). Such particles remain airborne for long periods and a large proportion would be expected to penetrate the respiratory tract (85). House dust from homes with a cat commonly contain high levels of Fel d I (86,87). However, the allergen is ubiquitous and low levels are found in many homes without a cat. Occasionally a house in which no cat is reported has high levels of cat allergen. It is known that this allergen is quite adherent, being found even on wall surfaces (88), so that it is almost certainly transported on clothing from houses with a cat to those without. This may explain why it has also been detected in public places (with levels reaching 5.2 μg/g) including schools, although the levels reported there were not very high (~0.5 μg/g) (89,90). It is assumed that the levels of Fel d I found in a house with a cat (i.e. ≥8 μg Fel d I/g of dust; levels as high as 1.5 mg/g have been reported) will give rise to symptoms. It is not known what level will give rise to sensitization; however, it seems likely that many children are sensitized by exposure to the levels often found in homes without a cat (i.e., between 1 and 8 μg/g).

## Dog

The study of allergens derived from dog has progressed more slowly, partly due to the diversity of dog allergens and partly because of the impression that sensitivity to dogs is a minor clinical problem. Until recently there has been no standardization of extracts and a large variation in the potency of extracts (91). There appear to be differences in the clinical response to specific breeds of dog, of which there are over 100 (92,93). Despite this, no true breed-specific allergens have been purified and a number of dog allergens have been shown to be common to several breeds (94–96). An international standard for dog extract has recently been established that contains a sufficient number (~20) and concentration of individual allergens to be useful in assessing extracts used clinically (97). One of these allergens (allergen 13) has been purified to homogeneity and renamed Can f I. It is thought to contain approximately 25% of the allergenic activity of dog hair and dander (24,98). It is now possible to measure this allergen in house dust (87,99). As with cat allergen, raised levels are found in schools and in occasional houses without a dog, suggesting that the allergen can be conveyed on clothing. There are anecdotes of sensitized individuals reacting in the presence of a dog owner without the animal being present (92).

## Rodents

The importance of pet rodents as a cause of sensitization and asthma has been known for many years. Many children keep rodents in their bedrooms, and in inner city areas wild mice or rats may be present throughout the house. The allergenicity of rodent allergens is dramatically illustrated by the number of animal handlers and scientists who become sensitized to urinary proteins (100). The urinary nature of mouse, rat, and guinea pig allergens is of importance because very large quantities accumulate in the animal's bedding (101,102). It is totally inappropriate to keep cages in a child's bedroom

### Others

While the above allergens appear to be the most potent, this does not mean that there are no other allergens, yet to be defined, present in the indoor environment. It is well known that some patients who show negative skin test reactions to a standard panel of allergens show positive skin test reactions to specially prepared extracts of their own dust ("autologous dust"). There may well be other sources of allergen; for example, fungi, algae, and possibly bacteria. The two most common indoor fungi are *Penicillium* and *Aspergillus*, although a great variety of fungal taxa have been reported (103). Ubiquitous outdoor fungi such as *Alternaria* and *Cladosporium* are also to be found indoors. The characterization of fungal allergens is technically difficult: fungi survive by enzymatic degradation of surrounding structures, and these enzymes also digest allergen extracts. In addition, different allergens may be released at various stages of fungal maturation and sera with high titers of antibodies to fungal allergens, suitable for use in allergen characterization, are difficult to obtain. An allergen from germinating *Aspergillus fumigatus* (Asp f I) has been characterized and sequenced, but appears not to be present in house dust (104,105).

The possibility of allergens derived from bacteria was once entertained, although little subsequent support emerged. However, secreted products from bacteria—endotoxins—are receiving considerable interest. Animal studies have shown that inhalation causes increasing airway hyperresponsiveness and inflammation in a dose-dependent fashion (106). Endotoxin is present in house dust and, while not an allergen, is capable of stimulating T cells in an antigen-nonspecific manner (a so-called superantigen) (107).

### Measurement

Indoor allergens can be measured using two-site monoclonal-antibody-based assays (enzyme-linked immunosorbent assay [ELISA] techniques) (22,23,25). Before their introduction it was only possible to count pets, mites, cockroaches, and mice (if you could catch them). The number of mites in house-dust specimens can be counted by a flotation or filter method.

These methods are still useful for identifying mite species and their viability; however, they are time consuming, and do not lend themselves to epidemiological studies. Using ELISA, allergen levels can be measured either in house dust (an extension of mite counting techniques) or in indoor air (108–110). Both sampling methods have advantages and disadvantages. The quantity of allergen in house dust is much higher than airborne levels: generally more than 1000 times higher (e.g., 30 μg/g in house dust and 30 ng/m$^3$ in airborne samples). The carpet, sofas, and bedding act as a reservoir for the allergen. Although there is some evidence that synthetic carpets may release less allergen that woolen ones, or even that different carpets are better for mite growth, this has proved difficult to confirm. Some allergens, notably those derived from the house-dust mite, are contained on large particles that become airborne with difficulty: in an undisturbed room the amount of airborne allergen is below the level of measurement. Airborne measurements, in theory, provide a direct measure of what is available for inhalation, especially when personal samplers are used. However, standardization of disturbance required for airborne sampling has not been achieved and the much simpler technique of collecting dust samples lends itself to both routine use and international comparison.

While these methods are used as research procedures, simple measuring techniques have been developed for patient use. The level of guanine, found in association with dust mite allergen in fecal pellets, can be measured with a dip stick, and correlates reasonably well with dust mite allergen levels (111). Samples of dust can be assayed for group I mite allergens by reference laboratories and methods are being developed to measure allergen levels directly by dip stick assays.

### Measurement of Sensitization

The degree to which a child is sensitized to an allergen can be measured by clinical or laboratory methods. It is important to remember that these tests only measure sensitization: they do not establish a causal relationship and certainly do not confirm the presence or absence of asthma. The ability of a child to recognize antigens initially lies with the T cells of the immune system, which then help B cells to proliferate and secrete antibodies. Allergens characteristically evoke an IgE response, which is thought to reflect repeated low-dose exposure. This immunoglobulin isotype is present in relatively low concentration in sera and binds to high-affinity receptors on mast cells and basophils. The immune response is considered to be antigen- (and allergen-) specific, so the total level of IgE is the summation of individual levels of allergen-specific IgE. Total IgE can be measured by ELISA or radioimmunoassay. Extreme values (e.g., IgE $<20$ or $>200$ IU/ml) are very useful in differentiating between children who are unlikely or likely to be sensitized to individual allergens. However, many values lie between the extremes and there is considerable overlap between the groups, rendering it a poor discriminating test. Serum values rise progressively throughout childhood, attaining a lifetime peak during puberty (112). An elevated IgE level has been shown (in a cohort of 562 children in New Zealand studied at age 11 years) to be strongly associated with the presence of diagnosed asthma, and even with nonspecific bronchial responsiveness to methacholine in asymptomatic children (113,114). No asthma was reported in children with an IgE <32 IU/ml, while 36% of those with an IgE >1000 IU/ml were diagnosed with asthma. These findings parallel those of a general population study of adults, which found similar results if IgE values were adjusted for age and sex (115). In Third World countries the mean serum IgE is elevated with regard to "Western" levels and asthma is not more frequent. However, a few studies have shown that asthmatic subjects have an even higher group mean than the population mean (116).

Sensitization to individual allergens can be measured by serologic measurement of allergen-specific IgE levels or by skin testing, which detects the presence of specific IgE bound to mast cells (117). Serum-specific IgE is measured by radioallergosorbent test (RAST) or modifications of this in vitro technique, in which the amount of IgE that binds to the allergen is detected by isotope-labeled anti-IgE (118,119). The results are expressed in either semiquantitative (neg, 1+, 2+, or 3+) or RAST units. The RAST unit we use represents approximately 0.1 ng IgE, while the Pharmacia RAST unit represents ~1.0 ng IgE antibody.

Skin testing is most commonly undertaken in children by the prick technique (117), in which the allergen is introduced epidermally using a 25-gauge needle. Mast cells, which are widely distributed in the skin, degranulate if relevant antibody is introduced and cross-links IgE antibodies. Degranulation results in the release of numerous cell mediators, principally histamine, resulting in a wheal response. The diameter of the wheal reflects the sensitization of skin mast cells and correlates with allergen-specific serum IgE levels, especially for wheals greater than 5 mm. Intradermal testing is sometimes used after negative or equivocal test results have been obtained with skin prick testing. Using this technique, a larger volume (at least 1000-fold) is injected intradermally; because of this it is essential to use diluted extracts. In effect, the skin reactivity is pushed harder to see if it can respond. Intradermal testing should be used with caution, since sufficient allergen is introduced to produce anaphylaxis in highly sensitized individuals, and deaths have been reported. It should not be used to diagnose food allergy and, in general, intradermal skin testing should only be used by clinicians trained in their use. Antihistamines affect the releasibility of histamine, and children should not be skin tested if they have taken these in the recent past (for the newer agents with longer half-lives, this can be as long as 4 weeks). There is also some concern over the lack of standardization of some allergen extracts used in skin testing. Examination of some commercially produced skin test extracts has shown wide variations in the quantity of allergen, including a 200-fold difference in the quantity of Bla g I between extracts, underscoring the need for allergen standardization.

There is no accepted threshold of a positive skin response in children, nor what should be regarded as a significant RAST level. Extreme reactions (a negative skin test, negative RAST or a 10 mm wheal, + + + RAST), pose no difficulty, with few false-positive or false-negative readings. However intermediate values are very common. For skin prick testing it is emerging that a skin wheal of 4 mm diameter in 12-year-old children is a useful working threshold (120,12). In longitudinal studies, values below this diameter could sometimes not be repeated on subsequent skin testing, whereas values of 4 mm or more were found to be reproducible. In younger children the wheal sizes regarded as significant are smaller: 3 mm in 5-year-old children and 2 mm in infants are commonly used. The validity of these responses needs further study. A recent recommendation was that a common limit of positivity (i.e., 3 mm wheal diameter) should be used (121). Positive skin reactions or elevated allergen-specific IgE to inhalant allergen is exceedingly rare in infants. It has been shown that skin reactivity to histamine increases from infancy to adolescence. In a population study, the presence of a 4 mm wheal to histamine (histamine hydrochloride 27 mg/ml) was found in 33% of children aged 0–3 years, 45% of those 4–5, 85% 6–9, 87% 10–14, and 100% 15–20 year (122). The wheal size regarded as positive for intradermal testing is somewhat larger, 6 × 6 mm (if enough allergen is introduced, any individual can show a nonspecific reaction). Serum RAST measures of ≥+ +, 2 Phadebar RAST Units (PRU) or ≥40 RAST units are usually taken as the threshold markers of sensitization.

## IMMUNOSPECIFIC TREATMENT

### Avoidance

The first step towards any solution is identifying the problem. Having demonstrated sensitization to a particular allergen, the next step is to answer whether the patient is exposed (ideally, exposure would also be measured). As individuals with hay fever realize, it is best not to be exposed unnecessarily to pollen allergens (i.e., the first line of treatment is avoidance). One distinct advantage when dealing with indoor allergens is that it is possible to modify the home environment greatly and reduce allergen exposure. However, it requires both the conviction of the physician and effort on the parents' behalf to effect these changes.

*House-Dust Mites*

Practical methods of reducing mite populations have been developed in recent years, as understanding of mite ecology has advanced. Mites are extremely vulnerable to dessication and can also be killed by extremes of temperatures (above 130°F and below 0°F). Reduction methods are based on two additional foundations: remove the habitat of mites and make what remains inhospitable to them. It has been shown that simply applying measures to a child's bedroom results in significant benefits, although ideally the whole apartment or house ought to be treated (49). In the bedroom, most attention should be directed to the bed, flooring, and furniture (Fig. 3). Mattresses and box springs should be encased. This not only contains the allergen but also deprives mites of an external source of humidity. The currently available bed covers, with a cotton outer cover and impermeable inner cover are a marked improvement in comfort over previously available

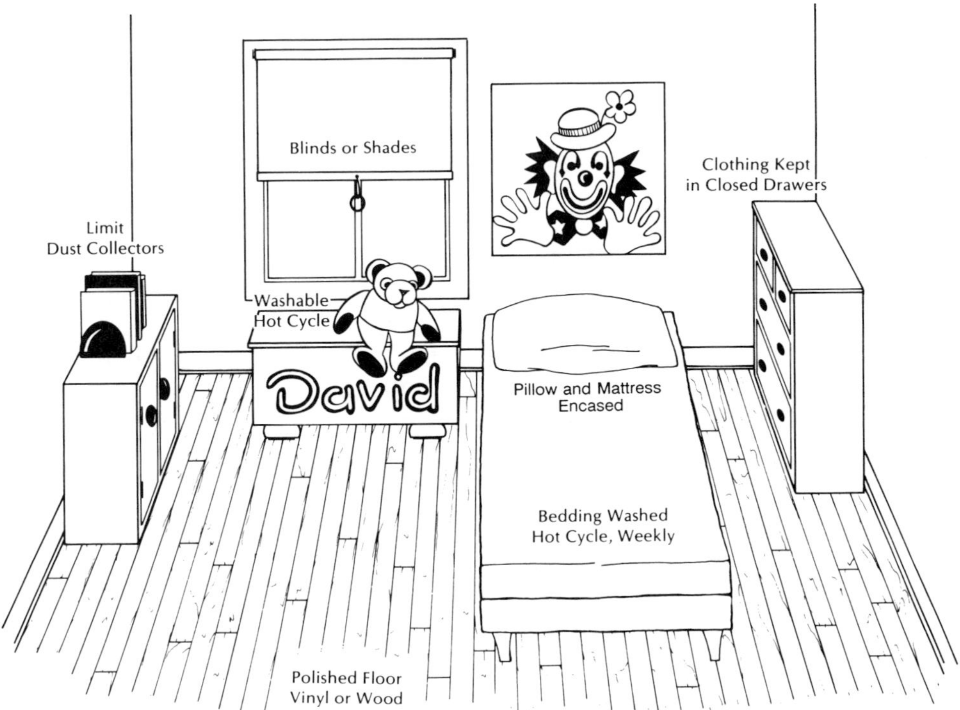


FIGURE 3 Methods for reducing house-dust mites in the bedroom.

polyethylene covers. Impermeable covers dramatically reduce the level of mite allergen; in one study this fell by 100-fold from 22.4 to 0.24 μg Der p I/g (123). Pillows should also be either encased, or washed at least every 2 weeks (although it is difficult to dry them completely) and renewed on a yearly basis. Sheets should be regularly washed in hot water (>130°F) to ensure mite killing. Biological washing powders, detergents, and economical wash cycles will wash out allergen but have little effect on mites. Blankets should be hot washable (e.g., cotton open cell design) and if duvets are used they should be encased or washed and regularly aired (sunlight assists in mite killing). The carpet should preferably be removed and replaced by vinyl or polished wooden floor boards. Vacuum cleaning removes loose dust but has no effect on the number of live mites in the carpet, and in fact some devices make large quantities of allergen airborne (124). It is best to use a vacuum cleaner with an efficient exhaust system that entraps allergen particles. Steam cleaning is inefficient at killing mites; they simply burrow deep into the carpet and are insulated from the heat. Carpets laid on concrete in a basement will always be damp enough to harbor large mite colonies, and it is best to move the bedroom to another room. In rented accommodations if it is impossible to remove the carpet, it can be covered by polyethylene sheeting, taped to the skirting board, or treated (see below). Furniture should not be fabric covered. Vinyl, leather, or plain wooden furniture is best. Curtains should either be hot washable or, preferably, removed and replaced with washable blinds. Bedroom clutter should be kept to a minimum, clothes hot washed frequently, and kept in a closet. Fabric toys should also be hot washed frequently. Surfaces should be damp dusted on a weekly basis to reduce dust. Ambient humidity can be reduced with air conditioning or dehumidifiers.

There has been some interest in acaricides (compounds that kill mites) and compounds that denature allergen (Table 2). Both benzyl benzoate and tannic acid are very effective in vitro, however, the difficulty of applying them so that they reach deep into the pile or padding of furniture reduces their effectiveness in hours.

### *Cockroaches*

Eradication of cockroaches is a formidable undertaking; they are capable of prodigious reproduction under ideal conditions. Professional help is probably required to eradicate them, not only in the affected apartment but also in neighboring ones since they are capable of quickly reinfesting a treated apartment from a nearby untreated one. No information is available on the effect of eradication methods on allergen levels.

### *Pets*

Families with atopic children should not acquire pets, those with one should preferably remove them, and if this cannot be done the pet should be

TABLE 2 Currently Available Acaricides and Allergen Denaturing Agents

| Chemical | Trade name | Mechanism | Form | Reference |
|---|---|---|---|---|
| Benzyl benzoate | Acarosan | Acaricide (used for scabies) | Powder (USA/ Europe) | 125 |
| Pyrethroids | Actomite | Insecticide/acaricide | Pressurized canister (Europe only) | 126 |
| Pirimiphos methyl | Actellic | Insecticide/acaricide | Not available for domestic use | 127 |
| Natamycin | Tymasil | Antifungal (reduces food supply) | Powder (Europe) | 128 |
| Tannic acid (3%) | Allergy control solution | Protein denaturing | Fluid (USA) | 129 |
| Liquid nitrogen | — | Kills mites by freezing | Liquid gas | 130 |
| Benzyl alcohol and tannic acid | D.M.S. spray | Acaricide and protein denaturant | Fluid (Australia) | 131 |
| Mixture of surface wetting agents and solvents | Allerex | Cleaning solution used with special vacuum cleaner | Fluid (Europe) | 132 |

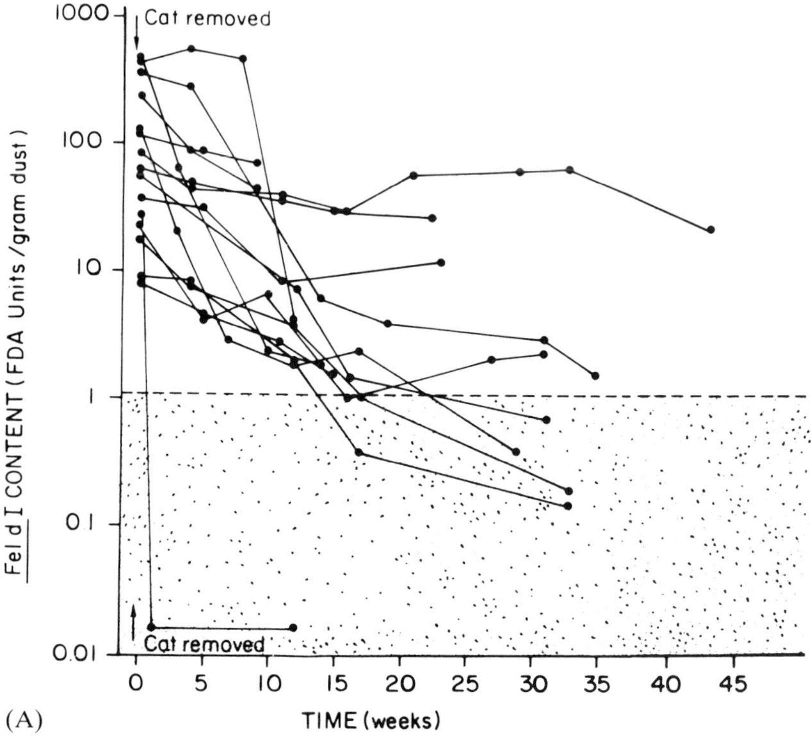


(A)

FIGURE 4 (A) Methods for reducing cat allergen (Fel d I): the effect of removal and of washing a cat. A. Content of serial dust samples obtained after cat removal. The dashed line represents the upper limit of cat allergen levels in control homes without a cat. (From Ref. 133.) (B) Airborne Fel d I content measured immediately before the cat was washed and during the 30 min after washing the cat. The dashed bar represents the range of initial values when the cat entered the room (n = 8). (From Ref. 134.)

washed frequently. Cats are not only a source of allergen but also a family member in many households. Many parents prefer to get rid of their doctor than the cat. If the cat cannot be removed, a poor second best is to ensure that the animal remains outdoors and certainly outside the child's bedroom. Removal of the cat does not, however, lead to immediate benefit. A study has shown that the allergen levels fall progressively and take up to 6 months to return to normal (133) (Fig. 4A). This reflects the very high levels that accumulate in carpets and upholstered furniture. Steam cleaning had little effect and only removal of the carpets and furniture had any dramatic effect. This should be explained to parents before the animal is removed,

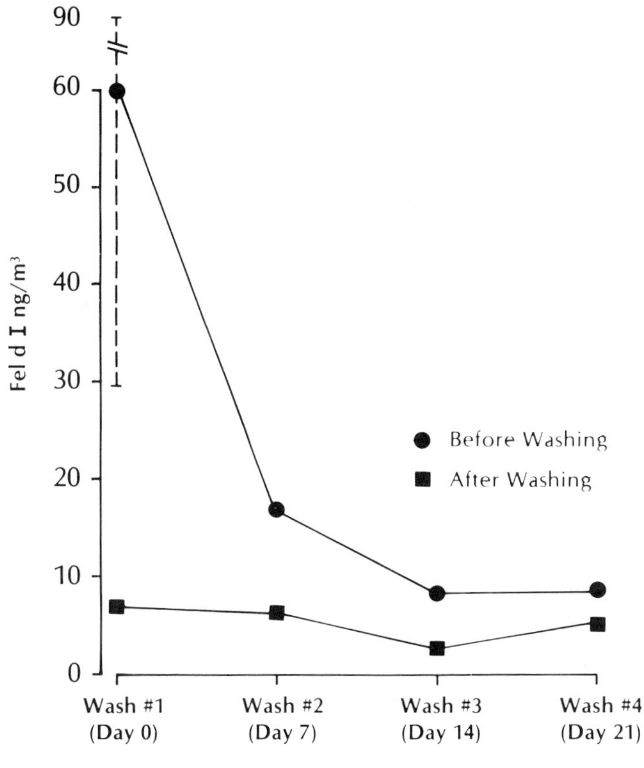


(B)

so that they are not disappointed by the slow improvement. It has recently been shown that simply washing the cat is sufficient to reduce dramatically the allergen coming off the cat (134). Simply pouring a liter of water over the cat on a weekly basis was sufficient. While dogs are regularly washed, cats are usually excluded from this regimen. It is best to introduce a washing regimen when cats are young. Current evidence would suggest that a large reduction of airborne cat allergen can be obtained by either removing the cat completely or by keeping it outdoors, or by having polished floors, no carpets, a minimum of upholstered furniture, a vacuum cleaner with a high-efficiency exhaust filter, air filtration, and washing the cat every week. Little evidence exists on the effect of the reduction of dog allergen levels following removal of the animal. The results would probably be the same as those found with cat allergen. To reduce the level of dog allergen, similar procedures as those proposed for cat, including regular washing, should be considered.

## Immunotherapy

Immunotherapy was originally introduced for seasonal hay fever, and multiple controlled trials have established its efficacy and safety for this disease. It consists of the administration of increasing quantities of allergen to which a child is sensitized, with a view to obtaining protection against natural allergen exposure. Noon first described this method of treatment for grass pollen rhinitis (135). His previous work with tetanus toxoid made him believe that a pollen toxin was responsible for allergic symptoms and that it would be possible to induce protection against it by immunizing with pollen extracts. He carefully assessed conjunctival sensitivity before each immunization, and only when blunting of the response occurred was the dosage of pollen administered increased. His anecdotal descriptions of "cure" of pollen rhinitis were impressive in an era before antihistamines or any effective medications were available. In the 1920s several cases were reported of patients successfully treated with house-dust extract for asthma. Indeed, several authors reported that immunotherapy was more effective for asthma than hay fever. Since the discovery of dust mites, controlled trials have been reported both in children (Table 3) and adults, with generally good results. However there are several reasons for being less enthusiastic about immunotherapy as a treatment for asthma than for hay fever. First, the controlled trials for asthma have not given consistently good results, and it is disappointing that immunotherapy has not been shown to produce a sustained reduction of bronchial hyperreactivity. Second, judging from reports from Australia, Europe, and the United States it appears that there is more risk of severe anaphylactic reactions in patients with asthma than in those with rhinitis. Avoidance measures are feasible with most of the major allergens associated with asthma while reduction of exposure to pollens is not possible.

Perhaps the biggest problem is to understand the factors influencing severe reactions. In the United States it is clear that patients with brittle or labile asthma are at greater risk (144). It is widely accepted that patients with hay fever have more reactions during the pollen season, suggesting that the increased reactivity produced by natural exposure increases the risk of a reaction to immunotherapy. In the case of asthma and house-dust mite or cat sensitivity, many children are exposed perennially, which may well be a factor increasing the risk of reactions. In addition, severe reactions that include bronchospasm are particularly difficult to treat. The obvious conclusion is that aggressive avoidance measures as well as pharmacologic anti-inflammatory treatment should be instituted before one considers immunotherapy. In addition, it has been recommended that added precautions should be taken including a 30 min (2 hr in the United Kingdom) observation period after injections, with measurement of respiratory func-

TABLE 3 Studies on Immunotherapy in Children Using Indoor Allergens

| | Year | Entry criteria | Duration | Extract | Improvement | | Number | |
|---|---|---|---|---|---|---|---|---|
| | | | | | Symptoms | Broncho provocation test | Active | Placebo |
| *House dust mite* | | | | | | | | |
| Warner (136) | 1978 | Strict[a] | 1 yr | Tryosine | Yes | Yes (late) | 27 | 24 |
| Wahn (137) | 1988 | Strict | 2 yr | Aqueous | NR | Yes | 24 | 0 |
| Van Bever (138) | 1989 | Skin test | 1 yr | Aqueous | | Yes (late) | 24 | |
| *Dog* | | | | | | | | |
| Valovirta (139) | 1984 | Strict | 1 yr | Alum adsorbed | n.s. | Yes | 15 | 12 |
| *Cat and Dog* | | | | | | | | |
| Bertelsen (140) | 1988 | Strict | 9 mo. | Alum adsorbed | NR | Yes | 14 | 13 |
| *Cockroach* | | | | | | | | |
| Kang (141)[b] | 1988 | Strict | 5 yr | Aqueous | Yes | NT | 11 | 2 |

[a]Strict: positive skin test, RAST test, and bronchial provocation to allergen.
[b]Adult study.
NT, not tested; NR, not reported; n.s., no significant differences between groups.
Source: Data based on Refs. 142 and 143.

tion using a peak flowmeter before injections and before the patient leaves the physician's office. Resuscitation facilities should also be available in case of anaphylaxis. In addition, all clinicians should have specific guidelines for withholding injections if a patient is wheezing, has had an asthma attack recently, or has required treatment with steroids within 1 month. Although immunotherapy can be effective in the right cases, it does not play a major role in the treatment of childhood asthma. Certainly it should not be considered until after avoidance measures and pharmacologic measures have been tried.

## CONCLUSION

Recent advances in allergen characterization has resulted in a clear understanding of the detrimental effect that allergens have on the lungs of children. While the association between sensitization to indoor allergens and asthma has been known since the 1920s, the other half of the relationship, that sensitization was itself dependent on exposure and that symptoms were dependent on subsequent re-exposure, could not be formally tested until techniques to measure these allergens were available. Measurement of allergens has revealed the presence of allergens in quantities harmful to sensitized children in many homes; the levels found in many children's beds and bedrooms should be considered a health hazard. The current recommendations to reduce allergen exposure are similar to the measures advocated in an age before effective pharmacologic treatments were available. There is increasing concern about the potential adverse influence of treatment with beta-agonists; whether this is intrinsic to the medication or because it allows greater exposure to allergen to occur without the protective effect of bronchoconstriction is uncertain. Many clinicians find themselves caught between the realization that undertreatment may be harmful in the short term and that overtreatment may be deleterious in the long term. Allergen avoidance provides some simple, rather unsophisticated, solutions to this dilemma. Allergen avoidance should be seen as the primary anti-inflammatory treatment for asthma and as an essential foundation of pharmacologic treatment: the former treating the cause of asthma and the latter treating its current symptoms. Reducing allergen exposure usually allows a reduction in the amount of medication required. Allergen avoidance, however, requires a degree of effort and commitment from the parents of asthmatic children that has become alien in the treatment of asthma in an era used to rapid bronchodilation and short-term improvement. It also requires of the physician a considerable degree of conviction, explanation, encouragement, and persistence.

## ACKNOWLEDGMENTS

This chapter was made possible by financial support from NIH grants AI-20565, AI-30840, AI-24687, and AI-24261, Fisons, Allergy Control Products, and the American Lung Association. We are also grateful to many of our colleagues for helpful conversations during the preparation of this chapter.


## REFERENCES


1. Smith E. *Disease in Children*, William Wood & Co., New York, 1884, p. 520.
2. Peat JK, Woolcock AJ. Sensitivity to common allergens: relation to respiratory symptoms and bronchial hyper-responsiveness in children from three different areas of Australia. *Clin Exp Allergy* 21:573–581, 1991.
3. Lau S, Falkenhorst G, Weber A, Werthman I, Lind P, Bucttner-Goetz P, Wahn U. High mite-allergen exposure increases the risk of sensitization in atopic children and young adults. *J Allergy Clin Immunol* 84:718–725, 1989.
4. Sarsfield JK. Role of house-dust mites in childhood asthma. *Arch Dis Child* 49:711–715, 1974.
5. Korsgaard J. Mite asthma and residency. A case-control study on the impact of exposure to house-dust mites in dwellings. *Am Rev Respir Dis* 128:231–235, 1983.
6. Di Nicolo R, Nelson RP, Fernandez-Caldas E, Trudeau W, Swanson M, Bonini LV, Perez A, Arthur P, Lockey R, Good RA. Allergen-specific IgE levels in children presenting to the emergency room with acute asthma. *J Allergy Clin Immunol* 87:1(2):234 (abstract), 1991.
7. Smith TF, Kelly LB, Heymann PW, Wilkins SR, Platts-Mills TAE. Natural exposure to house-dust mite of mite allergic children with asthma in Atlanta. *J Allergy Clin Immunol* 76:782–788, 1985.
8. Dekker H. Asthma und Milben. *Münch Med Wochensch* 515–516, 1928, (translated by Deaner WC. *Allergy Clin Immunol* 48:251–252, 1971).
9. Arruda LK, Rizzo MC, Chapman MD, Fernandez-Caldas E, Baggio D, Platts-Mills TAE, Naspitz CK. Exposure and sensitization to dust mite allergens among asthmatic children in São Paulo, Brazil. *Clin Exp Allergy* 21:433–439, 1991.
10. Smith JM, Disney ME, Williams JD, Goels ZA. Clinical significance of skin reactions to mite extracts in children with asthma. *Br Med J* 1:723–726, 1969.
11. Charpin D, Birnbaum J, Haddi E, Genard G, Lanteaume A, Toumi M, Faraj F, Van der Brempt X, Verloet D. Altitude and Allergy to house-dust mites: a paradigm of the influence of environmental exposure on allergic sensitization. *Am Rev Respir Dis* 143:983–986, 1991.
12. Sporik R, Holgate ST, Platts-Mills TAE, Cogswell JJ. Exposure to house dust mite allergen (Der p I) and the development of asthma in childhood: a prospective study. *N Engl J Med* 323:502–507, 1990.

13. Foucard T, Sjoberg O, A prospective 12-year follow-up study of children with wheezy bronchitis. *Acta Paediatr Scand* 73:577–83, 1984.
14. Wilson NM. Wheezy bronchitis revisited. *Arch Dis Child* 64:1194–1199, 1989.
15. Sporik R, Holgate ST, Cogswell JJ. Natural history of asthma in childhood—a birth cohort study. *Arch Dis Child* 66:1050–1053, 1991.
16. Platts-Mills TAE, de Weck AL. Dust mite allergens and asthma—a world wide problem. *J Allergy Clin Immunol* 83:416–427, 1989.
17. Bernton HS, McMahon TF, Brown H. Cockroach asthma. *Br J Dis Chest* 66:61–66, 1972.
18. Pollart SM, Reid MJ, Fling JA, Chapman MD, Platts-Mills TAE. Epidemiology of emergency room asthma in northern California: association with IgE antibody to rye grass pollen. *J Allergy Clin Immunol* 82:224–230, 1988.
19. O'Hollaren MT, Yunginger J, Offord KP, Somers MJ, O'Connell EJ, Ballard DJ, Sachs MI. Exposure to an aeroallergen as a possible precipitating factor in respiratory arrest in young patients with asthma. *N Eng J Med* 324:359–363, 1991.
20. Kang B. Study on cockroach antigen as a probable causative agent in bronchial asthma. *J Allergy Clin Immunol* 58:357–365, 1976.
21. Sears MR, Taylor DR, Print CG, Lake DC, Li QQ, Flannery EM, Yates DM, Lucas MK, Herbison GP. Regular inhaled beta-agonist treatment in bronchial asthma. *Lancet* 336:1391–1396, 1990.
22. Chapman MD, Heymann PW, Wilkins SR, Brown MB, Platts-Mills TAE. Monoclonal immunoassays for the major dust mite (*Dermatophagoides*) allergen, Der p I and Der f I and quantitative analysis of the allergen contact of mite and house dust extracts. *J Allergy Clin Immunol* 80:184–194, 1987.
23. Luczynska CM, Li Y, Chapman MD, Platts-Mills TAE. Airborne concentrations and particle size distribution of allergen derived from domestic cats (*Felis domesticus*). Measurements using cascade impactor, liquid impinger, and a two-site monoclonal antibody assay for Fel d I. *Am Rev Respir Dis* 141:361–367, 1990.
24. De Groot H, Goei KG, van Swieten P, Aalberse RC. Affinity purification of a major and minor allergen from dog extract: serological activity of affinity purified Can f I and of Can f I-depleted extract. *J Allergy Clin Immunol* 87:1056–1065, 1991.
25. Pollart SM, Mullins DE, Vailes LD, Hayden ML, Platts-Mills TAE, Sutherland WM, Chapman MD. Identification quantitation, and purification of cockroach allergens using monoclonal antibodies. *J Allergy Clin Immunol* 87:511–521, 1991.
26. Hill AB. The environment and disease: association or causation? *Proc R Soc Med* 58:295–300, 1965.
27. Warner JA, Little SA, Pollack I, et al. The influence of exposure to house dust mite, cat, pollen, fungal allergens in the home on primary sensitization in asthma. *Pediatr Allergy Immunol* 1:79–86, 1990.
28. Korsgaard J. Mite asthma and residency. A case-control study on the impact of exposure to house-dust mites in dwellings. *Am Rev Respir Dis* 128:231–235, 1983.

29. Holt PG, McMenamin C, Nelson D. Primary sensitization to inhalant allergens during infancy. *Pediatr Allergy Immunol* 1:3–13, 1990.
30. Warner JO, Price SA. Aero-allergen avoidance in the prevention and treatment of asthma. *Clin Exp Allergy* 20:15–19 (supplement), 1990.
31. Peat JK, Britton WJ, Salome CM, Woolcock AJ. Bronchial hyperresponsiveness in two populations of Australian schoolchildren. III. Effect of exposure to environmental allergens. *Clin Allergy* 17:297–300, 1987.
32. Miyatomo T, Oshima S, Ishizaki T, Sato S. Allergenic identity between the common floor mite (*Dermatophagoides farinae* Hughes 1961) and house dust as a causative agent in bronchial asthma. J Allergy 42:14–28, 1968.
33. Sporik R, Platts-Mills TAE, Cogswell JJ. Exposure and sensitization of children admitted to hospital with asthma to house dust mite allergen (Der p I). *J Allergy Clin Immunol* 87:1(2); 291 (abstract), 1991.
34. Platts-Mills TAE, Hayden ML, Chapman MD, Wilkins SR. Seasonal variation in dust mite and grass pollen allergen dust from the houses of patients with asthma. *J Allergy Clin Immunol* 79:781–791, 1987.
35. Dowse GK, Turner KJ, Stewart GA, Alpers MP, Woolcock AJ. The association between Dermatophagoides mites and the increasing prevalence of asthma in village communities within the Papua New Guinea highlands. *J Allergy Clin Immunol* 75:75–83, 1985.
36. McMenamin C, Girn B, Holt PG. Localisation of sites of IgE synthesis in vivo by Dot blot and Northern blot analysis of IgE-specific mRNA. ICACI 14:194 [abstr].
37. Martinez FD, Morgan WJ, Wright AL, Holberg CJ, Taussig LM. Diminished lung function as a predisposing factor for wheezing respiratory illness in infants. *N Eng J Med* 319:1112–1117, 1988.
38. Young S, Lee Souef PN, Geelhoed GC, Stick SM, Turner KJ, Landau LI. The influence of a family history of asthma and parental smoking on airway responsiveness in early infancy. *N Engl J Med* 324:1168–1173, 1991.
39. Mitchell I, Inglis H, Simpson H. Viral infections in wheezy bronchitis and asthma in children. *Arch Dis Child* 51:707–711, 1972.
40. Warner JO. Significance of late reactions after bronchial challenge with house dust mite. *Arch Dis Child* 51:905–911, 1976.
41. Aas K. Bronchial provocation tests in asthma. *Arch Dis Child* 45:221–228, 1970.
42. Cavanaugh MJ, Bronsky EA, Buckley JM. Clinical value of bronchial provocation testing in childhood asthma. *J Allergy Clin Immunol* 59:41–47, 1977.
43. M'Raihi L, Charpin D, Thibaudon M, Vervloet D. Bronchial challenge to house dust can induce immediate bronchoconstriction in allergic asthmatic patients. *Ann Allergy* 65:485–488, 1990.
44. Booij-Noord H, de Vries K, Sluiter HJ, Oriie NGM. Late bronchial obstructive reaction to experimental inhalation of house dust extract. *Clin Allergy* 2:43–61, 1972.
45. Djukanovic R, Roche WR, Wilson JW, Beasley CRW, Twentyman OP, Howarth PH, Holgate ST. Mucosal inflammation in asthma. *Am Rev Respir Dis* 142:434–457, 1990.

46. Bousquet J, Chanez P, Lacoste JY, Barndeon G, Ghavania N, Enander I, Venge P, Ahlstedt S, Simony-Lafontaine J, Godard P, et al. Eosinophilic inflammation in asthma. *N Engl J Med* 323:1033–1039, 1990.
47. Boner AL, Niero E, Antolini I, Valletta EA, Gaburro D. Pulmonary function and bronchial hyperreactivity in asthmatic children with house dust mite allergy during prolonged stay in the Italian Alps (Misurina 1756m). *Ann Allergy* 54:42–45, 1985.
48. Platts-Mills TAE, Tovey ER, Mitchell EB, Moszoro H, Nock P, Wilkins SR. Reduction of bronchial hyperreactivity during prolonged allergen avoidance. *Lancet* 2:675–678, 1982.
49. Murray AB, Ferguson AC. Dust-free bedrooms in the treatment of asthmatic children with house dust or house dust mite allergy: a controlled trial. *Pediatrics* 71:418–422, 1983.
50. Tattersfield AE. Effect of beta-agonists and anticholinergic drugs on bronchial reactivity. *Am Rev Respir Dis* 136:S64–68, 1987.
51. Vathenen AS, Knox AJ, Wisniewski A, Tattersfield AE. Time course of change in bronchial reactivity with an inhaled corticosteroid in asthma. *Am Rev Respir Dis* 143:1317–1321, 1991.
52. Robertson DG, Kerigan AT, Hargreave FE, et al. Late asthmatic responses induced by ragweed pollen allergen. *J Allergy Clin Immunol* 54:244, 1974.
53. Hughes AM. *The Mites of Stored Food and Houses*. Her Majesty's Stationary Office, London, 1976.
54. Arlian LG. Biology and ecology of house dust mites, *Dermatophagoides* spp. and *Euroglyphus* spp. *Immunol Allergy Clin North Am* 9:339–356, 1989.
55. Chapman MD, Platts-Mills TAE. Purification and characterization of the major allergen from *Dermatophagoides pteronyssinus*-antigen P1. *J Immunol* 125:587–592, 1980.
56. Heymann PW, Chapman MD, Aalberse RC, Fox JW, Platts-Mills TAE. Antigenic and structural determinants of Group II allergens (Der f II and Der p II) from house dust mites (*Dermatophagoides* spp). *J Allergy Clin Immunol* 83:1055–1067, 1989.
57. Heymann PW, Chapman MD, Platts-Mills TAE. Antigen Der f I from the dust mite Dermatophagoides farinae: structural comparison with Der p I from *D. pteronyssinus* and epitope specificity of murine IgG and human IgE antibody responses. *J Immunol* 137:2841–2847, 1986.
58. Heymann P, Farris H, Chapman M, Platts-Mills T. Proportion of human IgE antibody directed against group I and group II dust-mite allergens. *J Allergy Clin Immunol* 87:194 (abstract), 1991.
59. Tovey ER, Chapman MD, Platts-Mills TAE. Mite faeces are a major source of house dust allergens. *Nature* 289:592–593, 1981.
60. Dilworth RJ, Chua KY, Thomas WR. Sequence analysis of cDNA coding for a major house dust mite allergen, Der f I. *Clin Exp Allergy* 21:25–32, 1991.
61. Trudinger M, Chua KY, Thomas WR. cDNA coding the major mite allergen Der f II. *Clin Exp Allergy* 21:33–37, 1991.
62. Bernton HS, Brown H. Insect allergy—preliminary studies of the cockroach. *J Allergy* 35:506–513, 1964.

63. Bernton HS, Brown H. Cockroach allergy. II. The relation of infestation to sensitization. *South Med J* 60:852–855, 1967.
64. Twarog FJ, Picone FJ, Struck RS, So J, Colten HR. Immediate hypersensitivity to cockroach: isolation and purification of the major antigens. *J Allergy Clin Immunol* 58:357–365, 1976.
65. Mendoza J, Snyder FD. Cockroach sensitivity in children with bronchial asthma. *Ann Allergy* 28:159–163, 1970.
66. Morris EC, Smith TF, Kelly LB. Cockroach is a significant antigen for inner city children. *J Allergy Clin Immunol* 77:206 (abstract), 1986.
67. Gelber L, Pollart S, Chapman MD, Platts-Mills TAE. Serum IgE antibodies and allergen exposure as a risk factor for acute asthma. *J Allergy Clin Immunol* 85:193 (abstract), 1990.
68. Steinburg DR, Bernstein DI, Gallagher JS, Arlian L, Bernstein IL. Cockroach sensitization in laboratory workers. *J Allergy Clin Immunol* 80(4):586–590, 1987.
69. Thong YH, Omar A, Kok A, Robinson MJ. Skin reactivity to household aerollergens in children with bronchial asthma. *Singapore Med J* 17:90–91, 1976.
70. Pola J, Zapata C, Valdivieso R, Armentia A, Subiza J, Hinojosa M, Losada E. Cockroach asthma: case report and literature review. *Allergol Immunopathol* 16(1):61–65, 1988.
71. Lan JL, Lee DT, Wu CH, Chang OP, Yeh CL. Cockroach hypersensitivity: preliminary study of allergic cockroach asthma in Taiwan. *J Allergy Clin Immunol* 82(5 Pt 1):736–740, 1988.
72. Guerrier G. History of hunting . . . . to cockroaches. *Pediatrie* 43(7):607–608, 1988.
73. Pola J, Valdivieso R, Zapata C, Quirce S, Hinjosa M, Losada E. Specific bronchial challenge in cockroach asthma. *Allergol Immunopathol* 16(3):171–173, 1988.
74. Bell WJ. *The Laboratory Cockroach* Chapman and Hall, London, 1981.
75. Schou C, Lind P, Fernandez-Caldas E, Lockey RF, Lowenstein H. Identification and purification of an important cross-reactive allergen from American (*Periplaneta americana*) and German (*Blattella germanica*) cockroach. *J Allergy Clin Immunol* 86(6 Pt 1):935–946, 1990.
76. Pollart SM, Smith TF, Morris E, Gelber LE, Platts-Mills TAE, Chapman MD. Environmental exposure to cockroach allergens: analysis with a monoclonal antibody-based enzyme immunoassays. *J Allergy Clin Immunol* 87:505–510, 1991.
77. Ohman JL, Lowell FC, Block KJ. Allergens of mammalian origin III: Properties of a major feline allergen. *J Immunol* 113:1668–1677, 1974.
78. Ohman JL, Lowell FC, Bloch KJ, Kendall S. Allergens of mammalian origin V: properties of extracts derived from the domestic cat. *Clin Allergy* 6:419–428, 1976.
79. De Groot H, van Swieten P, van Leevwen J, Lind P, Aalberse RC. Monoclonal antibodies to the major feline allergen Fel d I. I. Serologic and biologic activity of affinity-purified Fel d I and of Fel d I-depleted extract. *J Allergy Clin Immunol* 82:778–786, 1988.

80. Bartholome K, Kissler W, Baer H, Kopietz-Schulte E, Wahn U. Where does cat allergen 1 come from? *J Allergy Clin Immunol* 76:503–506, 1985.
81. Charpin C, Mata P, Lavaut MN, Allasia C, Charpin D, Vervloet D. Immunochemical detection of Fel d I antigen in cat hair and skin: densitometric (SAMBA) and ultrastructural (scanning) studies. *J Allergy Clin Immunol* 87:1(2) (abstract), 1991.
82. Dabrowski AJ, van der Brempt X, Soler M, Seguret N, Lucciani P, Charpin D, Vervloet D. Cat skin as an important source of Fel d I allergen. *J Allergy Clin Immunol* 86:462–465, 1990.
83. Anderson MC, Baer H, Ohman JL. A comparative study of the allergens of cat urine, serum, saliva, pelt. *J Allergy Clin Immunol* 76:563–569, 1985.
84. Luczynska CM, Li Y, Chapman MD, Platts-Mills TAE. Airborne concentrations and particle size distribution of allergen derived from domestic cats (*Felis domesticus*). Measurements using cascade impactor, liquid impinger, and a two-site monoclonal antibody assay for Fel d I. *Am Rev Respir Dis* 141:361–367, 1990.
85. Findlay SR, Stotsky E, Leiterman K, Hemady Z, Ohman JL. Allergens detected in association with airborne particles capable of penetrating into the peripheral lung. *Am Rev Respir Dis* 128:1008–1012, 1983.
86. Chapman MD, Aalberse RC, Brown MJ, Platts-Mills TAE. Monoclonal antibodies to the major feline allergen Fel d I. *J Immunol* 140(3)812–818, 1988.
87. Wood RA, Eggleston PA, Lind P, Ingemann L, Schwartz B, Graveson S, Terry D, Wheller B, Adkinson NF. Antigenic analysis of household dust samples. *Am Rev Respir Dis* 137:358–363, 1988.
88. Wood RA, Mudd KE, Eggleston PA. The distribution of cat allergen on vertical surfaces. *J Allergy Clin Immunol* 85:226 (abstract), 1990.
89. Shamie S, Enberg R, Terry L, Ownby D. The consistent presence of cat allergen (Fel d I) in various types of public places. *J Allergy Clin Immunol* 85:226 (abstract), 1990.
90. Dreborg SKG, Munir AKM, Einarsson R. The level of Fel d I in school dust is sufficiently high to induce symptoms in asthmatics. *J Allergy Clin Immunol* 87:169 (abstract), 1991.
91. Moore BS, Hyde JS, Manaligod LM. A comparative study of allergens of canine origin. *Ann Allergy* 39:240–245, 1977.
92. Hooker SB. Qualitative differences among canine danders. *Ann Allergy* 2:281–288, 1944.
93. *The Complete Dog Book, An Official Publication of the American Kennel Club*, 15th edition. New York, 1976, p. 572.
94. Fagerberg E, Wide L, Diagnosis of hypersensitivity to dog epithelium in patients with asthma bronchiale. *Int Arch Allergy* 39:301–309, 1970.
95. Blands J, Lowenstein H, Weeke B. Characterization of extract of dog hair and dandruff from six different dog breeds by qualitative immunoelectrophoresis. Identification of the allergen by crossed radioimmunoelectrophoresis (CRIE). *Acta Allergol* 32:147–169, 1977.
96. Lindgreen S, Belin L, Dreborg S, Einarsson R, Pahlman I. Breed-specific dog dandruff allergens. *J Allergy Clin Immunol* 82:196–204, 1988.

97. Larsen JN, Ford A, Gjesing B, Levy D, Petrunov B, Silvestri L, Lowenstein H. The collaborative study of the international standard of dog, *Canis domesticus*, hair/dander extract. *J Allergy Clin Immunol* 82:318–330, 1988.
98. Schou C, Lowenstein H. Purification and characterization of the important dog allergen Can f I (Ag 13). *J Allergy Clin Immunol* 85:170 (abstract), 1990.
99. Schou C, Hansen GN, Lintner T. Assay for the major dog allergen Can f I. Investigation of house dust samples. *J Allergy Clin Immunol* 87:170 (abstract), 1991.
100. Platts-Mills TA, Longbottom J, Edwards J, Cockcroft A, Wilkins S. Occupational asthma and rhinitis related to laboratory rats: serum IgG and IgE antibodies to the rat urinary allergen. *J Allergy Clin Immunol* 79:505–515, 1987.
101. Walls AF, Longbottom JL. Quantitative immunoelectrophoretic analysis of rat allergen extracts. II. Fur, urine and saliva studied by cross radioimmunoelectrophoresis. *Allergy* 38:501–512, 1983.
102. Lorusso JR, Moffat S, Ohman JL. Immunologic and biochemical properties of the major mouse urinary allergen (Mus m I). *J Allergy Clin Immunol* 78:928–937, 1986.
103. Van Bronswijk JE. *House Dust Biology—For Allergists, Acarologists and Mycologists*. NIB Publishers, The Netherlands, pp. 151–164.
104. Arruda LK, Platts-Mills TAE, Fox JW, Chapman MD. *Aspergillus fumigatus* allergen I, a major IgE-binding protein, is a member of the mitogillin family of cytotoxins. *J Exp Med* 172:1529–1532, 1990.
105. Lamy B, Moutaouakil M, Latge JP, Davies J. Secretion of a potential virulence factor, a fungal ribonucleotoxin, during human aspergillosis infections. *Mol Microbiol* 5:1811–1815, 1991.
106. Michel O, Ginanni R, Duchateau J, Vertongen F, Le Bon B, Sergysels R. Domestic endotoxin exposure and clinical severity of asthma. *Clin Exp Allergy* 21:441–448, 1991.
107. Choi YW, Herman A, DiGiusto D, Wade T, Marrack P, Kappler J. Residues of the variable region of the T-cell receptor beta-chain that interact with *S. aureus* toxin superantigens. Nature 346:471–347, 1990.
108. Price JA, Pollock J, Little SA, Longbotom JL, Warner JO. Measurements of airborne mite allergen in homes of asthmatic children. *Lancet* 336:895–897, 1990.
109. Sakaguchi M, Inouye S, Yasueda II, Irie T, Yoshizawa S, Shida T. Measurements of allergens associated with dust mite allergy. II. Concentrations of airborne mite allergens (Der I and Der II) in the house. *Int. Arch Allergy Appl Immunol* 90:190–193, 1989.
110. Tovey ER, Chapman MD, Wells CW, Platts-Mills TAE. The distribution of dust mite allergen in the houses of patients with asthma. *Am Rev Respir Dis* 124:630–635, 1981.
111. Van der Brempt X, Haddi E, Michel-Nguyen, Fayon JP, Soler M, Charpin D, Vervloet D. Comparison of the ACAREX test with monoclonal antibodies for quantification of mite allergens. *J Allergy Clin Immunol* 87:130–132, 1991.

112. Kjellman N-IM, Johansson SGO. IgE and atopic allergy in newborns and infants with a family history of atopic disease. *Acta Pediatr Scand* 65:601–607, 1976.
113. Sears MR, Burrows B, Flannery EM, Herbison GP, Hewitt CJ, Holdaway MD. Relation between airway responsiveness and serum IgE in children with asthma and in apparently normal children. *N Engl J Med* 325:1067–1071, 1991.
114. Sears MR, Burrows B, Flannery EM, Herbison GP, Hewitt CJ, Holdaway MD. Airway hyperresponsiveness in children is related to serum total IgE even in the absence of asthma and atopic disease. *Am Rev Respir Dis* 143(4):19 (abstract), 1991.
115. Burrows B, Martinez FD, Halonen M, Barbee RA, Cline MG. Association of asthma with serum IgE levels and skin-test reactivity to allergens. *N Engl J Med* 320(5):271–277, 1989.
116. Alshishtawy MM, Abdella AM, Gelber LE, Chapman MD. Asthma in Tanta, Egypt: serological analysis of total and specific IgE antibody levels and their relationship to parasite infection. *Int Arch Allergy Appl Immunol* (in press).
117. Pepys J. Skin testing. *Br J Hosp Med* 14:412–417, 1975.
118. Wide L, Bennich H, Johansson SGO. Diagnosis of allergy by an in vitro test for allergen antibodies. *Lancet* 2:1105–1107, 1967.
119. Ceska M, Eriksson R, Varga JM. Radioimmunosorbent assay of allergens. *J Allergy Clin Immunol* 49:1–9, 1972.
120. Peat JK, Salome CM, Woolcock, AJ. Longitudinal changes in atopy during a 4 year period: relation to bronchial hyperresponsiveness and respiratory symptoms in a population sample of Australian schoolchildren. *J Allergy Clin Immunol* 85:65–74, 1990.
121. Dreborg S. Bronchial hyper-reactivity and skin sensitivity. Editorial. *Clin Exp Allergy* 231A:529, 1991.
122. Skassa-Brociek W, Manderschied JC, Michel FB, Bousquet J. Skin test reactivity to histamine from infancy to old age. *J Allergy Clin Immunol* 80(5):711–716, 1987.
123. Owen S, Morganstern J, Hepworth J, Woodcock A. Control of house dust mite antigen in bedding. *Lancet* 335:396–397, 1990.
124. Kalra S, Owen SJ, Hepworth J, Woodcock A. Airborne house-dust mite antigen after vacuum cleaning. *Lancet* 336:449 (letter), 1990.
125. Bischoff E, Fischer A, Liebenberg B. Assessment and control of house dust mite infestation. *Clin Ther* 12:216–220, 1990.
126. Charpin D, Birnbaum J, Haddi E, N'Guyen A, Fondarai J, Vervloet D. Evaluation d'un acaricide ACARDUST dans le traitement de l'allergie aux acariens. Rev Fr Allergol 30:149–155, 1990.
127. Mitchell EB, Wilkins S, Deighton J, Platts-Mills TAE. Reduction of house dust mite allergen levels in the home: use of the acaricide pirimiphos-methyl. *Clin Allergy* 15:235–240, 1985.
128. Saint-George-Gridelet D de, Kneist FH, Schober G, Penaud A, van Bronswijk JEMH. Lutte chimique contre les acariens de la poussiere de maison. *Notes Prelim Rev Franc Allergol* 12:216–220, 1988.

129. Miller JD, Millar A, Luczynska C, Rose G, Platts-Mills TAE. Effect of tannic acid spray on dust mite allergen levels in carpets. *J Allergy Clin Immunol* 83:262 (abstract), 1989.
130. Colloff MJ. Use of liquid nitrogen in the control of house dust mite populations. *Clin Allergy* 16:41–47, 1986.
131. Green WF, Nicholas NR, Salome CM, Woolcock AJ. Reduction of house dust mites and mite allergens: effects of spraying carpets and blankets with Allersearch DMS, an acaricide combined with an allergen reducing agent. *Clin Exp Allergy* 19:203–207, 1989.
132. Mitchell E (in prep.)
133. Wood RA, Chapman MD, Adkinson NF Jr, Eggleston PA. The effect of cat removal on allergen content in the household-dust samples. *J Allergy Clin Immunol* 83:730–734, 1989.
134. De Blay F, Chapman MD, Platts-Mills TAE. Airborne cat allergen (Fel d I): environmental control with the cat in situ. *Am Rev Respir Dis* 143:1334–1339, 1991.
135. Noon L. Prophylactic inoculation for hay fever. *Lancet* 1:1572, 1911.
136. Warner JO, Price JF, Soothill JF, Hey EN. Controlled trial of hyposensitization to Dermatophagoides pteronyssinus in children with asthma. *Lancet* 2:912–915, 1978.
137. Wahn U, Schweter C, Lind P, Lowenstein H. Prospective study on immunologic changes induced by two different *Dermatophagoides* extracts prepared from whole mite culture and mite bodies. *J Allergy Clin Immunol* 82:360–370, 1988.
138. Van Bever HP, Stevens WJ. Suppression of the late asthmatic reaction by hyposensitization in asthmatic children allergic to house dust mite (*Dermatophagoides pteronyssinus*). Clin Exp Allergy 19:399–404, 1989.
139. Valovirta E, Koivikko A, Vanto T, Viander M, Ingeman L. Immunotherapy in allergy to dog: a double blind clinical study. *Ann Allergy* 53:85–88, 1984.
140. Bertelsen A, Anderson JB, Christensen J, Ingeman L, Kristensen T, Ostergaard PA. Immunotherapy with dog and cat extracts in children. *Allergy* 44:330–335, 1989.
141. Kang BC, Johnson J, Morgan C, Chang JL. The role of immunotherapy in cockroach asthma. *J Asthma* 25:205–218, 1988.
142. Ohman JL. Allergen immunotherapy in asthma: evidence for efficacy. *J Allergy Clin Immunol* 84:133–140, 1989.
143. Bousquet J, Hejjaoui A, Michel FB. Specific immunotherapy in asthma. *J Allergy Clin Immunol* 86:292–305, 1990.
144. Reid M, Lockey R, Turkletaub P, Platts-Mills TAE. Survey of fatalities from skin testing and immunotherapy. (submitted).

# 19

# Food Hypersensitivity and Asthma in Children

**S. ALLAN BOCK**

*National Jewish Center for Immunology and Respiratory Medicine and*
*University of Colorado Health Sciences Center*
*Denver, Colorado*

## INTRODUCTION AND DEFINITIONS

This chapter considers a simple question with a complicated answer: Does food ingestion precipitate airway obstruction (asthma) and, if so, by what mechanism? On the surface this would seem to be a fairly straightforward question that could be answered by a simple approach. Feed the child a food and see if he or she wheezes. The reader who has tried this approach will recognize its futility. Asthma is too complex an illness to be approached in this fashion. This chapter will be limited to data pertinent to this question that have been obtained using double-blind placebo-controlled food challenges. Any other method of patient evaluation is subject to bias and the effect of emotions on the lower airway.

Terminology in this field is not uniform and there is some disagreement concerning appropriate definitions. I favor the following terms. Adverse reaction to food is the best generic term to use when referring to symptoms associated with food ingestion for which the mechanism is not known. Food hypersensitivity should be reserved for those reactions in which it can be shown that the immune system is definitely or highly likely to be playing a role. Hypersensitivity is preferred to allergy because the term allergy has been so misused and abused when applied to food reactions. Symptomatic hypersensitivity is present when symptoms occur during food ingestion and the immune system can be shown to be making a specific response. Asymptomatic hypersensitivity exists when no symptoms occur during food ingestion, but the immune system can be shown to be making a specific response. Food intolerance should be reserved for carbohydrate malabsorption (e.g., lactose intolerance). Other modifiers such as toxicologic, pharmacologic, and psychological may be useful in certain circumstances, but at present their use is often imprecise. The term idiosyncratic does not have a precise definition.

## INCIDENCE AND PREVALENCE

Determining the incidence and prevalence of food hypersensitivity that induces airway obstructive symptoms has been fraught with difficulty. Investigators who have studied this subject have generally examined food allergy in general as opposed to food-induced wheezing specifically. Even in studies in which food ingestion and wheezing have been associated with each other, suboptimal methodology has been used to confirm the relationship. The number of subjects in whom food-induced wheezing has been proven by double-blind placebo controlled food challenges has been quite small. Studies that have used proper techniques have not really approached the question of prevalence or incidence. The most honest answer to the question, "What is the incidence or prevalence of food induced wheezing?"

is "Unknown." Solving the methodologic problems involved in studying large populations of patients in order to gain a proper answer to the question awaits future research. All that can be safely said at this time is that the existing studies have found wheezing to be unusual in food-hypersensitive individuals, and that wheezing as the sole symptom of a food allergic reaction is rare.

## RESPIRATORY SYMPTOMS

Respiratory symptoms, including asthma, are frequently attributed to food ingestion. Yet respiratory symptoms as the sole manifestation of food hypersensitivity or even in concert with cutaneous and gastrointestinal symptoms are not common. In reviewing the presentation of food-associated symptoms in over 550 children evaluated at the National Jewish Center, several patterns of management of respiratory reactions have become clear (1–3). The most obvious are those patients in whom severe allergic reactions (anaphylaxis) have been accompanied by wheezing and measurable decreases in pulmonary function parameters. These patients are always the most impressive and garner the most attention, but are uncommon in actual practice. A second pattern is seen in those children in whom wheezing is a frequent occurrence and parents and/or physicians have acquired the habit of associating symptoms with ingested food(s) and removing the food(s) from the diet without proper challenge testing. A third pattern involves youngsters with asthma who are placed on elimination diets, who experience improvement, and in whom the very restricted diet is then maintained for long periods of time without challenging the true association between food and symptoms. The fourth common pattern is represented by the numerous subjects we have evaluated who previously have had many food skin tests applied and then have restricted diets prescribed based upon the skin testing without actually having challenged the importance of those foods in the production of symptoms. Except for the first group, parents and children who have been subjected to diets based upon vague associations are often confused and frustrated. Depending upon the status of the asthma control, they vacillate between strict adherence to the diet and liberal ingestion of incriminated foods without being comfortable with either approach. Children with asthma are subjected to enough restrictions in their lifestyles without also being victims of haphazard dietary recommendations.

Review of 367 children who came to the National Jewish Center with the chief complaint of asthma revealed that 257 (70%) had a history of specific foods being associated with the initiation of asthma symptoms. Of these 257, 163 (63%) had some symptom produced during positive double-blind placebo-controlled food challenges (DBPCFC). Fifty-seven of 257 children (22%) with these positive DBPCFCs exhibited wheezing as one of the symptoms. Five of 257 patients (2%) had wheezing as the only symptom. Another 203 children underwent DBPCFC because of a history of food-associated symptoms in whom wheezing was not suspected of being precipitated by food ingestion. Six (3%) of these 203 children had wheezing as one of the elicited symptoms, but in 5 of 6 the wheezing was quite mild. None of these children had wheezing as the only symptom elicited.

Thus, one can see that wheezing is commonly attributed to food ingestion but much less frequently proven to be caused by food ingestion. Wheezing produced during DBPCFC rarely occurs in children without asthma.

Other investigators have found results similar to those cited above: that asthma as the sole manifestation of a food hypersensitivity reaction is uncommon. Furthermore, even in conjunction with other symptoms, wheezing has not been a frequent finding during properly controlled food challenges. Onorato et al. began with a clinic population of 300 patients, adults and children (4). Of this entire group only six subjects had asthma during a food challenge and all six of these were children (age range, 4–17 years). Three of the six had a reaction to at least one food in which wheezing was the only symptom, while in the other three patients skin or gastrointestinal symptoms accompanied the wheezing. Wheezing was triggered by egg, wheat, and corn.

Novembre et al. studied 140 children using DPBCFC to confirm asthma elicited by food ingestion (5). Asthma occurred in eight children (age range, 2–9 years) but only one child was reported to have wheezing as the sole symptom.

Sampson has published several studies covering different aspects of the patients with atopic dermatitis whom he has investigated (6–10). In each of his studies some of his patients have exhibited respiratory symptoms as well as skin symptoms during their positive DBPCFCs. The number of patients experiencing wheezing during challenge in these studies has been about 20%. These patients, like those in investigated at the National Jewish Center, have had other respiratory symptoms in addition to wheezing. Many in both groups have had gastrointestional symptoms. Burks also reported respiratory symptoms including wheezing in some of this DBPCFC-positive patients with atopic dermatitis (11). Host and Samuelsson challenged five children with multiple cow milk preparations and provoked wheezing in addition to other symptoms in some (12).

Although this is less common, children and adults have been reported to wheeze following inhalation of foods. This has been best documented in adults with occupational diseases such as baker's asthma and in seafood workers. In some of these subjects the food may be ingested without problem but when the food is inhaled, symptoms are produced. The situation in children seems to be somewhat different and has been less well characterized. A few of the youngsters we have evaluated reportedly wheeze when they ingest the incriminated food and/or inhale it. It is not easy to document the latter observation using blinded methodology. This phenomenon has been reported most often with the inhalation of wheat flour. Wheat flour is easily suspended in air and therefore may provoke airway obstruction by inhalation as well as by ingestion. We tend to discount the frequency which parents report wheezing in their asthmatic children when "someone opens a jar of peanut butter." We have tested the "open peanut butter jar" hypothesis in a blinded fashion and have been unable to reproduce any symptoms with the open jar directly behind the child. On the other hand, some children have such marked aversions to foods to which they are allergic that merely seeing the food is likely to precipitate bronchospasm.

## ONSET OF SYMPTOMS

It has been commonly reported by patients that wheezing reactions due to foods develop hours to days after ingestion as well as within minutes of food consumption. Invariably these histories of delayed reactions seem to grow more vague as the time from ingestion to onset of wheezing increases. In the studies using DBPCFC cited above (1–12), one finds that the only confirmed reactions occurred within minutes to hours except for a few of the patients reported by Hill et al. (13). Since Hill's subjects represent a somewhat different segment of the population (younger age) than subjects reported by other authors, and since many of his subjects have been studied openly, although under observation, these data need to be confirmed by other investigators.

It is worth noting that late-phase reactions in the lung (i.e., the biphasic reaction after food challenge) that have so often been noted following allergen inhalation challenge have not been unequivocally reported after food ingestion. Although some authors have claimed that late-phase reactions can be produced following food ingestion, these observations have not been rigorously tested using controlled challenges and unbiased observations. We have triggered an asthmatic reaction exhibiting a biphasic pattern in a young adult reacting to a DBPCFC with cottonseed protein (14). However, treatment with bronchodilators was administered after the immediate onset of symptoms and this phenomenon was observed in only a single subject. Further work needs to be undertaken in this area because one would suspect that late-phase reactions should be found following food reactions.

## MECHANISMS

At present only IgE has been strongly associated with the food-induced production of wheezing. Perusal of the studies cited above reveals that the vast majority of children reacting to foods during DBPCFC had a positive skin test. Unfortunately this does not prove that IgE-mediated release of mediators is the responsible biochemical mechanism. Nevertheless, the presence of IgE as detected by skin testing, radioallergosorbent assay (RAST), enzyme-linked immunosorbent assay (ELISA), or leukocyte histamine release in association with DBPCFC-induced symptoms is strong associative support for the notion that IgE plays a significant role in the production of these symptoms. Perhaps further research will demonstrate that IgE is necessary but not sufficient for the production of food-induced immediate hypersensitivity reactions. Many children who lose their clinical reactivity over time continue to have IgE demonstrable in skin or serum, which we have termed asymptomatic hypersensitivity.

Some adverse reactions to foods appear to involve the immune system and are either not IgE mediated or IgE may be playing an as yet unidentified role in the process. The best studied of these reactions are the enteropathies (gluten-sensitive enteropathy, cow milk and soy protein enteropathies). This group of illnesses does not involve the lung. A rare and less well-characterized syndrome that does involve the lung is chronic lower respiratory disease associated with antibodies to cow's milk in the serum. This illness, known as Heiner's syndrome, has been reported with varying consistency (15). Infants with this illness exhibit pulmonary infiltrates and pulmonary hemosiderosis. They present with anemia, failure to thrive, and chronic lung disease. Hemosiderin-laden macrophages have been found in the gastric material aspirated from the stomach and in lung biopsy specimens. The detection of precipitating antibodies to cow's milk led the original investigators to remove cow's milk from the diet, following which they noticed an improvement in the lung condition of their subjects. Our understanding of this condition would be improved if these youngsters were subjected to more systematic and prolonged observation to determine the true role of cow milk proteins and to determine whether other food proteins can produce chronic pulmonary changes in children with "idiopathic" lung disease.

## DIFFERENTIAL DIAGNOSIS

The differential diagnosis (Table 1) of food hypersensitivity as it pertains to the lung constitutes a shorter list than when considerations of adverse reactions to food include skin and gastrointestinal manifestations. Conditions such as lactose intolerance and food intoxication do not involve chest

TABLE 1 Differential Diagnosis of Adverse Reactions to Foods Affecting the Lung

| |
|---|
| Hypersensitivity/allergy (immune system involvement) |
| Psychological reactions (strongly held beliefs) |
| Pulmonary infiltrates with hemosiderosis, precipitating antibodies to milk (Heiner's syndrome) |

symptoms. Asthma as it may be precipitated by food and Heiner's syndrome has been mentioned above. The major remaining chest symptom that may be associated with or attributed to food ingestion is chronic cough without evidence of airway obstruction. Allergic cough due to food has not been easily demonstrated. In the studies undertaken, cough triggered by food ingestion is usually accompanied by wheezing and measurable airway obstruction indicating asthma. We have seen patients with chronic cough who were thought to have asthma who have had a tic or habit blamed on food. In these children the cause of the cough is psychological. These patients are often difficult to diagnose and treat because the patient and family members are often very attached to the notion that food is the culprit.

## EVALUATION

### History

The most important component of the evaluation of any patient complaining of an adverse reaction to food is the DBPCFC (16). To undertake a challenge, the history (Table 2) must be obtained in a precise and detailed manner. Usually in medicine the detailed history establishes the diagnosis but in subjects complaining of food allergy the history is used to design the food challenge. For each food the following information must be ob-

TABLE 2 History to be Obtained from a Patient Complaining of Asthma Due to Food

| |
|---|
| Description of symptoms |
| Timing from ingestion to onset of symptoms |
| Quantity of food required to produce symptoms |
| Most recent occurrence |
| Approximate number of occurrences |
| Associated symptoms |

tained. First the patient is asked to describe the symptoms precipitated by the food. Then he or she is asked about the timing between ingestion and onset of symptoms. The least amount of food that has recently triggered symptoms is determined so that a starting dosage for challenge may be chosen. The characteristics of the most recent reaction and its proximity to the present are especially important. If the history of reaction is in the distant past, it is useful to try and determine whether the patient has been accidentally ingesting the food in some hidden fashion, thus obviating the need for any further evaluation.

### Laboratory Testing

Various methods of testing have been used to identify more precisely subjects with true food hypersensitivity. Despite many studies in many different centers, no one has yet found an in vivo or in vitro test capable of replacing the blinded food challenge. However, a number of studies have found that detection of IgE can be useful in directing the evaluation of children who complain of adverse reactions to foods (17–19). Despite many attempts to replace the skin test, it remains the most cost-effective method by which to detect food protein antibodies of the IgE class. Properly applied and interpreted prick/puncture skin tests using verified extracts efficiently identify patients with food-specific IgE. This information is then used to determine which subjects need blinded challenges and which subjects should undergo open challenges with little chance of either a positive reaction or a severe reaction. Studies by both Sampson and our center have shown that allergy skin tests have a high negative predictive accuracy; that is, when skin tests are negative, children rarely exhibited symptoms during objective food challenges (1–3,6–11,17–19). By contrast, the positive skin test *only detects* the presence of antibody and therefore the positive predictive accuracy is not very high, especially for some foods commonly incriminated in the production of adverse food reactions.

The RAST assay is nearly equivalent in sensitivity to the skin test for the detection of IgE but it has not been found to be quite as sensitive as the skin test and is much more expensive and therefore not nearly as cost-effective (19). RAST should be reserved for special circumstances in which skin tests cannot be performed. Rare patients will have such severe atopic dermatitis that their skin cannot be ameliorated sufficiently for skin testing to be undertaken. We have skin tested many children with a history of food anaphylaxis using the prick/puncture test without ever triggering a severe systemic reaction. RAST testing in many laboratories may be subject to problems of quality control. In patients with *elevated total IgE* and *elevated specific IgG* to the food protein sought, the reported levels may be inaccurate. It is crucial for the physician requesting this test to be familiar with the laboratory in order to avoid these pitfalls. Measurement of leukocyte histamine release suffers from similar limitation.

Most other tests used for the diagnosis of food hypersensitivity have never been properly correlated with blinded food challenges, although some detect biochemically significant compounds. This is true of the immune complexes formed between food proteins and antibodies and also of IgG4 antibodies to food proteins. Although both of these tests may eventually prove useful, at present they should be regarded as experimental. Other tests such as the cytotoxic food test and applied kinesiology for the diagnosis of food hypersensitivity should not be used. Dilution–titration skin testing for the diagnosis of food hypersensitivity has likewise never been confirmed as having scientific validity and should not be used at all except under experimental protocols to investigate its place in this field.

A number of other techniques are under investigation in the development stage at university centers.

## Food Challenges

Only one test unequivocally determines whether a patient is having an adverse reaction to a food, no matter what the mechanism: DBPCFC (16). This procedure was first systematically applied to food allergy by May (1) and has been described in a number of publications by authors at a number of institutions (1–12). Although often disparaged, it has been found to be very useful by investigators and clinicians alike when its use has been assiduously pursued.

A complete description of the procedure is beyond the scope of this chapter, but a few important comments about DBPCFC must be made. Of the available challenge procedures in allergy, it is the only one that actually reproduces the natural exposure that patients experience. For this reason the results are unequivocal in the vast majority of situations. Because asthma is an illness subject to emotional influences, challenges must be administered blindly and a placebo must be used. It is not necessary in all situations for the challenge to be double-blind, but single-blind challenges are subject to bias by the observer, whose bias may influence the patient. It is fortunate that most children do not believe that they are allergic to foods and thus their natural bias is less apt to influence the interpretation of the results than is the bias of adults. In general, children believe they are not allergic to foods until proven otherwise, whereas the converse seems to be the case in adults.

With older children it is particularly important and illuminating to garner their opinion about the purported reaction in their parents' absence. Children often acquiesce to their parents' opinion about the negative effect of certain food when in the presence of their parents. However, the action of these children when they are with their peers or alone is often contrary to the parents' opinion, but is usually correct.

Any number of vehicles have been used to hide or disguise foods and the possibilities are only limited by the imagination of the people arranging the challenge. About one new vehicle is introduced into our center each year based upon the need to overcome the resistance of recalcitrant subjects. Table 3 lists a number of vehicles used for food challenge at our center and at others. Challenges may be administered in clinical research centers, clinics, hospital emergency rooms, and doctors' offices. Although challenges of anaphylactically sensitive subjects garners a great deal of attention, most physicians who undertake food challenges are usually testing vague or mild symptoms and refute far more histories than they confirm. Challenges are administered by starting with a small amount of the incriminated food and then having the patient ingest incrementally increasing amounts at intervals suggested by the history. Spirometry is measured before the procedure begins and after each challenge. If the spirometry decreases by 15–20% or if other symptoms appear, the challenge is discontinued and is interpreted as being positive. If the challenge is negative up to 8 g of dried food (40–60 g of wet food) when ingested in a single dose, the food is ingested openly by the patient who has first been told that the DBPCFC has been negative. The procedure is not complete until it has been demonstrated that the suspect food can be ingested in usual portions prepared in a usual fashion. Food challenges should be administered with the same precautions undertaken for patients receiving allergy injections, specifically in the presence of a physician and with emergency treatment available in the very unlikely event of a marked systemic reaction. In more than 2000 food challenges in various settings we have needed to administer emergency treatment to patients during less than 10 challenges. This remarkable safety record is due to the precautions taken, the use of incremental challenges, and the presence of excellent nursing personnel to monitor the challenges.

TABLE 3 Vehicles Used in Food Challenges

| | |
|---|---|
| Capsules | Hamburger |
| Infant formulas | Tuna fish |
| Applesauce | Popsicles |
| Milk shakes | Tapioca–fruit mixture |
| Grape juice | Lentil soup |
| Grape-flavored ice cream | |

## MANAGEMENT

### Avoidance

At this time the management of food hypersensitivity is avoidance of the offending food and regular reintroduction by challenge. Because avoidance is the only treatment that is really effective in persons with food hypersensitivity it is very important that all food culprits be confirmed as rigorously as possible so that the child is on the least stringent elimination diet possible.

Natural history studies have illustrated that children "outgrow" their food hypersensitivity reactions with regularity when the foods involved are egg, milk, soy, and wheat. Allergic reactions to peanuts seem to be more likely to persist. Because the rate of loss of food hypersensitivity may be as much as 25–30% per year for many foods, it is crucial that prolonged elimination diets lasting for years be avoided so that children and their families do not have to endure the endless strain that accompanies these diets. Regular reintroduction of the food should be done using blinded food challenges as described. These interval challenges are easy to perform with the results of the original challenge used as a guide to starting dosage, incremental increase, timing between doses, and expected symptoms (20–22).

There are currently no data on the natural history of food hypersensitivity specifically examining children whose only symptom is wheezing due to food ingestion. However, guidelines used for interval challenges from the extant studies may be applied to the patients discussed in this chapter. Although different authors propose varying recommendations, certain general intervals may be recommended. For young children with equivocal or mild reactions, the suspect food may be reintroduced in 1–3 months. If the second challenge is positive, an interval of 3–6 months is reasonable. For more severe reactions and depending upon the age of the child, the food challenge should occur 6–12 months after the initial reaction. For severe or anaphylactic reactions, the challenge may be repeated every 1–2 years until it is clear that the problem is resolving or that it appears likely to be lifelong. One may reasonably ask why patients with a history of anaphylaxis should be challenged at all. The answer is that we do know that some children do outgrow their anaphylactic reactions (23). Since we do not know with certainty which children will lose which food hypersensitivity reactions, and because we do know that the majority of children with food hypersensitivity do have food-induced accidents, it seems reasonable to arrange for them to have their reactions under supervision in a safe setting. It is most gratifying to both parents and physicians when it is observed that a youngster is no longer having serious reactions to a food that has long been under careful scrutiny. These problems cause considerable anxiety for parents and lead to social problems for both parents and their children. We may hope that someday we will have a test to predict whether symptomatic hypersensitivity is abating or persisting.

## Medication

Three classes of medication have been used to treat children with food hypersensitivity: corticosteroids, antihistamines, and disodium cromoglycate. Corticosteroids are often required to treat children with asthma but have never been shown even in these children to have a significant impact on the food-induced wheezing or urticaria that occur during food hypersensitivity reactions. At present they should be reserved for use in children with food-induced gastrointestinal reactions of a severe nature, such as eosinophilic gastroenteropathy with protein loss and growth failure.

Antihistamines have never been systematically studied as a preventive treatment for food hypersensitivity for respiratory or other symptoms and should be regarded as a probably ineffective and currently experimental. Over the years we have administered food challenges to some children while they were taking antihistamines and they had reactions to the foods despite the medication. These studies have not been specifically undertaken in children with only food-induced asthma.

Disodium cromoglycate (DSCG) has been studied in a number of centers as a preventive measure for food hypersensitivity. However, very few of these studies have been properly controlled and many of the patients in these studies were not proven to have food hypersensitivity before the treatment was administered. The best controlled study to date (10) did not show DSCG to be effective for the prevention of food-induced atopic dermatitis. In our center some children have been studied while receiving inhaled DSCG and it did not prevent their food-induced asthmatic reactions. However, a study examining the effect of both inhaled and oral DSCG might be useful if there were more subjects with pure food-hypersensitivity-induced asthma to evaluate. At this time the oral form of DSCG should be viewed as an experimental treatment for asthma due to food hypersensitivity and should only be administered under experimental protocols.

Injection therapy has never been shown to be effective for the prevention of food-induced asthma during controlled trials and should be viewed as an experimental treatment worthy of study but only under properly controlled protocols in approved trials. This is a treatment whose time may come, but its current use in large numbers of patients, most of whom do not have food hypersensitivity, is to be deplored.

## NATURAL HISTORY AND PREVENTION

The natural history of food hypersensitivity has two aspects: the development of food-induced symptoms and the loss of reactivity as the child grows. The latter aspect has been covered above with regard to clinical observations and attempts to evaluate the process systematically. At this time there does not appear to be any effective way to accelerate the loss of clinical food hypersensitivity unless studies demonstrate that avoidance for specified intervals of time really does hasten the loss of the problem. At present we really do not understand what it means biologically for a youngster to "outgrow" food hypersensitivity.

The development of food hypersensitivity is also poorly understood at present. However, there is a large and growing body of work examining whether dietary and environmental manipulations can prevent or delay the onset of atopy and, probably most importantly, asthma. Detailed review and analysis of this subject would require a chapter devoted solely to this subject and many of the studies do not specifically examine, in a critical manner, whether these children develop asthma. Also, many of the studies suffer from serious methodologic problems. This has been critically and excellently reviewed by Zeiger, and his group has performed one of the best controlled studies on the subject (24,25). One may summarize the extant work by noting that very few if any children have been shown, during controlled trials, to have had the probable development of asthma prevented by dietary manipulation. It is possible that some youngsters have the onset of their asthma delayed by dietary alterations during infancy but this too has not been definitively demonstrated.

## CONSIDERATIONS FOR THE FUTURE

The critical reader of this chapter will have noted numerous lacunae in our present knowledge of this subject. Many of these areas are under active study and others will be in the future. One important area continues to be observation of the various symptoms. As noted earlier, the frequency of food-hypersensitivity-induced asthma seems to be quite low. Of the hundreds of children challenged in controlled settings with food, even children with asthma, elicitation of wheezing has been infrequent. It is important to try to continue to confirm or refute this observation. Efforts aimed at the total prevention of asthma by dietary manipulation of infant diet and other means are continuing. We must learn more about the mechanism of food-induced asthma; what mediators and cells are involved; if there is a late-phase reaction; and whether the airway reactivity changes after a positive reaction as occurs with inhaled allergen. At present, despite claims to the contrary, controlled studies have not been able to identify late or delayed (many hours or days) onset of symptoms after food challenge; however, it is important for investigators and clinicians to continue to evaluate critically and examine rigorously these claims in properly controlled studies. Finally, we need better treatment other than avoidance for those children with asthma induced by food hypersensitivity. Several centers around the world are now developing experimental protocols to treat food-allergic patients whose lifestyle is significantly altered by their food allergy and for whom ingestion of forbidden foods would make their lives immeasurably better. We can only hope that these studies will shed light on the mechanism of food hypersensitivity and identify a safe and effective treatment.

## REFERENCES

1. May CD. Objective clinical and laboratory studies of immediate hypersensitivity reactions to foods in children. *J Allergy Clin Immunol* 58:500–515, 1976.
2. Bock SA, Lee WY, Remigio LK, May CD. Studies of hypersensitivity reactions to foods in infants and children. *J Allergy Clin Immunol* 62:327–334, 1978.
3. Bock SA, Atkins FM. Patterns of food hypersensitivity during sixteen years of double-blind placebo-controlled food challenges. *J Pediatr* 86:387–392, 1990.
4. Onorato J, Merland N, Terral C, Michel FB, Bousquet J. Placebo-controlled double-blind food challenge in asthma. *J Allergy Clin Immunol* 78:1139–1146, 1986.
5. Novembre E, de Martino M, Vierucci A. Foods and respiratory allergy. *J Allergy Clin Immunol* 81:1059–1065, 1988
6. Sampson HA. Role of immediate food hypersensivity in the pathogenesis of atopic dermatitis. *J Allergy Clin Immunol* 71:473–480, 1983.
7. Sampson HA, Jolie PL. Increased plasma histamine concentrations after food challenges in children with atopic dermatitis. *N Engl J Med* 311:372–376, 1984.
8. Sampson HA, McCaskill CC. Food hypersensitivity and atopic dermatitis: evaluation of 113 patients. *J Pediatr* 107:669–675, 1985.
9. Sampson HA, IgE-mediated food intolerance. *J Allergy Clin Immunol* 81:495–504, 1988.
10. Burks AW, Sampson HA. Double-blind placebo-controlled trial of oral cromolyn in children with atopic dermatitis and documented food hypersensitivity. *J Allergy Clin Immunol* 81:417–423, 1988.
11. Burks AW, Mallory SB, Williams LW, Shirrell MA. Atopic dermatitis: clinical relevance of food hypersensitivity reactions. *J Pediatr* 113:447–451, 1988.
12. Host A, Samuelsson, EG. Allergic reactions to raw, pasteurized, and homogenized/pasteurized cow milk: a comparison. *Allergy* 43:113–118, 1988.
13. Hill DJ, Shelton MJ, Hosking CS. Manifestations of milk allergy in infancy: clinical and immunologic findings. *J Pediatr* 109:270–276, 1986.

14. Atkins FM, Wilson M, Bock SA. Cottonseed hypersensitivity: new concerns over an old problem. *J Allergy Clin Immunol* 82:242–250, 1988.
15. Heiner DC, Sears JW, Kniker WT. Multiple precipitins to cow's milk in chronic respiratory disease. *Am J Dis Child* 103:634–654, 1962.
16. Bock SA, Sampson HA, Atkins FM, Zeiger RS, Lehrer S, Sachs M, Bush RK, Metcalfe DD. Double-blind placebo-controlled food challenge (DBPCFC) as an office procedure: a manual. *J Allergy Clin Immunol* 82:986–997, 1988.
17. Bock SA, Buckley J, Holst A, May CD. Proper use of skin tests with food extracts in diagnosis of hypersensitivity to food in children. *Clin Allergy* 7:375–383, 1977.
18. Bock SA, Lee WY, Remigio LK, May CD. Appraisal of skin tests with food extracts for diagnosis of food hypersensitivity. *Clin Allergy* 8:559–564, 1978.
19. Sampson HA, Albergo R. Comparison of results of skin test, RAST and double-blind placebo-controlled food challenges in children with atopic dermatitis. *J Allergy Clin Immunol* 74:26–33, 1984.
20. Bock SA. The natural history of food hypersensitivity. *J Allergy Clin Immunol* 69:173–177, 1982.
21. Bock SA, Atkins FM. The natural history of peanut allergy. *J Allergy Clin Immunol* 83:900–904, 1989.
22. Sampson HA, Scanlon S. Natural history of food hypersensitivity in children with atopic dermatitis. *J Pediatr* 115:23–27, 1989.
23. Bock SA. Natural history of severe reactions to food in young children. *J Pediatr* 107:676–680, 1985.
24. Zeiger RS. Development and prevention of allergic disease in childhood. In:Middleton E, Reed CE, Ellis EF, Adkinson NF, Yunginger JW (eds.), *Allergy: Principles and Practice*. C.V. Mosby, St. Louis, pp. 930–968, 1988.
25. Zeiger RS, Heller S, Mellon MH, Forsythe AB, O'Connor RD, Hamburger RN, Schatz M. Effect of combined maternal and infant food-allergen avoidance on development of atopy in early infancy: a randomized study. *J Allergy Clin Immunol* 84:72–89, 1989.

# 20

# Psychological Impact of Childhood Asthma

**THOMAS L. CREER**

*Ohio University*
*Athens, Ohio*

References to asthma occur thoughout history (1). Potential relationships between psychological factors and asthma have been debated during the entire period, although arguments have generated considerable heat and little resolution. The reason for the debate is not to deny that psychological factors are involved in childhood asthma; no one seriously questions this assumption since there is too much prima facie evidence to that suggest interactions exist between psychological or behavioral factors and asthma. The debate heats up in attempting to describe the exact nature of these relationships and interactions. Inflammation of the argument occurs primarily because of two major factors. First, many investigators, particularly behavioral scientists, fail to recognize the heterogeneity and complexity of factors involved in the pathogenesis, course, and manifestations of asthma. Busse and Reed (2) suggest that the disorder involves a complex interaction of genetic, environmental, psychosocial, physiological, and molecular biological factors. The exact contribution of each set of variables, let alone the delineation of the role of relationships between and among variables to either a specific patient's asthma or to a given attack, is beyond our knowledge. Second, many investigators claim the existence of causal relationships between variables thought to affect asthma and the disorder itself. The search for causal links has proven elusive; there is no evidence to suggest that the quest will change to any degree in the foreseeable future. Nevertheless, it is too great a temptation to many investigators who, despite their stated intentions in describing their research, gradually slip into describing "links" between variables and, eventually to describe events "causing" other events.

## LEVELS OF EXPERIMENTATION

The function of science is the search for general laws to explain the empirical events the scientist is investigating. According to Braithwaite (3), science should allow us to synthesize information concerning separate events and to make reliable predictions about future events. To do so, we rely upon the scientific method. The method is composed of four cyclical steps that may be executed repeatedly to solve a scientific problem (4): observing a phenomena; formulating tentative explanations or statements of cause and effect; further observing or experimenting to rule out alternative interpretations; and revising and refining the explanations. In describing research on the relationships of psychological variables to childhood asthma, it is pertinent to consider three levels of research: demonstration, correlation, and experimental (5). The most basic, demonstration, provides an empirical statement of the "if . . . then" variety for single values of the variables in question. Demonstration is important in science, observe Johnston and Pennypacker (5), because it often reveals the operation of a process or procedure that has not been fully defined and quantified. No controlled experimental manipulations are involved, and demonstration fails to explain fully the phenomenon in question. In this paradigm, events are seen as associated with other events. Demonstration has provided valuable insights into the mechanisms underlying asthma, including Sir John Floyer's description of exercise-induced asthma (1). As will be noted, it has not generated similar insights into the relationship of psychological or behavioral variables and asthma.

The second level of scientific research, correlation, requires the identification and measurement of multiple values of the variables being investigated (5). From such information, statements such as "when X occurs, Y occurs," can be made and tested for accuracy. Repeated observation and confirmation of a particular correlation permit speculation about the probable mechanism relating the two sets of observations. Johnston and Pennypacker (5) point out that "the utility of the correlational approach is directly proportional to the precision and sensitivity of the measurement involved because the form of experimentation consists solely of measurements" (p. 26). This form of experimentation has produced much of our knowledge of the relationship between psychological or behavioral variables and asthma (6), as well as medical knowledge about the disorder.

A final type of research (experimental or functional relation) is a refinement of a "co-relation" in that two classes of variables—independent and dependent—are involved (5). An independent variable is one that exists independently of asthma or asthma-related phenomena; its presence in no way depends upon the dependent variable. The existence of the dependent variable, on the other hand, depends on the influence exerted by the independent variable. For example, in confirming asthma, a methacholine challenge might be used. Methacholine is the independent variable; the measurable change in respiration that occurs with inhalation of methacholine is the dependent variable. Johnston and Pennypacker (5) note that a functional relation "is a quantitative statement of the dependent relation between two types of variables, usually expressed as $y = f(x)$ where x is the independent variable or argument of the function and y is the dependent variable" (p. 27). Demonstrating functional relations requires a specific mode of experimentation; the independent variable must be manipulated or controlled, (e.g., administering methacholine) and the resulting impact on the dependent variable observed, (e.g., assessing respiratory responses). It is difficult to demonstrate a functional relation with respect to psychological factors or behavior associated with asthma, although there is experimental evidence that certain behaviors are functionally related to asthma (6).

The brief description of the three types of experimental paradigms provides an outline of the research described in the remainder of the chapter. It furnishes a framework for discussing studies on the interaction of psychological or behavioral factors to asthma, as well providing the reader with a conceptual basis for considering the merit of any given investigation.

## DEMONSTRATION RESEARCH

Demonstration resembles an experiment but lacks the features of a true experiment, namely an experimental design (4). In childhood asthma, demonstration research has generally taken the form of anecdotal reports. Demonstration research can be useful in that it may provide topics that might be of interest in a formal investigation. However, demonstrations do not show causal relationships. Demonstration research and childhood asthma will be illustrated by briefly describing three types of research based on psychoanalytic theory, parentectomy, and learning factors.

### Psychoanalytic Theory

Thomas French and Franz Alexander were psychoanalysts who worked together at the Chicago Institute of Psychoanalysis. Their monograph on psychogenic factors in 1941 (7) had a major impact upon research on childhood asthma. They offered four observations based upon a review of the anecdotes of other writers and their personal experience with 27 asthmatic patients; these conclusions were that asthmatic patients are subject to a universal conflict between an infantile dependent attachment to their mothers and other emotional attitudes (especially sexual–genital wishes) that are incompatible with and threaten such a dependent attitude; asthma attacks are related to a suppressed cry by the patient for his or her mother; the asthmatic patient has a unique personality; and psychotherapy, particularly psychoanalysis, will alleviate their symptoms. Later, Alexander (8) expanded upon these premises by proposing the nuclear conflict theory. The theory holds that each psychophysiological disorder is associated with certain unconscious emotional conflicts. This hypothesis is based on the belief that an individual's repressed psychic energy can be discharged directly to affect the autonomic nervous system, leading to an impairment of body functions. Using asthma as an example, DiMatteo (9) pointed out that asthma is believed to be caused by unresolved dependency needs, particularly with respect to a child's mother. The obstruction that defines asthma is "believed to *be*, not just to be *like*, a suppressed cry for the mother as a reaction to the threat of separation" (9, p. 288).

French and Alexander stimulated considerable research in the three decades following publication of their monograph (7). Scientific findings have, however, repudiated their basic observations (with the exception of their first premise, which, like most tenets of psychoanalysis, is untestable). For example, despite a large number of investigations directed towards the topic, no one has found a personality pattern unique to children with asthma (10–12). The effect of psychoanalysis in improving symptoms of asthma has never been demonstrated (10–12), nor has the hypothesis that asthma is a repressed cry for a child's mother. In investigating the relationship between crying and asthma, Purcell (13) reported that many children realized crying triggered their asthma; hence, they made every effort to avoid crying and, in turn, the provocation of asthma. Two legacies remain from the monograph by French and Alexander (7). The first is that despite evidence to the contrary, many behavioral scientists still present the theory proposed by French and Alexander as if it were valid (e.g., 9). In many instances, failure to abandon the theory in the face of contradictory data has served to impede collaboration between behavioral and medical or biological scientists. Second, the work of French and Alexander (7) served to create and perpetuate many myths about childhood asthma; as noted in the earlier edition of this book (14), this sadly remains the major legacy of the work by French and Alexander (7).

## Parentectomy

In 1930, M. Murray Peshkin (15) appealed for the creation of a residential treatment center for children with intractable asthma. His plea was based on his observations of 41 children with the disorder. Of these youngsters, 23 of 25 who had been absent from home for periods extending from 2 months to more than a year experienced remission of their asthma during the time they were away from their families. No improvement was observed, however, in 16 children with asthma of equal severity who remained at home. Peshkin labeled the process of separating asthmatic children from their parents "parentectomy," an approach to the treatment of childhood asthma he championed for the remainder of his life (16).

As a consequence of Peshkin's appeal, a residential treatment facility for children with asthma was established in 1940 at what was called the Jewish National Home for Asthmatic Children. The name of the facility was subsequently changed to the Children's Asthma Research Institute and Hospital (CARIH) and, later, to the National Asthma Center; it was generally referred to as CARIH or the "Home" until the facility was closed and demolished in 1981. During the early days of its existence, data were gathered at CARIH that supported Peshkin's hypothesis of the therapeutic role of parentectomy. Peshkin (17) presented data indicating that 98% of the youngsters treated at CARIH between 1953 and 1955, irrespective of age, sex, and duration of illness, experienced a complete remission of their asthmatic symptoms. These gains, he continued, were maintained when the children returned home. The significance of the finding was short-lived, however, in that from 1958 to 1959 complete remission of asthma was noted in only 28% of children admitted to CARIH (18). By 1969, Falliers (18) further reported that the number of youngsters showing complete remission of their asthma symptoms with admission to CARIH declined to 12%. The number of these children, labeled *rapid remitters*, declined even more in the years that followed. This was reflected during the final decade of its existence when the term rapid remitter almost disappeared from the vocabulary of the CARIH staff; there simply were no residents who fit the label (19).

The question can be asked: Why did the asthma of children later admitted to CARIH fail to remit when rapid remission was common in the early days of the facility? Renne and Creer (12) suggest a number of reasons, but three are prominent. First, children with more severe asthma were admitted to the facility; as noted by Falliers (18), the number of rapid-remitting children was inversely related to the number of steroid-dependent youngsters admitted to CARIH. Second, it is questionable whether the children whose asthma rapidly remitted actually had the disorder according to the more stringent criteria for diagnosing asthma that developed over the course of CARIH's history. It would be unlikely, speculated Renne and Creer (12), that many of the rapid remitters would be diagnosed as having asthma if verification were based on a methacholine challenge. Finally, Renne and Creer (12) suggested that many of the children who exhibited asthma that rapidly disappeared upon their admission to CARIH may have acquired learned respiratory responses that mimicked asthma. This explanation by no means weakens the findings of Peshkin (15–17); rather, it suggests a more appropriate mechanism for the phenomenon of rapid remitters.

## Learning Factors

Parallel with research that tested psychoanalysis and parentectomy, the period was rife with investigations spurred by learning theory. Of the hundreds of studies that emerged during the first half of the century, one fact seemed clear: two kinds of learning, classic conditioning and operant conditioning, occur. Classic conditioning, emanating from the work of Pavlov (20), involved pairing an unconditioned stimulus (UCS) known to produce an unconditioned reaction (UCR) with a neutral stimulus that failed to produce a similar response. Through repeated pairings of the UCS and the neutral stimulus, an association was formed so that with presentation of the once neutral stimulus, now referred to as a conditioned stimulus (CS), there was a conditioned response (CR) similar to but not identical to the UCR elicited by the UCS. This type of conditioning, formed by pairing a UCS with what becomes a CS, could account for respiratory changes acquired through learning. In operant conditioning, introduced by Skinner (21), the emphasis is upon the stimulus or response that follows a response emitted by the organism. Since the association is between the emitted behavior and the stimulus or response that follows it, a stimulus or class of stimuli, referred to as a discriminative stimulus or discriminative stimuli, may set the occasion for the emission of operant behavior.

It was speculated as late as the 1960s that operant conditioning played no role in the acquisition or maintenance of learned respiratory behaviors (22). Two developments occurred in the next two decades, however. First, the distinction between operant and classic conditioning became blurred. It was gradually recognized that respondent and operant behaviors represent a continuum along which the probability varies that a particular response will be produced by a particular stimulus (23). Second, it became apparent that building grand theories to account for learning produced disillusionment; such theories were conceived to account for all learning with a simple set of principles, but they became increasingly fragmented over time (24). As a result, learning theory is no longer as powerful an impetus for conducting research as it once was. Similar disillusionment occurred with respect to theorizing about psychological factors and asthma: only a few comprehensive theories involving emotional reactions and the autonomic system have been put forward to account for asthma in recent years (e.g., 25 and 26). It was noted in the earlier edition of this book (14) that it was unlikely that such theories would stimulate research to any extent; this statement remains true today.

In the past two decades, a literature on patients who present learned respiratory behaviors has accumulated. This literature is based upon observations of the behaviors of patients; hence, it represents demonstration research. The behaviors often mimic symptoms of asthma, but are probably the result of some combination of classic and operant conditioning principles. Examples of such behavior in patients include sneezing (27–28), coughing (29–30), and wheezing (31–33). To many physicians, these symptoms represent full-blown asthma attacks; therefore, the episodes are treated in a manner similar to genuine attacks. There are two differences between asthma and learned responses, however. First, asthma can be dismissed as the correct diagnosis when a thorough medical examination, sometimes involving a bronchial challenge, is performed and negative results are obtained. Second, learned respiratory behaviors may be altered through application of a variety of behavioral and psychological techniques including positive reinforcement (30), negative reinforcement (29), punishment (27), and counseling (31). Since learned respiratory responses represent a pattern that can be misdiagnosed as asthma, it is of importance to physicians; it is likely, for example, that patients who experienced a rapid remission of asthma-like symptoms with a change in their environment possibly exhibited learned respiratory behaviors (11). Removal from positive reinforcement resulted in extinction of the symptoms; this is an explanation for the success of parentectomy with so many patients. At the same time, the fact that learned respiratory responses are altered by psychological procedures reaffirms that the condition is not asthma.

## CORRELATIONAL RESEARCH

Bordens and Abbott (4) point out that in correlational research the main interest of the scientist is to determine whether variables covary and, if so, to establish the direction of the observed relationship. Establishing that a correlation exists between two variables permits scientists to predict from the value of one variable the probable value of the other variable. The variable used to predict is called the predictor variable; the variable whose value is being predicted is called the criterion variable. Bordens and Abbott (4) caution that while predictor and criterion variables are analogous to independent and dependent variables, there is an important difference: whereas you can establish with a certain confidence whether an independent variable *causes* change in a dependent variable, you can only show that predictor variables *predict* changes in criterion variables.

Creer and Kotses (6) observed that much of our current knowledge of the relationship of psychological or behavioral factors to asthma is correlational in nature. This is reflected in investigations on behavioral stimuli correlated with the precipitation of asthma attacks, as well as behavioral and psychological consequences of the disorder. Correlational research is represented in two areas of research: psychological or behavioral side effects of asthma drugs and medication compliance.

### Psychological or Behavioral Side Effects of Asthma Medications

In the past decade, a number of studies have been conducted to analyze the relationships between asthma medications and psychological or behavioral changes; many of these investigations were summarized in the previous edition (14). The current review will summarize the more current research concerning theophylline, corticosteroids, and beta-agonist drugs.

#### *Theophylline*

A number of studies were directed at analyzing the correlation of theophylline consumption and changes in psychological or behavioral measures. In the earlier edition, it was emphasized that no resolution had been achieved in interpreting the claims and counterclaims that emerged from this research (14). As a result, there was considerable debate about whether theophylline should be prescribed for childhood asthma. The situation has settled considerably in the past 5 years. Contributing to the current situation were critical reviews of the scientific merit of previous investigations; better-designed and executed investigations; and more cautions and valid interpretations of the resulting data.

Studies investigating the correlation of theophylline with psychological or behavioral performance were critiqued by Creer and colleagues (34,35). In the first review (34), 10 studies were evaluated in accordance with 12 criteria. In general, the studies were found to be strong with respect to six standards: use of appropriate experimental designs, including control procedures; application of standardized assessment procedures; inclusion of a broad spectrum of valid and reliable dependent measures; recruitment of enough subjects for appropriate parametric statistical procedures to be used; application of acceptable standards for interpreting results; and interpretation of data in a reasonable and appropriate manner. Overall, the studies were weak with respect to five criteria: descriptions of how the asthma of subjects was confirmed; application of unbiased recruitment and random assignment; selection of subjects from similar populations with respect to classification, severity, and treatment of asthma; control over extraneous variables, including medication compliance; and concern regarding the clinical significance of findings. None of the studies met one criterion: the collection of sufficient follow-up data to rule out normal fluctuations of asthmatic symptoms or medication effects. Based on their review, Creer and his co-workers (34) concluded that there was no evidence that any psychological or behavioral changes correlated with the taking of theophylline were indicative of a learning disorder. Furthermore, they cautioned, there was absolutely no evidence to indicate that any of the data proved that the hyperactive-like behaviors reported by a number of investigators met the standards required for the diagnosis of an attention deficit hyperactivity disorder (ADHD). The critique concluded by outlining a methodology for examining children with asthma when it is suspected that they may react negatively to theophylline. Investigations using such procedures would, it was suggested, permit physicians to tailor medication regimens better for patients.

In the second critique, Creer and Gustafson (35) extended the earlier review, as well as reiterating conclusions made in that critique (34). In addition, Creer and Gustafson (35) emphasized that there appear to be individual differences among asthmatic children who take theophylline for their asthma; in particular, they stressed, there is a subgroup of children who are particularly sensitive to xanthine-based products, including theophylline. To predetermine which children could have difficulties, Creer and Gustafson (35) offered five recommendations. First, they suggested that a thorough history of a patient's use of xanthines be obtained before theophylline is prescribed. This suggestion was made because products that contain caffeine, consumed by children in the form of soda pop and chocolate, could interact with theophylline and intensify behavioral side effects. Second, it was proposed that tighter control be established over extraneous variables or factors that may affect the behavior under investigation. In particular, the need to monitor the consumption of other xanthine products, such as chocolate or soft drinks, as well as medication compliance was emphasized. Third, Creer and Gustafson (35) stressed that valid and reliable psychological and behavioral techniques be used to screen patients before they are put on theophylline. A number of instruments, especially those that assess behavior and motor performance, can be used for this purpose (36,37). Fourth, it was suggested that more refined xanthine challenge tests be developed and implemented; this recommendation could also help detect youngsters likely to experience behavioral side effects as a consequence of taking theophylline. Finally, it was recommended that patients taking theophylline be observed for longer periods of time in their natural environments. This type of field study could yield considerable information about any naturally occurring changes in a patient's psychological or behavioral performance that result from taking theophylline (or any other asthma medication, for that matter).

Better designed and executed studies have recently been conducted to correlate theophylline with psychological or behavioral indices (38–40); more research on the topic is planned. A prototype study on the relationship between asthma and behavioral or psychological factors was reported by Schlieper and colleagues (40). This well-conceived study featured a double-blind, randomized, crossover paradigm for assessing the effects of theophylline on behavior, mood, and cognitive processing. Thirty-one children, ages 8–12 years, with moderate asthma were randomly assigned to a 10 day theophylline trial followed by placebo, or to a placebo followed by theophylline experimental conditions (separated by a 2 day washout period). Theophylline plasma concentrations to assess compliance and pulmonary function tests were measured throughout the study. A wide variety of valid and reliable measures developed to assess cognitive functions, as well as self-report measures, were administered at baseline and after each medication test. In addition, behavioral ratings were obtained from parents and teachers. Results of the study showed that theophylline had no effect on attention or activity level as determined by parents' and teachers' ratings. Children's self-reports also showed no changes in their mood; no significant differences were found on measures of cognitive functioning.

Schlieper and her colleagues (40) reported large individual differences in sensitivity to theophylline. They noted that although most of their subjects tolerated theophylline well, children who already had attentional or achievement problems appeared vulnerable to adverse effects.

Finally, recent studies have been cautious in interpreting their results. Instead of the shrill alarmist interpretations that did little more than frighten children and their parents, more recent studies have been characterized by careful interpretation and reporting of findings. Almost all investigators realize that the relationship between theophylline and psychological or behavioral variables is complex; furthermore, there is the recognition that delineating the parameters of individual responses to theophylline must be a focus of future studies (35,40,41). All investigators would likely agree with Ellis (42,43) who emphasized that when used correctly, theophylline has a role in the treatment of asthma for many children.

### *Corticosteroids*

After almost 30 years, renewed interest has been directed at determining the relationship between corticosteroids and psychological or behavioral variables. Two studies were described by Bender and colleagues (44,45). In the first investigation (44), 27 children with severe asthma, aged 8–16 years, were evaluated when they were receiving high (61.5 mg/day) or low (3.33 mg/day) dosages of steroids. A number of valid and reliable measures were used to assess attention, impulsivity, hyperactivity, motor control, verbal memory, and mood. Results indicated that when receiving the high dosage of steroids, subjects reported increased depression and anxiety symptoms; they were also less proficient on a test of long-term verbal memory. No low-steroid differences were found on the other measures of attention, impulsivity, hyperactivity, or motor control In a second study, Bender and co-workers (45) evaluated 32 children (mean age, 14 years) with severe asthma throughout the course of receiving a short-term "burst" of prednisone. On high-steroid days (mean dose = 61.4 mg), the children reported more symptoms of anxiety and depression; they also showed diminished verbal memory relative to low-steroid days (mean dose, 6.97 mg). No dose-related changes were noted with measures of hyperactivity, attention, impulsivity, or fine motor control. In this second study, Bender and colleagues (45) also examined six subject variables: age, socioeconomic status, severity score, intelligence quotient (IQ), child global assessment score, and family global assessment score. No significant results were found with the initial five subject variables, although significant findings indicated that as children increasingly demonstrated emotional difficulty or were from dysfunctional families, they were more likely to experience negative psychological changes associated with high-dose steroids. However, these latter findings must be interpreted with some caution since no validity or reliability data have been published concerning either the child or family global assessement scales.

### *Beta-Agonists*

Mazer and colleagues (46) examined the role of albuterol on the fine-motor performance of asthmatic children in a double-blind, crossover trial. Twenty children, aged 4–14 years, were tested after the administration of either albuterol aerosol or a placebo. There were three dependent variables: fine-motor abilities in response speed, visual–motor control, and speed and dexterity; tremor; and postural adjustment. No significant differences were found in fine-motor skills after administration of either albuterol or placebo; a significant increase in tremor and postural adjustment occurred after administration of albuterol. The authors concluded that the increase in tremor was not of the magnitude to suggest that major educational adjustments were required for those receiving albuterol, however.

In conclusion, the findings on theophylline, corticosteroids, and beta-agonist medications suggest that all are correlated in varying degrees with some behavioral or psychological change. Because individual differences exist in the changes that occur among patients, physicians may wish to consider these effects in tailoring a medication regimen for a given child.

## Medication Compliance

Compliance with medication regimens in children with asthma can be plotted along a continuum ranging from total compliance to total noncompliance. In 10 studies in which a biochemical assay or marker was used to assess compliance, the range went from 2% to 100%; the average rate of compliance was 43% (47). Much of the variance among studies is due to methodologic differences: low rates of compliance were found in randomly selected patients who sought medical attention during attacks and high rates of compliance were found in selected groups of children who volunteered for investigations. Range effects are created by scores at both extremes. Floor effects occur when rates of compliance approach their lowest possible level. At this point, it would be impossible to determine if a program designed to increase compliance would have the opposite effect and decrease the behavior; no lower rates are possible. On the other hand, ceiling effects occur when compliance rates approach their highest possible value. In these instances, the beneficial effects of a program designed to increase compliance cannot be determined; no higher rates are possible.

Studies of medication compliance in childhood asthma have relied upon correlational procedures. Of particular interest in this chapter are variables thought to be related to compliance (or, perhaps more appropriately, noncompliance); monitoring methods; altering treatment regimens; and patient education.

### *Compliance Variables*

A number of variables have been reported as correlated with medication compliance and childhood asthma (6,11,47–51). These are enumerated in Table 1. These have been classified into six categories of variables: patient; parent; physician; medication and prescribing; asthma; and contextual. Most of these variables are self-explanatory; thus, the discussion will only highlight the various categories.

Patient Variables. Three types of patient variables are described: beliefs and expectancies, behaviors, and memory decay. We know less about patient beliefs and expectancies than any set of patient variables (47,51). Part of our lack of knowledge is because despite their importance, the variables tend to be ignored in assessing compliance. This is especially true of the perceived social stigma many patients attach to taking asthma medications, particularly in public, and the tendency of patients to weigh the perceived costs of asthma medications (e.g., expense, side effects, etc.) against what they see as potential gains (e.g., amelioration of asthma). As a result, some patients are compliant when symptomatic but noncompliant when asymptomatic. Age-related beliefs are prominent when patients are adolescents: almost all go through a period where they are noncompliant in order to "prove" that they do not require asthma medications, particularly those medications prescribed on a prophylactic basis. Compliant or, more accurately, noncompliant behaviors are recognized by all physicians. What are often overlooked are variables related to memory. Arkes (52) has repeatedly found that memory is a major impediment to appropriate clinical judgment and decision-making. Thus, the frequently used reason for failing to take medications ("I forgot") is not always an excuse. Memory may be less of a factor in the taking of maintenance medications; patients usually fail to take all doses that are prescribed, but this behavior is to be expected when medications are taken over a period of time (47). Memory contributes more to noncompliance when patients take medications as needed for occasional attacks. Unless a patient has posted instructions on exactly how he or she should manage asthma, the sequence to be followed in treating an episode is apt to be forgotton (47,51).

Parent Variables. These include beliefs and expectations, behaviors, and memory decay. Most are self-explanatory. A difference between child and parent beliefs revolve around myths about asthma (47,51). Many parents, particularly fathers, hear from their co-workers or relatives that children always outgrow asthma, that the disorder is never serious or life-threatening,

TABLE 1 Variables Correlated with Medication Compliance in Children with Asthma

- Patient Variables
  - Beliefs and expectations
    - Indifference or apathy
    - Lack of understanding of asthma or medications
    - Past experience with asthma or medications
    - Perceived social stigma about taking medications
    - Misinterpretation of attack severity
    - Age-related beliefs
    - Perceived costs versus gains in taking medicine
  - Behaviors
    - Failure to have medications available for use
    - Taking of incorrect dosages of medicine for asthma
      - Overuse of medicine
      - Underuse of medicine
      - Erratic use of medicine
    - Refusal or vomiting of medicine
  - Memory decay
- Parent Variables
  - Beliefs and expectations
    - Indifference or apathy towards asthma
    - Lack of understanding of asthma or medications
    - Perceived social stigma about taking asthma medicine
    - Misinterpretation of attack severity
    - Myths about asthma and asthma drugs, including overreaction to medication side effects
    - Perceived costs versus gains in taking asthma medications
  - Behaviors
    - Failure to obtain or to refill medications as prescribed
    - Failure to monitor child's asthma or taking of medications
    - Failure to provide appropriate dosages of asthma medications
    - Failure to provide reinforcement to child for compliance behaviors
  - Memory decay
- Physician Variables
  - Communication Deficits
    - Failure to provide complete or adequate instruction
    - Failure to establish communication with patients or their parents
    - Failure to explain medication side effects
  - Behaviors
    - Failure to monitor medication use
    - Failure to analyze medication-taking behaviors of children
    - Failure to prescribe correct medicine or dosages of asthma medicines
    - Failure to perceive severity of attack
    - Failure to reinforce compliant behavior
  - Memory decay

TABLE 1 Continued

| |
|---|
| Medication and Prescribing Variables |
| Medication variables |
| Taste of medicine |
| Expense of medicine |
| Side effects of medicine |
| Incomplete labeling or dispensing of medicine |
| Delivery method |
| Prescribing variables |
| Schedule for taking medications |
| Prescribing multiple medications |
| Failure to explain difference in maintenance vs. PRN medicines |
| Duration of medication use |
| Asthma variables |
| Intermittent, variable, and reversible nature of asthma |
| Lack of naturally occurring reinforcement for compliance |
| Contextual variables: Environmental and social factors that affect compliance |

or that asthma is a psychosomatic disorder. Fathers tend to be more antagonistic towards medical care because physicians and other medical personnel cannot provide a quick "cure" for asthma.

Physician Variables. Communication deficits, behaviors, and memory decay are noted. Communication deficits are self-explanatory; it is unlikely that medical personnel who treat asthma are different from personnel who treat other diseases or physical disorders. The behavior of physicians is also not unique to asthma. Two variables are noteworthy: failure to analyze patient behaviors and to reinforce compliant behavior. Physicians often fail to learn about behaviors exhibited by children with asthma, particularly adolescents, who begin to smoke or experiment with illicit substances. Because these substances interfere with asthma medications, it is imperative that physicians know of such patient behaviors. Failure to reinforce patients for being compliant is common among medical personnel (47), perhaps in part because they are preoccupied with attempting to enhance medication compliance in patients who are noncompliant. Finally, memory decay influences clinical judgments and decision making (47,51). It is likely that memory decay is less a variable in allergists or other physicians who specialize in treating asthma. Specialists in asthma were recently shown to be more effective in treating asthma (53); memory decay of the steps required to manage asthma would be less of a factor in these physicians than it would be in those who treat asthma on an occasional basis.

Medication and Prescribing Variables. Most of these variables are self-explanatory. The fewer medications required by the patient, the better should be compliance; similar results should be anticipated if drug doses are taken so as to fit into the patient's normal routine (49). Two variables should be discussed in greater detail: delivery method and failure to explain the difference between maintenance and as needed medications. The proper use of an inhaler or nebulizer requires the coordination of behavioral skills on the part of the patient. Unless patients are taught to perform these skills correctly, medications taken via these routes are apt not to have the desired effect. The difference between maintenance and as needed medications is often unclear to patients (51). As a consequence, they may attempt to use a prophylactic medication during attacks, when such drugs could exacerbate the episode. Failure to differentiate between the two types of medicines is often misunderstood by medical personnel who are not that familiar with asthma and its treatment; in these cases, there is little effort to clarify the types of drugs for patients.

Asthma Characteristics. Since asthma is an intermittent condition, patients discover that attacks do not always occur when they are noncompliant. In these cases, the patients may be reinforced for noncompliant behavior. Severe attacks may also occur when patients are compliant. Here, patients may believe that compliant behaviors are punished; there simply is no reinforcement in the form of attack avoidance that they anticipate as a consequence of their behavior.

Contextual Variables. Contextual variables include the stimulus events that exert general control over other stimulus–response interactions (54). With asthma, these events may include stimuli that establish how a child is going to respond to an attack. If youngsters are at home, they may immediately take steps to abort the episode. If involved in a game with their peers, they may ignore warning signs of asthma and fail to seek assistance while the episode is mild. Contextual variables are prominent in medication compliance; we have not as yet, however, directed the research attention to them that they merit.

### *Monitoring Medication Use*

Monitoring compliance serves two functions: it provides information about the degree of compliance and improves patient compliance. A number of techniques have been used including patient self-reports, telephone monitoring, physician auditing, and quantitative assessment.

Self-Report Measures. Reports from patients represent the most or least reliable data gathered about their asthma and medication use (55). Some patients know more about their attacks and how they are controlled than anyone, including their physicians. Data collected by these patients are apt to be the most accurate information available. Other patients, however, fail to observe and record reliable information about themselves; this can result in invalid interpretations based upon their data (55). Increasing evidence indicates patients can be taught to observe and record accurate information about their asthma. Data gathered by patients in their homes and recorded in asthma diaries, attack forms, and medication charts have been demonstrated to correlate highly with independent observations of trained professionals (37). It must be emphasized that such information is gathered only when patients are well-versed in observation and recording skills, and when they are motivated to monitor their behavior. It should be noted that accurate information is usually collected regarding only a few categories of operationally defined behaviors within specified periods of time (55). It is easy to overwhelm patients by asking them to observe and record too much information about their behavior over long periods of time. Their monitoring behavior usually deteriorates under these conditions.

Telephone Monitoring. Weinstein and Cuskey (56) found that weekly telephone calls were effective in monitoring compliance in patients with asthma. Telephone calls permitted physicians and their staffs to gather invaluable information from patients; at the same time, the calls served to prompt patients to comply with medication instructions. The caveat noted earlier, however, should be reiterated: self-monitoring is apt to become ineffective if carried out over a prolonged period of time.

Auditing Medications. Spector (49) advocated the periodic auditing of all medications (including over the counter [OTC] drugs) and vitamins by asking asthmatic patients to bring everything with them when they visited their physicians. This procedure reveals whether patients consume products that could interfere with asthma medications; in addition, Spector (49) observed that the procedure prompted patients to fill their prescriptions.

Quantitative Assessment. A number of approaches have been taken to quantitatively assess compliance in patients with asthma. Many of these procedures were introduced by pharmaceutical companies to monitor use of medications being tested.

The pill count technique involves counting the pills taken by a patient over a period. It is a direct, observable, and quantifiable way to assess compliance; the procedure, however, does not definitively indicate whether the patient actually took the medicine since pills can be discarded before an appointment with the physician (47,51).

Canisters containing inhaled medications can be weighed to assess the volume of a medication taken over a given period. The method is direct, objective, and yields quantifiable data. Its weakness is that any changes do not ensure that patients actually inhaled the medication; they could have discharged several bursts into the air instead of their airways (47,51).

Serum or salivary assays can be performed to determine the level of a medication in a patient's blood. The methods are objective, direct, and yield quantifiable data. Weaknesses of the approach are that patients have variable rates of absorption, metabolism, and elimination of asthma medications; interactions between the drug being measured and other substances; timing of the measurement; and reluctance of parents to have blood drawn from their children (47,51).

A riboflavin tracer can be added to a medication to assess compliance (47). The approach is objective, direct, and provides quantifiable data; its weaknesses are the same as those described for serum and salivary assays (47,51).

The Nebulizer Chronolog (NC) is a device that encircles a nebulizer or metered-dose inhaler like a glove; it is small, light, and easy to carry. Each inhalation triggers a microswitch. The memory unit of the instrument stores a record of each activation accurate to within 4 min of use; up to 256 activations can be stored at any one time (49). The strengths of the instrument are that it provides direct, objective, quantifiable data. Weaknesses are the expense of the NC and its interpreter and printer, the mechanical reliability of the device, and the potential for patients to discharge the nebulizer or MDI without actually inhaling the medication (47,51). The latter was recently demonstrated in a study by Mawhinney and colleagues (57), who found compliance was poor in two studies where the NC was used with adults with asthma. It is likely that similar data would be obtained with asthmatic children if the NC were used to assess compliance.

The Medication Event Monitoring System (MEMS) involves a container with a computer chip embedded in its cap. Each time the cap is removed, the day and time of its removal are recorded. As with the NC, the cap requires a translator and printer. Strengths of the MEMS are that it yields direct, objective, quantifiable data; weaknesses include the cost of the MEMS and related equipment, as well as the possibility that medications can be removed but not taken by patients (47,51).

### *Altering Treatment Regimens*

At times, the easiest way to improve compliance is to change a patient's treatment regimen (47,49–51). Methods to enhance compliance include decreasing the complexity of a regimen by prescribing fewer drugs and fewer doses of a given medication, discontinuing ineffective or unnecessary drugs, and decreasing the duration of therapy. Gearing a treatment regimen to a patient's lifestyle can also improve compliance. Spector (49) suggested that the latter aim may be achieved by having patients take medications with naturally occurring events, such as taking a drug with each regularly timed meal. Negotiation should be used with children to decide when medications are taken; a written contract, stipulating the agreement achieved between a patient and his or her physician, should result from such negotiation. Contracts should also stipulate the reinforcement that is contingent upon compliance. With younger children, TV viewing is an excellent reinforcement; use of the family automobile is a potent reinforcer with older adolescents.

### *Patient Education*

Patient education is another method that can be used to improve medication compliance. Physicians can incorporate different methods of teaching including the use of written and audiovisual materials, verbal instruction, and cues and reminders. Considerable educational materials are available through pharmaceutical firms; other educational programs can be obtained through such organizations as the American Lung Association. The importance of compliance must be thoroughtly explained in a warm, genuine, and emphatic manner. In discussing the importance of compliance, physicians should emphasize the practicality of the behavior in terms patients and their parents understand. At all times, it is suggested that medical jargon be avoided and patient interactions encouraged.

Potential side effects of prescribed drugs should be described to patients and their parents. Experience indicates that ignorance of side effects promotes not only noncompliant behavior but also a tendency on the part of children and their parents to perceive other physical changes as due to a medication when they are caused by another factor (11).

It is important to demonstrate the correct use of inhalers and nebulizers when required. Thereafter, it is important periodically to ask patients to demonstrate how they use a drug-dispensing instrument. Other interactions with the patient, including providing feedback and assessing patient comprehension or recall of instructions, should occur during regular office visits (49). Key elements of compliance should also be reviewed periodically. Finally, as noted earlier, it is important that constant support and reinforcement be provided to patients. Social reinforcement from physicians can be invaluable in maintaining compliance in children with asthma and their parents (47,51).

In summary, correlation research involves gathering data on two or more variables across subjects or time periods. The states of the variables are simply observed or measured "as is" and, as Bordens and Abbott (4) point out, are not manipulated. Despite these limitations, correlational research is useful in that it provides a method for identifying potential causal relationships during the early stages of an area of study, determining relationships when variables cannot or should not be manipulated, and describing how variables relate to one another in the real world (4). Knowledge of these relationships, as well as their ability to permit us to make predictions, clarify our understanding of the interactions between behavioral or psychological variables and asthma.

## EXPERIMENTAL DESIGNS

Bordens and Abbott (4) explain that experimental research has two defining characteristics: manipulation of an independent variable and control over extraneous variables. An independent variable is a variable whose levels are chosen and set by the experimenter; values are referred to as levels of the independent variables. The dependent variable is the measure selected for the study; this could be differences in pulmonary function as a result of the administration of a medication. If a causal relationship exists, the value of the dependent variable will be a function, to some extent, of the level of the independent variable.

Extraneous variables are variables that are not of interest to us, but that may affect the phenomena we investigate. If allowed to vary on their own, extraneous variables can produce uncontrolled changes in the dependent variable. Bordens and Abbott (4) warn that this may result in two consequences. First, uncontrolled variability may make it difficult or impossible to detect effects of the independent variable. For example, this could be another substance taken by subjects that interacts with and modifies the effect of an asthma medication. Second, uncontrolled variability may produce chance differences across levels of the dependent variable. These differences could make it appear as though the independent variable produced effects when it did not. Extraneous variables are controlled in two ways. The first is to hold extraneous variables constant. As will be described, this is often impossible to achieve. The second technique is to randomize the effects of extraneous variables across treatments. This procedure is typically followed; it is further required by assumptions of parametric statistical techniques.

There are three types of experimental designs: between-subjects, within-subjects, and single-subject. In addition, combinations of these designs are used in asthma research. Each design will be described.

### Between-Subjects Designs

In between-subjects designs, different groups of subjects are randomly assigned to levels of the independent variable. Manipulating an experimental variable is usually as simple as exposing one group of subject to a treatment (the experimental group) and the other to the same conditions minus the treatment (the control group). Between-subjects designs can be classified according to the number of groups required (two groups or multigroup), the number of independent variables manipulated (single factor or multifactor), the way in which subjects are assigned to groups (random assignment or matching), and the number of dependent variables (univariate or multivariate). The application of between-subjects designs in research on behavioral or psychological factors and asthma will be illustrated by describing three topics: educational and self-management programs, relaxation and biofeedback, and judgment and decision-making.

### *Educational and Self-Management Programs*

These programs are described in Chapter 21; current comments focus on the designs of these studies. Three suggestions are offered for future research. First, a critique of nearly two dozen educational and self-management programs for childhood asthma found that, overall, positive findings were reported with application of the programs (58,59). However, a weakness in a majority of the studies was the failure to follow guidelines for unbiased subject recruitment and random assignment. The guidelines are critical to experimental designs; they fulfill assumptions underlying the parametric statistical procedures used to analyze data gathered in such investigations.

A second suggestion is to tighten control over extraneous variables. A prominent variable concerns continuity in the medical care provided to patients. It is imperative that subjects be recruited from a single source or, an aim more likely to be achieved, from physicians who share a common philosophy and comparable skills in treating asthma. It was noted earlier that significant differences result when patients with asthma, including children, are treated by either allergists or general care physicians (53). Differences in the management by physicians may be resolved by the random assignment of patients treated by different physicians across treatment and control groups. However, the variable of physician differences in managing asthma could be too potent to control through randomized assignment; in these cases, any effects of an education or self-management program would be obscured by the effect of medical management. A related question was posed by Miklich and his colleagues (60): How can medication use be held constant over the course of a behavioral or psychological study? Since medications are a concurrent independent variable, any change in drugs could produce interference with the application of behavioral or psychological treatment. Control over this variable is left to the random assignment of patients to treatment and control groups; as Miklich and his co-workers (60) cautioned, however, it is virtually impossible to control the variable over a period of time even under the best of situations (e.g., in a residential treatment facility).

A third question concerns whether the between-subjects design is the best paradigm for the evaluation of education and self-management programs. It is appropriate if the desire of the investigator is to assess changes in patient knowledge as a result of the introduction of an independent variable. It may not be appropriate, as will be argued, if the aim is to assess knowledge of self-management skills and the subsequent application of these competencies over time.

### *Relaxation and Biofeedback*

Teaching children with asthma to relax is a staple of most behavioral intervention programs. Relaxation is important in that it may prevent the exacerbation of an attack in progress, an outcome that can prove infectious to parents or personnel attempting to treat the episode. Perhaps a more significant value of relaxation, however, is that it assists patients to think of and perform steps necessary to control attacks. By remaining calm, children can make an invaluable contribution to the management of their asthma (61).

A recent study by Kotses and colleagues (62) analyzed the long-term effects of biofeedback-induced relaxation on asthma in children. Twenty-nine children with a confirmed diagnosis of asthma were randomly assigned to either a treatment or control group. Fifteen children in the treatment group received biofeedback training as the independent variable. The groups were balanced with regard to the gender and age of subjects. A number of asthma dependent measures were used, including lung function, and self-reported asthma severity, medication use, and frequency of attacks. Results indicated that the children who received biofeedback exhibited higher pulmonary function scores, more positive attitudes towards asthma, and lower chronic anxiety during the follow-up period. Children in the experimental and control groups, however, did not differ on self-rated asthma severity, medication use, or frequency of attacks; there also were no changes in self-concept.

The investigation by Kotses and co-workers (62) was noteworthy because of the significant improvement linked to biofeedback in forced expiratory volume (FEV), forced vital capacity (FVC) scores. The finding followed an earlier study by Miklich and colleagues (60) who reported improved FEV in 1 sec (FEV-1) following relaxation training with and without biofeedback. Data from both investigations prompt the conclusion that biofeedback training contributes to the self-control of asthma. For this reason, such a procedure would be a valuable addition to any self-management program (62).

### *Judgment and Decision-Making*

Between subjects-designs can be used to conduct informal analyses of data from two sources. An example is the content analysis of judgment and decision-making skills of physicians and patients. Data from two studies were recently compared (63): in the first investigation (64), three scenarios describing typical cases of childhood asthma were composed by an experienced allergist. The scenarios were then presented to three groups of subjects with instructions to use a decision-making matrix to indicate treatment steps they would take to manage the patients' asthma. Subjects included 30 second-year medical students; 30 allergists; and 7 physicians who, because of their standing among their peers, were considered the Gold Standard. The latter group proved different from the other groups with respect to more requests for additional information about patients described in the scenarios, the generation of more treatment options, and greater consideration of the consequences of their actions. Information gathered from this group of participants served as one data set.

The second data set was gleaned from participants in a self-management program, Living with Asthma (65). In particular, information was gathered from a subset of participants who described their responses to asthma on a report of an attack episode form. The form, as well as data gathered with the instrument, has excellent reliability and validity (37). The questionnaire includes information on stimuli perceived as correlated with the onset of attacks; where and when the episodes occurred; and the sequential order of steps performed to control attacks. A total of 84 families with an asthmatic child completed an average of 13.03 report of attack/episode forms. These participants were referred to as the Gold Standard patients.

Data from the Gold Standard physicians and patients were compared. Out of the content analysis emerged 12 judgment rules or strategies employed by both groups. Not all physicians or patients used all of the rules all of the time; however, all employed the strategies most of the time. The rules that governed their management of asthma are enumerated in Table 2. Since the majority of these rules are self-explanatory, readers interested in a more detailed discussion are referred to the article by Creer (63). Of interest here is that the analysis of responses by physicians and patients

TABLE 2 Judgment Rules or Strategies Common to Gold Standard Physicians and Patients

| |
|---|
| Considered each patient and/or asthma attack as separate experiment |
| Were thoughtful and cautious |
| Perceived events as correlated with, not causative of, asthma and attacks |
| Avoided preconceived notions of the treatment of asthma and individual attacks |
| Showed greater awareness of attacks, treatments, and potential outcomes |
| Generated number of testable treatment alternatives |
| Consistently referred to personal data base in making decisions |
| Adjusted treatment to fit perceived severity of asthma |
| Did not misperceive severity of attacks |
| Thought in terms of probabilities in considering treatment outcomes |
| Were not overconfident |
| Did not rely heavily on memory in treating asthma |

Source: Adapted from Ref. 63.

yielded similar findings. The information provides the opportunity to generate hypotheses on the topic of judgment and decision-making by physicians and patients that can be tested in a more rigorous manner.

## Within-Subjects Designs

Within-subjects designs differ from between-subjects designs in that only one group of subjects may be involved (4). Subjects receive all levels of the independent variable; a within-subjects design thus requires fewer subjects per study. As can occur in a between-subjects design, as many levels of the independent variable may be included as needed. The design permits subjects to be matched with themselves, the only form of matching feasible in a long-term study of childhood asthma. Another advantage is that within-subjects variance excludes error variance caused by subjects' differences; in this situation, the analysis will have more power. A disadvantage is that within-subjects designs have less power than equivalent between-subjects designs when the dependent variable is related to subject differences (4). Carryover effects may also occur, although these are usually dealt with in asthma research by counterbalancing treatment conditions.

Within-subjects designs have proven useful in the investigation of behaviors related to asthma. Examples include their application with panic, the overuse of hospital facilities by asthmatic children, and analyzing steps sequentially taken by patients to manage their asthma.

### *Panic*

There are children with asthma who panic during their attacks (11,46,66). The label of panic covers a broad spectrum of individual behaviors: at one end of the continuum, children constantly complain that they require more of a prescribed medication or that the drug they take is ineffective. They often appear frightened and agitated, a pattern that is contagious to those around them (including parents or members of a treatment staff). At the other end of the continuum, there are patients who appear opposite to the above description. They remain silent and frozen in their beds; they will not ask for help even when required, but can lapse into unconsciousness unless carefully monitored.

In investigating the pattern, Creer and Renne (66) asked nurses and other medical personnel to list the behaviors they thought constituted panic. A broad array of responses was reported. Those items listed by more than one individual were included on a checklist of behaviors; the series of items served as a dependent measure. A dozen children described as panicking according to the checklist were treated with an independent variable: systematic desensitization by reciprocal inhibition (67). With this procedure, children were seen individually for training in muscle relaxation and to obtain descriptions of the stimuli they thought induced their panic. Most of the descriptions provided by the children were based on an especially severe attack they had suffered at home with their families; usually, the attack was frightening not only to the child but also to his or her parents. The material provided by the children was recast into hierarchies composed of separate items, with the stimulus provoking the least amount of reported anxiety placed at the bottom of a hierarchy and the stimulus that generated the greatest amount of reported anxiety at the top.

Following training in muscle relaxation, the children were asked to imagine the fear-arousing items they described in their hierarchies. Items were presented in order from the item that generated the least amount of anxiety through the items that elicited the greatest amount of anxiety. The juxtaposition of relaxation and anxiety apparently produced by the imagined stimuli led to a diminution and extinction of the panic as reported by nurses and attending medical personnel. Appropriate responses to asthma later were reported by their parents when the children returned to their homes. Long baseline and follow-up periods differentiated this paradigm from a single-group uncontrolled outcome design. In this manner, systematic desensitization became a vital tool in the arsenal of methods to treat panic; when applied, the technique can virtually eliminate the commonly reported pattern of panic in almost any patient with asthma.

### *Hospital Overuse*

Creer (68) initially referred to the pattern of children attempting to be admitted or to remain hospitalized when their asthma symptoms had cleared as *malingering*. However, the term has so many connotations that the words *hospital overuser*, suggested by Hochstadt and colleagues (69), is preferred. The behavior was originally altered in a single-subject design format (68,70). Baseline data were gathered on both frequency and duration of hospital admissions in children described as overusers of the hospital. After data were gathered, the children were exposed to a time-out procedure. This involved making the hospital environment dull by removing television, limiting reading materials to school texts, and reducing interactions with peers. The procedure was applied both during each hospitalization (68) or on a less frequent, aperiodic basis (70). The results were the same: a dramatic reduction in the number and duration of hospitalizations of children thought to overuse the hospital. Hochstadt and colleagues (69) used a time-out procedure in a within-subjects design; the subjects were 7 children, including 6 boys between the ages of 8 and 12 years, and a 13-year-old girl. The results of the time-out procedure were: the mean length of stay for the children was reduced from 18.3 days in the year before intervention to 9.0 after intervention; and the mean time required for children to reach optimal peak flow values decreased from 9.8 days to 4.8 days.

These changes were statistically significant at the 0.01 and 0.05 levels, respectively. Although constituting a sharp decrease, the mean interval between hospitalizations of 48.9 days before the study to 85.3 days during the study was not statistically significant.

*Sequential Performance of Asthma Management Steps*

Within-subjects designs permit an analysis of the attack management performance of subjects. An illustration is provided in a study by Baum and Creer (71). The major purpose of this investigation was to determine if compliance could be improved as a result of patient education (it was not). However, of equal interest was the sequential performance of steps required to bring an attack under control in the group who received patient education. Data gathered on the report of attack episode form served as the dependent variable. Before exposure to intervention, 29% of the children said they informed an adult as the initial step in their management of their attacks; following intervention, only 4% reported this as their initial step. At the same time, attempting to escape from the precipitating stimulus increased from 24% to 73%, respectively, when data gathered before and after intervention were compared. Pre- and postintervention changes were also noted in the taking of medication, with children introducing asthma medications as a second or third step rather than as the first step they took to manage attacks. This content analysis of data provided preliminary information as to how children manage asthma and, in particular, how management strategies change with patient education.

## Single-Subject Designs

Single-subject designs have been the backbone of behavioral research (54). Characteristics of the single-subject design include individuals being observed under each of several phases, with multiple responses recorded in each phase. The procedure followed involves extensive observations during the baseline phase to obtain a standard against which any changes due to the independent variable can be compared; subjects remaining in each phase until a stability criterion is met; and all subjects being observed under all phases, with each treatment phase repeated at least twice. The repetition, or intrasubject repetition, establishes the reliability of the findings; multiple subjects can be included to provide intersubject replication to establish the generality of findings across subjects (4,54).

Single-subject designs have been instrumental in developing many of the behavioral and phychological procedures used with childhood asthma. These include procedures for managing hospital overuse, panic, inappropriate social behaviors, and maladaptive academic behaviors (11). Components of self-management for childhood asthma were developed and tested in large part through the application of single-subject designs; this forms the background for the current plethora of educational and self-management programs designed for the disorder (72). Examples of a single-subject design, with multiple subjects, included studies that shaped appropriate use of pressurized nebulizer (73) and the reduction of phobic behaviors (11) in children with asthma.

### *Use of Pressurized Nebulizer*

Renne and Creer (73) observed that children with asthma often did not use the intermittent positive pressure breathing (IPPB) machine correctly. As a consequence, they did not receive the benefit of dispensed medications that should have occurred. The procedure used to change the behavior involved the following steps. First, the behavior of the children was analyzed. It was determined that there had to be a synthesis of three behaviors in order for the equipment to be used correctly: eye fixation, facial posturing, and diaphragmatic breathing. Eye fixation was defined as a child looking at the dial on the apparatus whenever the mouthpiece was inserted into his or her mouth. The response is not necessary to operate the machine; however, eye fixation ensured that the youngsters received immediate feedback on their performance, that they were not distracted by sounds or other stimuli about them, and that they attended to operating the machine. Facial posturing was defined as holding the mouthpiece at a 90 degree angle to the face, with the lips firmly secured around the mouthpiece. The children were asked not to puff out their cheeks, but to inhale the medication into their lungs. Diaphragmatic breathing was defined as distention of the abdominal wall upon inspiration and contraction upon expiration. This indicated that the child was inhaling the nebulized medication.

The procedure employed by Renne and Creer (73) entailed a multiple baseline design in which baselines were obtained on all three behaviors and sequentially shaped. Results indicated that the procedure was highly effective in teaching asthmatic children to use the IPPB machine; the multiple baseline permitted the strategy to be assessed convincingly. Two consequences occurred as a direct result of this training. First, it was demonstrated that the children required less medication after they were taught to use the IPPB machine correctly. The mean treatment effectiveness was calculated to 41% prior to intervention; effectiveness rose to 82% for the same children following training. Second, the method of teaching children to use the IPPB machine appropriately was readily taught to nurses who routinely began to instruct children to use IPPB equipment effectively.

### *Phobic Behaviors*

A number of types of phobic behaviors, ranging from fears of a specific stimulus such as needles, to fears of a general stimulus, such as the hospital environment, have been observed in children with asthma (10,74). The technique used to change the behavior is systematic desensitization by reciprocal inhibition. Creer (11) described the following three stages of the procedure: the first stage entailed teaching the child to discriminate his or her muscle sensations, to determine whether these feelings denote tension or relaxation, and, consequently, to relax on self-cue; the second stage involved obtaining an account of the stimuli provoking the phobia, such as fears of needles or being hospitalized; and the third stage involved having the children relax while imagining materials presented from the hierarchies developed from their statements. Systematic desensitization, as applied in a single-subject design, was effective in all cases of phobic behaviors presented by children with asthma.

## COMBINATION DESIGNS

According to the aims of the investigator, research designs can be merged into various combinations. Three combination designs have special relevance to the investigation of psychological or behavioral variables and childhood asthma: between-subjects and within-in subjects design; correlational and single-subject design; and between-subjects and single-subject design.

### Between-Subjects and Within-Subjects Design

Some research questions can best be answered with an approach that combines elements of these different design options (4). There is no better example than the design and evaluation of self-management programs for childhood asthma. Two factors dictate use of the combined design: The first factor is the heterogeneous and complex nature of asthma. This issue nullifies the matching of subjects with asthma; consequently, it argues against using only between-subjects designs. The noted pulmonary physician, T.J.H. Clark, described problems that arise in between-subjects research, and emphasized that "patients should wherever possible be used as their own controls and comparisons between subjects should be kept to a minimum" (75, p. 226). As the argument for tailoring treatment regimens for individual patients gains greater currency, this question can be asked: Why do we accept this argument for treatment yet continue to pool the same assortment of patients into a common category for research purposes? Statistical procedures manage much of the variability, but not all. Furthermore, as pointed out earlier, it may not control for all extraneous factors in a study.

The second factor is created by the learning/performance dichotomy and related assessment issues. Learning refers to changes that occur in a person due to educational instruction. The assessment of learning, in turn, requires specific dependent measures. In a typical self-management program, this would involve measuring the patients' knowledge of asthma and how they can contribute to management of the program before and after training. Performance, on the other hand, refers to the patients' translation of what they learn into behavior. Assessment requires a second set of specific dependent measures to measure performance variables as executed by patients over a period of time. Assessment of performance is complicated by two factors: what is taught to patients is unlikely to be performed immediately because of the intermittent nature of asthma (this weakens the bridge between learning and performance); and many psychological variables, particularly those that assess the patients' confidence in their abilities to manage asthma (e.g., self-efficacy) change only with successful performance of self-management strategies. Judgment and decision-making skills also change only with the successful performance of self-management strategies.

To investigate self-management programs successfully, it is recommended that a between-subjects and within-subjects combination design be employed. The design permits the investigator to use a between-subjects design to assess whether patients learn the knowledge and skills they require to help manage their asthma. Subjects can be randomly assigned to a treatment and a waiting-list control group; comparison can be made following training with the experimental group. Subjects in the experimental group would then serve as their own control in a within-in subjects design; this permits subjects to serve as their own control for the duration required in self-management studies (at least a year). An additional advantage of the design is that patients in the waiting-list control can then be trained by either serving as an intervention group in a between-subjects design or as their own control in a within-subjects design. A result is often a significant retention of subjects for the period required to obtain adequate follow-up data (65). The combination between-subjects and within-subjects design represents an excellent strategy for the development and evaluation of second-generation self-management programs for childhood asthma.

### Correlation and Between-Subjects Design

This design features a combination of correlation procedures with the experimental options provided by a between-subject design. This is reflected in the following two-stage research. The first stage involves determining what stimuli are correlated with and predict the probability that a child will experience an attack. The initial research on prediction of asthma employed the peak flowmeter with a correlational design. Taplin and Creer (76) showed that by determining the base rate or prior probability of a child's attacks, they could enter peak flow values into a conditional probability equation and improve by 300% the prediction that the child would have an asthma attack within a specified period. Harm and co-workers (77) refined the procedure with a larger sample of children and demonstrated almost a 500% improvement in the predictability of asthma attacks by using peak flow rates. Risk factor data on asthma have been gathered on other variables including medication compliance (11,77), exercise (77), mold, pollen, and temperature change (78) to predict the likelihood of attacks in asthmatic patients; all have proven efficacy in attack prediction in individual patients. Not all predictors are the same for all patients: Stout and co-workers (78) found that of 17 patients, increased attacks were significantly correlated with mold in 2 patients, temperature change in 1 patient, pollen count in 1 patient, and both temperature change and pollen in 1 patient. These findings underscore the need to determine exactly what stimuli are correlated with the asthma of each individual patient.

Research on attack prediction has two implications (61). First, it can be immediately used by physicians not only to refine predictions of the future attacks of individual patients but also to tailor preventive strategies to allow patients to avoid some attacks. Second, as a long-term goal, tactics can be developed to permit a child to predict, on the basis of changes he or she detects through self-monitoring, the probability of future attacks. The use of prediction, obtained through correlational procedures, was combined by Kotses and his colleagues (79) into a self-management program that included a between-subject design. Eight patients were asked to monitor their asthma through the use of self-report measures. Baseline data revealed which stimuli appeared correlated with the patients' attacks; this was entered into a probability equation to determine the probability that the stimuli would produce asthma within a prescribed period of time.

Following the determination of the stimuli correlated with their asthma, Kotses and co-workers (79) developed a set of individualized self-management recommendations for each individual. These recommendations were given to four subjects who were randomly selected as the self-management group: specific suggestions concerning asthma medications, triggers, and symptoms. The remaining four subjects made up the control group. Results indicated that each individual in the experimental group experienced a decrease in the frequency of their asthma; there was an average decrease in attacks of 22% between baseline to the follow-up period. Only one subject in the control group showed a similar decrease. Severity ratings of attacks showed a comparable decrease for subjects assigned to the control group. Kotses and colleagues (79) concluded that gathering information about a patient's asthma and then tailoring a program to that individual represents a blueprint for future asthma self-management programs and for health care in general. It also represents another type of second-generation self-management program for childhood asthma.

**Between-Subjects and Single-Subject Design**

The emphasis of self-management programs is beginning to shift from the development and evaluation of educational materials (this aim has been achieved) to assessing processes involved in the self-management of asthma. This was illustrated in describing the previous two types of combination designs. In addition to the use of these designs, an aim of second-generation programs is to conduct a precise analysis of specific behaviors sequentially performed by individual patients to manage their asthma. Behaviors include not only self-monitoring but also judgment and decision-making skills applied by patients in selecting and performing competencies tailored for each individual.

To determine specific behaviors performed by patients in self-management, the format requires a combination of between-subjects and single-subject design. Two separate stages are involved. In the first, or acquisition, stage, patients will be taught about asthma and how it should be managed. Like past programs, the instruction can be provided and evaluated with a between-subjects design; unlike past programs, however, instruction will be brief and cover only basic knowledge of asthma and self-management. Dependent measures for assessing acquisition of knowledge will be used in the stage.

Stage two will emphasize analyzing the precise sequence of steps executed by individual patients to manage each of their attacks over a period of time. Obtaining this information requires more refined self-report measures, as well as closer monitoring of self-management skills by investigators. Developing procedures to determine how patients use personal data bases to make judgments and decision-making with respect to their asthma will be particularly challenging. Ways to assess the sequential performance of behaviors of individual patients requires more sophisticated dependent measures than are currently used in self-management programs; many of these measures will likely be similar to those used in field studies of asthmatic children in the naturalistic environment (11). In addition, second-generation self-management programs will require the development and evaluation of more sophisticated outcome measures. Besides assessing indices of morbidity, there is a need for quality of life measures to detect changes that occur as a result of a patient making a contribution to the control of his or her asthma through the performance of self-management skills.

The combination of between-subjects and single-subject design has two advantages over other designs. First, it permits comparisons to be made between experimental and control subjects in acquiring knowledge of asthma and its management. This feature is currently the backbone of much of the research conducted in asthma. Second, the combined design will allow investigators to achieve Clark's (75) suggestion that subjects should serve as their own controls. The procedure has other advantages: it allows momentary fluctuations to average out since a large number of observations will be collected from each subject; it controls incidental factors that may contribute to unwanted variability; and it permits investigators to focus their attention on powerful variables whose effects can be detected against the remaining background of uncontrolled variability (4). The suggested design is complex and will produce considerable behavioral data. At the same time, however, the design can capture the heterogeneous and complex nature of behaviors and their relationship to childhood asthma.

## CONCLUSIONS

The chapter has reviewed a number of behavioral or psychological factors related to childhood asthma. These have been described within the framework of three commonly used research designs: demonstration, correlational, and experimental. The use of combinations of these designs was also illustrated by discussing topics of interest to both behavioral and medical scientists. It is hoped that the conclusion voiced in the earlier edition of the book will remain valid: "Careful investigation is rapidly replacing untestable theory in accounting for psychological and behavioral factors and asthma. The result is a synthesis of medical and behavioral knowledge that, when applied, promises greater hope to the millions of children afflicted with asthma (19, p. 367)."

## ACKNOWLEDGMENT

Preparation of this chapter was supported, in part, by grant 32538 from the National Heart, Lung, and Blood Institute and by an Academic Challenge Award from the State of Ohio. The author is indebted to Harry Kotses, Ph.D., for his suggestions and comments.

## REFERENCES

1. McFadden ER Jr, Stevens JB. A history of asthma. In: Middleton E Jr, Reed CE, Ellis EF (eds.), *Allergy: Principles and Practice*, 2nd ed., St. Louis: CV Mosby Co., 1983, pp. 805–809.
2. Busse WW, Reed CE. Asthma: Definitions and pathogenesis. In: Middleton E Jr, Reed CE, Ellis EF, Adkinson NF Jr, Yunginer JW (eds.), *Allergy: Principles and Practice*, 3rd ed., C.V. Mosby, St. Louis, 1988, pp. 969–998.

3. Braithwaite RB. *Scientific Explanations*, Harper & Row, New York, 1953.
4. Bordens KS, Abbott BB. *Research Design and Methods: A Process Approach*, 2nd ed., Mayfield Publishing, Mountain View, CA, 1991.
5. Johnston JM, Pennypacker HS. *Strategies and Tactics of Human Behavioral Research*, Lawrence Erlbaum Associates, Hillsdale, NJ, 1980.
6. Creer TL, Kotses H. An extension of the Reed and Townley conception of the pathogenesis of asthma: the role of behavioral and psychological stimuli and responses. *Pediat Asthma Allergy Immunol*. 2:169–184, 1988.
7. French TM, Alexander F. Psychogenic factors in brochial asthma. *Psychosom Med Monogr*. 4, 1944.
8. Alexander F. *Psychosomatic Medicine*, Norton, New York, 1950.
9. DiMatteo MR. *The Psychology of Health, Illness, and Medical Care*, Brooks/Cole Publishing, Pacific Grove, CA, 1991.
10. Purcell K, Weiss JH. Asthma. In: Costello CC (ed.), *Symptoms of Psychopathology*, John Wiley & Sons, New York, 1970, pp. 597–623.
11. Creer TL. *Asthma Therapy: A Behavioral Health Care System for Respiratory Disorders*, Springer, New York, 1979.
12. Renne CM, Creer TL. Asthmatic children and their families. In: Wolraich ML, Routh DK (eds.), *Advances in Developmental and Behavioral Pediatrics*, vol. 6. Jai Press, Greenwich, CT, pp. 41–81.
13. Purcell K. Distinctions between subgroups of asthmatic children: children's perceptions of events associated with asthma. *Pediatrics* 31:486–494, 1963.
14. Creer TL. Psychological and neurophysiological aspects of childhood asthma. In: Tinkelman DG, Falliers CJ, Naspitz CK (eds.), *Childhood Asthma: Pathophysiology and Treatment*, Marcel Dekker, Inc., New York, 1987, pp. 341–371.
15. Peshkin MM. Asthma in children. IX. Role of environment in the treatment of a selected group of cases: a plea for a "home" as a restorative measure. *Am J Dis Child* 39:774–781, 1930.
16. Peshkin MM. Intractable asthma in children. In: Weiss EB, Segal MS (eds.), *Bronchial Asthma: Mechanisms and Therapeutics*, Little Brown, Boston, 1976, pp. 957–970.
17. Peshkin MM. Intractable asthma of childhood rehabilitation at the institutional level with a follow-up of 150 cases. *Int Arch Allergy* 15:91–112, 1959.
18. Falliers CJ. Treatment of asthma in a residential center: a fifteen-year study. *Ann Allergy* 20:513–521, 1970.
19. Creer TL, Ipacs J, Creer PP. Changing behavioral and social variables at a residential treatment facility for childhood asthma. *J Asthma* 20:11–15, 1983.
20. Pavlov IP. *Conditioned Reflexes: An Investigation of the Physiological Activity of the Cerebral Cortex*. Oxford University Press, London, 1927.
21. Skinner BF. *The Behavior of Organisms: An Experimental Analysis*. Appleton-Century-Crofts, New York, 1938.
22. Kimble GA. *Hilgard and Marquis' Conditioning and Learning*. Appleton-Century-Crofts, New York, 1961.
23. Catania AC. *Contemporary Research on Operant Behavior*. Scott, Foresman, Glenview, IL, 1968.

24. Hill WF. *Learning: A Survey of Psychological Interpretations*. 5th ed. Harper & Row, New York, 1990.
25. Miklich DR. Chronic homoestatic vagal efferent activity turndown: a theory of asthma. *Med Hypothesis* 3:226–234, 1977.
26. Knapp PH, Mathe AA. Psychophysiologic aspects of bronchial asthma. In: Weiss DB, Segal MS, Stein M (eds.), *Bronchial Asthma: Mechanisms and Therapeutics*, 2nd ed. Little, Brown, Boston, 1985, pp. 914–931.
27. Kushner M. The operant control of intractable sneezing. In: Spielberger CD, Fox R, Masterson R (eds.), *Contributions to General Psychology: Selected Readings for Introductory Psychology*, Ronald Press Co., New York, 1968, pp. 361–365.
28. Weiner D, McGrath K, Patterson R. Factitious sneezing. *J Allergy Clin Immunol* 75:741–745, 1985.
29. Alexander AB, Chai H, Creer TL, Miklich DR, Renne CM, Cardoso R. The elimination of chronic cough by response suppression shaping. *J Behav Ther Exp Psychiatry* 4:75–80, 1973.
30. Lavigne JV, Davis AT, Fauber R. Behavioral management of psychogenic cough: alternative to the "bedsheet" and other aversive techniques. *Pediatrics* 87:532–537, 1991.
31. Christopher KL, Wood RP III, Ecberg RC, Blazer FB, Raney RA, Southrada JF. Vocal cord dysfunction presenting as asthma. *N Engl J Med* 308:1566–1570, 1983.
32. Downing ET, Braman SS, Fox MJ, Corrao WM. Factitious asthma: physiological approach to diagnosis. *JAMA* 248:2878–2880, 1982.
33. Rodenstein DO, Francis C, Stanescu DC. Emotional laryngeal wheezing: a new syndrome. *Am Rev Respir Dis* 127:354–356, 1983.
34. Creer TL, Kotses H, Gustafson KE, Wigal JK, Wagner MD, Westlund RE, Trusel CS. A critique of studies investigating the association of theophylline to psychologic or behavioral performance. *Pediatr Asthma Allergy Immunol* 2:169–184, 1988.
35. Creer TL, Gustafson KE. Psychological problems associated with drug therapy in childhood asthma. *J Pediatr* 115:850–855, 1989.
36. Creer TL, Psychological and behavioral assessment of childhood asthma. Part I: Psychological instruments. *Pediatr Asthma Allergy Immunol* 5:317–328, 1991.
37. Creer TL. Psychological and behavioral assessment of childhood asthma. Part II: Behavioral approaches. *Pediatr Asthma Allergy Immunol* 6:21–34, 1992.
38. Furukawa CT, DuHamel TR, Weimer L, Shapiro GG, Pierson WE, Bierman CW. Cognitive and behavioral findings in children taking theophylline. *J Allergy Clin Immunol* 81:83–88, 1988.
39. American Academy of Allergy and Immunology Study Group. Treatment of mild to moderate asthma: comparison of aerosol beclomethasone and oral theophylline. *Am Rev Respir Dis* 143:A625, 1991.
40. Schlieper A, Alcock D, Beaudry P, Feldman W, Leikin L. Effect of therapeutic plasma concentrations of theophylline on behavior, cognitive processing, and affect in children with asthma. *J Pediatr* 118:449–455, 1991.

41. Weinberger M, Lindgren S, Bender B, Lerner J, Szefler S. Effects of theophylline on learning and behavior: reason for concern or concern without reason? *J Pediatr* 111:471–474, 1987.
42. Ellis EF. Asthma in infancy and childhood. In: Middleton E Jr, Reed CE, Ellis EF, Adkinson NF Jr, Yunginer JW (eds.), *Allergy: Principles and Practice*, 3rd ed., C.V. Mosby, St. Louis, 1988, pp. 969–998.
43. Ellis EF. Asthma: current therapeutic approach. *Pediatr Clin North Am* 35:1041–1052, 1988.
44. Bender BG, Lerner JA, Kollasch E. Mood and memory changes in asthmatic children receiving corticosteroids. *Am Acad Child Acolesc Psychiatry* 27:720–725, 1988.
45. Bender BG, Lerner JA, Poland JE. Association between corticosteroids and psychologic change in hospitalized asthmatic children. *Ann Allergy* 66:414–419, 1991.
46. Mazer B, Figueroa-Rosario W, Bender B. The effect of albuterol aerosol on fine-motor performance in children with chronic asthma. *J Allergy Clin Immunol* 86:233–238, 1990.
47. Creer TL. Medication compliance and childhood asthma. In: Epstein L, Johnson S, Kessell W, Krasnegor NA, Yaffe SJ (eds.), *Developmental Aspects of Health Compliance Behavior*. Lawrence Erlbaum Associates, Hillsdale, NJ, in press.
48. Sublett JL, Pollard SJ, Kadlec GJ, Karibo JM. Non-compliance in asthmatic children: a study of theophylline levels in a pediatric emergency room population. *Ann Allergy* 43:95–97, 1979.
49. Spector SL. Is your asthmatic patient really complying? *Ann Allergy* 55:552–556, 1985.
50. Spector SL, Lewis CE, Feldman CH, Haynes RB, Hindi-Alexander M, Kinsman RA, Menendez RA, Sbarbaro JA. Workshop 6: compliance factors. *J Allergy Clin Immunol* 78:529–533, 1986.
51. Creer TL. Medication compliance and asthma. *J Respir Dis* 12:543–548, 1991.
52. Arkes HR. Impediments to accurate clinical judgment and possible ways to minimize their impact. *J Consult Clin Psychol* 49:323–330, 1981.
53. Zieger RS, Heller S, Mellon MH, Wald J, Falkoff R, Schatz M. Facilitated referral to asthma specialist reduces relapses in asthma emergency room visits. *J Allergy Clin Immunol* 87:1160–1168, 1991.
54. Sulzer-Azaroff B, Mayer GR. *Behavior Analysis for Lasting Change*. Holt, Reinhart and Winston, Inc., Ft. Worth, 1991.
55. Creer TL, Winder JA. Asthma. In: Holroyd KA, Creer TL (eds.), *Self-Management of Chronic Disease. Handbook of Clinical Interventions and Research Medicine*. Academic Press, New York, 1986, pp. 29–55.
56. Weinstein AG, Cuskey W. Theophylline compliance in asthmatic children. *Ann Allergy* 54:19–24, 1985.
57. Mawhinney H, Spector SL, Kinsman RA, Siegel SC, Rachelefsky GS, Katz RM, Rohr AS. Compliance in clinical trials of two nonbronchodilator, antiasthma medications. *Ann Allergy* 66:294–299, 1991.

58. Wigal JK, Creer TL, Kotses H, Lewis PD. A critique of 19 self-management programs for childhood asthma. Part I. The development and evaluation of the programs. *Pediatr Asthma Allergy Immunol* 4:17–39, 1990.
59. Creer TL, Wigal JK, Kotses H, Lewis PD. A critique of 19 self-management programs for childhood asthma. Part II. Comments regarding the scientific merit of the programs. *Pediatr Asthma Allergy Immunol* 4:41–55, 1990.
60. Miklich DR, Renne CM, Creer TL, Alexander AB, Chai H, Davis MH, Hoffman A, Danker-Brown P. The clinical utility of behavior therapy as an adjunctive treatment for asthma. *J Allergy Clin Immunol* 60:285–294, 1977.
61. Creer TL. The application of behavioral procedures to childhood asthma: current and future perspectives. *Patient Ed Counsel* 17:9–22, 1991.
62. Kotses H, Harver A, Segretto J, Glaus KD, Creer TL, Young GA. Long-term effects of biofeedback-induced facial relaxation on measures of asthma severity in children. *Biofeedback Self-Regul* 16:1–21, 1991.
63. Creer TL. Strategies for judgment and decision-making in the management of childhood asthma. *Pediatr Asthma Allergy Immunol* 4:253–264, 1990.
64. Marion RJ, Creer TL, Arkes HR, Kotses H. The treatment of asthma: A decision-making approach. Paper presented at World Congress on Behavior Therapy and 17th Annual Convention, Association for the Advancement of Behavior Therapy, Washington, December 10, 1983.
65. Creer TL, Backial M, Burns KL, Leung P, Marion RJ, Miklich DR, Morrill C, Taplin PS, Ullman S. Living with asthma. I. Genesis and development of a self-management program for childhood asthma. *J Asthma* 25:335–362, 1988.
66. Creer TL, Renne CM. Panic in asthmatic children. Unpublished data presented in Creer TL. The synthesis of medical and behavioral sciences with respect to bronchial asthma. In: Ader R, Weiner H, Baum A (eds.), *Experimental Foundations of Behavioral Medicine: Conditioning Approaches*. Lawrence Erlbaum Associates, Hillsdale, NJ, 1988, pp. 111–158.
67. Wolpe J. *Psychotherapy by Reciprocal Inhibition*. Stanford University Press, Stanford, 1958.
68. Creer TL. The use of a time-out from positive reinforcement procedure with asthmatic children. *J Psychosom Res* 14:117–120, 1970.
69. Hochstadt N, Shepard J, Lulla SH. Reducing hospitalizations of children with asthma. *J Pediatr* 97:1012–1015, 1980.
70. Creer TL, Weinberg E, Molk L. Managing a problem hospital behavior: malingering. *J Behav Ther Exp Psychiatry* 5:259–262, 1974.
71. Baum D, Creer TL. Medication compliance in children with asthma. *J Asthma* 23:49–59, 1986.
72. Decker JL, Kaliner MA. *Understanding and Managing Asthma*. Avon Books, New York, 1988.
73. Renne CM, Creer TL. Training children with asthma to use inhalation therapy equipment. *J Appl Behav Anal* 9:1–11, 1976.
74. Creer TL, Renne CM, Christian WP. Behavioral contributions to rehabilitation and childhood asthma. *Rehab Lit* 37:226, 1976.

75. Clark TJH. Definition of asthma for clinical trials. *J Dis Chest* 71:225–226, 1977.
76. Taplin PS, Creer TL. A procedure for using peak expiratory flow rate data to increase the predictability of asthma episodes. *J Asthma Res* 16:15–19, 1978.
77. Harm DL, Kotses H, Creer TL. Improving the ability of peak flow rates to predict asthma. *J Allergy Clin Immunol* 76:688–694, 1985.
78. Stout C, Kotses H, Carlson BW, Creer TL. Predicting asthma in individual patients. *J Asthma* 28:41–47, 1991.
79. Kotses H, Stout C, Wigal JK, Carlson B, Creer TL, Lewis P. Individualized asthma self-management: a beginning. *J Asthma* 28:287–289, 1991.

# 21

# Asthma Self-Management Programs for Children

**KATHLEEN CONBOY**

*Children's Hospital of Buffalo*
*Buffalo, New York*



The concept upon which asthma self-management programs is based is the premise that individuals can benefit from becoming involved in their own health care. Self-care has been defined as those activities initiated or performed by an individual family or community in the hope of achieving, maintaining, or promoting maximum potential for good health (1). Asthma, as a common chronic disease, lends itself well to the application of self-care practice. There is a consensus among health care providers who treat children with asthma that the more the family knows about the disease, the better the child will do. Since asthma is the most common chronic disease of childhood and is responsible for more school absences (about 25%) (2), hospital admissions (3), and emergency room visits than any other chronic illness, implementation of asthma self-management programs is very likely to have substantial payoff in terms of reduced morbidity, mortality, and savings of health care dollars.

During the past decade, there has been considerable interest and research into health education programs that emphasize patient involvement in their own care, especially as they apply to those with chronic, disabling diseases (4).

## ASTHMA MORBIDITY, MORTALITY, AND SELF-MANAGEMENT

Despite advances in our understanding of the pathophysiology and management of asthma, morbidity has not significantly decreased. In fact, the number of hospitalizations for asthma has actually increased as has the mortality rate. From 1979 to 1987, hospitalizations of children with asthma, ages 0–17 years, increased on the average of 4.5% per year (5). Asthma is the most frequent cause of hospitalization for children, responsible for 11–17% of all children hospitalized in urban communities in the United States (3). During the 1970s, asthma mortality for both children and adults ages 5–34 decreased by approximately 7.8% per year. However, during the 1980s, this trend reversed and mortality has increased by 6.2% per year. The rate of increase was greatest in children aged 5–14 years and somewhat slower in those aged 15–34 years. From 1980 to 1987 the total deaths from asthma in the United States increased from 2,891 to 4,360. This represents a 31% increase in mortality rate from 1.3:100,000 to 1.7:100,000 (6). Retrospective studies of deaths from asthma have shown a substantial lack of information on the part of the patients and parents concerning the disease and its appropriate management (7). While intuitively reasonable, it has not been established that teaching self-management principles will reduce asthma mortality but the hypothesis merits serious consideration. Outcome evaluation of the success of asthma education programs suggests that families benefit by acquiring knowledge about asthma that better enables them to cope with the illness with less fear and stress and greater confidence in their skills to manage various aspects of the disease. Children enrolled in the programs, for the most part, have decreased morbidity, less utilization of emergency departments and hospital resources, and improved school attendance and achievement.

## WHAT IS ASTHMA SELF-MANAGEMENT?

Some health professionals prefer the term *cooperative care/cooperative management* to the term *self-management* because it includes the role of the physician, nurse, and other health care professionals in the program, whereas the term *self-management* might be interpreted to mean that the patients are "on their own." Critics of the self-care concept fear that implementing self-care may delay medical diagnoses, promote faddist treatments, and divert resources from medical care and research (4).

It is important to emphasize that the purpose of self-care is not to replace the traditional medical care model but rather to expand it to include patient/family participation. Cooperative management simply means the working together of all those individuals concerned with promoting the health of children with asthma. The goal of self-care in asthma is to teach families how to make informed decisions about their child's asthma with the assistance of their physician and the health care providers involved. Teaching can be done in the physician's office on a one-to-one basis, in group programs conducted after office hours, or in a school setting.

## EXISTING ASTHMA EDUCATION PROGRAMS

At the Children's Hospital of Buffalo, education of the family regarding self-care or cooperative-care skills includes individual (or group) instruction in the pathophysiology of asthma, recognition (by child and parents) of symptoms that trigger the disease, what to do if these symptoms occur, which drugs to use when, discussion of adverse drug effects, and recognition of when to call for professional assistance.

Many asthma education programs have been developed and published during the past decade (Table 1). Among them are several programs obtainable from the National Heart, Lung and Blood Institute, the American Lung Association, and the Asthma and Allergy Foundation of America. A comprehensive review of five of these programs was published in the *Health Education Quarterly* (8) (Open Airways [9], Living with Asthma [10], Air Power [11], Air Wise [12], and Superstuff [13]). Implicit in all programs is the belief that children can take more responsibility for management of their asthma. All the programs involve the parents and use examples of interactive skills to translate medical advice into practice in the family's daily life. The programs also emphasize the partnership of the children, the parents, and the physician and health care provider. Each program is unique, however, so some brief highlights will be mentioned here. Three other asthma education programs, Asthma Care Training (ACT), Childhood Asthma: Learning To Manage (CALM), and the Self-Care Rehabilitation Program in Pediatric Asthma will also be discussed.

TABLE 1 Comparison of Asthma Education Programs

| | Living with Asthma | Air Wise | Open Airways | Air Power |
|---|---|---|---|---|
| Teaching mode | Groups | One-on-one | Groups | Groups |
| Age range | Children 7–13 and parents | Children 9–13 | Children 4–7, 8–14, parents | Children 8–13 and parents |
| Leaders needed | Two | One | Two to three | Two |
| Number of sessions | Eight | Four to six | Seven | Four |
| Target groups | Rural, anyone | Hard-to-manage | Low education, low socio-economic status | Anyone |
| Place of use | Anywhere | Doctor's office | Anywhere | Anywhere |

Source: Modified from Ref. 7.

### Open Airways

This group program was developed at the Columbia–Presbyterian Medical Center in New York. The program was designed for and tested among inner city families and the language, both English and Spanish, is simple. Open Airways discusses asthma triggers that may be particularly relevant to the urban environmental conditions (e.g., cockroach allergy). The program provides families with the instruction and skills necessary to follow an asthma treatment plan. The curriculum is based on group dynamics, and children and families learn asthma management skills from each other. A teacher acts primarily as a group discussion leader, but also corrects any misinformation that may be expressed by group members. Open Airways encourages group support and suggests new ways of dealing with asthma-related problems. An interesting teaching tool involves a series of stories about families with asthma-related problems that class participants try to solve. Sessions with younger children often use puppets to act out such stories. Open Airways is unique in that it can be used for children 4–7 years of age. The six or seven educational sessions can coincide with clinic visits, which appears to increase compliance.

Open Airways was tested among 310 families for a year, and results showed that the experimental group took significantly more steps to manage their asthma than they had before the program (14). Although there

| Superstuff | ACT | CALM | Self-rehabilitation program for pediatric asthma |
|---|---|---|---|
| Families | Groups | One family | Groups |
| Children and parents | Children 7–12 and parents | Children 2–19, parents and physician | Children 2–5 and 6–14 |
| None | Two | None | Two |
| As needed | Three | Ad lib | Six |
| Literate | Hispanic version available | Literate | Preschoolers and school aged children |
| Anywhere | Anywhere | Anywhere | Anywhere |

was no decrease in the use of acute care services between the entire experimental group and the control group, health care utilization was significantly reduced within a subgroup of children who had been hospitalized one or more times for asthma during the year before completing the program. One year before enrolling in the program, the experimental group had 7.8 emergency room (ER) visits compared with 3.96 the year after enrollment in the program (a reduction of 3.84 visits), while the control group had 8.1 ER visits the year before, and 8.04 the year after (a reduction of 0.06 visits) ($p < 0.05$). The experimental subgroup also achieved an average yearly decrease of 1.0 hospitalization compared with 0.31 fewer hospitalizations in the control group. Enrollment in the program was also associated with a decrease in health care costs (15).

## Living with Asthma

Living with Asthma was developed at the National Asthma Center in Denver by Thomas Creer and his colleagues (10). It is a seven-session group program for children and their families. Children and parents meet separately and each group learns basic information and skills presented in a manner appropriate to their developmental level. In the first two sessions, information about asthma, its management, and medications is provided.

The remaining sessions focus on methods for encouraging the development of self-management behaviors. Living with Asthma focuses on teaching asthma skills to children and providing parents with the knowoledge and behavior modification skills to help their children take over management responsibility. A number of teaching techniques are used including lectures, discussions, role-playing, decision making, problem solving, and modeling. Learning materials include games, illustrated notebooks, situation cards, Marvin Marvelous stories, and Dr. Q's Newsletters. Should teenagers become involved in this program, materials from the parents' manual can be used and adapted to reflect the concerns of adolescents. Living with Asthma was evaluated among families in Colorado. Long-term results were pooled for 125 families randomized into experimental and control groups. Not only did observed measures of asthma clinical status (peak flow rates) improve, but there was also a significant decrease in school absenteeism. There were 17.5 school days missed, which decreased to 6.4 days a year after the program (16). In a subgroup of nine families, health care costs were reduced by 66% as a result of participation in the program (17).

### Air Wise

Air Wise was developed at the American Institute for Behavioral Research in Palo Alto, California, based upon work done by Jacobs and colleagues. They studied what doctors, nurses, parents, teachers, and children themselves reported as things that children actually did or do that affect their asthma. The program provides one-to-one teaching and can be carried out in the doctor's office or in the hospital. Designed for children 9–13 years of age with difficult-to-manage asthma, the teaching approach is targeted to the specific needs of the patient. After interviewing the child, the teacher selects a program from among 25 objectives. The teacher then builds on what the child already knows and establishes priorities in terms of what he or she needs to know. After each session, the children, parents, and doctor meet to discuss the results in a cooperative management fashion. The self-management curriculum is directed toward four objectives: prevention of asthma attacks, management of symptoms, taking medications, and dealing with one's self and others as related to asthma. In the pilot evaluation, 17 children participated. Prior to participation in the program, both groups had similar rates of ER utilization. In the year after enrollment in the program, ER use decreased from 3.2 visits in the experimental group to 0.3 visits in the control group (18).

### Air Power

Air Power is a group program in which children are taught the basics of asthma self-management in four 1-hr sessions. The program is taught to small groups of children and their parents (three to six families per group). Each group attends separate sessions simultaneously. There are three components to each session: information-giving, group problem solving, and relaxation training. The underlying philosophy is based on a social learning theory that proposes that individuals are motivated to change their behavior when they have a sense of being in control of their environment. This suggests that self-management behaviors will be performed by children if they have the knowledge, skills, and motivation. The content of the parents' sessions parallels that of the children, and the parents learn to assist their children to become effective managers for much of their asthma care. The program was tested among 180 children in a health maintenance organization (19). The frequency of independent self-management behavior, as reported by the parents, increased after the program. The evaluators considered that this demonstrated a successful transfer of responsibility from parents to child, with no loss in the degree of asthma control (19).

### Superstuff

Another program that has been widely disseminated is Superstuff, produced under the auspices of the American Lung Association. Superstuff comes in a prepackaged kit containing a newsletter for parents and various teaching materials for children and may be used at home or in a group setting. For children it teaches the basics of asthma: what it is, how to avoid triggers, early warning signs, and how to make decisions. These concepts are taught through stories, puzzles, games, quizzes, and a recording. The parents' magazine has articles, for example, on coping with asthma, how to talk to physicians and teachers, and how to handle emergency situations. Since Superstuff is a self-contained learning module, it may also be used as a supplemental take-home tool to other group programs. When Superstuff was evaluated among 321 families, the experimental group missed significantly fewer days of school after participation in the program (20). If Superstuff is given to families for home use, the physician and nurse must monitor its use. The children and parents should regularly be asked what they have learned and encouraged to ask questions. This helps to keep the lines of communication open and encourages the family to use self-management skills.

### Asthma Care Training

Asthma Care Training (ACT) is a group program developed at the University of California at Los Angeles. In the recently revised 3 week program, children ages 8–12 and their parents meet in separate groups for 60 min and then together for 30 min to discuss their experiences. The message is that children with asthma are "in the driver's seat": they can take charge of their disease rather than be controlled by it.

In a trial of the original 5 week program curriculum, 76 children were randomized to either control or experimental groups and were evaluated for 1 year after completing the program (21). The control group and their parents received asthma education in a lecture format. The experimental group participated in the interactive ACT curriculum. The results showed that both groups showed equivalent increases in their knowledge about asthma and changes in their former beliefs; only the experimental group showed significant changes in self-reported compliance behaviors; and those given the experimental treatment had significantly fewer ER visits and days of hospitalization, leading to an average saving of $180 per child per year. Materials and information about this program are available from the Asthma and Allergy Foundation. ACT is available in both English and Spanish.

### Childhood Asthma: Learning to Manage

Childhood Asthma: Learning to Manage (CALM) is a home study program designed to educate children with asthma, their families, and physicians about managing asthma in the home (22) and was developed by IOX Assessment Associates in Los Angeles, California. Excellent illustrated manuals are available for prereaders (ages 1–7), preadolescents (ages 8–12), and teenagers (ages 13–19). It is the only program that specifically targets children in all age groups. It explains how to use a peak flowmeter, describes medications and their effects, asthma triggers, early warning signs, and prevention strategies. CALM shares the experience of others with asthma to promote confidence for active living and a cooperative relationship among children, parents, and physicians. Materials include a peak flowmeter (the program is also available without a peak flowmeter), peak flow record charts, an instructional guide for children, an information guide for parents, and a special supplement for physicians. CALM is currently under evaluation. The program is available from the Asthma and Allergy Foundation.

### Self-Care Rehabilitation Program in Pediatric Asthma

This program was developed at the University of Utah in cooperation with the American Lung Association of Utah (23) and is unique in that it offers a six-session group program for preschool children aged 2–5 years, which is a very important age in terms of need for asthma education. The children attend only sessions 2–5 while the parents attend all six 1 hr sessions. The school-age group program (6–14 years) has eight 90 min classes for both children and parents and is supplemented with Superstuff material for home study.

## ASTHMA IN SCHOOLS: PROBLEMS AND EDUCATIONAL SOLUTIONS

Schools can play an important role in asthma education programs but they often do not. Children with asthma (and many who have asthma but are undiagnosed [24]) encounter major problems in the school setting (25, 26). There is underrecognition of the signs and symptoms of asthma on the part of teachers and little knowledge of the disease. For example, nocturnal asthma, which keeps the child awake, will often make him sleepy in school, resulting in a reprimand and notes sent home to the parents. In particular, teachers lack information about medications used in treating the disease, for example, which are prophylactic and which are used to relieve an acute episode of bronchoconstriction (25). Few teachers have knowledge of the adverse effects of the drugs used (e.g., central nervous system stimulation with theophylline and oral adrenergic drugs, sleepiness caused by antihistamines given for coexisting allergic rhinitis). Precipitants of asthma, for example, irritants such as strong odors from floor cleaning solutions, chalk dust, and exercise, often go unrecognized. Physical education teachers in particular need to know the dangers of forcing a child with asthma to run laps around the school track. School policies differ enormously in terms of whether the child is permitted to carry and use an inhaler. The principal and not the school board often sets the rules in this regard, to the detriment of the child. Concerns about liability will more often that not be given higher priority than the child's best interest. In one published report, 70% of the parents communicated with the school about their child's asthma but had difficulty in getting the school staff to follow the medication treatment program (27). With increasing pressure on school budgets, school nurses have become a rapidly disappearing species. Children with asthma, who in times past might have been sent to the nurse's office for treatment of acute asthma, are now being sent home. Few teachers have sufficient information about asthma to inform other children in the class of the nature of their classmate's illness and the asthmatic child is often embarrassed and looked upon as sick and disabled. Instead of being a detriment to children with asthma, schools can be an important asset in terms of recognizing undiagnosed disease and decreasing morbidity, thus improving school attendance and academic performance (28, 29). Since schools receive funding based upon student attendance and asthma is responsible for one-quarter of all school absences due to chronic illness, this should be an incentive for the school system to become involved. Community campaigns against asthma, based in schools, have been shown to be successful in terms of lowered morbidity and significantly improved school attendance (30). At the Children's Hospital of Buffalo, pediatric nurse practitioners with special expertise in asthma have given seminars at school nurse association meetings and have been well received. Asthma education programs such as ACT lend themselves to presentations in evening sessions at schools with the participation of school teachers.

There are a number of resources available to school personnel who wish to learn more about asthma. An excellent monograph entitled Asthma in the School—Improved Control with Peak Flow is available through the Asthma and Allergy Foundation for the cost of mailing. The book provides an outline for a faculty workshop and sample letters from physicians and parents to school personnel illustrating information that needs to be communicated. A list of resources is available through the Asthma and Allergy Foundation, the American Lung Association, the National Heart, Lung and Blood Institute, the National Jewish Center for Immunology and Respiratory Medicine, and Mothers of Asthmatics. The Asthma and Allergy Foundation has also produced a videotape entitled Cooperative Care in Schools, which is available on loan or for purchase.

## REFERENCES

1. Goldstein RA, Green LW, Parker S. Self-management of childhood asthma. *J Allergy Clin Immunol* 72(5):522–525, 1983.
2. Evans R, et al. National trends in morbidity and mortality of asthma in the United States. *Chest* 91(6, suppl):65S–74S, 1987.
3. Parent JM, Homer CJ, Berwick DM, Woolf AD, Freeman JL, Wennberg JE. Variations of rates of hospitalizations of children in 3 urban communities. *N Engl J Med* 320:1183–1187, 1989.
4. Barry PZ, et al. Self-care programs: their role and potential. University of North Carolina at Chapel Hill, Health Services Research Center, 1980.
5. Gergen PJ, Weiss KB. Changing patterns of asthma hospitalization among young children 1979–1987. *JAMA* 264:1688–1692, 1990.
6. Center for Disease Control. Asthma/United States, 1980–1987. *MMWR* 39:493–497, 1990.
7. Strunk RO. Identification of the fatality prone subject with asthma. *J Allergy Clin Immunol* 83:477–485, 1989.
8. Krutzsch CB, et al. Childhood asthma management education. *Health Ed Q* 14(3):357–373, 1987.
9. National Heart, Lung and Blood Institute. Open Airways/Respiro Albierto: Asthma Self-Management Program. Bethesda, MD, 1984.
10. National Heart, Lung and Blood Institute. Living with Asthma. Part 1: Manual for Teaching Parents the Self-Management of Childhood Asthma. Part 2: Manual for Teaching Children the Self-Management of Asthma. Bethesda, MD, 1985.
11. National Heart, Lung and Blood Institute. Air Power: Self Management of Asthma Through Group Education. Bethesda, MD, 1984.
12. National Heart, Lung and Blood Institute. Air Wise: Self-Management of Asthma through Individual Education. Bethesda, MD 1984.

13. American Lung Association: Superstuff. Item #0317. Price: $10.00.
14. Clark NM, et al. Managing better: Children, parents and asthma. *Patient Ed Counsel* 8:27–38, 1986.
15. Clark NM, et al. The impact of health education on frequency and cost of health-care utilization by low-income children with asthma. *J Allergy Clin Immunol* 78:108–115, 1986.
16. Creer TL, Winder JA. Asthma. In: Holroyd KA, Creer TL (eds). *Self-Management of Chronic Disease. Handbook of Clinical Interventions in Research Medicine*. Academic Press, New York, 1986.
17. Marion R, Creer T, Reynolds R. Direct and indirect costs associated with the management of childhood asthma. *Ann Allergy* 54:1–4, 1985.
18. Wilson-Passano SR, McNabb WL. The role of patient education in the management of childhood asthma. *Prev Med* 14:670–687, 1985.
19. Wilson SR et al. Development and evaluation of self-management systems for children with asthma. Self-Manage and Co-Manage. Final report to the National Heart, Lung and Blood Institute. American Institutes for Research, Palo Alto, CA 1981.
20. Weiss JH, Hermalin J. The effectiveness of a self-teaching asthma self-management program for school-age children and their families. *Prev Human Serv* in press, 1987.
21. Lewis CE, Rachelefsky G, Lewis MA, et al. A randomized trial of ACT (Asthma Care Training for Kids). *Pediatrics* 74:478–486, 1984.
22. IOX Assessment Associates. Childhood Asthma: Learning to Manage (CALM). Los Angeles, CA.
23. Whitman N, Wesi D, Braugh FK, Welch M. A study of a self-care rehabilitation program in pediatric asthma. *Health Ed Q* 12:333–342, 1985.
24. Speight ANP, Lee DA, Hey EN. Underdiagnosis and undertreatment of asthma in childhood. *Br Med J* 286:1253–1255, 1983.
25. Bevis M., Taylor B. What do school teachers know about asthma?
26. Hill RA, Britton JR, Tattersfield AE. Management of asthma in schools. *Arch Dis Child* 62:414–415, 1987.
27. Freunderberg N, Feldman C, Clark NM, Maillman EJ, Valle I, Wasilewski Y. The impact of bronchial asthma on school attendance and performance. *J School Health* 50:522–526, 1980.
28. Mak H, Johnston P, Abbey H, et al. Morbidity and school absence caused by asthma and wheezing illness. *J Allergy Clin Immunol* 70:367–, 1982.
29. Parcel GS, Gilman SC, Nader PR, et al. A comparison of absentee rates of elementary school children with asthma and non-asthmatic schoolmates. *Pediatrics* 64:878, 1979.
30. Colver AF. Community campaign against asthma. *Arch Dis Child* 59:449–452, 1984.

# Glossary of Abbreviations

| | |
|---|---|
| ABG | Arterial blood gases |
| ABPA | Allergic bronchopulmonary aspergillosis |
| ACT | Asthma care training |
| ADCC | Antibody-dependent cellular cytotoxicity |
| ADHD | Attention deficit hyperactivity disorder |
| AgE | Main allergen of ragweed |
| AIA | Allergen-induced asthma |
| AMDGF | Alveolar macrophage-derived growth factor |
| AMPc | Cyclic adenosine monophosphate |
| APUD | Amine precursor, uptake and decarboxylation |
| ASA | Acute severe asthma |
| ATP | Adenosine triphosphate |
| B.U. | Breath unit |
| BAL | Bronchoalveolar lavage |
| BALT | Bronchus-associated lymphoid tissue |
| BDP | Beclomethasone diproprionate |
| BHR | Bronchial hyperresponsiveness |
| BPD | Bronchopulmonary dysplasia |
| BPI | Bactericidal/permeability-increasing protein |
| C | Compliance |

| | |
|---|---|
| CAL | Calibration factors |
| CALM | Childhood asthma: learning to manage |
| CARIH | Children's Asthma Research Institute and Hospital |
| CAT | Computorized tomography |
| CCA | Chipanzee coryza agent |
| CCK8 | Cholecystokinin |
| CD4 | T-helper lymphocyte |
| CD8 | T-suppressor lymphocyte |
| CF | Cystic fibrosis |
| COMT | Catechol-*O*-methyltransferase |
| COPD | Chronic obstructive pulmonary disease |
| CR | Conditioned reaction |
| CRGP | Calcitonin gene-related peptide |
| Crs | Total respiratory compliance |
| CS | Conditioned stimulus |
| DAD | Diffuse alveolar damage |
| DBPCFC | Double-blind, placebo-controlled food challenges |
| DSCG | Disodium cromoglycate |
| E | Elastance |
| ECF | Eosinophil chemotactic factor |
| ECP | Eosinophil cationic protein |
| ED | Emergency Department |
| EDN | Eosinophil-derived neurotoxin |
| EDRF | Endothelium-derived relaxant factor |
| EIA | Exercise-induced asthma |
| EIB | Exercise-induced bronchospasm |
| ELF | Epithelial lining fluid |
| ELISA | Enzyme-linked immunosorbent test |
| e-NANC | Excitatory nonadrenergic noncholinergic |
| EPO | Eosinophil peroxidase |
| ER | Emergency room |
| ETS | Environmental tobacco smoke |
| Fc RI | High-affinity Fc receptors |
| Fc RII | Lower-affinity Fc receptors |
| FEF25–75% | Slope of the curve from 25 to 75% of VC |
| FEV1 | Forced expiratory volume in 1 sec |
| FRC | Functional residual capacity |
| FVC | Forced vital capacity |
| G-6 PD | Glucose-6-phosphate dehydrogenase |
| GALT | Gut-associated lymphoid tissue |

| | |
|---|---|
| GER | Gastroesophageal reflux |
| GM-CSF | Granulocyte-macrophage colony-stimulating factor |
| GRP | Gastrin-releasing peptide |
| GSH | Reduced glutathione |
| GSSG | Oxidized glutathione |
| HEPA | High-efficiency particle air filter systems |
| HETEs | Hydroxyeicosatetraenoic acids |
| HLA | Histocompatibility genes |
| HPETE | Acyclic hydroperoxyeicosatetraenoic acid |
| IB | Ipratropium bromide |
| ICAM 1 | Intercellular cell adhesion molecule |
| ICD | International Classification of Diseases |
| ICU | Intensive care unit |
| IFN | Interferon |
| IL | Interleukin |
| IPPB | Intermittent positive-pressure breathing |
| LAR | Late-phase asthmatic reaction |
| LFA | Lymphocyte function-related antigens |
| LOH | Nontoxic lipid alcohol |
| LOOH | Lipid hydroperoxide |
| LRT | Lower respiratory tract |
| LT | Leukotriene |
| MAO | Monoamine oxidase |
| MBP | Major basic protein |
| MDI | Metered dose inhaler |
| MEMS | Medication event monitoring system |
| MHC | Major histocompatibility complex |
| MMEF | Maximum midexpiratory flow rate |
| MRI | Magnetic resonance imaging |
| NAAQS | National ambient air quality standards |
| NADPH | Nicotinamide adenosine diphosphate |
| NARES | Nonallergic rhinitis with eosinophilia |
| NC | Nebulizer chronolog |
| NCF | Neutrophil chemotactic factor |
| NE | Neutrophil elastase |
| NKA | Neurokinin A |
| $NO_2$ | Nitrous dioxide |
| NPY | Neuropeptide Y |
| OTC | Over the counter |
| P | Driving pressure |
| PAF | Platelet-activating factor |

| | |
|---|---|
| Pbox | Pletysmograph chamber pressure |
| $PC_{20}$ | 20% fall in $FEV_1$ after provocative challenge |
| $pCO_2$ | Partial pressure of $CO_2$ |
| PCW | Concentration of methacoline causing wheezing |
| PE | Physical education class |
| PEFR | Peak expiratory flow rate |
| PG | Prostaglandins |
| PMA | Premenstrual asthma |
| $pO_2$ | Partial pressure of $O_2$ |
| PUMP 1 | Putative metalloproteinase 1 |
| PV | Parainfluenza virus |
| PV | Pressure/volume curve |
| R | Resistance |
| RAD | Reactive airway disease |
| RAST | Radioallergosorbent test |
| Raw | Airway resistance |
| RDS | Hyaline membrane disease |
| RIA | Radioimmunoassay |
| Rrs | Total respiratory resistance |
| RSV | Respiratory syncytial virus |
| RV | Residual volume |
| $SAO_2$ | Oxygen saturation |
| SGaw | Specific conductance |
| SLPI | Secretory leukoprotease inhibitor |
| SOD | Superoxide dismutase |
| SP | Substance P |
| SRaw | Specific resistance |
| SRS-A | Slow-reacting substance of anaphylaxis |
| $T_e$ | Total expiratory time |
| $T_{me}$ | Peak tidal expiratory flow |
| T4 | T-helper lymphocyte |
| T8 | T-suppressor lymphocyte |
| TAO | Troleandomycin |
| TCR | T-cell receptor |
| TIMP | Tissue inhibitor of metalloprotease |
| TLC | Total lung capacity |
| TMV | Tracheal mucus velocity |
| TNF | Tumor necrosis factor |
| TXs | Thromboxanes |
| UCR | Unconditioned reaction |
| UCS | Unconditioned stimulus |

| | |
|---|---|
| URI | Upper respiratory infection |
| URT | Upper respiratory tract |
| VC | Vital capacity |
| VIP | Vasoactive intestinal peptide |
| $VO_2$ | Maximal oxygen uptake |
| V/Q | Ventilation/perfusion |
| VT | Tidal volume |
| Vtg | Thoracic gas volume |
| WHO | World Health Organization |

# Index

## B



## C

## D



## E

## F

## G



## H



## I

**K**



**L**

## M



## N

# About the Editors

DAVID G. TINKELMAN is Clinical Professor of Pediatrics at the Medical College of Georgia, Augusta, and a physician in private practice at the Atlanta Allergy Clinic, P.C., Georgia. A participant in many research projects, he is the author or coauthor of over 75 professional papers on asthma, Editor of the *Journal of Asthma*, and coeditor, with Charles K. Naspitz, of *Childhood Rhinitis and Sinusitis: Pathophysiology and Treatment* (Marcel Dekker, Inc.). He is Chairman of the Executive Committee of the Section of Allergy and Immunology (1990–1992) of the American Academy of Pediatrics, and a member of the American Academy of Allergy and Immunology, the American College of Allergy, and the American Thoracic Society. Dr. Tinkelman received the B.A. degree (1968) from Temple University, Philadelphia, Pennsylvania, and the M.D. degree (1972) from Hahnemann Medical College, Philadelphia, Pennsylvania.

CHARLES K. NASPITZ is Full Professor and Chief of the Division of Allergy, Immunology, and Rheumatology in the Department of Pediatrics at the Escola Paulista de Medicina in São Paulo, Brazil. A member of the American Academy of Allergy and Immunology and the American College of Allergy and Immunology, he is a past President of the Brazilian Society of Allergy and Clinical Immunology, a coeditor, with David G. Tinkelman, of *Childhood Rhinitis and Sinusitis: Pathophysiology and Treatment* (Marcel Dekker, Inc.), and the author or coauthor of more than 60 professional papers on allergy, particularly asthma, immunology, and rheumatology. Dr. Naspitz received the M.D. degree (1959) from the Escola Paulista de Medicina, São Paulo, and the M.Sc. degree (1967) in allergy and clinical immunology from McGill University, Montreal, Canada.